Lesions of the Scalp and Cranial Vault

Mehmet Turgut • Ali Akhaddar
Ahmet T. Turgut • Walter A. Hall
Editors

Lesions of the Scalp and Cranial Vault

State-of-the-Art Concepts

Springer

Editors
Mehmet Turgut
Department of Neurosurgery
Aydın Adnan Menderes University
Faculty of Medicine
Aydın, Türkiye

Ahmet T. Turgut
Department of Radiology
Ankara Medipol University
Faculty of Medicine
Ankara, Türkiye

Ali Akhaddar
Department of Neurosurgery
Avicenne Military Hospital of
Marrakech, Mohammed V University in
Rabat
Rabat, Morocco

Walter A. Hall
Department of Neurosurgery
State University of New York (SUNY)
Upstate Medical University
Syracuse, NY, USA

ISBN 978-3-031-88243-2 ISBN 978-3-031-88244-9 (eBook)
https://doi.org/10.1007/978-3-031-88244-9

This Springer imprint is published by the registered company Springer Nature Switzerland AG
The registered company address is: Gewerbestrasse 11, 6330 Cham, Switzerland

Contents

List of Contributors

Brahim Abdenbaoui Department of Neurosurgery, University Hospital of Fez, Fez, Morocco

Ali Akhaddar Department of Neurosurgery, Avicenne Military Hospital of Marrakech, Mohammed V University in Rabat, Rabat, Morocco

Abad Cherif El Asri Department of Neurosurgery, Mohamed V Military Hospital, University Mohammed V of Rabat, Rabat, Morocco

Hatim Belfquih Department of Neurosurgery, Avicenne Military Hospital of Marrakech, Cady Ayyad University, Marrakech, Morocco

Mohammed Benzagmout Department of Neurosurgery, Hassan II Hospital, Sidi Mohamed Ben Abdellah University of Fès, Fes, Morocco

Timothy Beutler Department of Neurosurgery, State University of New York (SUNY) Upstate Medical University, Syracuse, NY, USA

George H. Bourdages Department of Neurosurgery, State University of New York (SUNY) Upstate University Hospital, Syracuse, NY, USA

Alexander E. Braley Department of Neurosurgery, State University of New York (SUNY) Upstate Medical University, Syracuse, NY, USA

Servet Çelik Department of Anatomy, Ege University Faculty of Medicine, İzmir, Türkiye

Bogdan-Marius Corbu Department of Neurosurgery, Nordstadt Hospital KRH, Hannover, Germany

Dan Draytsel Norton College of Medicine, State University of New York (SUNY) Upstate Medical University, Syracuse, NY, USA

Srinivas Dwarakanath Department of Neurosurgery, National Instiute of Mental Health and Neurosciences, Bengaluru, Karnataka, India

Fedi Ercan Department of Gynecology and Obstetrics, Aydın Adnan Menderes University Faculty of Medicine, Aydın, Türkiye

Ersen Ertekin Department of Radiology, Hitit University Faculty of Medicine, Çorum, Türkiye

Christine E. Fuller Department of Pathology, State University of New York (SUNY) Upstate Medical University, Syracuse, NY, USA

Vaitsa Giannouli Aristotle University of Thessaloniki, Thessaloniki, Macedonia, Greece

Grahame C. Gould Department of Neurosurgery, State University of New York (SUNY) Upstate Medical University, Syracuse, NY, USA

Ferdi Gülaştı Department of Anesthesiology and Reanimation, Aydın Adnan Menderes University Faculty of Medicine, Aydın, Türkiye

Fuyou Guo Department of Neurosurgery, The First Affiliated Hospital of Zhengzhou University, Zhengzhou, Henan, China
International Joint Laboratory of Nervous System Malformation, Zhengzhou, Henan, China

Pengfei Guo Department of Burn and Reconstruction, The First Affiliated Hospital of Zhengzhou University, Zhengzhou, Henan, China

Walter A. Hall Department of Neurosurgery, State University of New York (SUNY) Upstate Medical University, Syracuse, NY, USA

Meryem Himmiche Department of Neurosurgery, University Hospital of Tangiers, Tangier, Morocco

Haydn Hoffman Department of Neurosurgery, State University of New York (SUNY) Upstate Medical University, Syracuse, NY, USA

Brody Hooper Department of Neurosurgery, State University of New York (SUNY) Upstate Medical University, Syracuse, NY, USA

Mohammed Amine Houssa Department of Plastic Surgery, El Hassani Hospital, Nador, Morocco

Josué Kazayi Ilunga Department of Neurosurgery, University Hospital of Fez, Fez, Morocco

Muhammad S. Jalal Department of Neurosurgery, State University of New York (SUNY) Upstate Medical University, Syracuse, NY, USA

Joseph Kedra Department of Neurosurgery, State University of New York (SUNY) Upstate Medical University Hospital, Syracuse, NY, USA

Emine Meliknur Kılıç Department of Civil Law, İzmir Bakırçay University Faculty of Law, İzmir, Türkiye
Program of Private Law Doctorate, Dokuz Eylül University Institute of Social Sciences, İzmir, Türkiye
Department of Civil Law, Trier University Faculty of Law, Trier, Germany

Kubilay Doğan Kılıç Department of Histology and Embryology, Ege University Faculty of Medicine, İzmir, Türkiye
Leibniz Institute for Evolution and Biodiversity Science, Museum für Naturkunde, Berlin, Germany

Katja Kniese Department of Neurosurgery, Nordstadt Hospital KRH, Hannover, Germany

Sotirios Kottas Papanikolaou General Hospital, Thessaloniki, Macedonia, Greece

George W. Koutsouras Department of Neurosurgery, State University of New York (SUNY) Upstate University Hospital, Syracuse, NY, USA

Satish Krishnamurthy Department of Neurosurgery, State University of New York (SUNY) Upstate Medical University, Syracuse, NY, USA

Rajiv Mangla Department of Radiology, State University of New York (SUNY) Upstate Medical University, Syracuse, NY, USA

Arya Nabavi Department of Neurosurgery, Nordstadt Hospital KRH, Hannover, Germany

Farideh Nejat Department of Neurosurgery, Children's Hospital Medical Center, Tehran University of Medical Science, Tehran, Iran

Sahar Ebrahem Orif Department of Anatomy and Embryology, Mansoura University Faculty of Veterinary Medicine, Mansoura, Egypt
Department of Stem Cell, Ege University Institute of Health Sciences, İzmir, Türkiye

Marouane El Ouahabi Department of Neurosurgery, University Hospital of Fez, Fez, Morocco

Hanish Polavarapu Department of Neurosurgery, State University of New York (SUNY) Upstate Medical University, Syracuse, NY, USA

Gökhan Sargın Department of Rheumatology, Aydın Adnan Menderes University Faculty of Medicine, Aydın, Türkiye

Sinem Sarı Department of Anesthesiology and Reanimation, Aydın Adnan Menderes University Faculty of Medicine, Aydın, Türkiye

Kossi Kouma Félix Segbedgi Department of Neurosurgery, Hôpital DOGTA LAFIE, Lomé, Togo

Cameron Shuman Department of Neurosurgery, State University of New York (SUNY) Upstate Medical University, Syracuse, NY, USA

Sophia Silas College of Medicine, State University of New York (SUNY) Upstate Medical University, Syracuse, NY, USA

Dengpan Song Department of Neurosurgery, The First Affiliated Hospital of Zhengzhou University, Zhengzhou, Henan Province, China
International Joint Laboratory of Nervous System Malformation, Zhengzhou, Henan Province, China

Nikolaos Syrmos Aristotle University of Thessaloniki, Thessaloniki, Macedonia, Greece
Human Performance and Health, Master Science Program, Aristotle University of Thessaloniki, Thessaloniki, Macedonia, Greece
Papanikolaou General Hospital, Thessaloniki, Macedonia, Greece
European Association of Neurosurgical Societies (EANS), Thessaloniki, Macedonia, Greece

Daphne J. Theodorou Department of Radiology, General Hospital of Ioannina, Ioannina, Greece

Ahmet T. Turgut Department of Radiology, Ankara Medipol University Faculty of Medicine, Ankara, Türkiye

Ali Çağlar Turgut Department of Histology and Emryology, Aydın Adnan Menderes University Institute of Health Sciences, Aydın, Türkiye
Department of Radiology, Ege University Faculty of Medicine, İzmir, Türkiye

Mehmet Turgut Department of Neurosurgery, Aydın Adnan Menderes University Faculty of Medicine, Aydın, Türkiye
Department of Histology and Embryology, Aydın Adnan Menderes University Institute of Health Sciences, Aydın, Türkiye

Yaşar Barış Turgut Internal Medicine Clinic, Aydın State Hospital, Aydın, Türkiye

Yiğit Uyanıkgil Department of Histology and Embryology, Ege University Faculty of Medicine, İzmir, Türkiye
Department of Stem Cell, Ege University Institute of Health Sciences, İzmir, Türkiye

Qiying Wang Department of Plastic Surgery, The First Affiliated Hospital of Zhengzhou University, Zhengzhou, Henan Province, China

Zheng Yang Department of Plastic Surgery, The First Affiliated Hospital of Zhengzhou University, Zhengzhou, Henan Province, China

Part I

General Characteristics of Lesions of the Scalp and Calvarium

Editor's Summary

In this "Part I: General Characteristics of Lesions of the Scalp & Calvarium," there are a total of six chapters describing the definitions and classifications, history, developmental anatomy and histology, regeneration, clinical presentation, and imaging features of these lesions. Given the variation of the tissues that comprise the scalp and calvarium, there can be a significant challenge to develop an organized and comprehensive presentation of this information due to the heterogenous nature of these lesions. The first of the chapters in this section (Chap. 1) defines and classifies the different types of lesions that can involve the scalp and calvarium. A historical perspective of these lesions in provided in the second chapter of this section (Chap. 2). In the third chapter (Chap. 3), the authors present the developmental anatomy and histology of those tissues comprising the lesions of the scalp and calvarium. The regenerative ability of the scalp and calvarium is discussed in the fourth chapter of this section (Chap. 4). The final two chapters of this section are directed at more of the clinical aspects of the lesions of the scalp and calvarium. With Chap. 5, a description of the different ways in which these lesions can present to the clinician is presented, whereas the last remaining chapter (Chap. 6) provides a detailed portfolio of the different imaging features of those lesions that are seen to involve the scalp and calvarium.

1 Definitions and Classifications for Lesions of the Scalp and Calvarium

Ali Akhaddar

1.1 Introduction

Scalp and cranial vault lesions include a wide range of pathologic entities with various topographic localizations, clinical manifestations, and imaging features. The majority of scalp disorders and superficial cutaneous and/or subcutaneous lesions are encountered in dermatologic practice. However, most deep scalp lesions and cranial vault diseases are managed by neurosurgeons as well as by craniofacial and plastic surgeons [1–15].

Generally, most scalp and cranial vault lesions are fortunately benign or are of little concern. However, some lesions are more worrying, especially when red flag symptoms/signs are present such as rapid growth of a mass, neurologic deficits, infectious symptoms, or a lesion discovered in the context of a known history of malignancy. Correct identification of the nature of the lesion and its relationship with cranial, extracranial, and intracranial structures is a key point for the surgeons' ability to discuss the best therapeutic approach for each case. Some lesions can be left alone with no follow-up, while others need aggressive treatment with surgical resection, radiation, and/or chemotherapy.

Due to their high variability, it is not always easy to categorize lesions of the scalp and calvaria. Many classifications have been proposed in the literature, mostly related to topographic locations, imaging features, histopathologic categories, specific populations, or clinical findings [9, 11, 15–22]. However, there are no standardized classifications.

An inventory of the most common scalp and calvarial lesions and pseudo-lesions encountered in neurosurgical practice is given in this chapter according to the anatomic locations and origins of the lesions. However, pure dermatologic, hair, and cutaneous/subcutaneous lesions are out of our scope and will not be discussed in this section.

1.2 Definitions

The scalp and skull vault can be affected by a wide variety of lesions and abnormalities that present differently in this location compared to other parts of the human anatomy. In addition, normal variants which may be mistaken for pathology, sometimes called pseudo-lesions, are also important to consider [17, 23–25].

To better understand scalp and cranial vault lesions in neurosurgical practice, it is important to recognize their pathologic nature and to specify their exact 3D topographic localization. A high index of suspicion needs to be kept in mind in order to achieve an appropriate diagnosis and to enhance the ability to discuss the best therapeutic option for each case. Indeed, different courses can

A. Akhaddar (✉)
Department of Neurosurgery, Avicenne Military Hospital of Marrakech, Mohammed V University in Rabat, Rabat, Morocco
e-mail: akhaddar@hotmail.fr

M. Turgut et al. (eds.), *Lesions of the Scalp and Cranial Vault*,
https://doi.org/10.1007/978-3-031-88244-9_1

be proposed for action: patient reassurance, simple survey, biopsy for pathologic confirmation, conservative treatment, or complete surgical resection with or without reconstruction.

These lesions may only concern the anatomical region of the skull or scalp or both of them. For example, the scalp-based lesions may involve the outer table while transdiploic lesions of the skull may invade the scalp. More seriously, deep intracranial extensive forms can co-exist (see below about topographic classification of the scalp and cranial vault lesions).

In this perspective, understanding the anatomy of the scalp and cranial vault is essential for the correct clinical and imaging interpretation of various lesions that occur in these locations (Fig. 1.1) [24, 27].

The scalp is the soft tissue that covers the bones of the cranial vault from the external occipital protuberance and superior nuchal line posteriorly to the orbital margins anteriorly and is laterally anchored by each ear. Classically, the scalp is described to have five layers (Fig. 1.2) which can be remembered by the mnemonic acronym SCALP from superficial to deep as:

- S: *Skin* (divided into a very thin external epidermis and a thicker inner dermis) with numerous hair follicles and sebaceous glands.
- C: *Connective tissue* (containing nerves, lymphatics, and vessels). It is a dense subcutaneous layer that connects the skin to the epicranial aponeurosis.
- A: *Aponeurosis* (epicranium or galea or deep fascia). It is a tendon-like structure that connects the frontalis/orbicularis, temporalis, and occipitalis muscles.
- L: *Loose connective tissue* (subgaleal space). It permits the mobility of the scalp on the underlying cranial vault. It provides the plane access to the surgical scalp flap.
- P: *Pericranium* which is the "external periosteum" of the skull bones. It can be separated from the bones except near the suture lines.

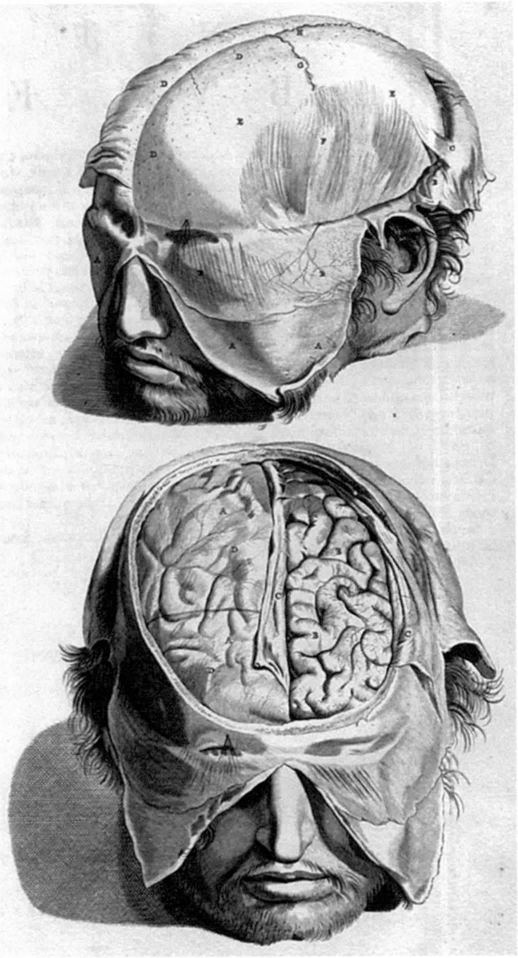

Fig. 1.1 Illustration from Bidloo's Anatomica humani corporis (edited in 1685). Table 5 shows a dissection of the cranial vault and scalp in the first figure (up) and the dura mater and brain parenchyma in the second (down) (This publication was in the public domain) [26]

The Cranial Vault (also known as Calvaria or Calvarium) is the superior and posterior part of the skull (or neurocranium) that surrounds and encloses the brain and is formed from several plates of bone separated by suture joints (Fig. 1.3). These flat bones comprise:

- Median frontal bone
- Paired parietal bones
- The squamous part of the paired temporal bones
- Tips of the greater wings of the paired sphenoid bones.
- Median occipital bone.

The calvarial bones are formed of two cortical layers of compact bone (the inner and outer tables) with spongious bony tissue between them (the dip-

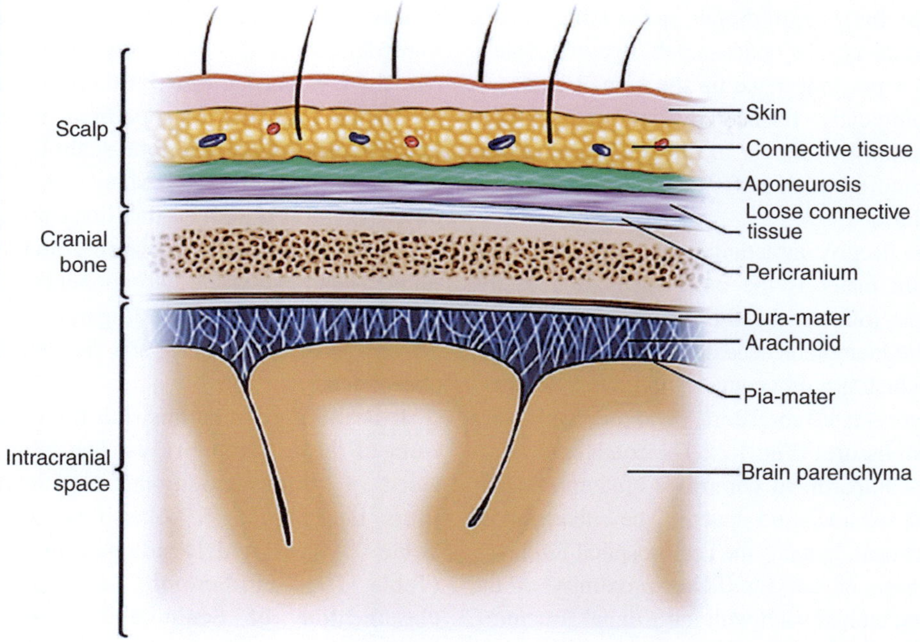

Fig. 1.2 Schematic drawing showing the different layers of the scalp, cranial bone, meninges, and brain parenchyma (Reproduced from Akhaddar, A. (2016). Pathophysiology and Anatomical Spreads of Infection. In: Cranial Osteomyelitis. Springer, Cham. https://doi.org/10.1007/978-3-319-30268-3_5; with permission)

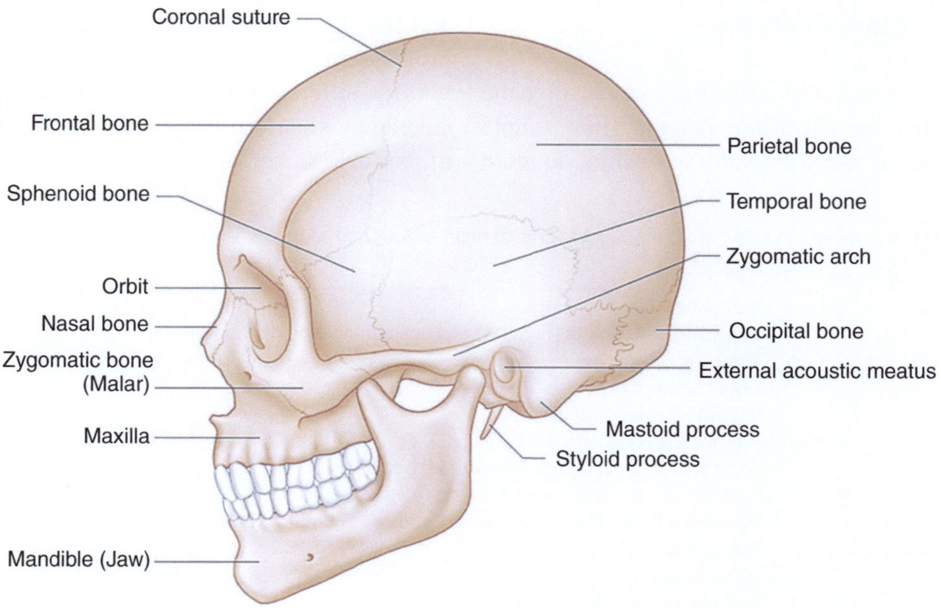

Fig. 1.3 Schematic drawing showing the lateral extracranial view of the skull bone (Reproduced from Akhaddar, A. (2016). Pathophysiology and Anatomical Spreads of Infection. In: Cranial Osteomyelitis. Springer, Cham. https://doi.org/10.1007/978-3-319-30268-3_5; with permission)

loe). The thickness of diploic space varies greatly between the type of bones and the age of people.

The bones that make up the cranial vault are embryologically formed by intramembranous ossification, in contrast to the skull base (chondrocranium), which is formed by endochondral ossification.

More deeply, intracranial structures are found. The dura mater is the outer membrane of the meninges followed by the arachnoid (a delicate avascular membrane beneath the dura), and the pia mater which is a thin connective tissue membrane that covers the cerebral cortex and even penetrates the brain fissures (Fig. 1.2). The contiguous intracranial compartment comprises epidural, subdural, and subarachnoid spaces. The subarachnoid compartment contains the cerebrospinal fluid.

Because of the significant proximity of the scalp and cranial vault with intracranial structures, the gravity of the scalp and cranial vault lesions is related to their intracranial extensions and potential neurologic complications [1, 17, 23, 24].

1.3 Classifications

A wide variety of abnormalities can involve the scalp and the calvarium ranging from simple incidental findings or painless swelling to more serious intracranial involvement with neurologic deficits, so it is not always easy to categorize these abnormalities. Furthermore, injuries can range from simple superficial abrasion or limited linear fracture to total scalp loss or penetrating foreign bodies. Many classifications have been proposed in the literature, mostly related to topographic locations, imaging features, histopathologic components, specific populations, or clinical findings [7, 11, 15–23, 28–34]. However, there are no standardized classifications.

It is difficult to summarize the large spectrum of these lesions in just one table. In the spirit of simplification and clarification for users, the "*pathologic*" classification given in Table 1.1 was widely adopted in this book (Table 1.1). Furthermore, a "*topographic*" classification of Scalp and Cranial vault Lesions based on the location of the lesion and its extension was summarized in Table 1.2 (Table 1.2).

There are some similarities between types Ib and IIb, types IIc and IIIa, as well as types Ic and IIIc; however, the sense of the topographic progression of the disease (outward or inward or both) is different and should be taken into consideration when managing patients with lesions of the scalp and cranial vault.

Table 1.1 Pathologic classification of scalp and cranial vault lesions and anatomic variants

Category of lesions	Type of lesions
Congenital	– Sinus pericranii – Congenital skull defect (Fig. 1.4) and congenital skull depression – Cutaneous ectopic brain – Dermal sinus tract – Intradiploic arachnoid cyst – Aplasia cutis congenita (Fig. 1.5) – Cutis Verticis Gyrata (Cyclist's Helmet Scalp) (Fig. 1.6) – Cephaloceles: meningoencephalocele, meningocele, atretic cephalocele, gliocele – Craniosynostosis: non-syndromic or "isolated" craniosynostosis versus syndromic craniosynostosis – Cranial bifidum – Craniopagus Conjoined Twins
Anatomic variants	– Abnormal arachnoid/pacchionian granulations – Dilatated/prominent venous channels and lakes (emissary veins) – Hyperostosis frontalis interna – Bilateral thinning of the parietal bones – Normal ageing calvarium – Enlarged parietal or biparietal foramina – Fontanelles (soft spots)

(continued)

Table 1.1 (continued)

Category of lesions	Type of lesions
Metabolic and rheumatologic	– Rickets – Hyperthyroidism – Hyperparathyroidism – Renal osteodystrophy – Acromegaly – Amyloidosis – Drug-induced hyperostosis – Osteogenesis imperfect – Chronic hemolytic anemia – Osteopenia – Thalassemia – Osteopetrosis
Traumatic	• No penetrating: scalp contusion, ulcers, skull fractures (Fig. 1.7), suture diastasis, cephalohematoma, subgaleal hematoma (Fig. 1.8), intraosseous hematoma, growing skull fracture/leptomeningeal cyst (Fig. 1.9), scalp nodules • Penetrating: laceration, wounds (Fig. 1.10), penetrating skull fractures (Fig. 1.11), craniocerebral injuries (Fig. 1.12), foreign bodies (Fig. 1.13), non-healing wounds (Figs. 1.14 and 1.15) • – Others: keloids (Figs. 1.16 and 1.17), pressure sore (bedsore) (Fig. 1.18), scalp necrosis (Fig. 1.19), flap osteonecrosis, granulomas, calcified/ossified epidural/subdural hematomas
Iatrogenic	– Burr holes – Bone flaps – Head-holders – Stereotactic frames – Cervical tractions tongs – Pseudomeningocele (Fig. 1.20) – Radionecrosis – Granulomas – Shunted hydrocephalus
Vascular	– *Scalp*: Ports wine stains, cirsoid aneurysm (Fig. 1.21), pseudoaneurysm, hemangioma – *Calvaria*: hemangioma (Fig. 1.22), aneurysmal bone cyst, arteriovenous malformation, venous malformation
Infectious	– Scalp abscesses (Fig. 1.23) – Osteomyelitis (Fig. 1.24)
Inflammatory	– Sarcoidosis – Langerhans cell histiocytosis (eosinophilic granuloma) (Fig. 1.25) – Collagenolytic (necrobiotic) granulomas – Chronic recurrent multifocal osteomyelitis – Cranial fasciitis – Other granulomas
Benign Neoplasms	– Lipoma (Fig. 1.26) – Giant pilar cyst (Fig. 1.27) – Dermoids, epidermoids (Fig. 1.28), and teratoid cysts – Neurofibroma – Desmoplastic fibroma – Myofibroma – Ossifying osteoma – Melanotic neuroectodermal tumor of infancy – Giant cell tumor – Lymphangioma – Hemangiopericytoma – Osteoma (Fig. 1.29) – Osteoblastoma – Meningioma (hyperostosis/ectopic) (Fig. 1.30)

(continued)

Table 1.1 (continued)

Category of lesions	Type of lesions
Malignant neoplasms	– Squamous (SCC) and basal (BCC) cell carcinomas (Fig. 1.31a) – Melanomas – Hematologic malignancies (lymphomas/leukemias) – Osteosarcoma (Fig. 1.31b) – Chondrosarcoma – Angiosarcoma – Fibrosarcoma – Ewing's sarcoma – Other sarcomas – Malignant peripheral nerve sheath tumors – Metastases (Figs. 1.32, 1.33, 1.34 and 1.35) – Plasmacytoma (Fig. 1.36) – Multiple myeloma – Meningiosarcoma (Fig. 1.37) – Glioma (Fig. 1.38) – Neuroblastoma
Others	– Paget's disease (osteitis deformans) – Fibrous dysplasia (Fig. 1.39) – Gorham disease – Parry-Romberg syndrome – Cleidocranial dysostosis (cleidocranial dysplasia) – Prominent Convolutional Marking (Copper-Beaten Skull) – Hamartoma – Frontal sinus mucocele

Table 1.2 Topographic classification of scalp and cranial vault lesions based on the location of the lesion and its extension

Types	Topographic location and possible extension
Type Ia	Limited to the scalp (Lesions may be subdivided according to their location within the scalp layers)
Type Ib	Scalp with cranial extension
Type Ic	Scalp with cranial and intracranial extension (extradural/intradural)
Type IIa	Limited to the cranial bone (Lesions may be subdivided according to their location within the cranial bone thickness)
Type IIb	Cranial bone with scalp extension
Type IIc	Cranial bone with intracranial extension (extradural/intradural)
Type IId	Cranial bone with scalp and intracranial extension
Type IIIa	Intracranial (brain/meninges) lesion with cranial bone extension
Type IIIc	Intracranial (brain/meninges) lesion with cranial bone and scalp extension

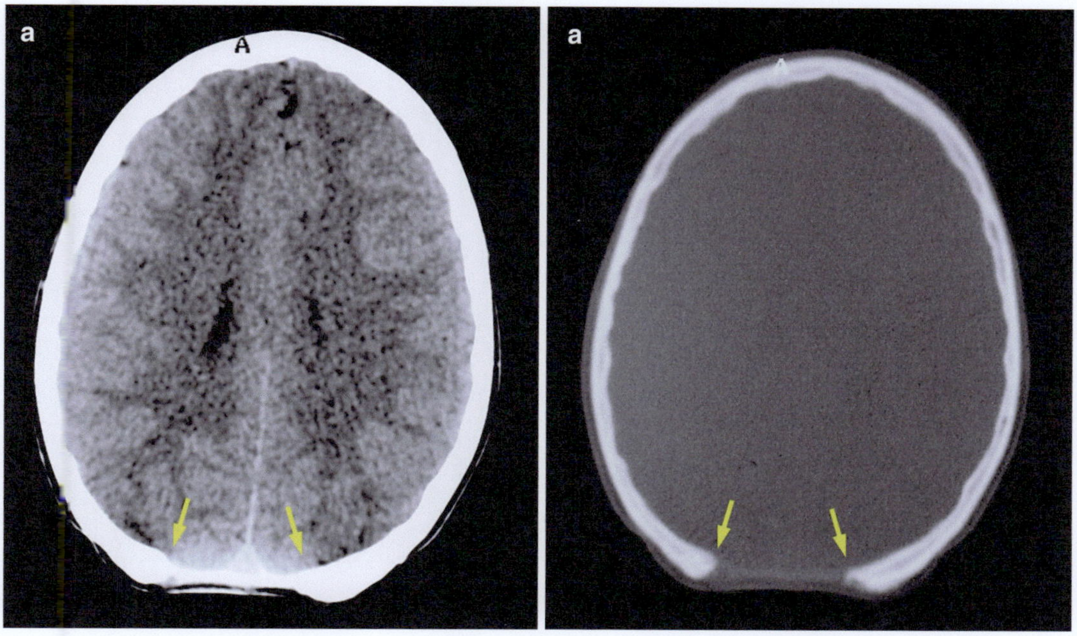

Fig. 1.4 Congenital skull defect of the posterior parietal area (arrows) as seen on axial CT-scan on parenchymal (**a**) and bone windows (**b**)

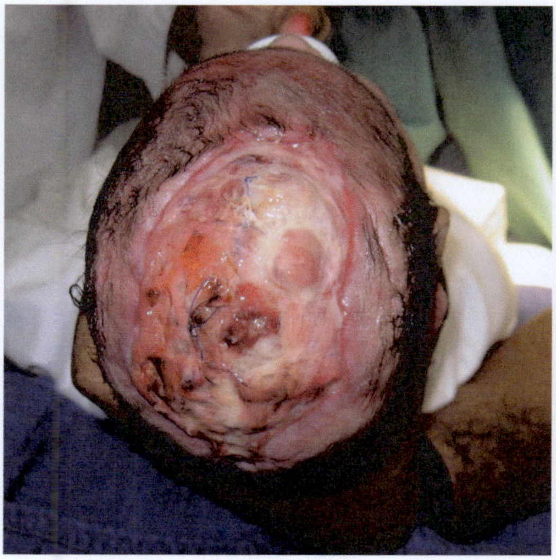

Fig. 1.5 Aplasia cutis congenital in a newborn

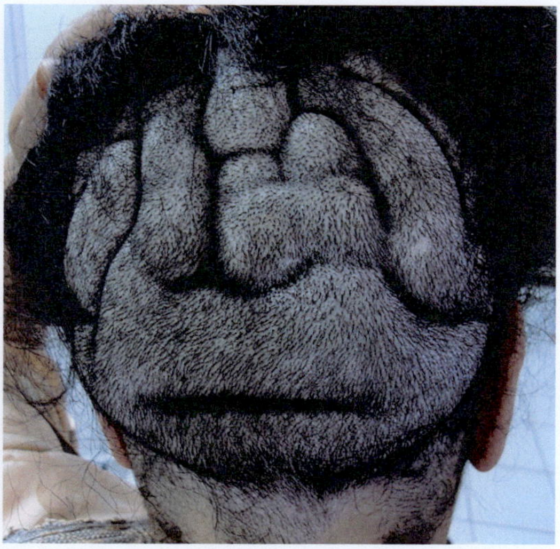

Fig. 1.6 Cutis Verticis Gyrata (Cyclist's Helmet Scalp) in a parieto-occipital view (Courtesy of Professor Adil Arrob, M.D)

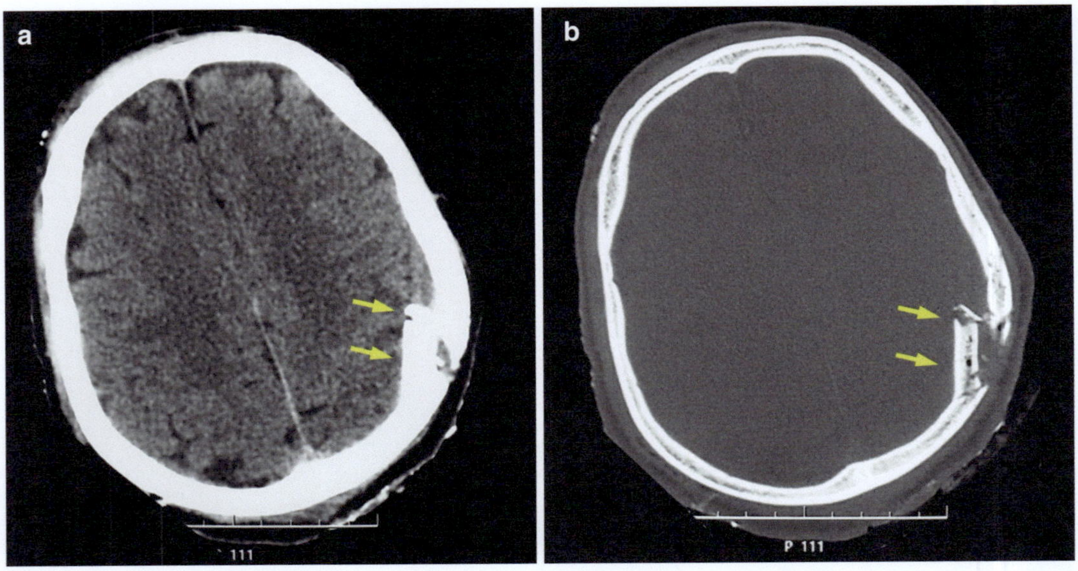

Fig. 1.7 Depressed parietal skull fractures (arrows) as seen on axial CT-scan, parenchymal (**a**) and bone windows (**b**)

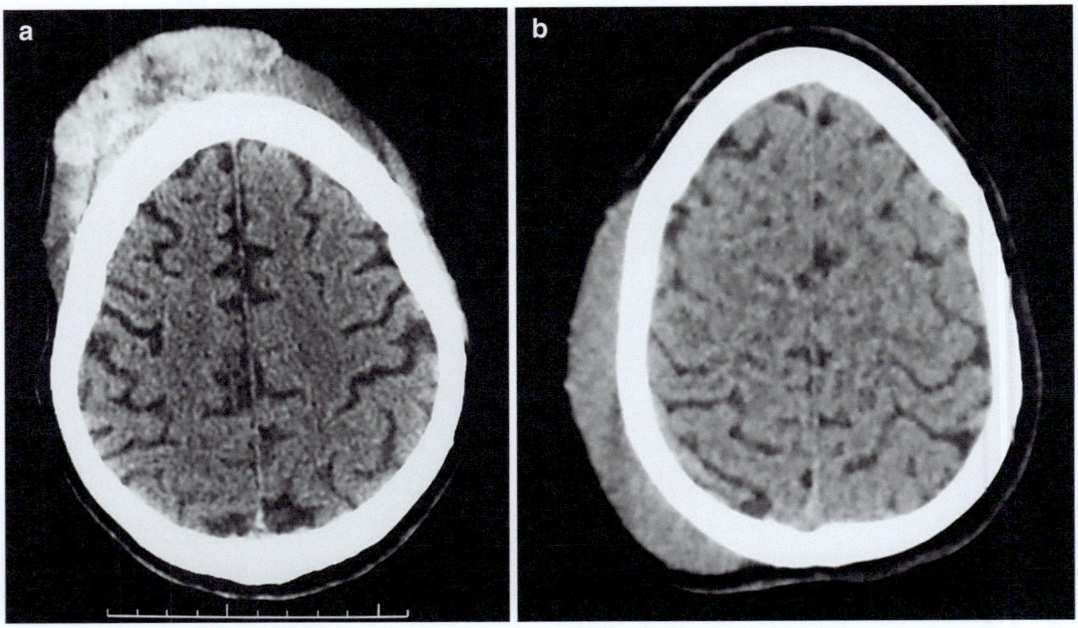

Fig. 1.8 Subgaleal hematomas as seen on axial CT-scan (**a**, **b**). Frontal post-traumatic (**a**) and fronto-parietal spontaneous hematoma due to coagulation disorders (**b**)

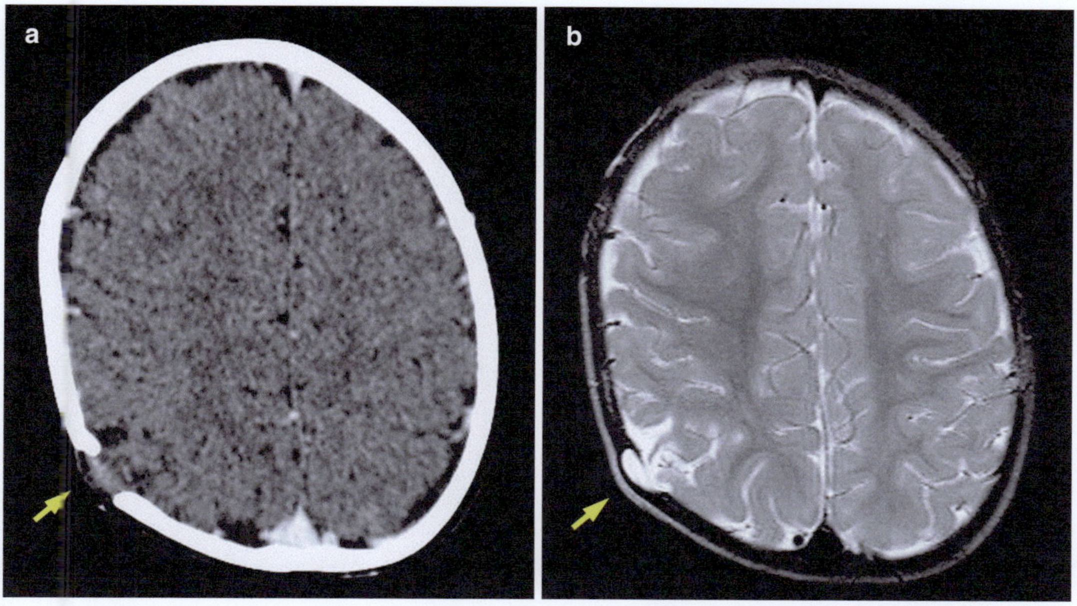

Fig. 1.9 Growing skull fracture/leptomeningeal cyst of the right posterior region (arrows) as seen on axial CT-scan (**a**) and T2-weighted MRI (**b**)

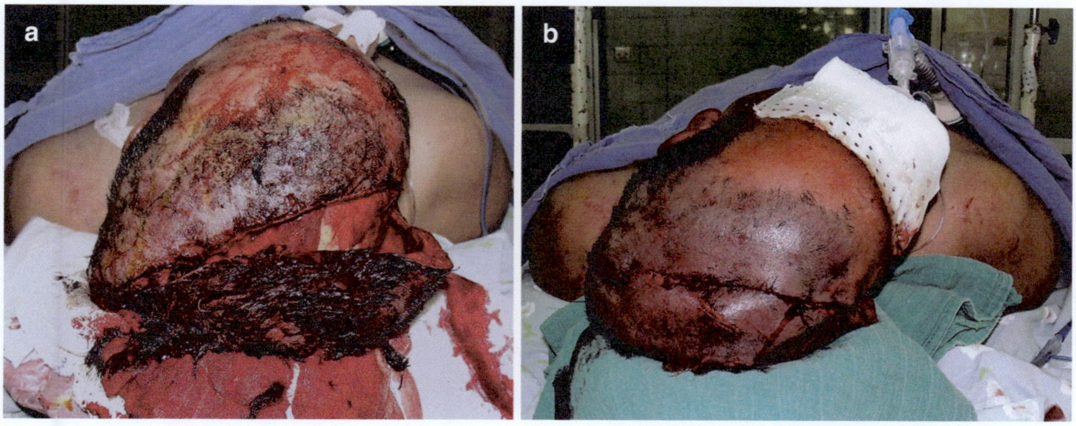

Fig. 1.10 Large scalp wound with laceration (**a**, **b**)

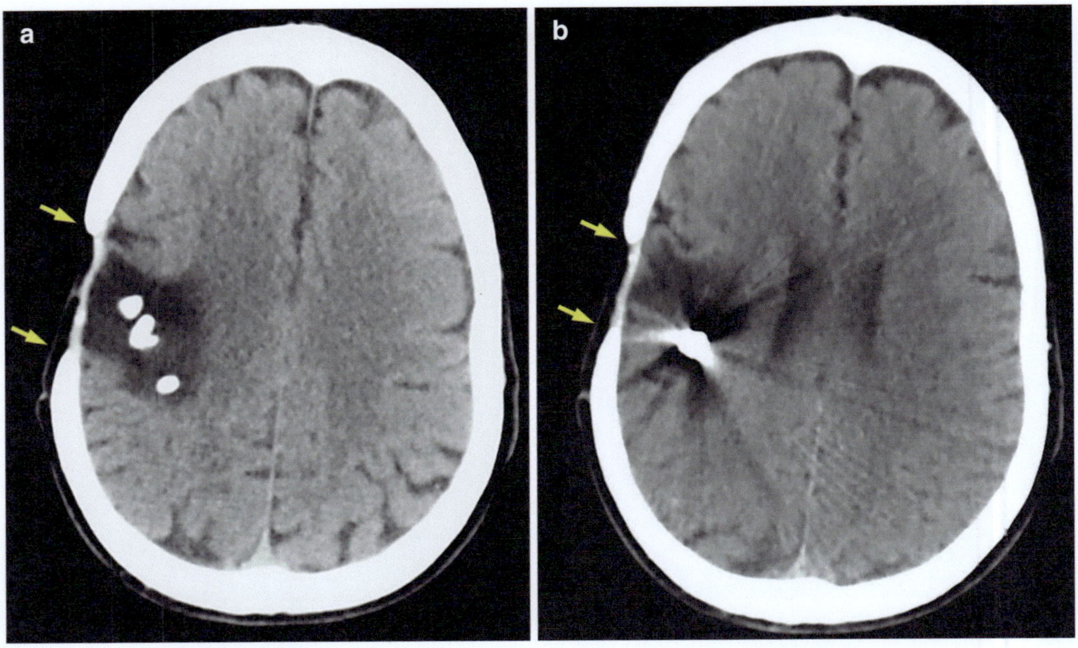

Fig. 1.11 Fronto-parietal craniocerebral injury: there is a post-traumatic cranial defect (arrows) with intracerebral bone and foreign bodies as seen on axial CT-scan (**a**, **b**)

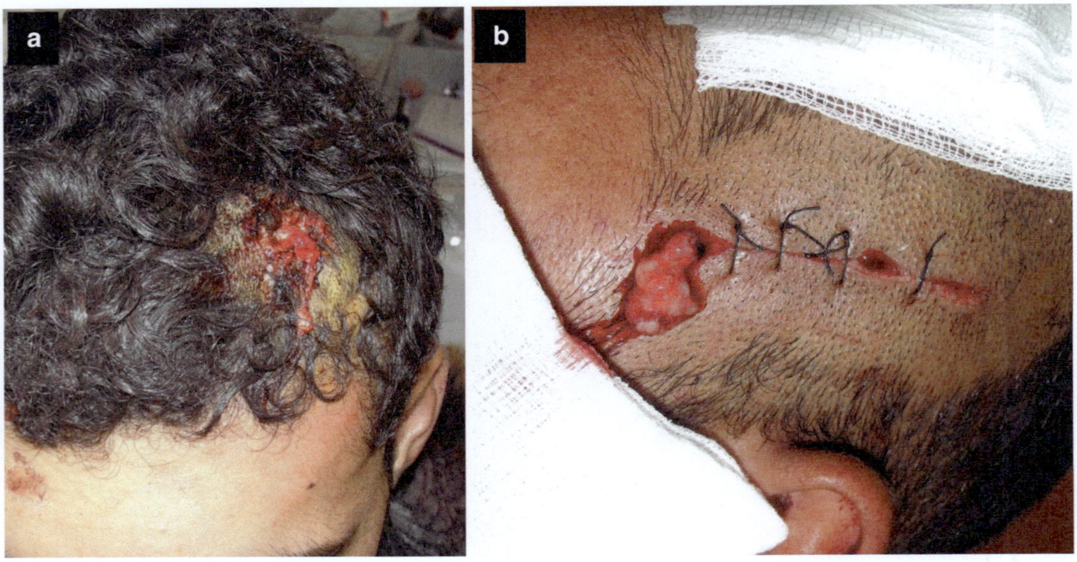

Fig. 1.12 Open head injury with extracranial extrusion of brain matter in two injured patients (**a**, **b**)

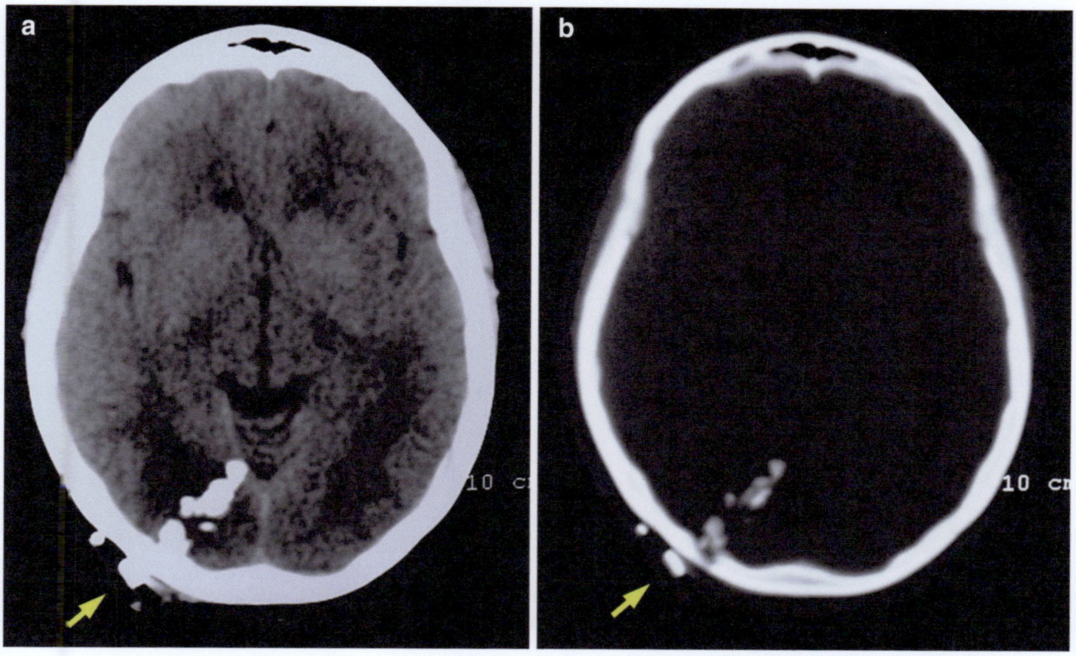

Fig. 1.13 Axial CT-scan on parenchymal (**a**) and bone windows (**b**) showing a penetrating perieto-occiptal cranio-cerebral injury with subgaleal (arrows) and intracerebral foreign bodies

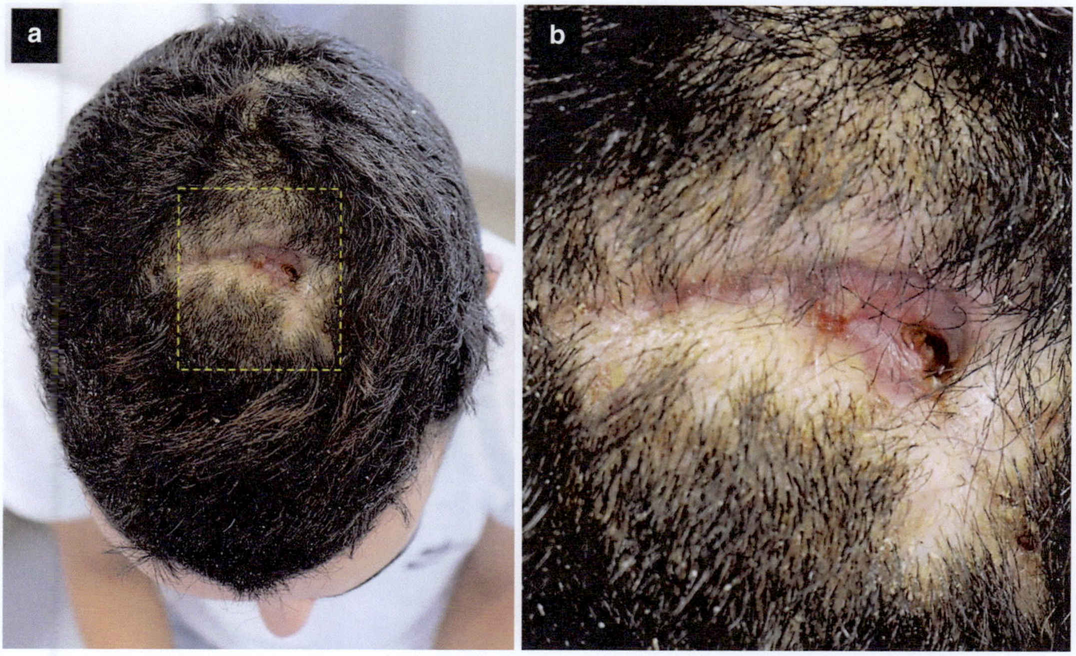

Fig. 1.14 Clinical pictures of post-traumatic non-healing wound (**a**, **b**)

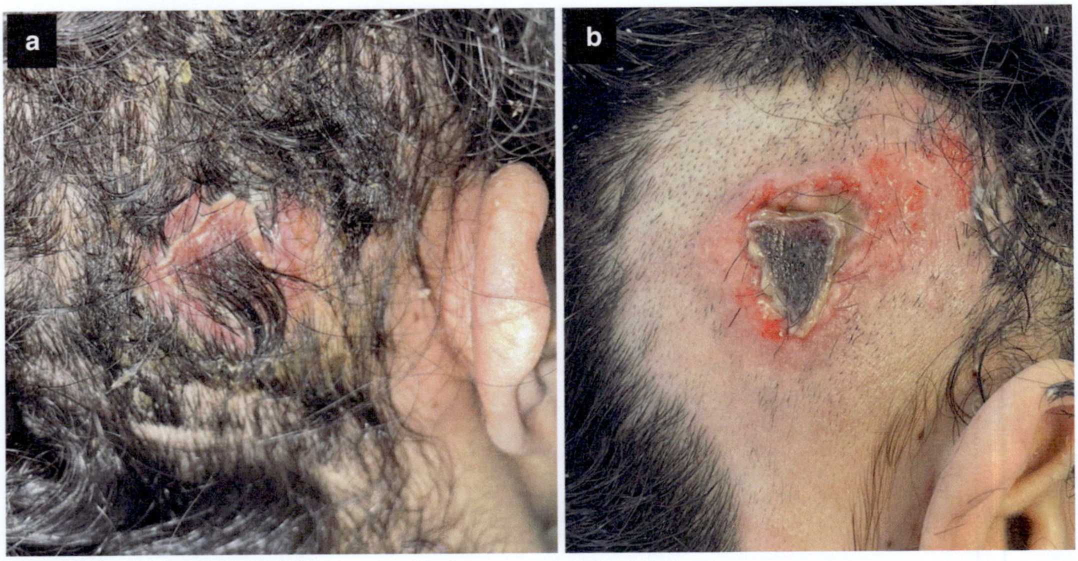

Fig. 1.15 Clinical pictures of post-traumatic neglected non-healing wound before (**a**) and after shaving (**b**) (Courtesy of Doctor Achraf Moussa, M.D). Note that the wound was hidden by hair

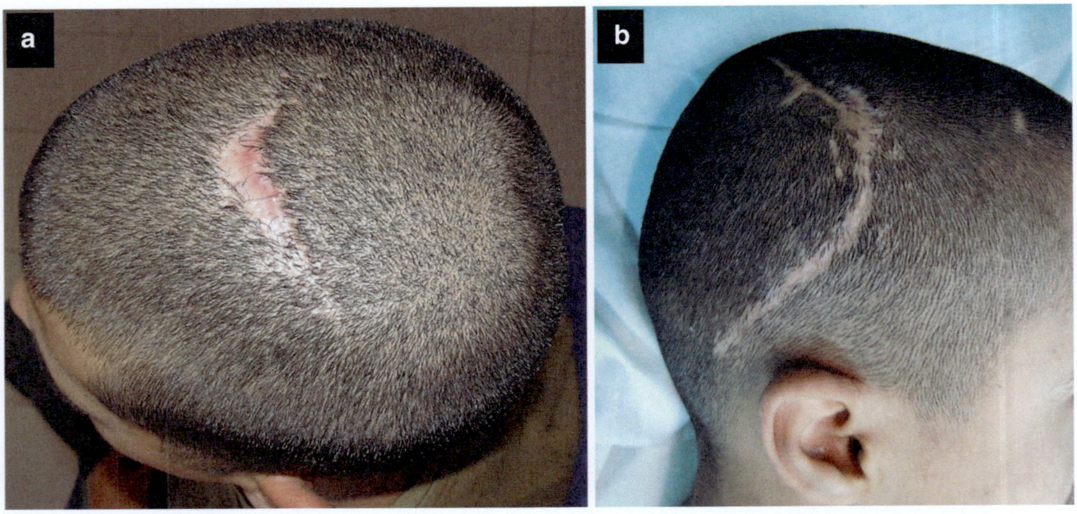

Fig. 1.16 Frontal (**a**) and parieto-occipital keloid scars (**b**) (**b**: Courtesy of Professor Adil Arrob, M.D)

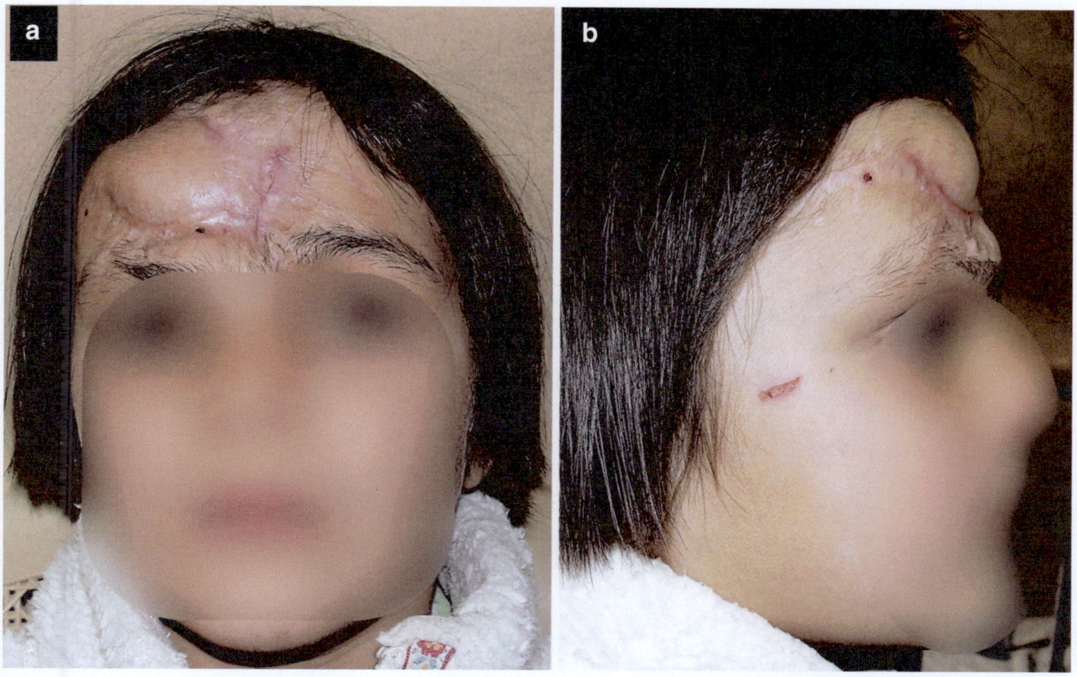

Fig. 1.17 Frontal hypertrophic keloid scars (**a**, **b**)

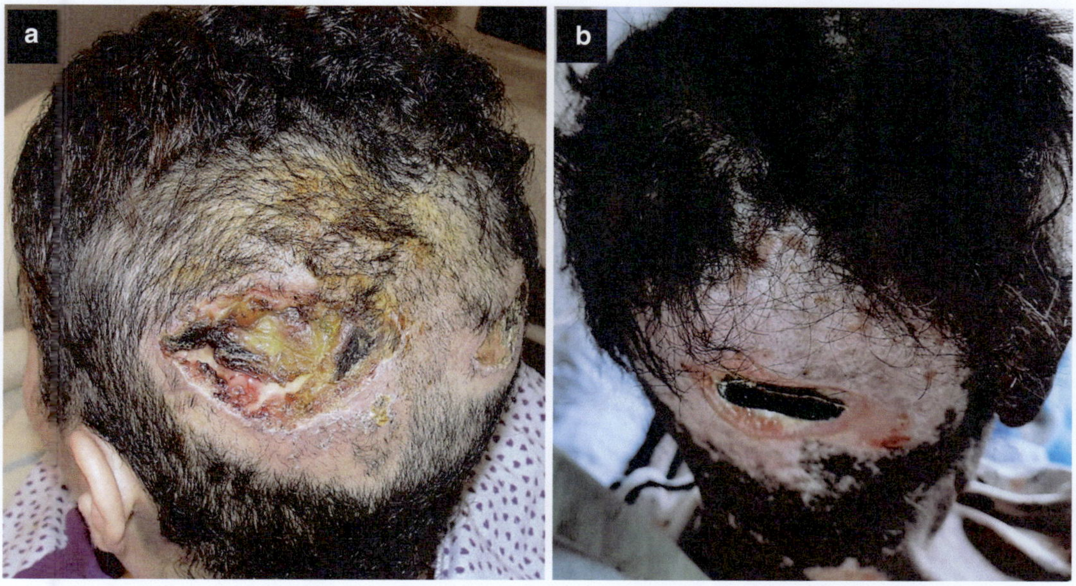

Fig. 1.18 Pressure sore (bedsore) of the parieto-oocipital area in two patients (**a**, **b**). (**b**: Courtesy of Professor Adil Arrob, M.D)

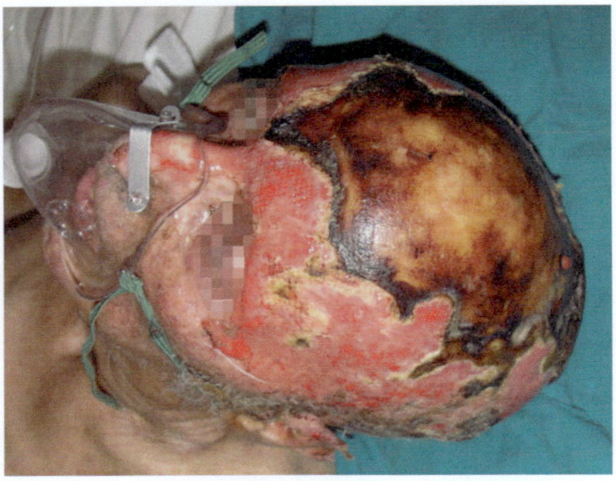

Fig. 1.19 Large scalp necrosis due to high voltage burn (electrocution)

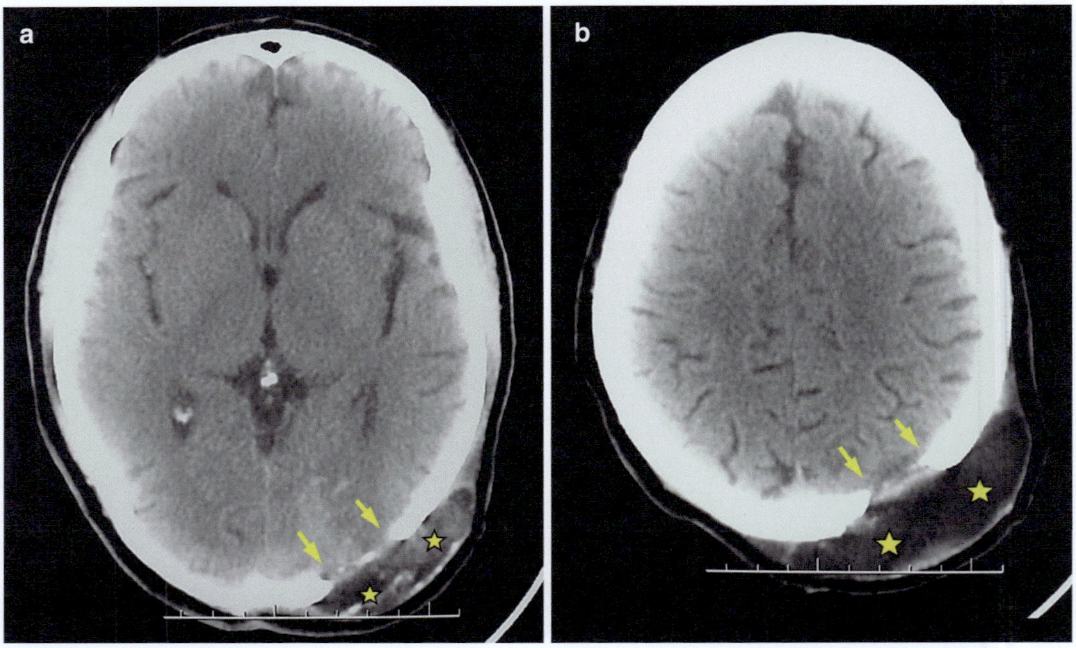

Fig. 1.20 Post-operative parieto-occipital pseudomeningocele as shown on axial CT-scan (**a**, **b**). Note the skull bone defect (arrows) and the extracranial cyst (star)

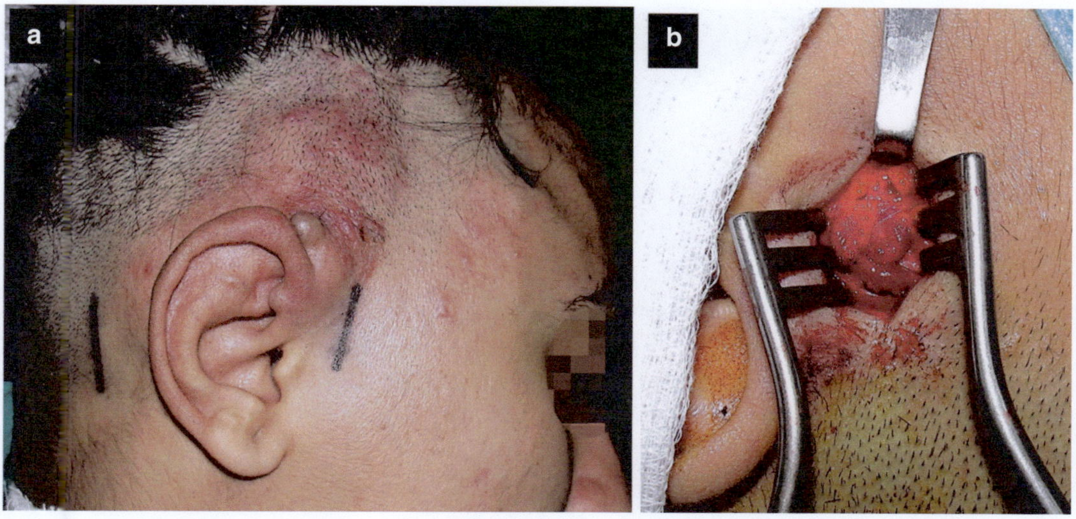

Fig. 1.21 Temporal arterio-venous malformation of the scalp (cirsoid aneurysm) (**a**, **b**). Note the subcutaneous ectatic blood vessels (**b**)

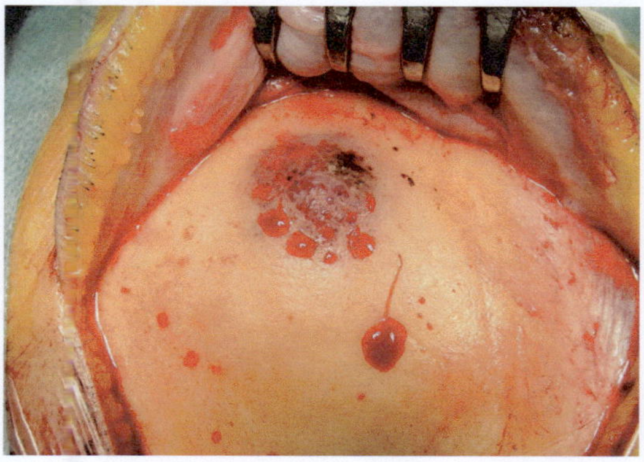

Fig. 1.22 Frontal intraosseous hemangioma: operative view

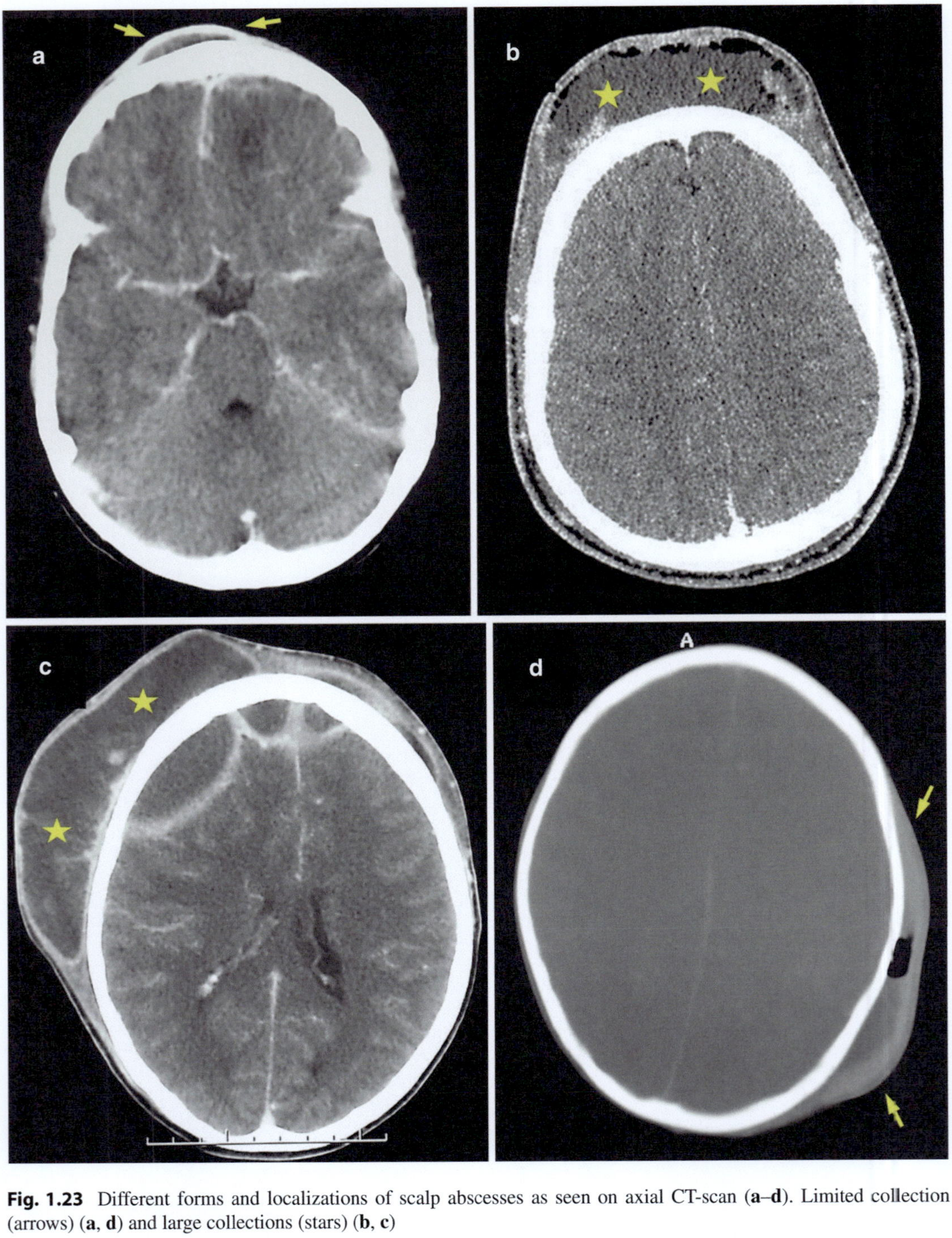

Fig. 1.23 Different forms and localizations of scalp abscesses as seen on axial CT-scan (**a**–**d**). Limited collection (arrows) (**a**, **d**) and large collections (stars) (**b**, **c**)

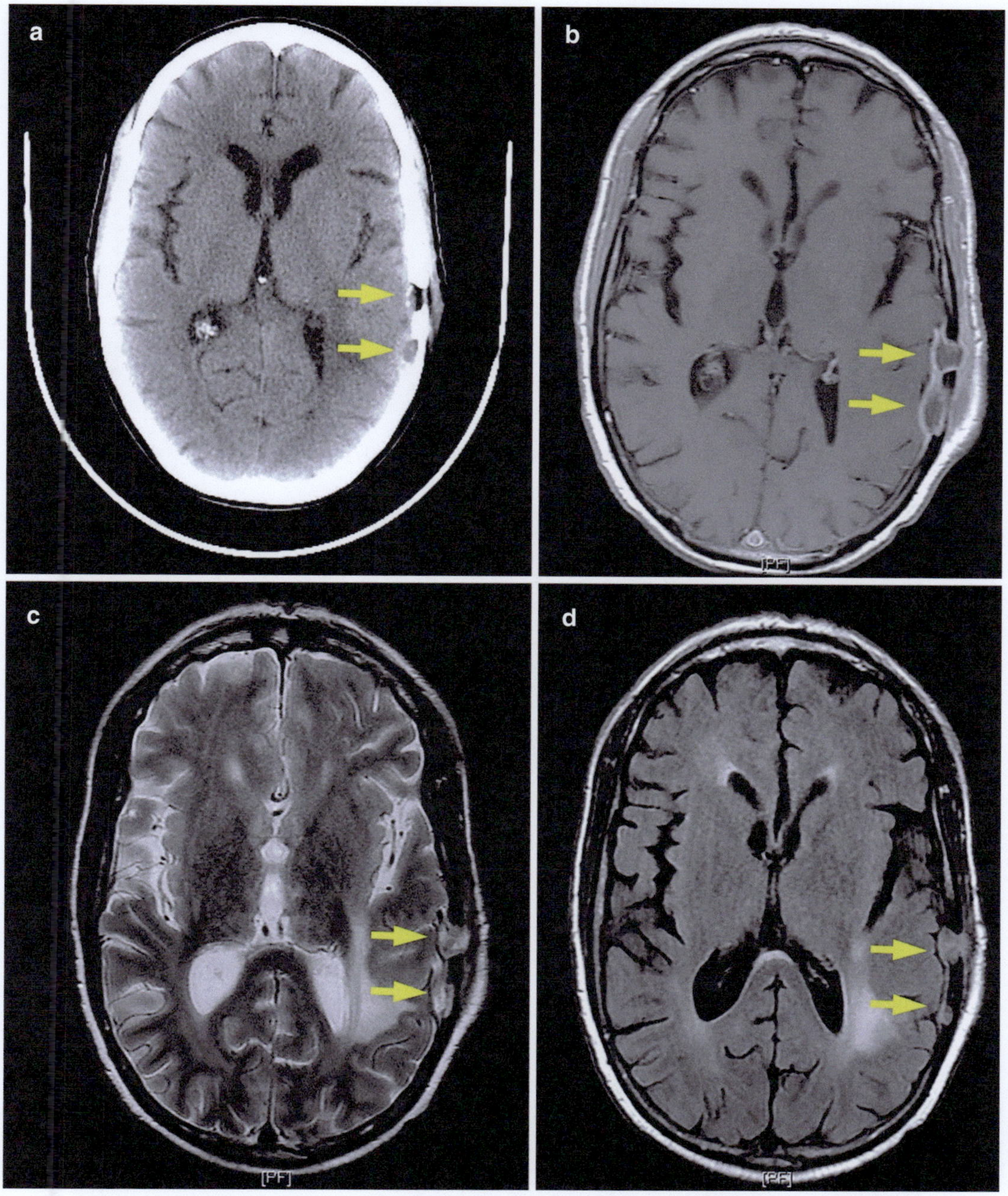

Fig. 1.24 Temporo-parietal cranial osteomyelitis as seen on axial CT-scan (**a**) and post-gadolinium T1- (**b**) and T2-weighted MRI (**c**) as well as on FLAIR sequences (**d**)

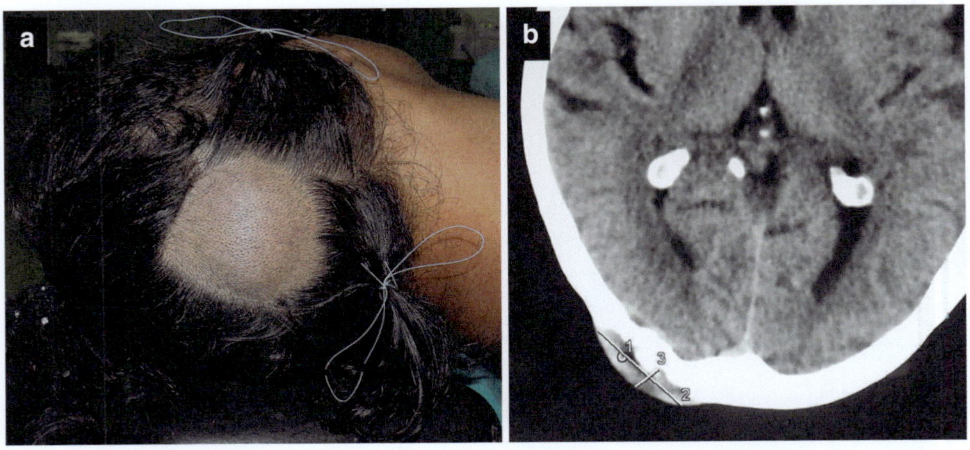

Fig. 1.25 Clinical picture showing an occipital eosinophilic granuloma (**a**). The same lesion on axial CT-scan (**b**)

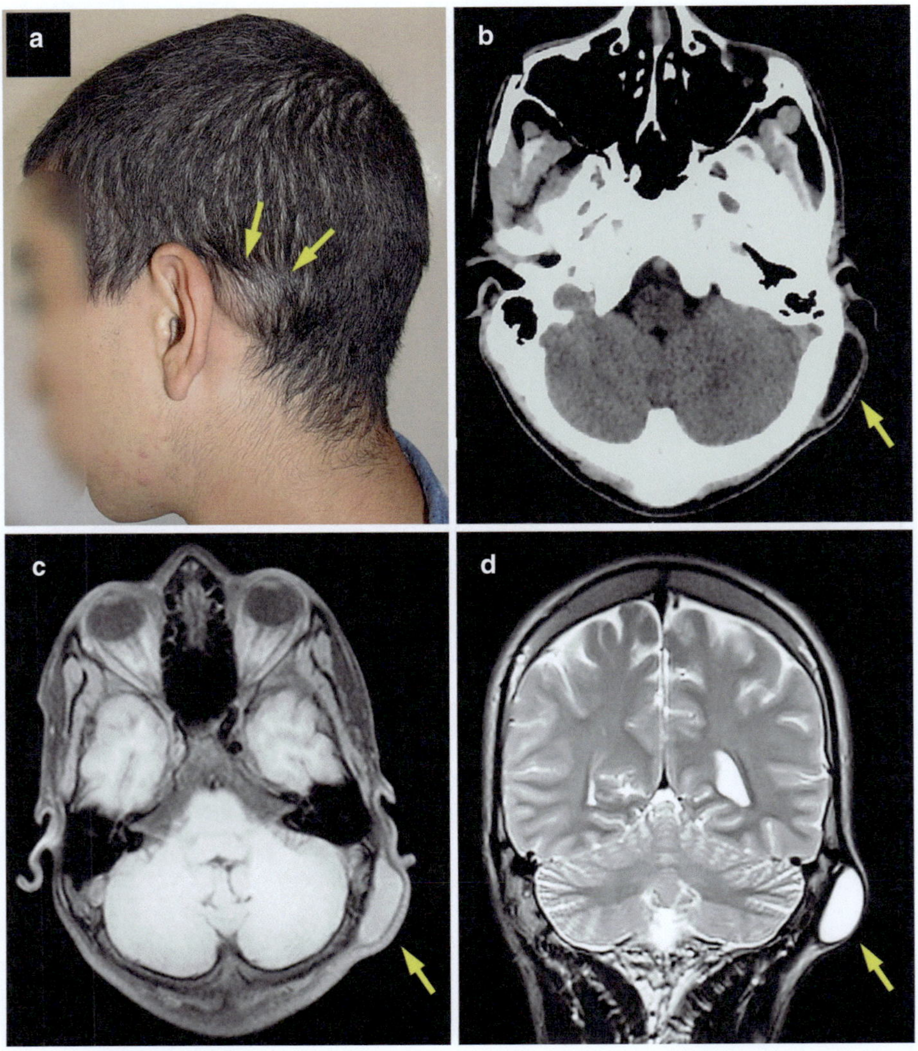

Fig. 1.26 Clinical picture showing a retroauricular lipoma (arrows) (**a**). The same lesion on axial CT-scan (**b**) and T1-weighted MRI (**c**) as well as on coronal T2-weighted MRI (**d**) (arrow)

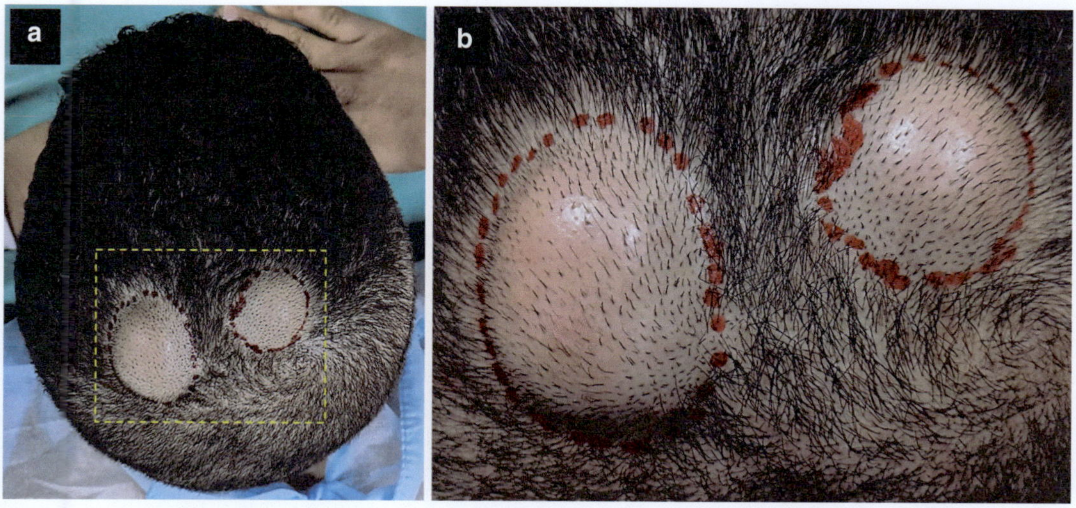

Fig. 1.27 Clinical picture of bilateral pilar cysts of the parietal area (**a, b**) (Courtesy of Professor Hatim Belfquih, M.D)

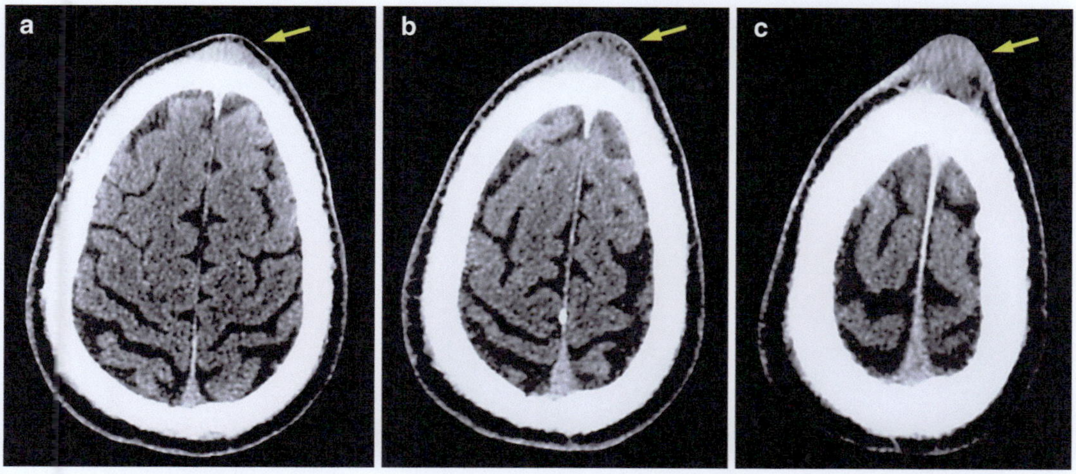

Fig. 1.28 Frontal epidermoid cyst as seen on axial CT-scan (**a–c**)

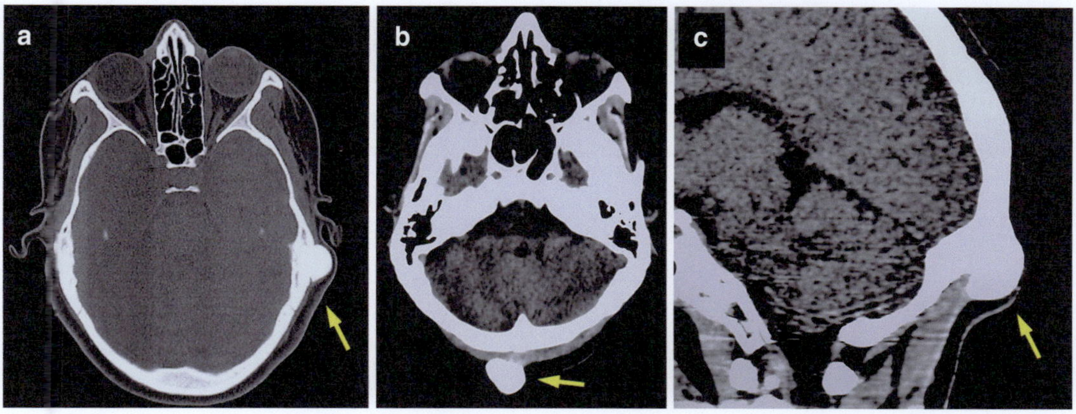

Fig. 1.29 Temporal (**a**) and occipital (**b, c**) osteomas (arrows) as seen on axial (**a, b**) and sagittal reconstruction (**c**) CT-scan

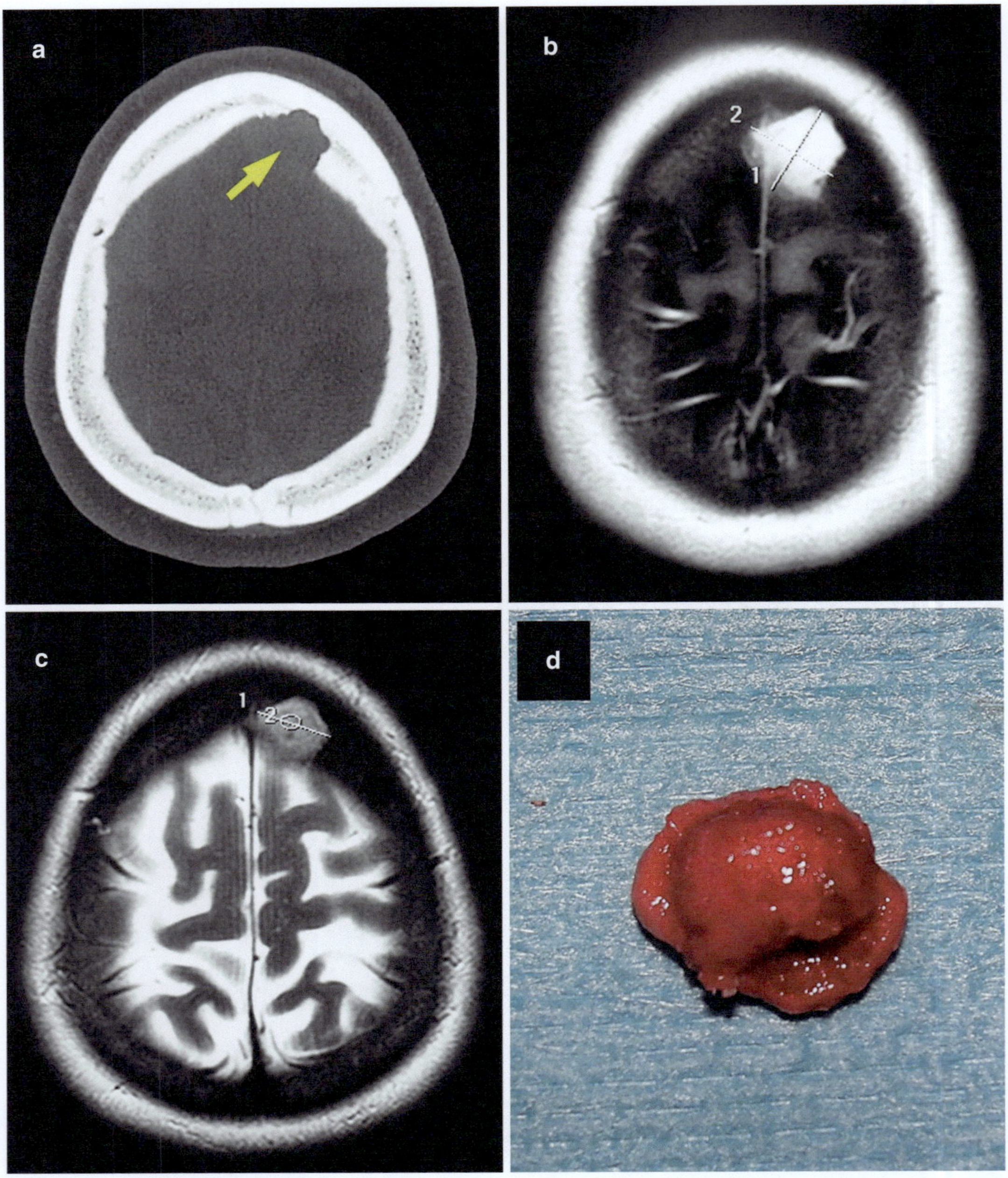

Fig. 1.30 Frontal extradural intraosseous meningioma (arrow) as seen on axial CT-scan (**a**), post-gadolinium T1- (**b**) and T2-weighted MRI (**c**). Macroscopic appearance of the ectopic meningioma after its resection (**d**)

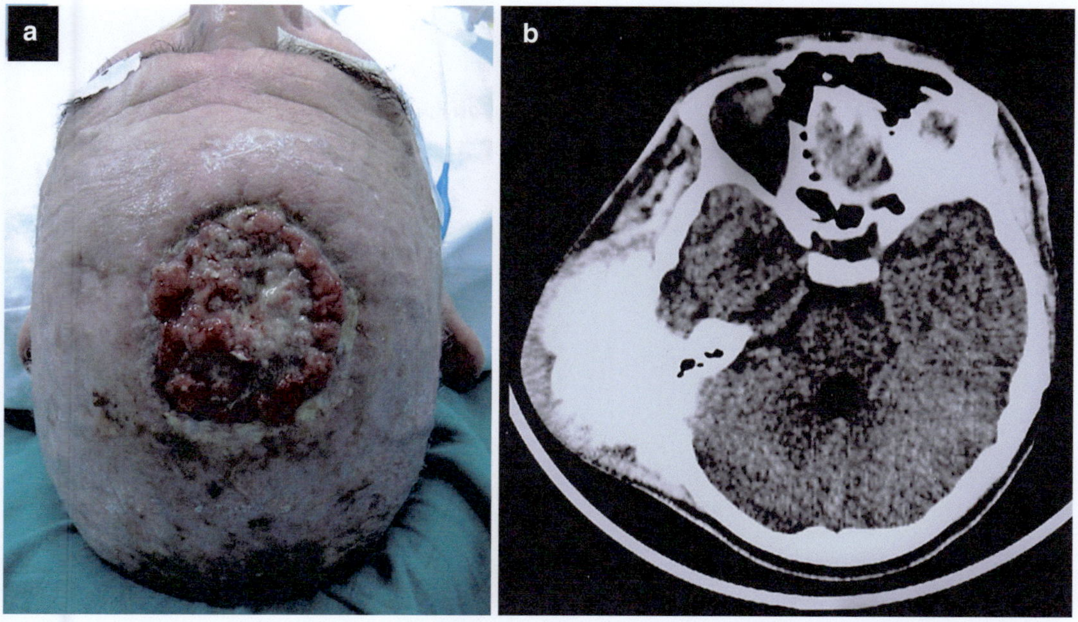

Fig. 1.31 Clinical picture of a basal cell carcinoma at the vertex (**a**) (Courtesy of Professor Adil Arrob, M.D). Temporal osteosarcoma as seen on axial CT-scan (**b**)

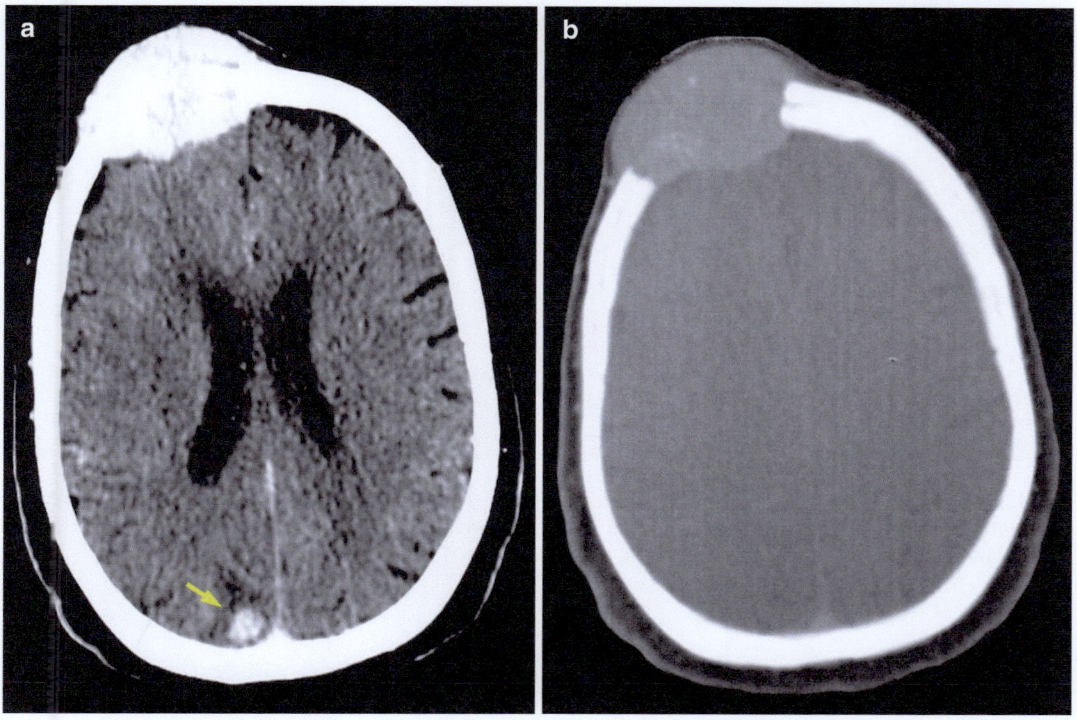

Fig. 1.32 Transdiploic frontal metastasis with extracranial and intracranial extension as seen on axial CT-scan on parenchymal (**a**) and bone (**b**) windows. Note the concomitant brain metastasis (arrow)

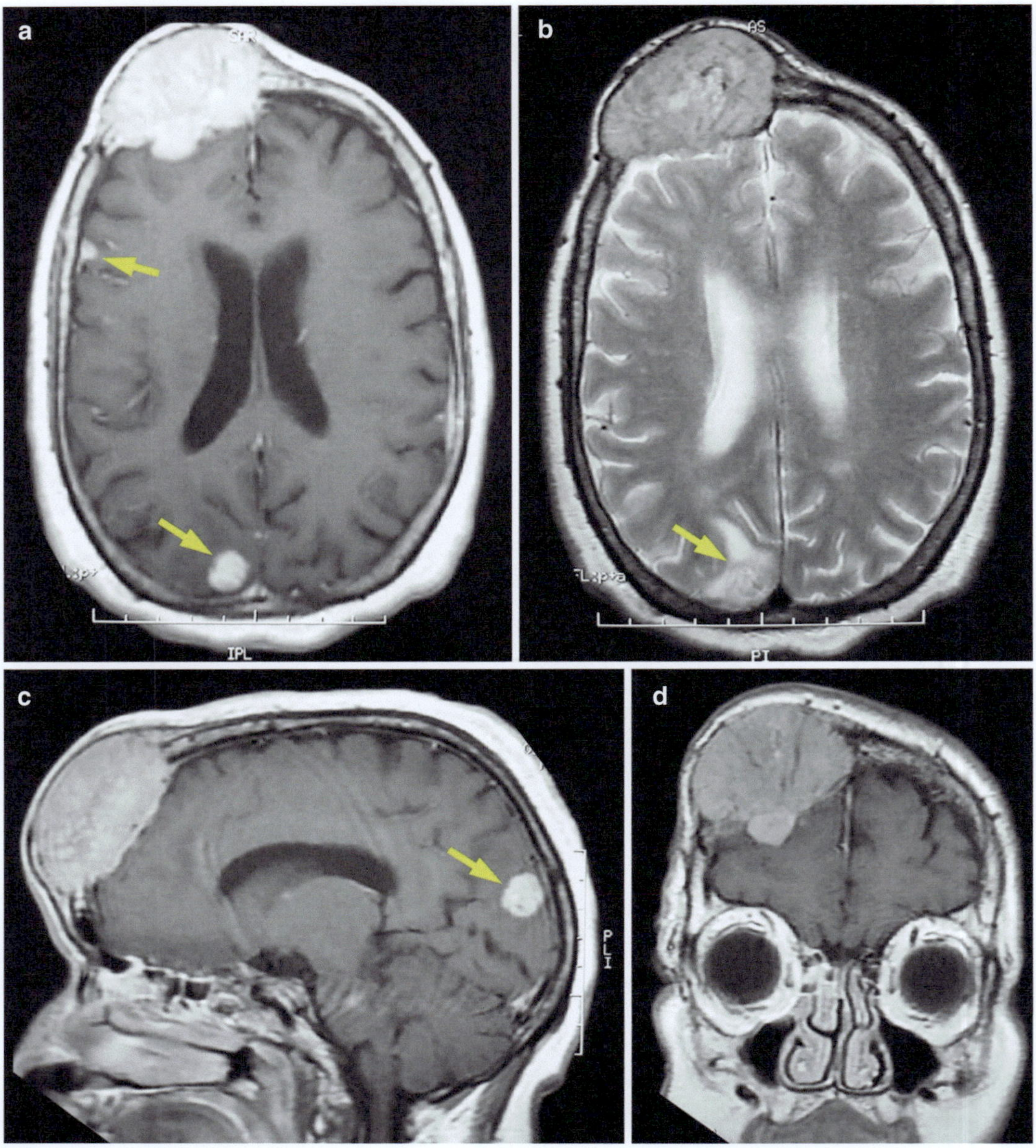

Fig. 1.33 Transdiploic frontal metastasis with extracranial and intracranial extension as seen on axial post-gadolinium T1- (**a**) and T2-weighted MRI (**b**) as well as on sagittal (**c**) and coronal (**d**) post-gadolinium T1-weighted MRI. Note the concomitant brain metastases (arrow)

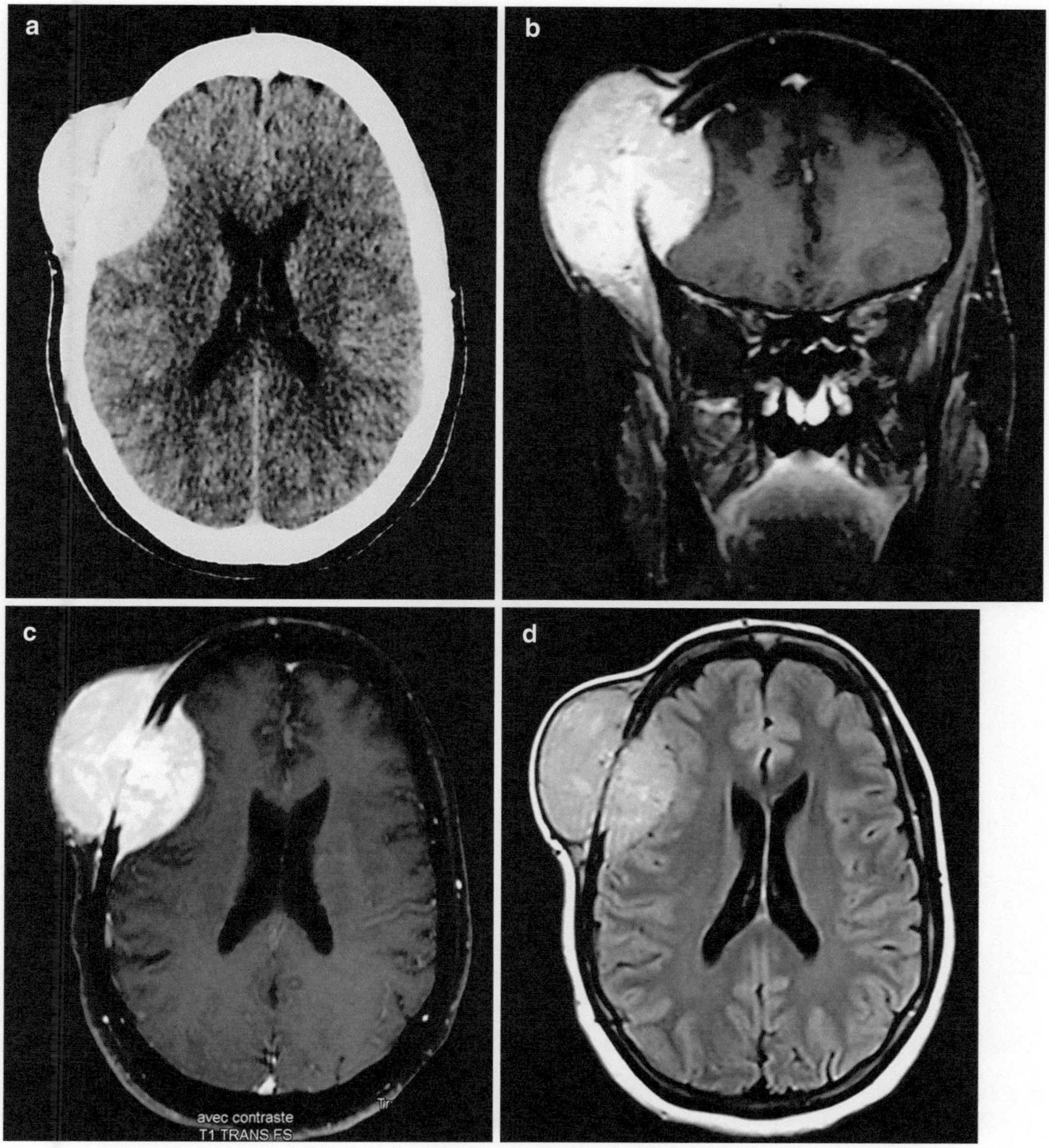

Fig. 1.34 Transdiploic fronto-temporal thyroid metastasis with extracranial and intracranial extension as seen on axial CT-scan (**a**) and post-gadolinium T1- (**b**), coronal post-gadolinium T1-weighted MRI (**c**) as well as on axial FLAIR sequences (**d**)

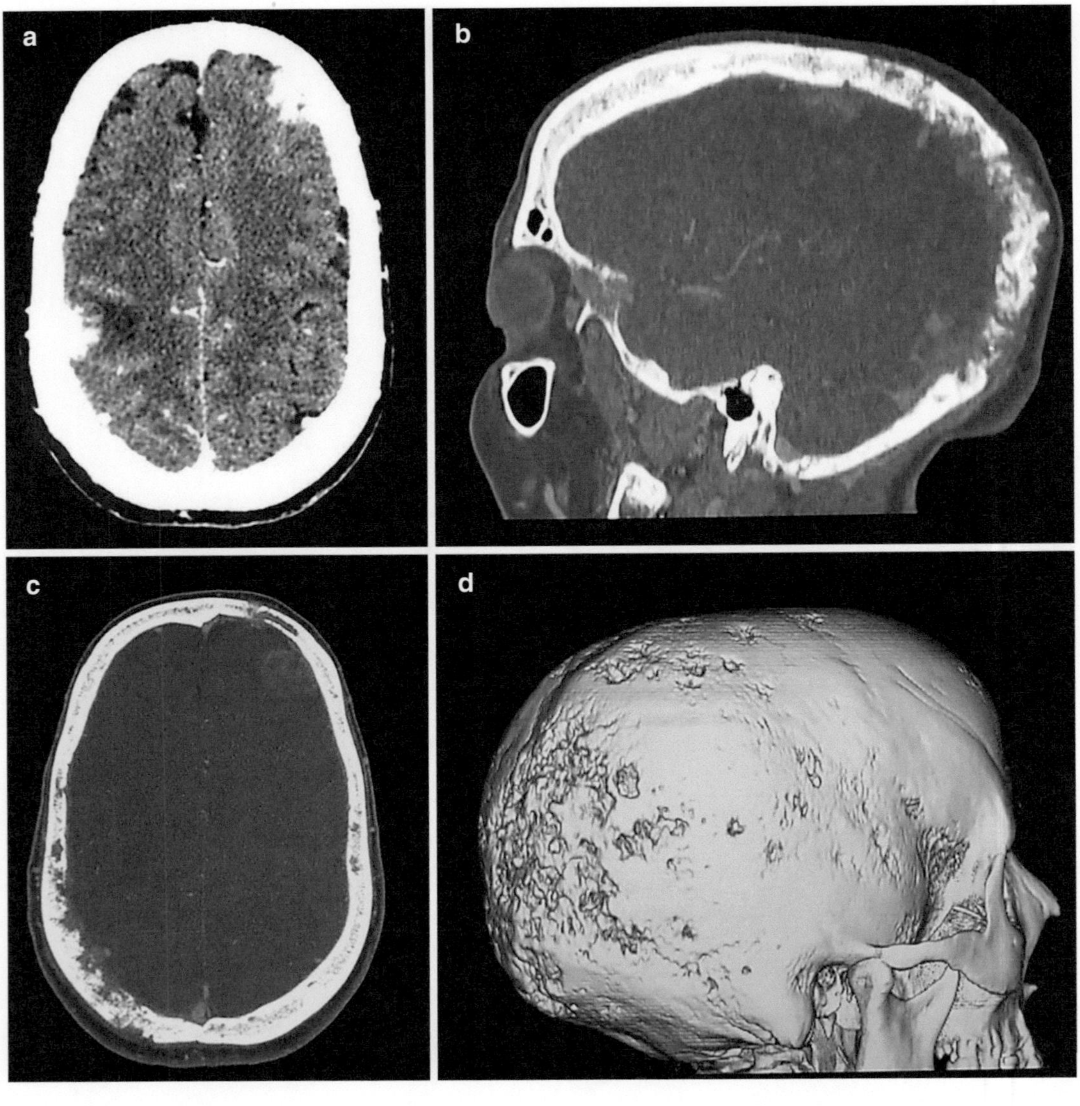

Fig. 1.35 Multiple craniocerebral breast metastases as seen on axial (**a, b**) and coronal reconstruction (**c**) CT-scan as well as on 3D CT-scan (reformatted volume-rendered) (**d**)

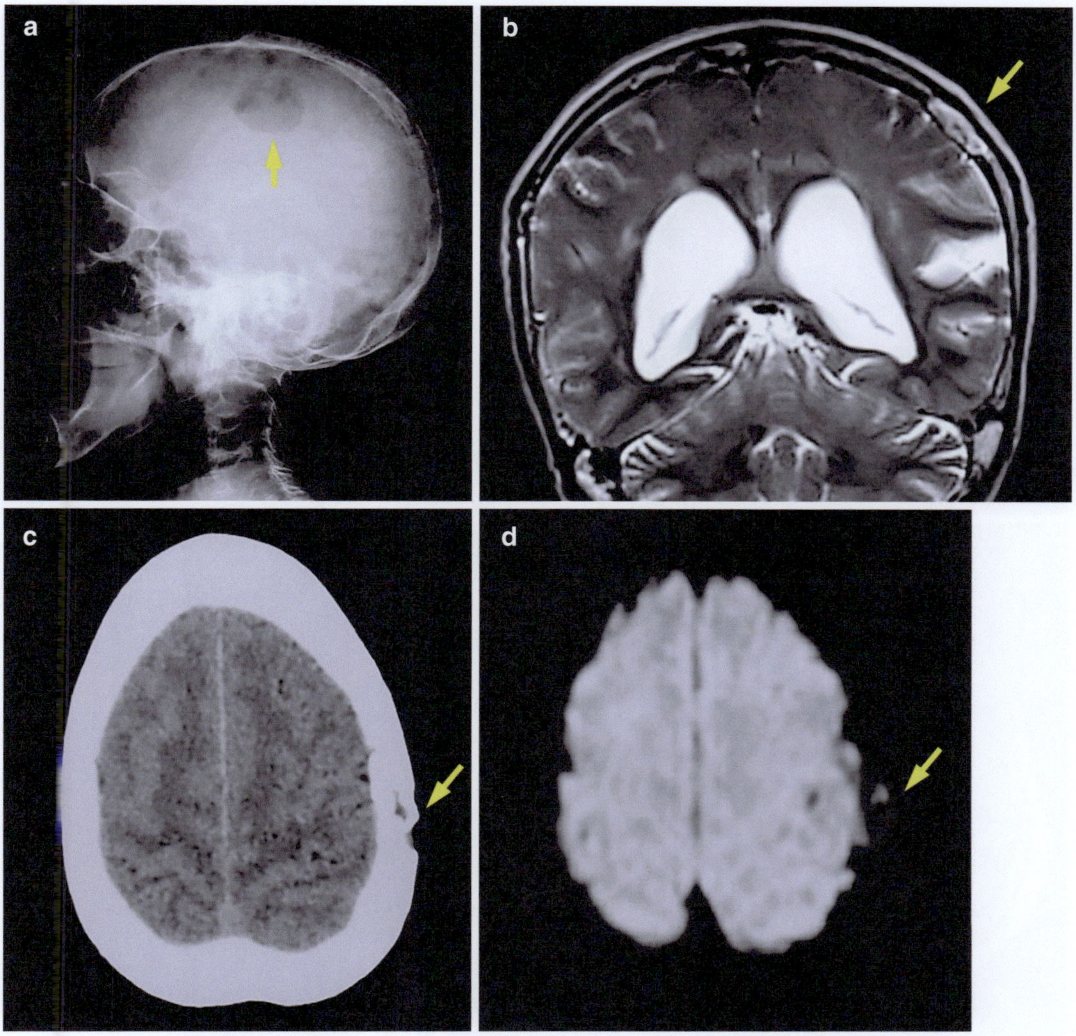

Fig. 1.36 Solitary plasmacytoma of the parietal vault (arrows) as seen on lateral plain radiography (**a**), axial CT-scan (**b**), coronal T2-weighted MRI (**c**), and on diffusion weighted-sequences DWI (**d**)

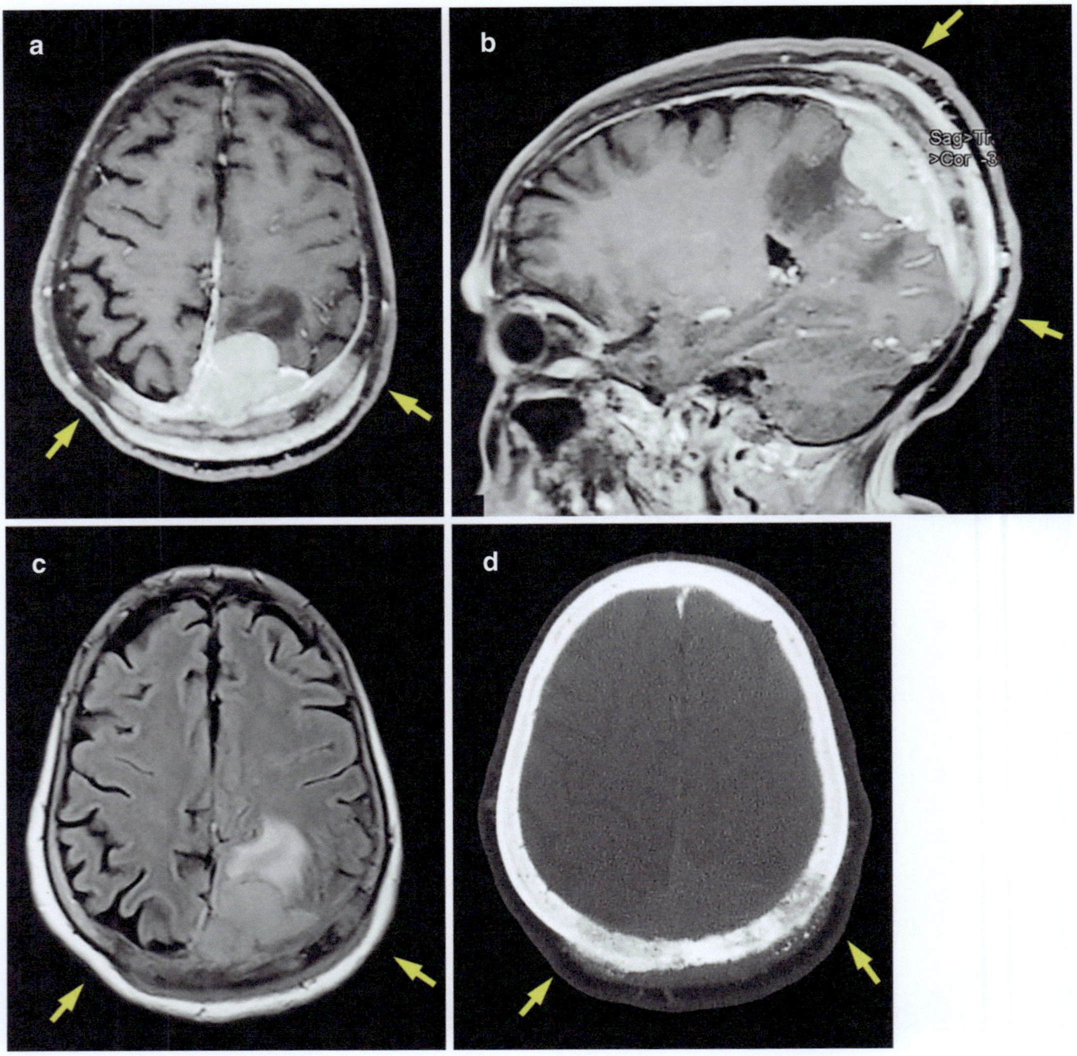

Fig. 1.37 Intracranial parieto-occipital meningiosarcoma with dural venous sinus involvement and extracranial extension (arrows). Axial (**a**) and sagittal (**b**) post-gadolinium T1-weighted MRI, axial FLAIR sequence MRI (**c**), and axial CT-scan (**d**)

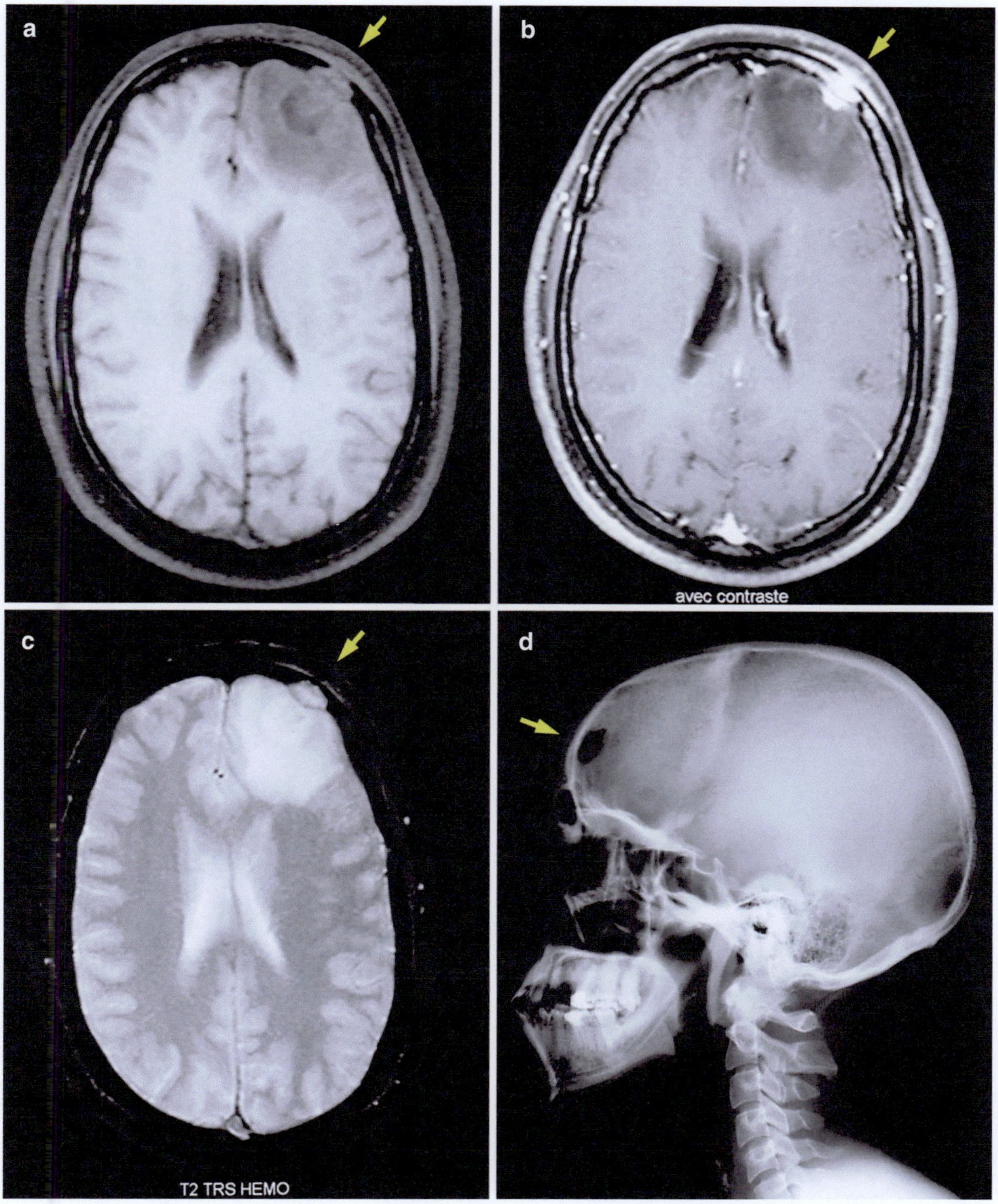

Fig. 1.38 Frontal astrocytoma with adjacent cranial bone and extracranial extension (arrows). Axial T1-weighted MRI before (**a**) and after (**b**) gadolinium injection. Axial T2-weighted MRI (**c**) and lateral cranial plain radiography (**d**)

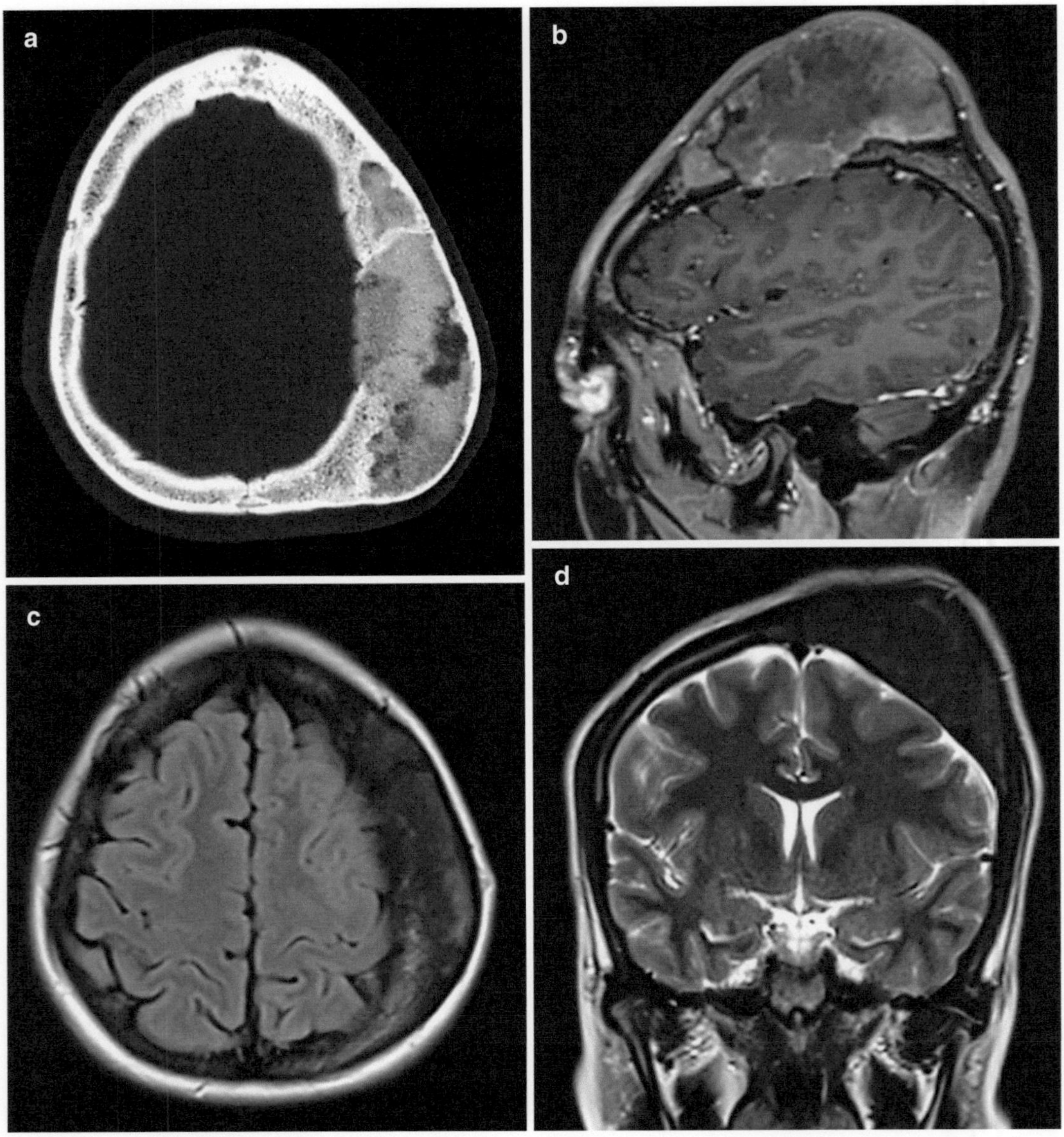

Fig. 1.39 Fronto-parietal fibrous dysplasia as seen on axial CT-scan on bone window (**a**), sagittal post-gadolinium T1-weighted image (**b**), axial FLAIR sequence (**c**), and on coronal T2-weighted MRI (**d**)

1.4 Conclusion

The unique morphology of the human scalp and skull provides a fertile ground for a variety of pathologies to evolve at any age. There are multiple temptations to establish a classification system for scalp and cranial vault lesions, most depending on their histopathologic findings, topographic locations, size of the lesions, imaging appearances, clinical data, or even patients' age. An agreement between the different practitioners (especially anatomopathologists, radiologists, dermatologists, neurosurgeons, maxillofacial, and plastic surgeons) is needed in order to establish a consensus classification.

Knowledge of a wide differential diagnosis of the scalp and calvarial lesions and familiarity with the anatomy of the scalp and cranial vault bones is paramount to localizing the exact anatomical position of the lesion, and accordingly the most likely pathologic entity.

References

1. Akhaddar A, editor. Cranial osteomyelitis. Diagnosis and treatment. 1st ed. Cham: Springer International Publishing; 2016. https://doi.org/10.1007/978-3-319-30268-3.
2. Akhaddar A. Scalp abscesses. In: Atlas of infections in neurosurgery and spinal surgery. 1st ed. Cham: Springer International Publishing; 2017. https://doi.org/10.1007/978-3-319-60086-4_3.
3. Akhaddar A, Albouzidi A, Elouennas M, Boucetta M. Nonsuppurative calvarial thickening: a new form of Garré disease? J Neurosurg. 2009;110(4):808. https://doi.org/10.3171/2008.3.17458.
4. Akhaddar A, Gazzaz M, Kadiri B, Lrhezzioui J, Boucetta M. Giant epidermoid cyst of the skull with extra and intracranial extension. A case report. J Neuroradiol. 2002;29(3):193–9.
5. Akhaddar A, Jiddane M, Chakir N, El Hassani R, Bellakhdar F. Cerebellar abscesses secondary to occipital dermoid cyst with dermal sinus: case report. Surg Neurol. 2002;58(3–4):266–70. https://doi.org/10.1016/s0090-3019(02)00847-9.
6. Attri G, Maurya VP, Srivastava AK, Behari S, Bhaisora KS, Sardhara J, et al. Calvarial lesions: a tertiary centre's experience over fifteen years. Neurol India. 2021;69(3):650–8. https://doi.org/10.4103/0028-3886.319236.
7. El Asri AC, Akhaddar A, Baallal H, Boulahroud O, Mandour C, Chahdi H, et al. Primary lymphoma of the cranial vault: case report and a systematic review of the literature. Acta Neurochir. 2012;154(2):257–65. https://doi.org/10.1007/s00701-011-1124-0.
8. Gupta S, Sharma G, Sajeevan S, Raut SN, Ahuja R, Joseph D, et al. Varied clinical presentation and management of calvarial metastases. Asian J Neurosurg. 2022;17(4):631–4. https://doi.org/10.1055/s-0042-1757626.
9. Howard BM, Manupipatpong S, Dion JE, Tamargo RJ, Gailloud P, Hui FK. Classification and management considerations for intraosseous dural arteriovenous fistulae. Neurosurgery. 2023;93(2):387–98. https://doi.org/10.1227/neu.0000000000002423.
10. Karki M, Roka YB. Surgical excision of cirsoid aneurysm of the scalp: case series and review of the literature. World Neurosurg. 2021;155:e600–4. https://doi.org/10.1016/j.wneu.2021.08.102.
11. Nasi-Kordhishti I, Hempel JM, Ebner FH, Tatagiba M. Calvarial lesions: overview of imaging features and neurosurgical management. Neurosurg Rev. 2021;44(6):3459–69. https://doi.org/10.1007/s10143-021-01521-5.
12. Omofoye OA, Huynh T, Jhun R, Ashfaque H, Cronk K. Primary intraosseous meningioma of the calvarium: a systematic review. Clin Neurol Neurosurg. 2020;199:106283. https://doi.org/10.1016/j.clineuro.2020.106283.
13. Prior A, Anania P, Pacetti M, Secci F, Ravegnani M, Pavanello M, et al. Dermoid and epidermoid cysts of scalp: case series of 234 consecutive patients. World Neurosurg. 2018;120:119–24. https://doi.org/10.1016/j.wneu.2018.08.197.
14. Tan AP, Rasheed S, Sidpra J, Lim MC, James G, Oztekin O, et al. An algorithmic clinicoradiological approach to paediatric cranial vault lesions: distinguishing normal variants from pathologies. Br J Neurosurg. 2021;7:1–14. https://doi.org/10.1080/02688697.2021.1919599.
15. Yoon SH, Park SH. A study of 77 cases of surgically excised scalp and skull masses in pediatric patients. Childs Nerv Syst. 2008;24(4):459–65. https://doi.org/10.1007/s00381-007-0523-2.
16. Amaral L, Chiurciu M, Almeida JR, Ferreira NF, Mendonça R, Lima SS. MR imaging for evaluation of lesions of the cranial vault: a pictorial essay. Arq Neuropsiquiatr. 2003;61(3A):521–32. https://doi.org/10.1590/s0004-282x2003000400001.
17. Barnett RR, Piazza MG, Elton SW. Pediatric neurosurgery in primary care: masses of the scalp and skull in children. Pediatr Clin N Am. 2021 Aug;68(4):743–57. https://doi.org/10.1016/j.pcl.2021.04.003.
18. Colas L, Caron S, Cotten A. Skull vault lesions: a review. AJR Am J Roentgenol. 2015;205(4):840–7. https://doi.org/10.2214/AJR.14.13415.
19. Garfinkle J, Melançon D, Cortes M, Tampieri D. Imaging pattern of calvarial lesions in adults. Skeletal Radiol. 2011;40(10):1261–73. https://doi.org/10.1007/s00256-010-0971-8.
20. Morcillo Carratalá R, Capilla Cabezuelo ME, Herrera Herrera I, Calvo Azabarte P, Dieguez Tapias S, Moreno de la Presa R, et al. Nontraumatic lesions of the scalp: practical approach to imaging diagnosis: neurologic/head and neck imaging. Radiographics. 2017;37(3):999–1000. https://doi.org/10.1148/rg.2017160112.
21. Pons Escoda A, Naval Baudin P, Mora P, Cos M, Hernandez Ganan J, Narvaez JA, et al. Imaging of skull vault tumors in adults. Insights Imaging. 2020;11:23. https://doi.org/10.1186/s13244-019-0820-9.
22. Yalçin O, Yildirim T, Kizilkiliç O, Hürcan CE, Koç Z, Aydin V, et al. CT and MRI findings in calvarial non-infectious lesions. Diagn Interv Radiol. 2007;13(2):68–74.
23. Gomez CK, Schiffman SR, Bhatt AA. Radiological review of skull lesions. Insights Imaging. 2018;9(5):857–82. https://doi.org/10.1007/s13244-018-0643-0.
24. Hayman LA, Shukla V, Ly C, Taber KH. Clinical and imaging anatomy of the scalp. J Comput Assist Tomogr. 2003;27(3):454–9. https://doi.org/10.1097/00004728-200305000-00027.
25. Sathishkumar D, Ogboli M, Moss C. Classification of aplasia cutis congenita: a 25-year review of cases presenting to a tertiary paediatric dermatology department. Clin Exp Dermatol. 2020;45(8):994–1002. https://doi.org/10.1111/ced.14331.
26. Bidloo G. Medicinae Doctoris & Chirurgi, Anatomia Hvmani Corporis: Centum & quinque Tabvlis Per artificiosiss. G. De Lairesse ad vivum delineates,

Demonstrata, Veterum Recentiorumque Inventis explicata plurimisque, hactenus non detectis, Illvstrata. Amesterdam (Netherlands) : Sumptibus Viduae Joannis à Someren, Haeredum Joannis à Dyk, Henrici & Viduae Theodori Boom; 1685.
27. Sharman AM, Kirmi O, Anslow P. Imaging of the skin, subcutis, and galea aponeurotica. Semin Ultrasound CT MR. 2009;30(6):452–64. https://doi.org/10.1053/j.sult.2009.08.001.
28. Chlebicka I, Stefaniak AA, Gawdzik A, RygaŁ A, Matusiak Ł, Szepietowski JC. Scalp lesions referred for surgical procedures: single-center 5-year experience in Southwestern Poland. In Vivo. 2020;34(5):2733–8. https://doi.org/10.21873/invivo.12095.
29. Haenssle HA, Winkler JK, Fink C, Toberer F, Enk A, Stolz W, et al. Skin lesions of face and scalp - classification by a market-approved convolutional neural network in comparison with 64 dermatologists. Eur J Cancer. 2021;144:192–9. https://doi.org/10.1016/j.ejca.2020.11.034.
30. Kawaguchi M, Kato H, Matsuo M. CT and MRI features of scalp lesions. Radiol Med. 2019;124(10):1049–61. https://doi.org/10.1007/s11547-019-01060-6.
31. Lloret I, Server A, Taksdal I. Calvarial lesions: a radiological approach to diagnosis. Acta Radiol. 2009;50(5):531–42. https://doi.org/10.1080/02841850902795274.
32. Mitra I, Duraiswamy M, Benning J, Joy HM. Imaging of focal calvarial lesions. Clin Radiol. 2016;71(4):389–98. https://doi.org/10.1016/j.crad.2015.12.010.
33. Ugga L, Cuocolo R, Cocozza S, Ponsiglione A, Stanzione A, Chianca V, et al. Spectrum of lytic lesions of the skull: a pictorial essay. Insights Imaging. 2018;9(5):845–56. https://doi.org/10.1007/s13244-018-0653-y.
34. Willatt JM, Quaghebeur G. Calvarial masses of infants and children. A radiological approach. Clin Radiol. 2004;59(6):474–86. https://doi.org/10.1016/j.crad.2003.12.006.

History of Calvarial Lesions

2

Nikolaos Syrmos, Vaitsa Giannouli, Sotirios Kottas, and Mehmet Turgut

2.1 Ancient Period

The approaches into the calvarial lessons are closely related to the development of the Medicine, as autonomous science, since the primitive–ancient periods of the Humanity in Earth and of the Neurosurgery as medical discipline.

The first documented Medical physician and also the first Neurosurgeon of the Medical History was the Hellenic Hippocrates of Kos (460–370 BC), who performed trephinations, the so called holes in the head—“τρυπανισμοί” in order to treat various skull pathologies, including the calvarial lesions, during his medical and scientific career. He used various instruments, from copper of bronze and innovative techniques in order to perform his interventions and has also good surgical results, also documented in his various books.

In his marvelous book, regarding the cranio-cerebral injuries, “περί κεφαλής τραυμάτων,” an accurate description of his surgical technique was performed. He was also an excellent teacher and they teach his students, “μαθητές,” how to operate and treat similar cases (Medical School of Hippocrates-Ιπποκράτειος Ιατρική Σχολή) [1–6] (Fig. 2.1). Also in other parts of the world, such as South America, Peru, there are documented cases of trephinations in order to ameliorate the quality of patients’ life with various skull and calvarial lesions. In the Museum of Gold in Lima, we can found also examples of surgical cases of “gold” cranioplasty after surgical operations for cranial-calvarial lesions [3–10].

N. Syrmos (✉)
Aristotle University of Thessaloniki, Thessaloniki, Macedonia, Greece

Human Performance and Health, Master Science Program, Aristotle University of Thessaloniki, Thessaloniki, Macedonia, Greece

Papanikolaou General Hospital, Thessaloniki, Macedonia, Greece

European Association of Neurosurgical Societies (EANS), Thessaloniki, Macedonia, Greece
e-mail: milanako76@yahoo.gr

V. Giannouli
Aristotle University of Thessaloniki, Thessaloniki, Macedonia, Greece

S. Kottas
Papanikolaou General Hospital, Thessaloniki, Macedonia, Greece

M. Turgut
Department of Neurosurgery, Aydın Adnan Menderes University Faculty of Medicine, Aydın, Türkiye

Department of Histology and Embryology, Aydın Adnan Menderes University Institute of Health Sciences, Aydın, Türkiye

M. Turgut et al. (eds.), *Lesions of the Scalp and Cranial Vault*,
https://doi.org/10.1007/978-3-031-88244-9_2

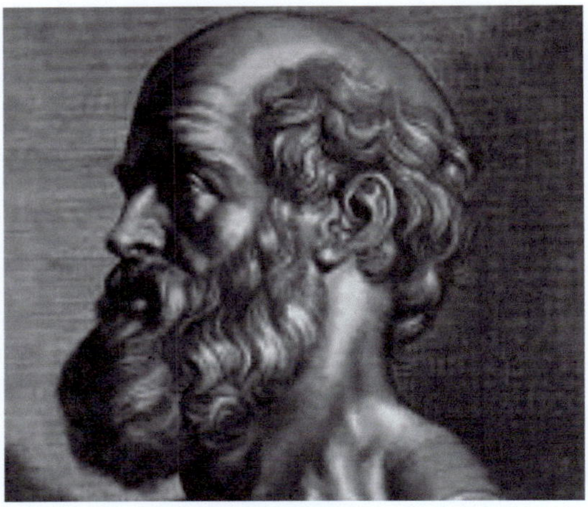

Fig. 2.1 Hippocrates of Kos 460–370 BC

2.2 Hellenic-Roman-Islamic Era

Galen of Pergamon (131–201 BC) was a skilled surgeon and anatomist of his era. He managed to improve the materials of his surgical instruments and he managed to perform surgical operations for various skull and calavarial lesions. He used in the beginning of his career primitive materials (stone, glass, chert) but he was able to change them into newly solid technology for his period (iron, bronze, cooper) in order to ameliorate both his surgical results and mainly, the safety of his patients [1–6] (Fig. 2.2).

The Arabs physicians, Avicenna (980–1037) and Albucasis (936–1013), codify the current surgical instrumentation and the apply innovative techniques in order to face with success the bleeding during operations regarding skull and calvarial lesions [1–6].

Paul of Aegina (625–690) was the scientist who documented by his studies, the works and the scientific efforts of Hippocrates, Galen, Avicenna, and Albucasis efforts in order to manage optimal results in the management of skull and calvarial lesions [3–10].

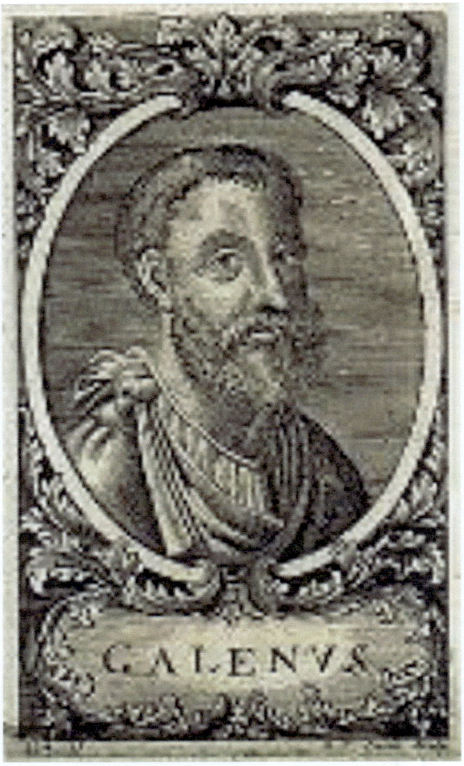

Fig. 2.2 Galen of Pergamon 131–201 BC

2.3 Medioeval Era

During this period, the approaches into the skull and calvarial pathology and traumatiology were performed under the concept of "hammer and chisel" technique. No significant improvement was performed during this period.

In this period, the surgeon was seen such as barber who performed procedures in the human skull-calvarium under minimal anesthesia. Antiseptic procedures were also primitive and cruel. The surgical results were controversial [1–6].

2.4 Reinassance Period

Hans Von Gersdorf (1455–1529), from Germany, introduce the so called tripod -style tool in order to perform accurate trephinations, for a variety of cranial and calvarial pathologies [1–6].

Jacopo Bergario da Capri (1460–1530) managed to publish a book with colored illustrations with the treatment of various skull-calvarial lesions [3, 4, 10–12] (Fig. 2.3). He described various surgical techniques and diverse instruments through the ages before and during his era. He performed anatomical dissections and he managed to treat various calvarial lesions for his patients.

Andrea Della Croce was a Venetian talented physician and surgeon (Fig. 2.4). He published a book with a series of surgical interventions with his modified surgical instruments in order to treat a variety of calvarial lesions, with success [1–6].

Peter Lowe (1550–1610) published a surgical manual in English language, a true innovation for the scientific community of his era, because the majority of the medical literature, until his effort, was published, in Latin language. In his work, an accurate illustration of many neurosurgical instruments was performed in order to achieve optimal surgical results for various calvarial pathological entities [3–12]. He performed also a Historical Vignette with all the achievements of the previous physicians, through the ages in the field of cranial pathology and terminology [1–6].

William Clowes the elder (1544–1604), a successful Military doctor, published a text-book with his surgical armamentarium, capable to perform surgical operations in the Human calvarial area [1–6] (Fig. 2.5).

John Woodall (1570–1643) proposed a new trephination system adopted and evolved by the French surgeon Rene Garengeot (1788–1841) in order to treat cranial pathology and traumatiology [1–6] (Fig. 2.6).

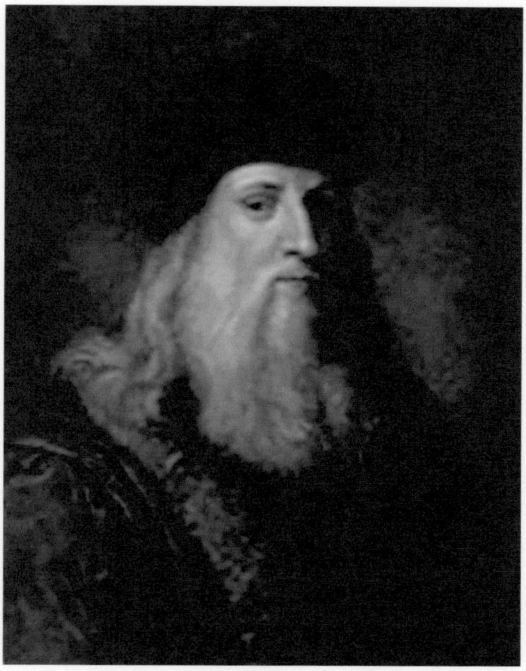

Fig. 2.3 Jacopo Berengario da Carpi 1460–1530

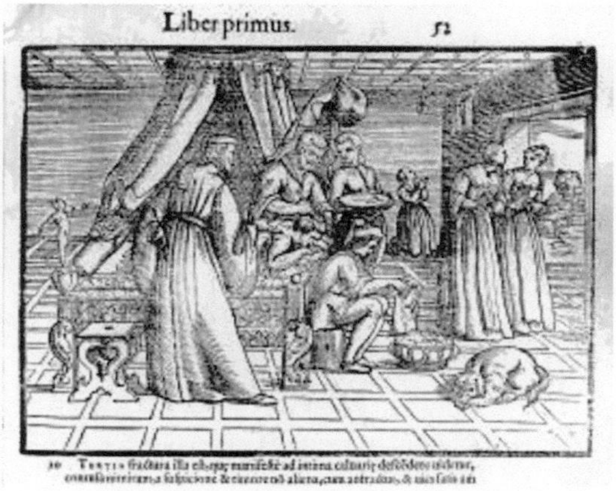

Fig. 2.4 Image from the book of Andrea della Croce

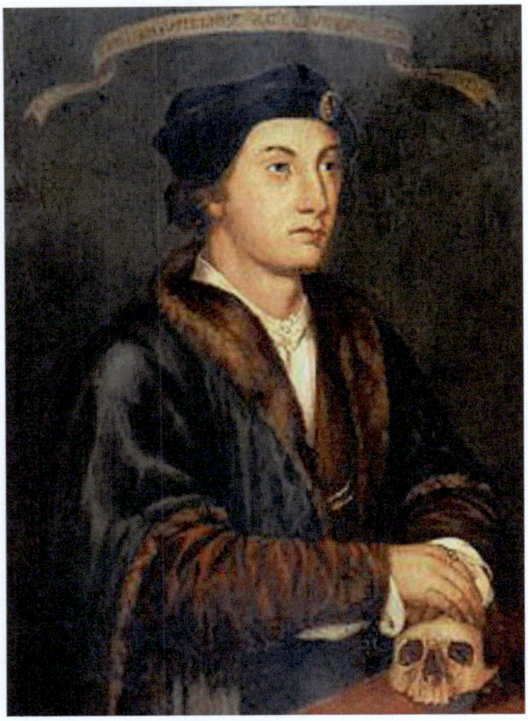

Fig. 2.5 William Clowes the Elder (1544–1604)

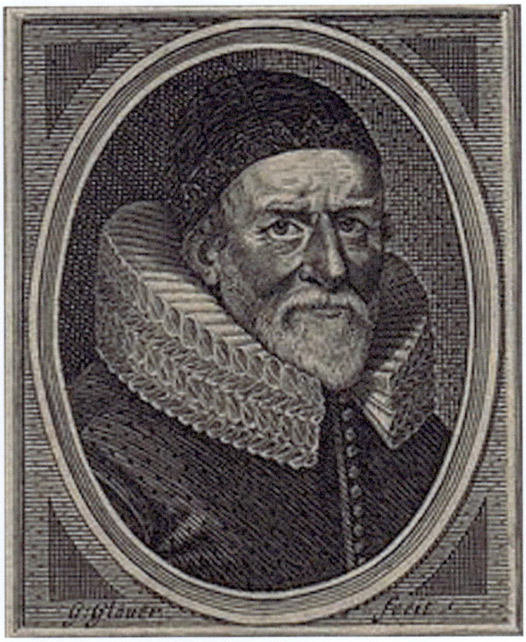

Fig. 2.6 John Woodall (1570–1643)

2.5 Eighteenth Century

It is the so called Travelling neurosurgical sets era. Many surgeons across Central Europe (England, France, Germany, Italy etc.) contributed in the development of these instruments, mainly using the "One hand performance style," allowing the physicians to do surgical interventions with a single hand. These sets were more flexible and smaller than the previous editions and they can travel together with the surgeons across Europe in order to expand Medical and Surgical knowledge [1–6].

Samuel Sharp (1709–1788) an English physician was one of the pioneer designers of these kinds of sets [1–6]. He was able to operate with success a variety of cranial and calvarial pathology in many patients, also of younger ages. He published a documented series of 60 cases, a huge number for his era [1–6].

Lorenz Heister (1683–1758) studied first under the auspices of the Anatomist Bernard Albinus and the Physician Herman Boerhaave and after he published a series of surgical and anatomical texts translated in many European languages [1–6]. He created a novel surgical set and he was able to perform with success many calvarial-cranial surgeries.

Percival Pott (1714–1788) also designed a tripod style trephination system in order to treat calvarial and cranial pathological entities [1–6] (Fig. 2.7).

Other trephination systems were designed by the Irish surgeon Samuel Goker, in 1791 and William Hey (1793–1797), in Leeds, England [1–6].

Charles Bell (1774–1842) published a marvelous book, with colored illustrations with almost all the surgical techniques of cranial approaches of his era [1–6]. He described also his technique of trephination in order to treat calvarial pathologies.

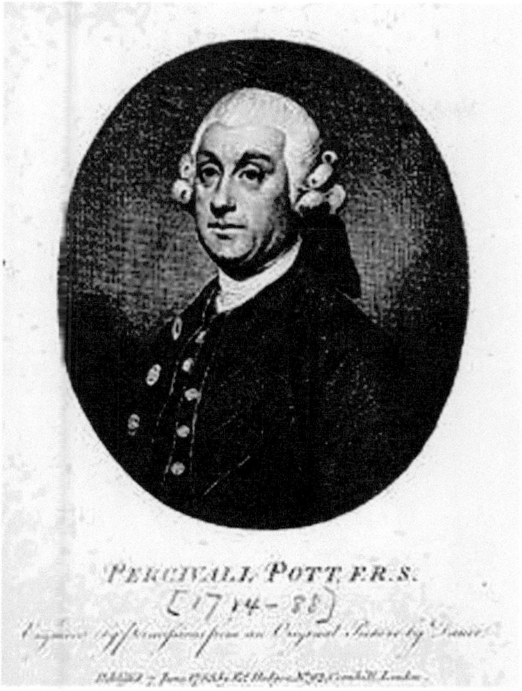

Fig. 2.7 Percivall Pott (6 January 1714–22 December 1788)

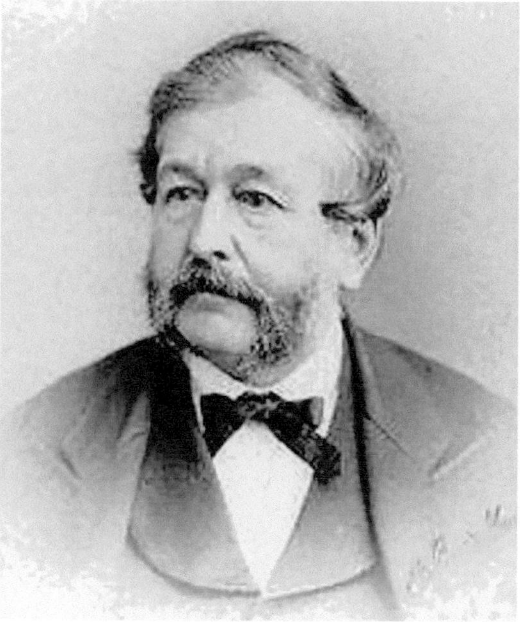

Fig. 2.8 Joseph Pancoast (November 23, 1805–March 6, 1882)

2.6 Nineteenth Century

The introduction in the current medical and surgical practice of the antisepsis concept by the Lord Joseph Lister was a very important step in order to perform better and safer approaches in order to treat skull and calvarial pathology [1–6]. In the same period, new anesthesia techniques, the so called painless surgery was performed in order to ameliorate the surgical results and the safety of patients and overall health.

Joseph Pancoast (1805–1882) published in 1844 a detailed textbook about his surgical techniques and his efforts to perform larger trephinations (Fig. 2.8).

By the end of the nineteenth century, more surgeons, all over the world, started to perform craniotomies and craniectomies instead of trephinations. These surgical and therapeutic options helped a lot in order to treat better the calvarial and the skull pathological entities. The so called Hammer and chisel technique was still a common used technique but still painful for the patient medical but also ethical approach. Many times it was also damaging for the brain morphology and brain functionality.

The introduction of osteoplastic flap was a true innovation for the cranial and calvarial surgery of this period. It was designed in order that the cranial bone was elevated upon a pedicle of overlying soft tissues. William Wagner was a pioneer of this technique [1–6].

Leonardo Gigli (1863–1908) designed his famous instrument in order to perform safer pubotomies (Fig. 2.9). Gigli was an obstetrician, but his idea to introduce a "jagged knife" find a perfect field of application in the human skull. The original design was developed, rapidly by the first ten years of his application and metal handles were included instead of the ebonies in order to be sterilized. Gigli instrument became rapidly also bidirective instead of the only one direction of his original form. It became, shortly more flexible in order to pass between two bur holes, a true evolution and revolution for the surgeons [1–6, 10–14].

Alfred Obalinski (1843–1898) from Poland was one of the major exponents in order to trans-

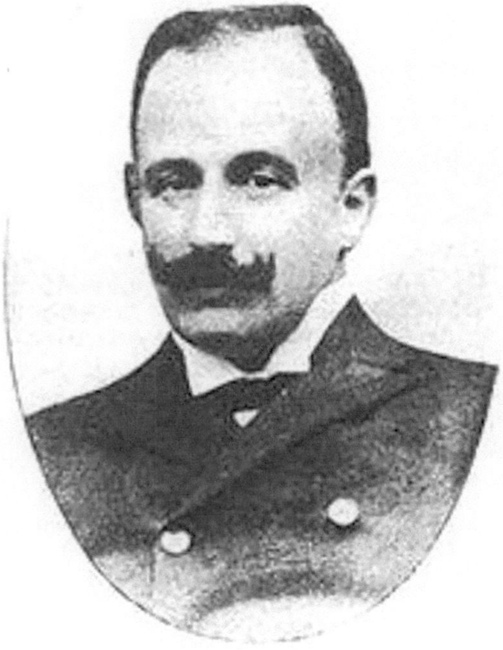

Fig. 2.9 Leonardo Gigli (30 April 1863–4 April 1908)

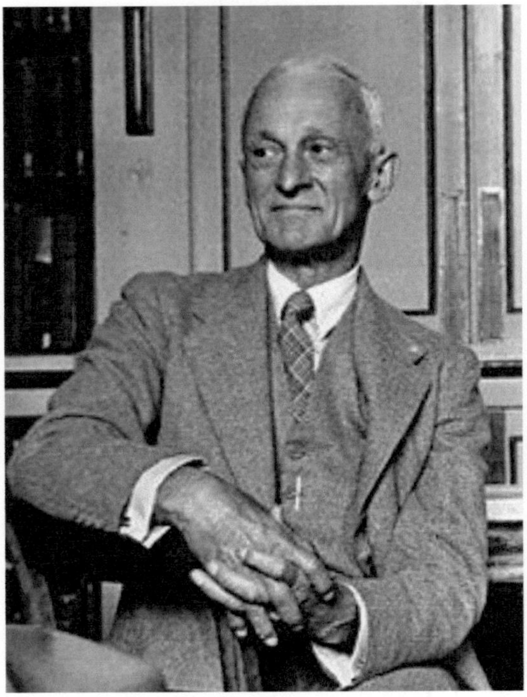

Fig. 2.10 Harvey Williams Cushing (April 8, 1869–October 7, 1939)

form the Gigli into one of the most famous, flexible and in the same time accurate instruments in the Neurosurgical History [3].

Eugen–Luis Doyen from France (16 December 1859–21 November 1916) also contributed in the transformation of Gigli from an obstetric tool into a unique neurosurgical arma [3].

In the late years of the nineteenth century and in the beginning of the twentieth, many surgeons performed larger cranial approaches in order to treat skull and calvarial pathologies [3].

- Fedor Krause (1857–1937), German pioneer surgeon and neurosurgeon.
- Antony Maxine Nicolas Cipaut, French pioneer surgeon and neurosurgeon.
- Thierry de Martel (1875–1940), from France.
- Charles Freizes, from Philapelphia, United States of America.

2.7 Neurosurgery as an Autonomous Medical Discipline

In the beginning of the twentieth century, Harvey Cushing (1869–1939) introduced new techniques for surgery of skull and calvarial lesions (Fig. 2.10). He became one of the foremost leaders and experts in the special field of neurosurgery as a result of his surgical and medical achievements. Under his significant influence and legacy, neurosurgery became a new and autonomous surgical discipline in the world [3, 15–20].

Walter Edward Dandy (1886–1946) was also an American pioneer neurosurgeon and scientist of his era, who managed to treat with success

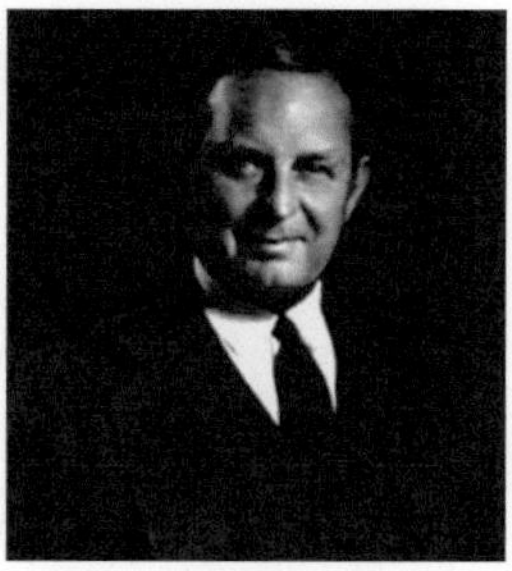

Fig. 2.11 Walter Edward Dandy (April 6, 1886–April 19, 1946)

various types of calvarial lesions, especially in young patients [3, 15–21] (Fig. 2.11).

2.8 The Establishment of Pediatric Neurosurgery

Antony (Toni) Raimondi was an American-Italian pioneer pediatric neurosurgeon.

In 1972, he hosted a reunion in Chicago attended by eleven neurosurgeons that later became the founding members of the International Society for Pediatric Neurosurgery (ISPN).

Many pediatric neurosurgeons, across the world, they perform surgical approaches in order to treat various calvarial pathologies such as [18, 21–26]:

- Anthony David Hockley (October 4th 1943–21st June 2009) in United Kingdom
- Concezio Di Rocco (1944) in Italy
- Jim T. Goodrich (April 16, 1946–March 30, 2020) in the United States of America and many others

2.9 The Modern Imaging Era

Godfrey Hounsfield (1919–2004), a biomedical engineer from England, contributed enormously into the management of calvarial–skull lesions towards the establishment of the computed axial computerized tomography (CT) in the early 70s.

Some years later the magnetic resonance imaging (MRI) scanning machine was introduced by Raymond Vahan Damadian (1936–2022), an American physician, medical practitioner.

With the CT SCAN and MRI SCAN, the neuroradiology-neuroimaging era became real, a very important tool in the armamentarium of the neurosurgeons and the pediatric neurosurgeons in the world. The modern imaging tools and the new up coming techniques provide much more details in order to evaluate and to treat the calvarial lesions. The new up coming three dimension technology (3D) is a further step in order to understand and treat better these pathologies [19–28].

2.10 Conclusion

Through the ages, many scientific efforts were performed in order to understand the anatomical, physiological, morphological, and structural approaches to the calvarial lesions. All of these contributions are demonstrations of the necessity of reciprocal interaction in order to achieve optimal, helpful, and useful results in performing more successful and safer neurosurgical and pediatric neurosurgery procedures. The modern era provides the tools in order to achieve better results.

References

1. Syrmos NC, Giannouli V, Kottas S, Turgut M. History of cranial subdural hematoma subdural hematoma: past to present to future management; 2021. p. 33–43.
2. Syrmos NC, Giannouli V, Turgut M. The sutures of the skull: a historical perspective the sutures of the skull: anatomy, embryology, imaging, and surgery, 2021, pp. 7–18.
3. Goodrich JT. How to get in and out of the skull: from tumi to "hammer and chisel" to the Gigli saw and the osteoplastic flap. Neurosurg Focus. 2014;36(4):E6. https://doi.org/10.3171/2014.2.FOCUS13543.
4. Syrmos N., Syrmos Chr History of Neurosurgery, 2010, Thessaloniki, Greece.
5. Cucu AI, Turliuc S, Costea CF, Perciaccante A, Bianucci R, Donell S, Scripcariu DV, Turliuc MD. The brainstem and its neurosurgical history. Neurosurg Rev. 2021;44(6):3001–22. https://doi.org/10.1007/s10143-021-01496-3.
6. Partiot C, Lepetit A, Dodré E, Jenger C, Maureille B, Liguoro D, Thomas A. Cranial trepanation and healing process in modern patients-bioarchaeological and anthropological implications. J Anat.

2020;237(6):1049–61. https://doi.org/10.1111/joa.13266.

7. Carod-Artal FJ, Vázquez-Cabrera CB. Paleopatología neurológica en las culturas precolombinas de la costa y el altiplano andino (II). Historia de las trepanaciones craneales [Neurological paleopathology in the pre-Columbine cultures of the coast and the Andean plateau (II). The history of cranial trepanations]. Rev Neurol. 2004;38(9):886–94. Spanish
8. Andrushko VA, Verano JW. Prehistoric trepanation in the Cuzco region of Peru: a view into an ancient Andean practice. Am J Phys Anthropol. 2008;137(1):4–13. https://doi.org/10.1002/ajpa.20836.
9. Giannouli V, Syrmos N. Information about Macedonian medicine in ancient Greece. Hell J Nucl Med. 2011;14(3):324–5.
10. Syrmos N, Ampatzidis G, Fachantidou A, Mouratidis I, Syrmos C. Historical back training in most important points of neurosurgery. Ann General Psychiatry. 2010;9(Suppl 1):S89. https://doi.org/10.1186/1744-859X-9-S1-S89.
11. Ugga L, Cuocolo R, Cocozza S, Ponsiglione A, Stanzione A, Chianca V, D'Amico A, Brunetti A, Imbriaco M. Spectrum of lytic lesions of the skull: a pictorial essay. Insights Imaging. 2018;9(5):845–56. https://doi.org/10.1007/s13244-018-0653-y.
12. Attri G, Maurya VP, Srivastava AK, Behari S, Bhaisora KS, Sardhara J, Verma PK, Nazar AH, Jaiswal S. Calvarial lesions: a tertiary centre's experience over fifteen years. Neurol India. 2021;69(3):650–8. https://doi.org/10.4103/0028-3886.319236.
13. Gomez CK, Schiffman SR, Bhatt AA. Radiological review of skull lesions. Insights Imaging. 2018;9(5):857–82. https://doi.org/10.1007/s13244-018-0643-0.
14. Nasi-Kordhishti I, Hempel JM, Ebner FH, Tatagiba M. Calvarial lesions: overview of imaging features and neurosurgical management. Neurosurg Rev. 2021;44(6):3459–69. https://doi.org/10.1007/s10143-021-01521-5.
15. Ligon BL. The mystery of angiography and the "unawarded" Nobel prize: Egas Moniz and Hans Christian Jacobaeus. Neurosurgery. 1998;43:602–11.
16. Cushing H. The special field of neurological surgery. Bulletin of the Johns Hopkins Hospital 16:77–87, 1905. Neurosurgery. 2005;57(6):1075. https://doi.org/10.1097/00006123-200512000-00002.
17. Sherman IJ, Kretzer RM, Tamargo RJ. Personal recollections of Walter E. Dandy and his brain team. J Neurosurg. 2006;105:487–93.
18. https://www.ispneurosurgery.org/ispn-history/
19. Bhattacharyya KB. Godfrey Newbold Hounsfield (1919–2004): The man who revolutionized neuroimaging. Ann Indian Acad Neurol. 2016;19(4):448–50. https://doi.org/10.4103/0972-2327.194414.
20. Damadian R, Zaner K, Hor D, DiMaio T. Human tumors detected by nuclear magnetic resonance. Proc Natl Acad Sci USA. 1974;71(4):1471–3. https://doi.org/10.1073/pnas.71.4.1471.
21. Gan YC, Hockley AD. Aneurysmal bone cysts of the cranium in children. Report of three cases and brief review of the literature. J Neurosurg. 2007;106(5 Suppl):401–6. https://doi.org/10.3171/ped.2007.106.5.401.
22. Prof. Anthony J. Raimondi. Childs Nerv Syst. 2000;16(8):464–75. https://doi.org/10.1007/s003810000375.
23. Di Rocco C, Schweder PM, Aziz TZ, Solanki GA, Rekate HL, Walker ML, Lewis E, Mazza C. Dr. Anthony David Hockley. Childs Nerv Syst. 2010;26(1):7–12. https://doi.org/10.1007/s00381-009-1010-8.
24. Frolov A, Lawson C, Olatunde J, Goodrich JT, Martin Iii JR. Sagittal craniosynostosis with uncommon anatomical pathologies in a 56-year-old male cadaver. Case Rep Pathol. 2019;2019:8034021. https://doi.org/10.1155/2019/8034021.
25. Dowling KA, Goodrich JT. Two cases of 16th century head injuries managed in royal European families. Neurosurg Focus. 2016;41(1):E2. https://doi.org/10.3171/2016.4.FOCUS15119.
26. Kobets AJ, Goodrich JT. The history of intracranial infections. Childs Nerv Syst. 2018;34(10):1849–57. https://doi.org/10.1007/s00381-018-3888-5.
27. Milham N, Schmutz B, Cooper T, Hsu E, Hutmacher DW, Lynham A. Are magnetic resonance imaging-generated 3Dimensional models comparable to computed tomography-generated 3Dimensional models for orbital fracture reconstruction? An in-vitro volumetric analysis. J Oral Maxillofac Surg. 2023;81(9):1116–23. https://doi.org/10.1016/j.joms.2023.05.015.
28. Ahmed M, Melaragno LE, Nyirjesy SC, von Windheim N, Fenberg R, Herster R, Sheldon A, Binzel K, Knopp MV, Herderick ED, VanKoevering KK. Higher computed tomography (CT) Scan resolution improves accuracy of patient-specific mandibular models when compared to cadaveric gold standard. J Oral Maxillofac Surg. 2023;81(9):1176–85. https://doi.org/10.1016/j.joms.2023.05.014.

3 Developmental Anatomy and Histology of the Scalp and Calvarium

Kubilay Doğan Kılıç, Sahar Ebrahem Orif, Ali Çağlar Turgut, Servet Çelik, and Yiğit Uyanıkgil

3.1 Introduction

3.1.1 Overview of the Scalp and Calvarium

The scalp consists of five different layers, recognizable by the acronym SCALP: Skin, Subcutaneous tissue, Galea Aponeurotica, Loose connective tissue, and Pericranium (Fig. 3.1). It is the thickest skin in the body and can be up to 8 mm thick. However, due to its hair-bearing nature in most individuals, the scalp can be difficult to reconstruct for aesthetic purposes.

The Galea aponeurotica extends forwards as the frontal muscle and backward as the occipital muscle, while at the sides it is seamlessly connected by the temporoparietal fascia. The pericranium blends with the deep temporal fascia towards the sides of the head.

It is worth noting that the scalp has limited elasticity, the galea aponeurotica has minimal elasticity and the pericranium is almost imperceptible in terms of elasticity. The areas encompassing the temporoparietal fascia, especially the parietal areas, exhibit the greatest mobility within the scalp [1].

Just above the Galea aponeurotica lies a well-vascularised subcutaneous layer. This strong blood supply allows local flaps to survive without distal tissue necrosis. The scalp receives its blood supply from arteries such as the supratrochlear, supraorbital, superficial temporal, posterior auricular, and occipital arteries, each of which has an accompanying vein. The supratrochlear and supraorbital arteries originate from the oph-

K. D. Kılıç (✉)
Department of Histology and Embryology, Ege University Faculty of Medicine, İzmir, Türkiye

Leibniz Institute for Evolution and Biodiversity Science, Museum für Naturkunde, Berlin, Germany
e-mail: kubilaydk@gmail.com

S. E. Orif
Department of Anatomy and Embryology, Mansoura University Faculty of Veterinary Medicine, Mansoura, Egypt

Department of Stem Cell, Ege University Institute of Health Sciences, İzmir, Türkiye

A. Ç. Turgut
Department of Histology and Emryology, Aydın Adnan Menderes University Institute of Health Sciences, Aydın, Türkiye

Department of Radiology, Ege University Faculty of Medicine, İzmir, Türkiye

S. Çelik
Department of Anatomy, Ege University Faculty of Medicine, İzmir, Türkiye

Y. Uyanıkgil
Department of Histology and Embryology, Ege University Faculty of Medicine, İzmir, Türkiye

Department of Stem Cell, Ege University Institute of Health Sciences, İzmir, Türkiye

M. Turgut et al. (eds.), *Lesions of the Scalp and Cranial Vault*,
https://doi.org/10.1007/978-3-031-88244-9_3

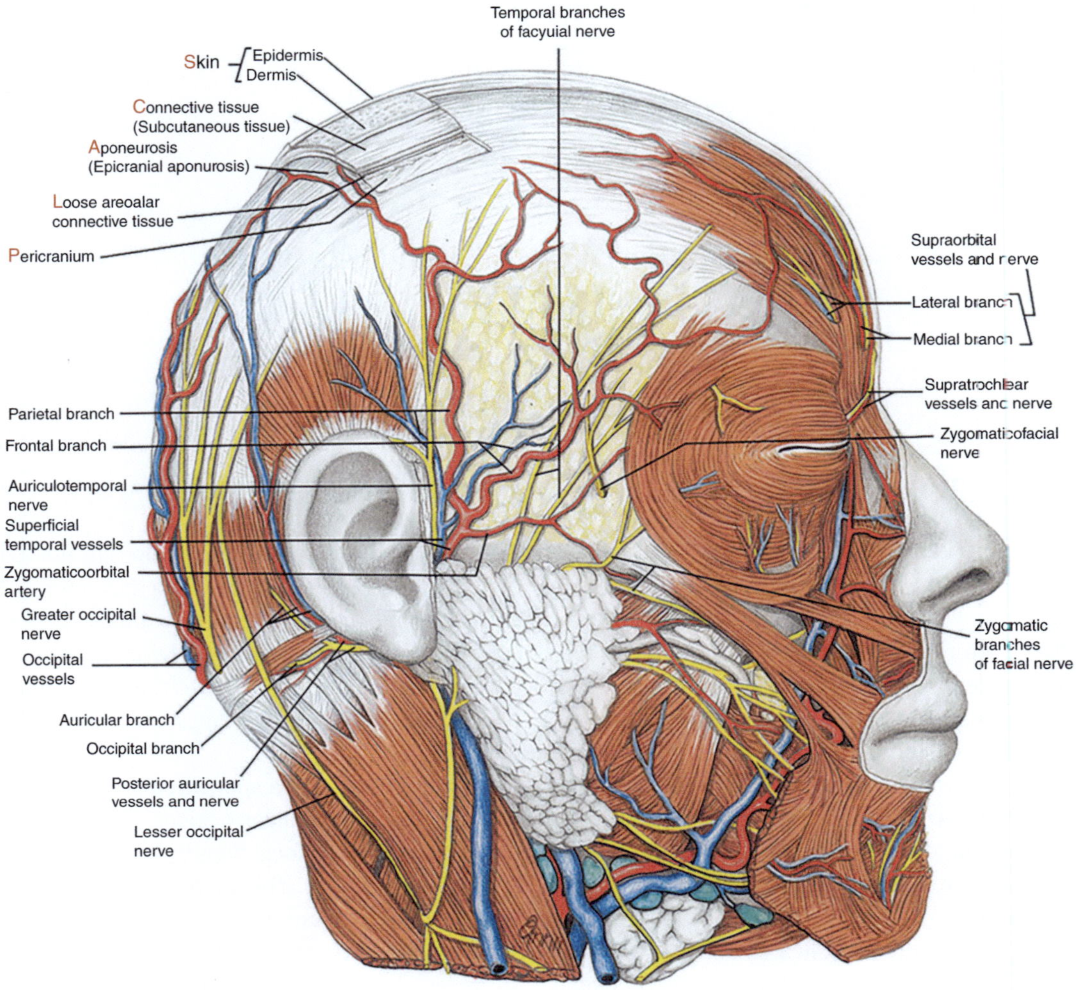

Fig. 3.1 Layers of SCALP, blood, and nerve supply of calvaria. Source: Bernhard N. Tillmann, Atlas der Anatomie des Menschen mit Muskeltabellen 3., überarbeitete und erweiterte Auflage, Springer-Verlag Berlin Heidelberg, 2016. Pg. 53 Oberfl. Leitungsbahnen, Speicheldrüsen **2.54** Oberflächliche Gesichtsregion, Hinterhauptsregion und Kopfschwarte, Ansicht von rechts-seitlich

thalmic artery, a branch of the internal carotid artery, while the remaining arterial supply comes from the external carotid artery [2].

Sensory nerves in the scalp are paired and include the supratrochlear (V1), supraorbital (V1), zygomaticotemporal (V2), auriculotemporal (V3), lesser occipital (C2-C3), and greater occipital (C2) nerves. The supraorbital and supratrochlear nerves serve the forehead and frontoparietal scalp. The zygomaticotemporal nerve supplies the area near the eyebrow and the temporal scalp up to the temporal line. The auriculotemporal nerve covers the lateral scalp, while the greater and lesser occipital nerves innervate the occipital region. In particular, the temporal branches of the facial nerve are found in loose areolar tissue on the deep surface of the temporoparietal fascia, following an imaginary line connecting the earlobe and a point 1.5 cm above the lateral eyebrow (known as the Pitanguy line). When dissecting this area, it is very important to stay deep in the superficial layer of the deep temporal fascia to avoid injury to the facial nerve [3].

The calvarium consists of bones formed by two processes: intramembranous ossification (for the frontal, parietal, and temporal bones) and endochondral ossification (for the occipital and sphenoid bones). The calvarium consists of three layers: an outer plate, a diploic space, and an inner plate. These layers develop in early childhood and most of the calvarium growth is completed by the age of 7 years [4].

3.1.2 Importance of Understanding Developmental Anatomy and Histology

Understanding the developmental anatomy and histology of the scalp and calvarium is very important for several reasons: The first is in clinical practice; in surgical procedures, surgeons performing cranial and scalp operations must have a deep understanding of the anatomy and histology of these regions to minimise complications and achieve successful outcomes. For trauma assessment knowledge of scalp and calvarial anatomy helps medical professionals evaluate and manage head injuries, including fractures and soft tissue injuries. Last, but not least, cosmetic procedures. Cosmetic and reconstructive surgeons rely on this knowledge to perform procedures such as hair transplants or craniofacial reconstruction [5].

The second is diagnostics and associated imaging. Radiology and imaging can be divided into two parts: radiologists use their knowledge of the anatomy of the scalp and calvarium to interpret imaging studies, such as CT scans and MRIs, to help diagnose various medical conditions, and histological understanding of pathology, which allows pathologists to identify and diagnose diseases or abnormalities, such as tumors or infections, in scalp and calvarium tissues. In this section, we will discuss histology as clearly as possible [6].

Trauma and forensic medicine can count for the public interest. In trauma cases or criminal investigations, forensic experts rely on their knowledge of the anatomy of the scalp and calvarium to determine the cause of injuries and to identify victims [7].

The last and most comprehensive subject is research and education. For research, developmental anomalies and disorders are the main concepts in birth defects. Understanding developmental anatomy can help in the diagnosis and management of congenital conditions affecting the scalp and calvarium [8]. Researchers also studying conditions such as craniosynostosis (premature fusion of skull sutures) or alopecia (hair loss) rely on a comprehensive understanding of developmental anatomy and histology to advance medical knowledge and treatment options. Cutting-edge technologies such as biomaterials and tissue engineering are essential for gaining knowledge about the underlying tissue structure and developing materials and techniques for regenerative medicine, including skull and scalp reconstruction [9, 10].

Appropriate training in developmental anatomy and histology is essential for medical and dental students, especially in medical and dental schools—we can also include veterinary medicine and life sciences—and ensures that they have a strong foundation for clinical practice and research.

The communication skills of future doctors with patients can also be influenced by this. Healthcare professionals can better explain conditions, procedures, and treatment options to patients when they have a thorough understanding of the anatomy and histology of the scalp and calvarium.

For the general public, this understanding can help prevent complications. A comprehensive knowledge of anatomy helps healthcare providers avoid damaging critical structures during medical procedures, reducing the risk of complications.

In summary, understanding the developmental anatomy and histology of the scalp and calvarium is crucial for healthcare professionals in various fields as it directly affects patient care, diagnosis, treatment, and research, as well as promotes safety and accuracy in medical practice.

3.2 Embryonic Origins of the Scalp and Calvarium

3.2.1 Formation of the Ectodermal and Mesodermal Layers

Embryonic development is a complex and meticulously regulated process that transforms a single fertilized egg into a fully formed human being. Central to this process is the differentiation of cells into various tissues and organs, and this includes the formation of complex and essential structures such as the scalp and calvarium, which protect and support the brain and provide a defining feature of human appearance.

Formation of the ectodermal layer: the embryonic ectoderm, one of the three main germ layers, plays a crucial role in the development of the scalp and calvarium. This layer is responsible for the emergence of the tissues that make up the outermost layer of the body, including the skin and nervous system [11].

The skin covering the head, including the scalp, is derived from the ectodermal layer. As the embryo undergoes gastrulation and neurulation, the ectoderm begins to fold and mold, eventually forming a multilayered structure. The outermost layer becomes the epidermis, which forms the visible surface of the scalp and the rest of the body. Within the epidermis, various structures such as hair follicles, sweat glands, and sebaceous glands develop. These contribute to the unique properties and functions of the scalp skin [12].

Nervous system formation beyond the skin, the ectoderm also gives rise to the nervous system. The central nervous system, including the brain, spinal cord, and cranial nerves, develops from this germ layer. Inside the calvarium, the brain is covered and protected by bony structures composed of mesodermal tissue, but the nervous tissue itself arises from the ectoderm. The complex structure and functions of the brain begin to develop during embryogenesis, setting the stage for the complex interaction between the nervous system and the bones of the skull within the calvarium [13].

The mesoderm is another primary germ layer that contributes significantly to the development of the scalp and calvarium. This layer specializes in forming connective tissues, muscles, and the skeletal system [14].

The mesodermal layer is responsible for producing the connective tissues that underlie the scalp. These connective tissues connect the scalp to the underlying skull bones. The dense fibrous tissue known as galea aponeurotic is an example of a structure formed from the mesodermal layer. It serves as a vital structural component that provides support and stability to the scalp [15].

The calvarium, which forms the upper part of the skull, is composed of several cranial bones. These bones, including the frontal, parietal, and occipital bones, are necessary to protect the brain. They develop from mesodermal tissue by a process known as intramembranous ossification. This process involves the transformation of mesenchymal cells into bone tissue and forms the hard but flexible structure of the calvarium. The skull bones fit together with sutures, allowing the skull to grow and expand during infancy and childhood.

Describing the complex processes by which the ectodermal and mesodermal layers contribute to the development of the scalp and calvarium is fundamental to understanding the anatomy and histology of these structures. It provides critical information about their function, potential developmental anomalies, and clinical significance in health, surgery, and research. Furthermore, this knowledge underlines the extraordinary complexity and precision of embryonic development in shaping the human body [16].

3.2.2 Role of Neural Crest in Development

The neural crest is a remarkable group of cells with a multitude of functions during embryonic development. Its influence on the formation of the scalp and calvarium is particularly noteworthy, as it underlies the complexity of craniofacial development.

Cranial Bone Formation: Neural crest cells, originating from the dorsal edge of the neural tube, play a pivotal role in cranial bone development. These cells migrate into the cranial region, where they undergo a highly coordinated process of differentiation and condensation. As they transform into mesenchymal cells, they contribute to the formation of the cranial bones, including the frontal, parietal, and occipital bones. This process, known as intramembranous ossification, results in the rigid yet adaptable structure of the calvarium, which is essential for protecting the brain [17].

Cranial Sutures and Fontanelles (Fig. 3.2): Neural crest cells are also involved in the formation of cranial sutures and fontanelles. Cranial sutures are fibrous joints that connect individual cranial bones, allowing for some degree of flexibility and growth during early development. Fontanelles are soft spots or gaps between the cranial bones in a baby's skull. They are crucial for accommodating the rapid brain growth that occurs in infancy. Neural crest-derived cells contribute to the development of the connective tissues within sutures and fontanelles, ensuring that the skull can expand harmoniously with the growing brain [18].

Influence on Cranial Nerves: Neural crest cells are not limited to bone and connective tissue formation; they also exert their influence on the development of cranial nerves. These nerves, some of which innervate the scalp, are integral for sensation, motor function, and the intricate

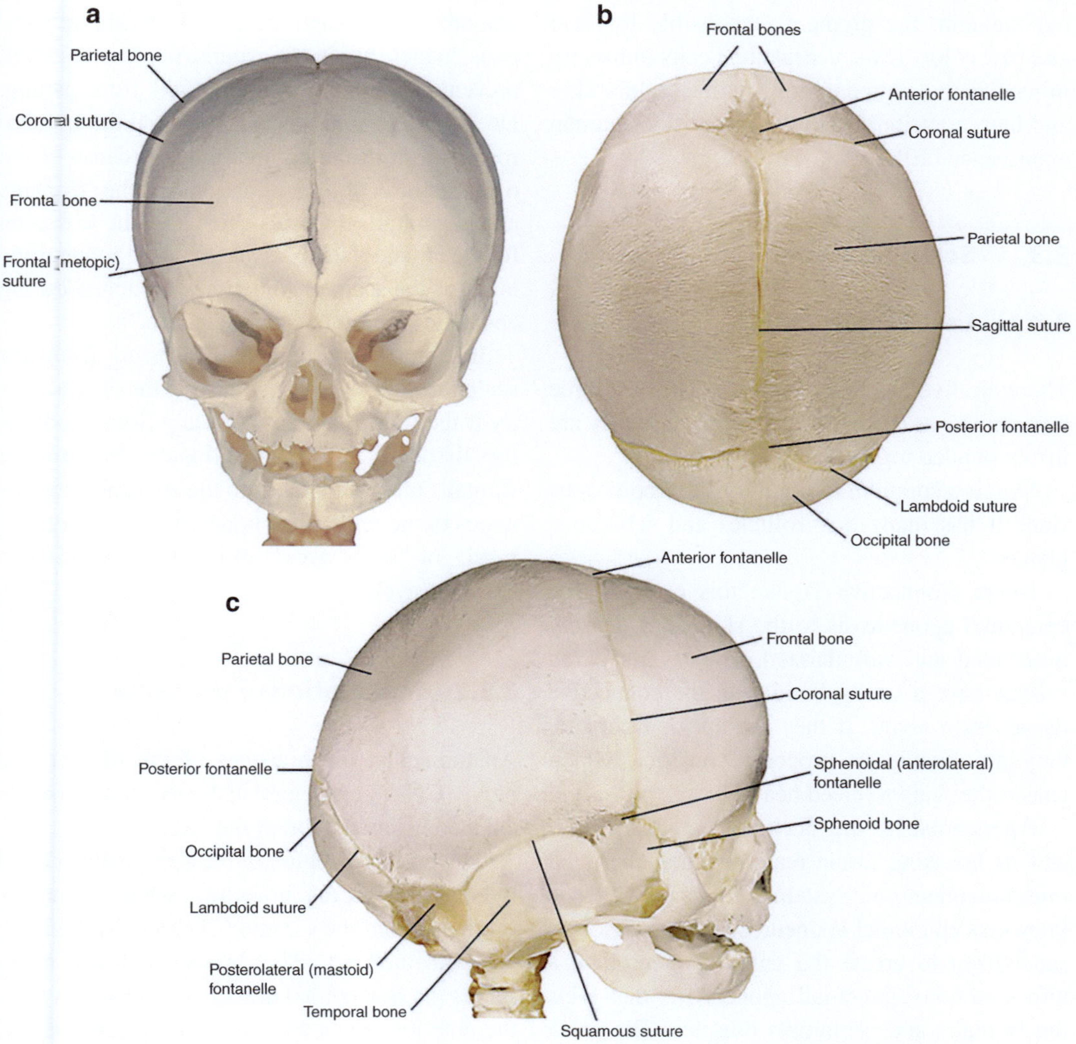

Fig. 3.2 Fontanelles of the skull of a fetus (seventh fetal month). (**a**) Anterior view, (**b**) Superior view, and (**c**) Right lateral view. Source: Bernhard N. Tillmann, Atlas der Anatomie des Menschen mit Muskeltabellen 3., überarbeitete und erweiterte Auflage, Springer-Verlag Berlin Heidelberg, 2016. Pg.21 Schädel: Osteogenese **2.1a-c** Schädel eines Feten (7. Fetalmonat), Skelett-Band-Präparat

neural connections within the cranial region. Neural crest cells contribute to the formation of cranial nerve ganglia, which are clusters of nerve cell bodies associated with cranial nerves. This contribution is fundamental for the proper functioning of cranial nerves that affect scalp sensation and motor control [19].

Melanocytes and Skin Pigmentation: While the primary role of neural crest cells in the context of the scalp and calvarium is centered on skeletal and neural tissue development, it is noteworthy that they also give rise to melanocytes. Melanocytes are responsible for producing melanin, the pigment responsible for skin and hair color. Thus, neural crest cells indirectly influence the pigmentation of the scalp's skin and hair, contributing to the diversity of human appearance [20].

3.3 Scalp Anatomy

3.3.1 Layers of the Scalp

There are five layers to the scalp. The first three layers move as a single structure because they are firmly bonded together.

Skin is a common location for sebaceous cysts since it has many hair follicles and sebaceous glands.

Dense Connective Tissue: this connects the epicranial aponeurosis to the skin. It is densely innervated and vascularized. The layer's blood vessels have a strong bond with the connective tissue. As a result, if they are cut or lacerated, they are unable to properly constrict, which causes the scalp to bleed heavily.

Aponeurosisis, the occipitofrontalis muscle, and its investing fascia make up the superficial musculoaponeurotic system of the scalp, which is known as epicranial aponeurosisis. This fascia is specialized to create the galea aponeurotica, a thin tendinous epicranial aponeurosis that joins the frontalis and occipitalis muscles. The galea attaches to the mastoid processes and the zygomatic arch before continuing into the temples and investing the auricular muscles. The facial nerve, cranial nerve (CN) VII, innervates the frontalis muscle, which is essential for brow and forehead motions and a key facial expression muscle.

Loose Areolar Connective Tissue is a thin layer of connective tissue that divides the epicranial aponeurosis from the periosteum of the skull.

Pericranium is the periosteum, the outer layer of the skull bones, and is home to numerous blood vessels, including emissary veins, which join the scalp veins to the diploic veins, and cerebral venous sinuses. At the suture lines, it blends into the endosteum (Fig. 3.3).

It's critical to comprehend the structure of the scalp when caring for individuals with scalp wounds, The strength of the underlying aponeurosis, which binds the wound borders together, prevents superficial scalp wounds from gaping. Deep scalp wounds gape, however, if the aponeurosis is torn in the coronal plane because of the opposite-direction contraction of the frontalis and occipitalis muscles. To assist in lessening forehead and facial wrinkles, this aponeurotic layer of the scalp is sometimes tightened during cosmetic surgery (such as "facelifts").

Infection may potentially spread from the scalp through emissary veins into the cranial cavity if the fourth layer of the scalp (loose connective tissue) is injured. Additionally, because the frontalis muscle inserts into the skin and subcutaneous tissue rather than bone, resulting in ecchymosis, or "black eyes," an infection or fluid can enter the eyelids.

3.3.2 Innervation of the Scalp

Anatomically, the branches of the fifth cranial nerve (CN-V) or the cervical nerve roots provide cutaneous innervation of the scalp.

The posterior region of the scalp is innervated by cervical plexus branches, which primarily originate from the C2 and C3 (lesser and greater occipital nerves). The lesser occipital nerve serves the skin behind the ear and originates from the anterior ramus (division) of C2. The skin of the occipital region is supplied by the greater occipital nerve, which originates from the posterior ramus of C2. The great auricular nerve, which emerges from the C2 and C3 anterior rami,

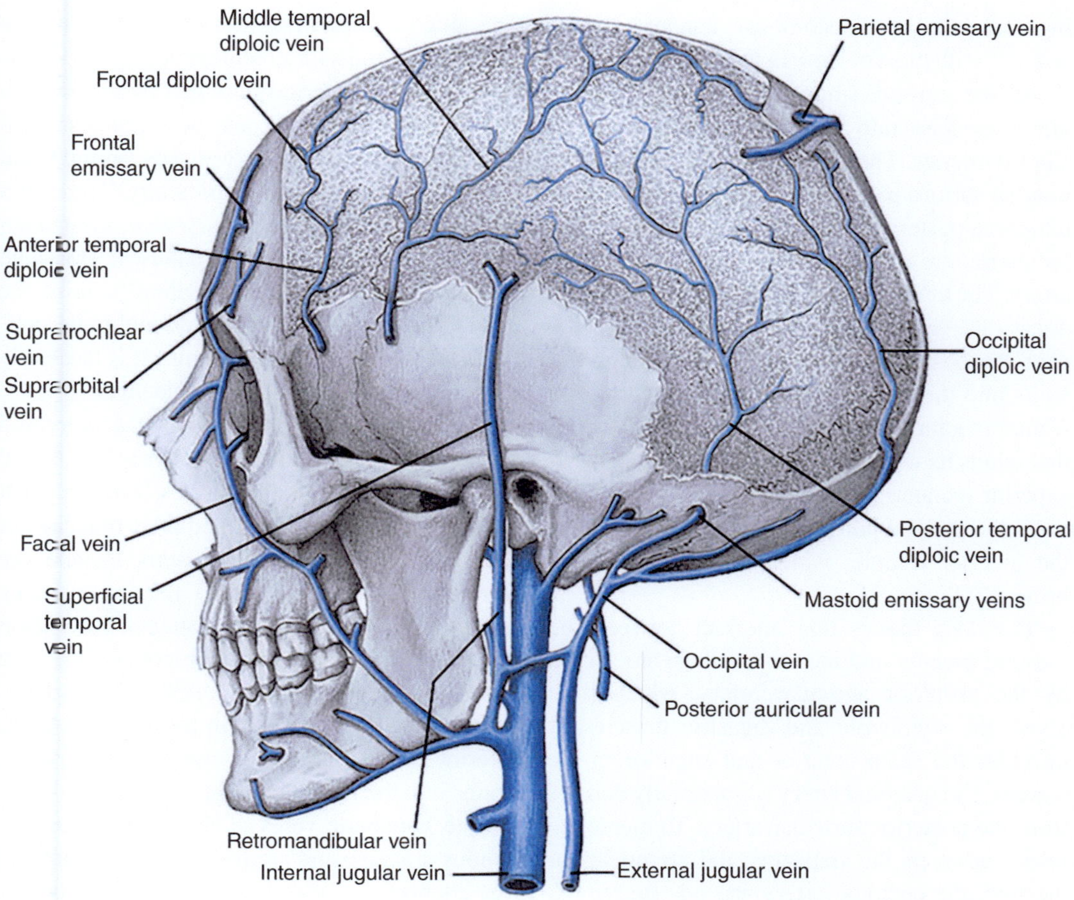

Fig. 3.3 Diploic and emissary veins with their connections to the superficial veins, view of the left side. Source: Bernhard N. Tillmann, Atlas der Anatomie des Menschen mit Muskeltabellen 3., überarbeitete und erweiterte Auflage, Springer-Verlag Berlin Heidelberg, 2016. Pg.106 Oberflächliches Venensystem · Hirnhäute, Subarachnoidalraum. **2.152** Vv. diploicae und Vv. emissariae mit ihren Verbindungen zu den oberflächlichen Venen, Ansicht der linken Seite

supplies the skin behind the ear and above the mandibular angle. The inferior occipital region's skin is supplied by the third occipital nerve, which originates from the posterior ramus of C3.

The anterior portion of the scalp is innervated by the supraorbital and supratrochlear nerves, which are derived from the first (ophthalmic) division of the trigeminal nerve (CN V-1). The supraorbital nerve especially supplies a large portion of the scalp between the anterolateral forehead and the vertex, while the supratrochlear nerve innervates the anteromedial forehead.

The lateral region of the scalp is innervated by the zygomaticotemporal and auriculotemporal nerves, which are branches of maxillary (CN V-2) and mandibular (CN V-3) divisions of the trigeminal nerve. The zygomaticotemporal nerve supplies the temple, and the auriculotemporal nerve, a branch of the mandibular nerve, supplies skin anterosuperior to the auricle.

3.3.3 Blood Supply of the Scalp (Arterial Supply, Venous Drainage, Lymphatic Drainage)

The common carotid artery, posterior intercostal arteries, and the terminal branches of the subclavian artery all send blood to the scalp. An amazing network of anastomoses connects these arteries, with most of them in the temporal region.

At the carotid sinus, the common carotid artery divides into the internal and external carotid arteries. They both produce branches that nourish various parts of the scalp. The superficial temporal, posterior auricular, occipital, and angular arteries are all offshoots of the external carotid artery. The terminal branch of the external carotid artery, the superficial temporal artery, crosses over the posterior aspect of the zygomatic and splits into the frontal and parietal branches. The frontal is a terminal branch with a winding path that winds its way across the temple in an anterosuperior manner. While the parietal branch provides the parietal portion of the scalp, it supplies the anterior temple, which is superior to the brows [21].

The deep tissues that intersect between the mastoid process and the ear cartilage are served by the posterior auricular artery, which rises above the stylohyoid and digastric muscles. It provides the scalp anterior and superior to the auricle. The occipital artery is proximally derived from the posterior auricular artery. To pierce the fascia between the trapezius and sternocleidomastoid, the occipital artery ascends superiorly. In addition to anastomosing with the superficial, posterior auricular arteries and the contralateral occipital artery, it tortuously ascends from that point and supplies the superficial fascia of the posterior scalp superior to the nuchal line [22].

A connection of vessels that also supply the trapezius and splenius capitis muscles supplies the posterior scalp inferior to the nuchal line. The transverse cervical and posterior intercostal arteries are the source of these blood vessels.

The supratrochlear and supraorbital arteries, which supply the anterior part of the scalp, are branches of the ophthalmic artery that arise from the internal carotid artery. Both arteries enter the skull through the supraorbital foramen, anastomose with their opposing arteries, and the superficial temporal artery to supply the majority of the anterior scalp [23].

Both superficial and deep venous systems receive drainage from the scalp. The corresponding arteries are followed by the superficial veins. The anterior superficial scalp is drained by the supraorbital and supratrochlear veins. The superficial scalp is posteriorly drained by the superficial temporal, occipital, and posterior auricular. The superficial temporal vein has parietal and frontal branches, just like the artery. Through a link with the parietal emissary vein, the frontal vein connects with the dural sinuses. This vein extends superiorly along the lateral side of the head, where it penetrates the cranium and connects to the superior sagittal sinus. It is located in the loose areolar connective tissue layer.

The deep scalp is drained by the pterygoid venous plexus. It is situated between the lateral pterygoid and temporalis muscles. The veins that make up the plexus are named after branches of the maxillary artery. These veins include the infraorbital, alveolar, middle meningeal, deep temporal, masseteric, sphenopalatine, buccinator, and pterygoid veins. Another connecting vein from the pterygoid plexus connects the cavernous sinus to the ophthalmic vein by passing via the inferior orbital fissure. In the end, the plexus drains into the maxillary vein.

The lymphatic veins of the scalp follow the venous drainage and are found in the subcutaneous connective tissue layer. The parotid nodes, which continue to drain through the deep cervical and submandibular lymph nodes, are typically the conduits through which the anterior regions of the scalp discharge. The occipital and posterior auricular (mastoid) lymph nodes receive drainage from the scalp posterior to the auricle. The occipital lymph nodes get drainage from the mastoid lymph nodes, which are located in the area of the scalp just posterior to the ear. The remainder of the posterior scalp is covered by the occipital lymph node drainage [24].

3.3.4 Hair Follicles and Associated Structures (Hair Shaft, Sebaceous Glands, Sweat Glands)

The hair follicle begins at the epidermis's surface. It spreads into the deep dermis and rarely into the subcutis for follicles of the hairs.

The infundibulum, isthmus, and lower follicle/inferior segment (which contains the bulb) are the three significant hair follicle segments that can be found on the head. The top part of the follicle is called the infundibulum segment. It extends from the epidermis's outermost layer to the sebaceous duct's entrance. The isthmus presents between the opening of the sebaceous duct and the bulge. From the bulge to the base of the follicle, the inferior segment of the hair follicle is then visible. The follicular matrix around the dermal papilla's top and sides is contained in the bulb, which is a part of this section.

Although hair follicles have a plain and simple shape, their functions and growth cycle are rather complicated. Alopecia areata1 and telogen effluvium are two examples of hair conditions that can develop as a result of major changes to the normal growth cycle of a hair follicle [25].

According to the Structure of Hair Follicles, these are the four most important structures in hair follicles, though there are numerous other parts as well. The papilla, connective tissue, and blood arteries that supply growing hair make up the papilla. It can be found at a hair follicle's very base. Genetic Matrix, cells make new hairs in the germinal matrix, commonly known as the "matrix," where matrix keratinocytes proliferate to form the hair shaft of growing hair as old hairs thin and fall out. It has the highest mitotic rate of any organ, and the lower portion of the hair follicle is where it is situated. The color of the hair shaft is provided by melanocytes, which are mixed up with the matrix cells. Bulb, the bulb is a spherical, bulb-shaped structure that surrounds the dermal papilla and the germinal matrix at the base of the hair follicle "stocking" and is nourished by blood vessels. This is the hair's living portion. In actuality, the hair that is visible above the skin's surface is dead. The bulb contains a variety of stem cell types that divide more quickly than any other type of cell in the body—every 23–72 h. Additionally, the bulb includes hormones that influence the development and structure of hair at various ages, including puberty and pregnancy [26].

Bulge, the isthmus, or central section of the hair follicle, is where the bulging region is situated. It has stem cells that divide and regenerate the sebaceous glands, the epidermis, and new hair follicles in addition to new hair. The insertion location for the arrector pili, a small band of muscular tissue, is likewise provided by the bulge. When you experience goosebumps, these muscles tense, which makes the hairs stand on end [27].

The hair shaft is composed of the medulla, or inner core. The cortex, which makes up the majority of the hair, is present around this. The shaft cuticle is made up of a single layer of cells that extends outward. The inner (internal) root sheath is then formed by three layers around the shaft cuticle. As the hair shaft emerges from the matrix, the inner sheath plays a significant role in structuring it. The inner sheath begins to keratinize from the outside in and will eventually fall off in mid-follicle, close to the isthmus. Afterwards, the entire hair shaft is enclosed by the external (outer) root sheath and the level of the isthmus is the premise layer of trichilemmal keratinization [28].

Sebaceous glands are holocrine glands strongly linked to hair follicles, especially in certain skin regions like the face. Except in places like the lips, where hair follicles are absent, these glands usually discharge straight onto the mucosa surface. Sebaceous glands release a lipid-rich sebum that shields the hair and gives the skin a hydrophobic barrier that can act as protection when activated by hormones like androgens [29].

According to the Hair Growth Cycle, the average rate of hair growth is around a half-inch per month or 6 inches per year; however, the pace varies from person to person. The three phases of the hair development cycle are anagen, catagen, and telogen. Anagen is the growing phase. While eyebrow hairs' anagen phase only lasts about 70 days, the anagen phase of typical scalp hair follicles lasts roughly 2–6 years. The size of anagen hairs varies as well, ranging from long, thick terminal hairs to short, pale vellus hairs. Vellus hair, which is nearly colorless, transforms into terminal hair throughout adolescence, which is darker and thicker [30].

Catagen is the regression phase. The hair follicle shrinks and the hair growth rate slows down over a few weeks. Two to three weeks pass during the catagen phase. Telogen is the phase of rest, which is around 3 months long. Hair stops growing after a few months and separates from the hair follicle. Old, dead hair is forced out while new hair begins to grow in its place. More hair enters the telogen phase and starts to fall out during stressful times. Humans typically lose 50–100 scalp hairs every day; however, stress can result in significantly more hair loss [31].

The sweat glands present in the scalp are eccrine glands, which are concentrated on the palms and soles in great numbers. The scalp has the third-highest density. Eccrine glands consist of "acrosyringium," an intraepidermal spiral duct, a dermal duct with a straight and coiled part, and a secretory tubule that is deeply coiled in the (hypo)dermis. The sweat pore is where the eccrine gland opens. Sweat is comprised of salt water and eccrine sweat glands release bicarbonate and potassium. Eccrine sweat glands are important for "thermoregulation" since they keep us both warm and cool. The surface cools down as a result of the body's heat being expended to evaporate the salt water that is secreted on it. Eccrine glands also become active in response to emotional stress (situations that cause fear, pain, or worry) or physical exercises [32].

3.4 Calvarium Anatomy

3.4.1 Structure of the Calvarium (Frontal Bone, Parietal Bones, Occipital Bone, Temporal Bones, Sutures of the Skull

The cranial vault (the skull vault, skullcap, or calvaria) is the space within the skull that protects the brain. The term "calvarium" (the neurocranium) is made up of the cranial vault and the base of the skull. The calvarium is the convex, dome-shaped part of the skull, which protects the brain's delicate tissues. The calvarium is made up of all the bones that surround the brain, except the jaw and cheek. The calvarium is frequently confused with the calvaria or the skullcap section of the calvarium. The coronal, lambdoid, and sagittal sutures connect these bones. The name "calvaria''is the Latin word for "skull.''The following flat bones make up the cranial vault: paired frontal bones, paired parietal bones, the squamous portion of the paired temporal bones, and the occipital bone's interparietal region (Fig. 3.4).

The frontal bone (Os Frontale) is the most anterior component of the superior skull and sits on top of the frontal lobe. The frontal crest is a ridge generated by the convergence of the two ridges of the superior sagittal sinus in the anterior squamous sec-

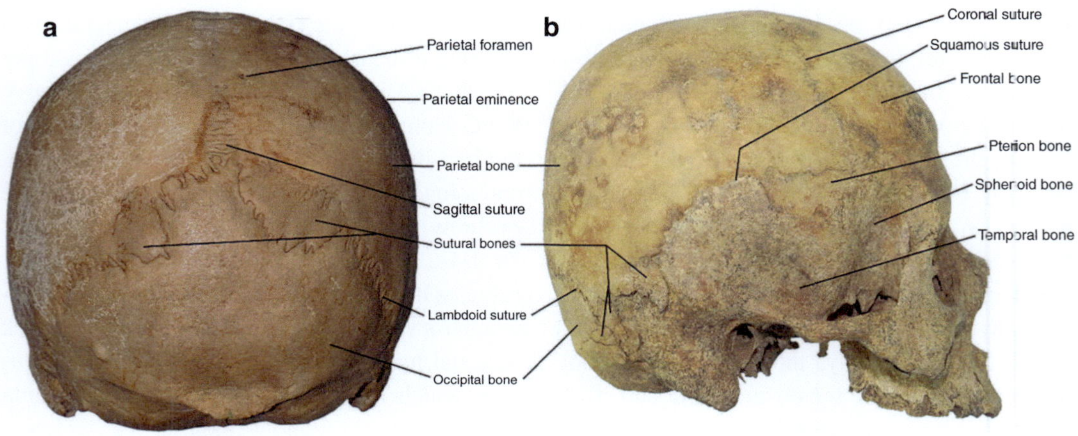

Fig. 3.4 Sutural bones of clavaria. (**a**) Sutural bones along the lambdoid suture, (**b**) Sutural bone along the anterior part of squamous suture, also known as pterion bone, and sutural bones long parietomastoid suture (With permission of Ege University Faculty of Medicine, Department of Anatomy)

tion of the frontal bone. At this stage, the dura fold that separates the two brain hemispheres (the falx cerebri) joins. The bone joins the sphenoid, zygomatic, and parietal bones in synarthrosis. The anterior pterion, which overlies the middle meningeal artery (a branch of the maxillary artery), is where these four bones articulate. The sphenoid fontanel is located here in infancy, allowing the bones of the skull to shift over each other to allow the head to pass through the birth canal. The frontal sinus, which protects the brain from direct skull trauma, is located in the frontal bone.

The parietal bone articulates with the frontal and occipital bones anteriorly and posteriorly. The bones are the skull's biggest bones, and they articulate in the midline via the sagittal suture. Underneath, the parietal lobe is engaged in sensory perception. Scaphocephaly is caused by the fusing of the sagittal suture too early. This bone is imprinted by meningeal arteries that run through the dura mater's material.

The squamous temporal bone, its outer convex surface offers attachment to the temporalis muscle and forms the temporal fossa boundary. The supramastoid crest (or temporal line) travels posterosuperiorly across its posterior section and connects to the temporalis fascia.

The zygomatic process is formed by the front aspect of the squamous temporal bone extending antero-inferiorly as well as laterally. The superior surface of the zygomatic process connects to the temporalis fascia, while the inferior surface is rough and thick, allowing the masseter muscle to adhere. The zygomatic process's posterior portion is divided into anterior and posterior roots. The anterior root is medially oriented and terminates in the rounded, cartilage-covered articular eminence that defines the anterior edge of the mandibular fossa. The posterior root extends from the external auditory meatus to the supramastoid crest [33].

The occipital bone is located in the back of the skull and articulates with the parietal bones superiorly while also forming the occipital condyles inferiorly. These condyles connect to the atlas' lateral masses. Atlas was the Greek titan who carried the skies; hence the C1 vertebra has been named after him.

The skull sutures:

The sagittal suture runs along the midline of the brain, from the coronal suture to the occipital bone in the back. The forward continuation of the sagittal suture, the metopic suture (Fig. 3.5), fuses at 1 year of age. Trigonocephaly is caused by premature fusion. The sutures of the skull are synarthrosis joints, which are related to gomphosis (tooth sockets), synchondrosis (a cartilaginous joint connected by hyaline cartilage), and synostoses. The sagittal suture is located in the mid-sagittal plane and splits both parietal bones superiorly.

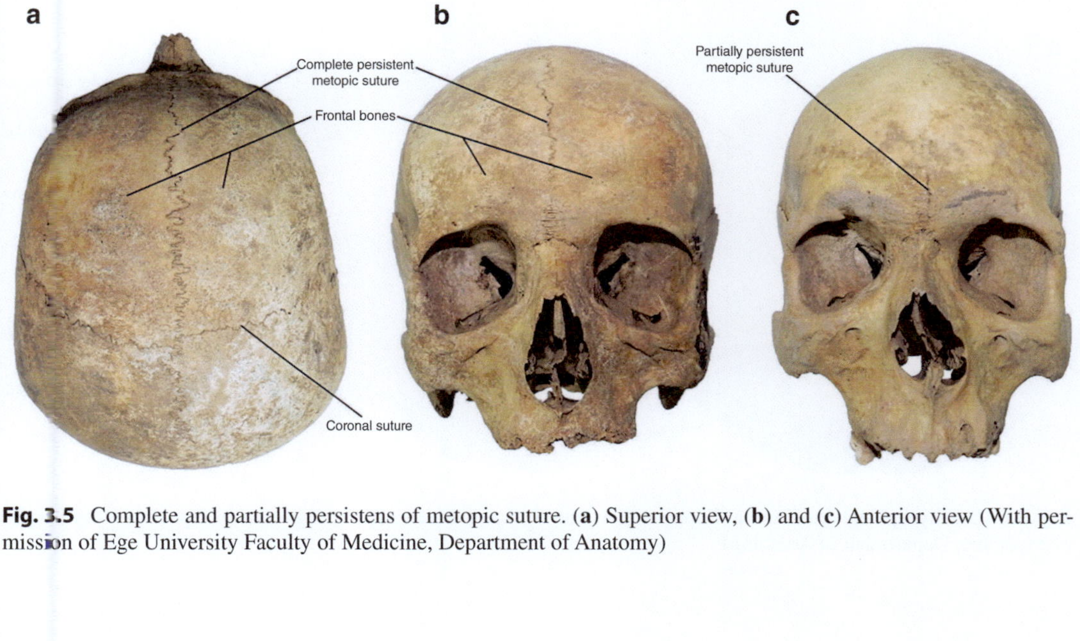

Fig. 3.5 Complete and partially persistens of metopic suture. (**a**) Superior view, (**b**) and (**c**) Anterior view (With permission of Ege University Faculty of Medicine, Department of Anatomy)

At roughly the age of 30, both parietal bones fuse, making it the last suture to fuse. The superior sagittal sinus is likewise covered by this suture.

The coronal suture runs roughly one-third of the way along the superior skull between the frontal bone and the two parietal bones. It fully fuses with the lambdoid suture at the age of 25.

The lambdoid suture connects the parietal bones superiorly and the occipital bones inferiorly, and fuses at the age of 25. It reaches from the back of the head to the posterior pterion. In infancy, the posterior pterion formed at the junction of the occipital, parietal, and temporal bones and was known as the mastoid fontanel.

The squamous suture connects the temporal bone to the parietal bone inferiorly and superiorly. It connects the anterior and posterior pterion.

There are also different types; for example a distinctive anatomical feature, the brachycephalic skull is characterized by its shortened and expanded dimensions relative to its length (Fig. 3.6). This phenomenon, measured by the cephalic index (ratio of maximum head width to maximum head length), typically occurs in individuals with a cephalic index exceeding 80. The etiology of brachycephaly involves a complex interaction of genetic and environmental factors. While genetic variations contribute to innate skull shapes, cultural practices such as head binding or shaping during infancy can also influence skull morphology. Anthropologists use cephalic index measurements to discern population characteristics and patterns of human migration. In forensic contexts, analysis of cranial features, including brachycephaly, aids in individual identification and understanding of historical demographics. Examination of the brachycephalic skull provides a nuanced perspective on human biodiversity, offering insights into evolutionary processes, cultural adaptations, and historical practices. This complex research advances our understanding of the multifaceted dynamics shaping human skull morphology across different periods and regions.

3.4.2 Fontanelles and Their Significance

Fontanelle is the outward curving of an infant's soft area (fontanelle).

Considerations of fontanelles: The skull is composed of several bones. The skull has eight bones and the face has 14 bones. They fuse to produce a solid, bony chamber that shields and supports the brain. The sutures are the points where the bones come together.

At birth, the bones are not firmly connected. This permits the skull to shift shape and pass through the birth canal more easily. The sutures solidify when minerals are supplied to them over time, firmly binding the skull bones together.

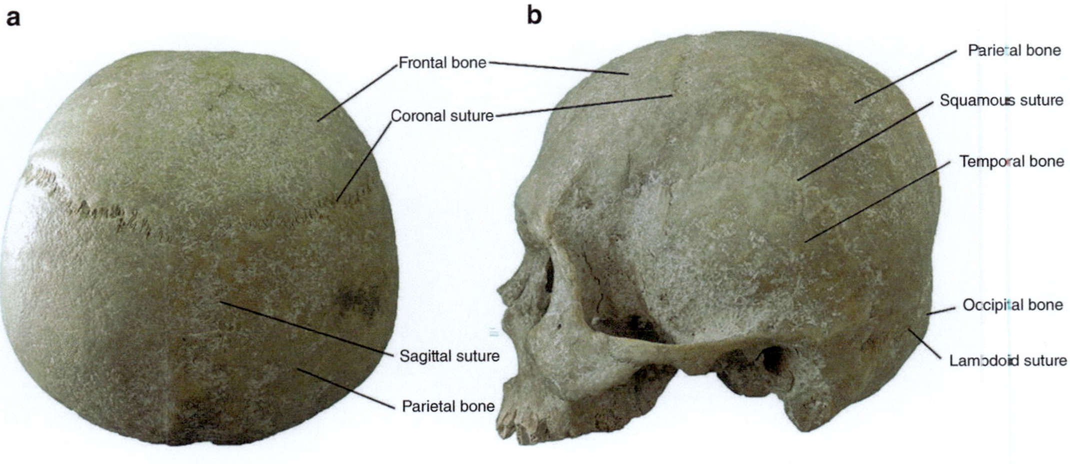

Fig. 3.6 Brachycephalic cranium. (**a**) Superior view and (**b**) Lateral view (With permission of Ege University Faculty of Medicine, Department of Anatomy)

A fontanelle (fontanel) is a membrane-covered "soft spot" formed by the junction of two sutures in an infant. During an infant's first year, the fontanelles enable brain and skull growth. A newborn's skull usually has numerous fontanelles. They are primarily seen on the top, back, and sides of the head. Fontanelles, like sutures, harden over time and become closed, solid bone structures.

The fontanelle in the back of the head (posterior fontanelle) usually closes by 1 to 2 months of age. The anterior fontanelle (at the top of the skull) usually closes from 7 to 19 months [34]. The mastoid fontanelle is a paired structure located at the junction of the temporal, parietal, and occipital bones. Furthermore, the mastoid fontanelle is known as the posterolateral fontanelle. These fontanelles can close between the ages of 6 and 18 months. The sphenoid fontanelle is also paired. It can be found on either side of the skull at the point where the sphenoid, parietal, temporal, and frontal bones meet. It is also known as the anterolateral fontanelle, and it closes about the sixth month after birth.

A third fontanelle between the anterior and posterior fontanelles is associated with disorders such as Down syndrome and prenatal illnesses such as rubella [35].

To the touch, the fontanelles should be firm and slightly folded inward. When fluid builds up in the brain or the brain swells, it causes increased pressure inside the skull, resulting in a tight or bulging fontanelle. The fontanelles may appear to bulge when the infant is sobbing, lying down, or vomiting. When the infant is in a peaceful, head-up position, they should return to normal.

3.4.3 Diploë and the Internal Structure of Cranial Bones

The term "diploe" refers to the spongy or cancellous portion of bone that exists between the hard outer cortical shell and the brittle inner shell (as in the skull). This term is typically applied to skull bones, but it can also refer to other short bones.

The diploic veins are a structure that lies within the diploe of the skull, between the inner and outer tables of the calvarium bone. The intracranial and extracranial venous systems are linked by these veins. They develop in size as they progress from youth to adulthood. The diploic cavity has been found as an additional location of cerebrospinal fluid (CSF) reabsorption [36].

In some situations, the vascular connection from the cortical surface and meninges into the superior sagittal sinus could render the diploic veins a route of infection. Sinusitis, for example, can cause major consequences if the infection travels to the cerebral area. Direct extension from infected sinuses or hematogenous dissemination by the diploic veins has been observed to cause intracranial problems. Complications of frontal sinusitis and their management [37].

The internal structure of the cranial bones:

The cranial cavity's inner surface is split into three discrete depressions. It is made up of three cranial fossae: anterior, middle, and posterior. Each fossa houses a separate portion of the brain. The anterior cranial fossa is the shallowest and superior of the three fossae. The fossa is made up of the frontal bone, the ethmoid bone, and the sphenoid bone's body and lesser wings. It houses the frontal lobe's antero-inferior part. The larger wings of the sphenoid bone and the temporal bone form the middle fossa. It is reported to be in the shape of a butterfly. It holds the pituitary gland and the temporal lobes are located in the two lateral sections of the fossa. The occipital bone and the posterior part of the temporal bones make up the majority of the posterior cranial fossa. It houses the brainstem and cerebellum, as well as the arteries and nerves that run through it.

3.4.4 Blood Supply to the Calvarium (Arterial Supply, Venous Drainage)

The common carotid arteries (anterior circulation) and vertebral arteries (posterior circulation) furnish the majority of the blood supply to the skull and its accompanying structures. The internal and external carotid arteries branch off the common carotid artery. The external carotid artery supplies the majority of blood to the skull bones and meninges. It runs along the side of the neck, with eight major branches feeding the skull and face's superficial structures. The most visible and clinically significant of these branches is the maxillary artery. The middle meningeal artery is a branch of the maxillary artery, and head injury at the pterion may result in extradural hematoma. The internal carotid artery passes through the neck without branching and penetrates the base of the skull, supplying intracranial tissues. The internal carotid and vertebral arteries join to produce the circle of Willis, a massive anastomosis, which is supported by the anterior communicating artery, two anterior cerebral arteries, two middle cerebral arteries, two posterior communicating arteries, two posterior cerebral arteries, and the basilar artery (superior continuation of the vertebral arteries).

The dural venous sinuses (such as superior sagittal, straight, and transverse sinuses) and superficial and deep veins of the head (such as cerebellar, facial, and cerebral veins) drain into the internal and external jugular veins bilaterally and eventually to the superior vena cava and right atrium of the heart [38].

Historically, lymphatic vessels were assumed to be absent from the brain and central nervous system. Some believe that cerebrospinal fluid (CSF) is connected to the lymphatic system and drains through the cervical lymph nodes. The recent discovery of a "glymphatic system," which is made up of a network of CSF, cerebral interstitial fluid, and meningeal vasculature, has thrown more light on this debate and is still being studied [39].

3.5 Histology of Scalp and Calvarium

3.5.1 Histological Composition of the Scalp Layers (Epidermis, Dermis, Subcutaneous Tissue, Connective Tissue Layers, Blood Vessels and Nerves)

The scalp, a complex structure covering the head region, is composed of numerous layers, each with different histological characteristics that contribute to its function and elasticity. Understanding the histological composition of these layers is essential to understanding the intricacies of scalp anatomy:

Epidermis: The outermost layer, the epidermis, is composed primarily of stratified squamous epithelium. The superficial skin of the scalp has a dark and warm environment filled with hair follicles and intense sebum production, making it prone to fungal infection. These different mycotic infections can cause varying degrees of itching, alopecia, inflammation, scaling, and scarring of the epidermis. The different infections are caused by different organisms, which determine what kind of treatment is required [14].

This epithelium consists of multiple cell layers, including:

– Stratum corneum: Composed of flattened, keratinized cells that provide a protective barrier against environmental factors. This layer is the major protective barrier against various external factors like microorganisms, toxic materials, and irradiation. In fact, it a barrier against loss of water, providing normal hydration of the scalp [40].

- Stratum granulosum: Contains granular cells that aid in keratinization. Both the stratum corneum and stratum granulosum form the primary barriers to skin protection. The stratum granulosum and stratum spinosum cells contain pigment particles as they migrate upwards. Eventually, all pigments present in the epidermis will be pushed upwards by exfoliation of the stratum corneum [41].
- Stratum spinosum: It consists of polygonal cells connected by desmosomes. The epidermis shows a regular maturation from the basal (germinative) layer of keratinocytes to the keratogenous layer towards the granular cell layer, the spinosum. It is very important to remember that in normal skin there is considerable morphological variation depending on topographic area and physiological variation depending on hormonal balance, sex, and age. The advanced stage is characterized by epidermal "psoriasiform hyperplasia" with regular acanthuses (thickening of the stratum spinosum) and regular elongation of the rete ridges and thinning of the supra-papillary plates. Mitotic activity is usually quite prominent, further indicating the hyperproliferative nature of this condition [42].
- Stratum basale: The deepest layer where keratinocytes divide and melanocytes produce melanin. The epidermis is considered to consist of the stratum basale, which contains O_2-consuming, CO_2-producing cells, and dead cells of the stratum corneum [43].

In addition to keratinocytes and melanocytes, Langerhans cells are present, contributing to the immune defense of the skin [44].

Collagen and elastin fibers provide strength and elasticity to the dermis.

- Dermis: Collagen and elastin fibers provide strength and elasticity to the dermis. The dermal papilla is localized at the base of hair follicles and has a critical role in the growth of hair and regulation of the activity of the follicle cells; The dermis, located beneath the epidermis, is a fibrous connective tissue layer rich in blood vessels, nerves, and various appendages [45] including:

- Hair follicles: The areas where hair growth takes place. Scalp hair follicles producing produce long hairs remain in the anagen phase for 2–8 years, while eyebrow hair follicles producing short hairs do so for only 2–3 months. The end of the anagen phase is controlled by fibroblast growth factor 5 and the vast majority of the people usually lose 50–150 scalp hairs per day. The telogen phase lasts 2–3 months and then the scalp follicles enter the anagen phase again and thus the cycle repeats. It is well-known that testosterone and dihydrotestosterone act through androgen receptors. As a rule, they increase the size of hair follicles in some androgen-dependent areas, including the beard area during puberty, although they can cause miniaturization of scalp follicles later in life [46].
- Sebaceous glands: secrete sebum, an oily substance that lubricates hair and skin. The human sebaceous glands can be found on the entire skin surface (except the palms and soles of the feet), but sebum secretion is highest on the scalp, face, chest, and back. Sebum is produced under hormonal control, the sebaceous glands are active at birth under the control of maternal androgens. Its size and sebum production decrease rapidly until the onset of puberty. At the onset of puberty, the sebaceous glands become active again, this time under the control of circulating androgens. The rate of sebum secretion increases throughout puberty, remains constant in the 20s and 30s, and decreases with age. During the active period of sebum secretion, the secretion rate is higher in men than in women. In men, this rate remains high for longer until the 50s and 60s, but in women, the secretion rate drops rapidly after menopause [47].
- Sweat glands: Produce sweat for thermoregulation. Some authors found that thermoregulatory sweating responses for the scalp region are increased in the hot-humid condition in contrast to the hot-dry condition. In particular, the vertex among the regions on the scalp surface was the least sensitive to changes in humidity and it has reported that porocarcinoma of the scalp is a very rare tumor [48, 49].

- Sensory receptors: Detect stimuli such as touch, temperature, and pain. The specific study explains the following lines. Frontal-Parietal Region: This region is primarily innervated by the ophthalmic division of the trigeminal nerve (cranial nerve V). The ophthalmic division is responsible for sensory input from the forehead and the upper part of the scalp. Occipital region: The occipital region is innervated by the occipital nerves arising from the second cervical root (C2). These nerves provide sensory innervation to the back of the scalp and the back of the head. Temporal Areas: The temporal areas on both sides of the head are innervated by the maxillary and mandibular divisions of the trigeminal nerve (cranial nerve V). The occipital nerves arising from the second and third cervical roots also contribute to the sensory input in these areas. Since potentials at a given distance from the stimulating electrodes tend to be similar for different depths, the depth of the nerve was expected to have minimal influence on the results. It was also predicted that sensory receptors would be effectively stimulated even at relatively large distances [50]. Nerves in the dermis transmit sensory information and control various physiological responses. Blood vessels and nerves traveling through the subcutaneous tissue contribute to overall scalp health and function. Nerves include sensory nerves that provide scalp sensation and motor nerves that control muscles, including those associated with hair follicles.

These nerves branch through various layers into the dermis, subcutaneous tissue, and deeper structures.

- Blood Vessels: The scalp is highly vascularized and has a complex network of arteries, veins, and capillaries. These vessels maintain tissue health by transporting oxygen, nutrients, and waste products. Blood vessels provide nutrients and oxygen and help regulate temperature. The arteries and veins supplying the scalp are located between the galea and the subcutaneous tissues. The blood supply of the scalp has extensive connections that allow the transfer of large scalp flaps that rely on a single blood vessel [51].
- Subcutaneous Tissue (Hypodermis): Below the dermis lies the subcutaneous tissue, composed mainly of adipose (fat) tissue. Since the hair follicle is located deep in the dermis, with its bulb in the hypodermis, detrimental age-related changes in the skin surrounding the scalp are likely to disrupt the hair follicle mechanism. The effects of these changes are unknown, but evidence suggests that scalp aging and hair follicle aging go hand in hand. In this paper, we summarize the evidence that the age-related changes observed in sun-exposed human skin also occur in the scalp skin and that these changes may play a contributory role in the aging hair phenotype [52].

Adipose tissue serves multiple functions, including insulation, energy storage, and cushioning. Brown fat acts as a thermogenic organ in many newborns. In humans, residual brown adipose tissue is most commonly found in the interscapular region, upper mediastinum, axilla, retroperitoneum, and neck [53].

- Connective Tissue Layers: The scalp contains several connective tissue layers that provide structural support and play key roles in its function:
- Galea aponeurotica: A dense, fibrous layer connecting the frontalis and occipitalis muscles and attaching to the periosteum of cranial bones. Loose areolar connective tissue: Beneath the galea aponeurotic, this tissue allows for mobility between the scalp and the underlying cranial bones. The loose areolar tissue or subgaleal fascia loosely connects the galea aponeurosis to the pericranium and allows the three superficial layers of the scalp to move over the pericranium. This layer is not normally seen on CT or MRI and is only detected pathologically. Histologically, it consists of a central dense collagenous layer surrounded by vascularised areolar tissue. In craniofacial and neurosurgical procedures, scalp flaps are raised along a relatively avascular plane [54, 55].

– Pericranium: The pericranium, the periosteum of cranial bones, is the fifth and deepest protective layer of the scalp. The pericranium is a dense membranous or fibrous layer loosely fused on its outer side with the galea aponeurotic, from which it is easily separated via the subgaleal space, and it is usually of similar thickness to the galea. It can be easily cut away from the outer layer of the skull as an intact layer [23].

A detailed understanding of the histological structure of the scalp is vital for healthcare professionals, including dermatologists, plastic surgeons, and neurosurgeons, as it informs diagnosis, treatment, and surgical procedures. Furthermore, this knowledge is invaluable in cosmetic procedures, providing the best results in hair transplantation, scalp reconstruction, and other interventions aimed at preserving both the structural integrity and aesthetics of the scalp and calvarium.

3.5.2 Histology of Cranial Bones (Compact Bone, Spongy Bone, Diploic Spaces, Periosteum)

The bones of the skull, which form the protective and structural skeleton of the calvarium (skullcap), exhibit a remarkable histological composition. These tissues combine to form robust yet complex structures that protect the brain and support various craniofacial functions. Let's explore the histology of the skull bones and examine their various components in meticulous detail:

– Compact Bone: Compact bone, also known as cortical bone, constitutes the outer layer of cranial bones and serves as a protective shield.
– Its microscopic structure comprises a dense network of structural units called osteons or Haversian systems. Each osteon comprises concentric lamellae surrounding a central Haversian canal, which houses blood vessels, nerves, and lymphatic vessels. Osteocytes, mature bone cells, reside in lacunae within the lamellae, connected via tiny canaliculi, facilitating nutrient and waste exchange. Compact bone provides strength and rigidity to cranial bones, enabling them to withstand external forces [56].
– Spongy Bone (Cancellous Bone): Below the compact bone layer, cancellous bone, also known as spongy bone, forms the inner part of the skull bones. Unlike compact bone, cancellous bone consists of a network-like structure of trabeculae, which are delicate bone plates. These trabeculae form a network of interconnected spaces that are usually filled with red bone marrow. The red bone marrow in cancellous bone is essential for hematopoiesis, the formation of blood cells. Cancellous bone offers structural support while maintaining a lighter and less dense composition compared to compact bone [57].
– Diploic Cavities: Specific to certain skull bones, such as the frontal and parietal bones, diploic cavities are centrally located within these flat bones. These cavities are characterized by the presence of cancellous bone and red bone marrow. Diploic cavities play a multifaceted role; they contribute to bone strength, support hematopoiesis, and optimize their functionality by helping to reduce the overall weight of the skull bones. Histologically, densification of the vessels and enlargement of the Virchow-Robinson spaces are described [58, 59].
– Periosteum: The periosteum provides a protective and functional cover by enveloping the outer surface of the skull bones. It consists of two main layers:

The outer fibrous layer, dense and tough, acts as a barrier against external influences.

An inner cellular layer rich in osteoprogenitor cells that contribute to bone growth and repair. Blood vessels within the periosteum supply the skull bones with the necessary nutrients and oxygen. This membrane is an integral part of cranial bone development during embryogenesis and plays a crucial role in bone repair after injury [60].

One specific study had the potential to change our view of to skull completely as explained here briefly. In humans, the functional roles and molecular structure of skull bone marrow and other types of bone marrow are less characterized. Although a limited number of 'omics studies on human bone marrow have been presented, a systematic characterization of the potential differences between different types of bone marrow and the possible differences under different conditions has not yet been performed. Even at the anatomical level, although the existence of human SMCs has been suggested using microCT, their detailed structure at the cellular level is still unclear.

They completed a systematic and comprehensive molecular analysis of the RNA and protein expression profiles of various bone marrow cells in mice and humans [61]. They performed batch and single-cell RNA sequencing and batch proteomic analyses on cells from six different bones, dura mater, and brains in mice [61]. These analyses were performed in three different conditions (native, middle cerebral artery occlusion, and sham-operated animals). Their data show that different bones have distinct molecular profiles [61]. In particular, the skull bone marrow has the most differentially expressed gene and ligand-receptor pairs, which are mostly related to migration and inflammation [61].

Understanding the intricacies of cranial bone histology is of great importance for healthcare professionals in various specialties, including neurosurgery, orthopedics, radiology, and pathology. This understanding provides the basis for accurate diagnosis, effective treatment, and informed decision-making in cases of cranial bone injuries, disorders, and anomalies. It is also indispensable for researchers investigating bone development, remodeling, disease, and surgical interventions and contributes to the advancement of craniofacial medicine and the improvement of patient care.

3.6 Developmental Changes Over Time

3.6.1 Changes in the Scalp and Calvarium During Development (Fetal Development, Childhood Development, Adult Changes)

The scalp and calvarium, integral components of the craniofacial region, undergo dynamic developmental changes throughout an individual's lifespan. These changes encompass complex processes of growth, maturation, and adaptation to the unique requirements of each developmental stage. Let's explore these remarkable transformations in greater depth:

1. Fetal Development

Formation of Cranial Bones: In the early stages of fetal development, the cranial bones begin to take shape. Neural crest cells, originating from the dorsal edge of the neural tube, migrate and condense to form the foundation of the cranial bones. Intramembranous ossification plays a pivotal role in this process. The embryonic development of the cranium and cranial suture complex extends to neural crest cell migration. This period is approximately between E19 and E38. Following neural crest migration, the calvarial mesenchyme originates from the paraxial mesoderm and the cranial neural crest; the boundaries between neural crest and bone undergo evolutionary changes [62]. Neural crest cells originating from the dorsal neural tube migrate and they are pulled by the expansion of the epidermis [62]. The mesenchyme of the frontal primordium forms the frontal bones and subsequent growth of the bone plates results in the formation of a "suture" [62]. BMP, Wnt, and SHH signals are vital during this process [17].

Cranial bone growth and brain enlargement: As the fetal brain undergoes rapid growth, it exerts pressure on the developing cranial bones. This effect shapes the growth of the cranial bones, especially in the fontanelle and suture areas. These open areas provide space for the brain to expand and bend during birth. The cranial vault, a vital component of the neurocranium, consists mainly of flat bones, including the paired frontal and parietal bones, the squamous portions of the temporal bone, and the interparietal portion of the occipital bone. These bones are formed by intramembranous ossification and their development extends from early embryogenesis to adulthood.

The embryonic phase, which occurs during the first 8 weeks of gestation, begins with the formation of mesenchymal cells through epithelial-mesenchymal transformation. Mesenchymal cells are derived from two sources: unsegmented paraxial mesoderm and cranial neural crest cells. The neurocranium, including both the chondrocranium and calvarium, develops from these mesenchymal populations, and the viscerocranium originates exclusively from neural crest mesenchyme [63].

The condensation of mesenchymal cells marks the beginning of cranial bone development, leading to the formation of the base of the ectomeningeal capsule. This early membrane formation represents the beginning of skull development. Later, the meninx primitiva, consisting of the endomeninx and ectomeninx layers, contributes to the formation of the cranial vault.

The fetal stage, from the end of the embryonic stage until birth, witnesses the intramembranous ossification of the primitive membranous skull. The cranial sutures play an important role in intramembranous bone growth during this stage. Various calvarial bones, such as the frontal, parietal, occipital, and temporal bones, undergo ossification through specific processes, leading to the formation of the cranial vault.

In the areas where the membranous bones approach each other, sutures are formed, corresponding to large dural reflections. These sutures function as growth zones and allow the cranial vault to expand as the brain grows. The sutures function by producing membranous bone at their edges, maintaining constant articulation between the bones while accommodating growth.

After birth, growth of the cranial vault combines sutural expansion, remodeling, and displacement due to brain enlargement. This dynamic process leads to differential growth of the various cranial bones, contributing to the complex shape of the human skull. In addition, the presence of fontanelles at birth allows some deformation during passage through the birth canal and then closes as bone deposition occurs along their edges [64].

Understanding normal cranial vault development is crucial to understanding craniosynostosis, in which early suture fusion disrupts the cranial growth process. This knowledge provides insight into the pathogenic mechanisms underlying craniosynostosis and informs potential interventions to address this condition.

In summary, prenatal development and growth of the cranial vault involve complex processes of mesenchymal cell formation, condensation, ossification, and suture formation [65].

Maturation of Scalp: Concurrently, the epidermis, dermis, and subcutaneous tissue layers of the scalp begin to form. Hair follicles develop, and melanocytes within the epidermis contribute to the pigmentation of the scalp and hair. Based on the studies regarding hair follicle development in normal fetuses and children, the hypothesis that the slope in the hair direction is secondary to the plane of tension applied to the skin by the growth of the underlying tissues during sub-growth of the hair follicles at about 10–12 weeks gestation [66]. The posterior parietal hair shaft has been interpreted as the focal point where growth tension is applied by the dome-like growth of the brain during hair follicle development [66].

Establishment of Blood Supply and Nerve Function: During fetal development, complex processes of vascularization and neural innervation in the scalp and skull bones emerge as crucial components. These processes are crucial for the supply of nutrients, the transport of oxygen, and the establishment of sensory functions in these vital areas. In this medical narrative, we embark on a detailed examination of the fascinating mechanisms underlying the formation of blood flow and nerve function in the developing scalp and skull bones.

Vascularization of the Scalp and Skull Bones: The formation of vascular networks in the scalp and skull bones occurs in the early embryonic stage. These channels, which are vital for sustaining life, originate from both mesodermal and ectodermal areas within the developing embryo [24].

In the third week of gestation, a crucial milestone is reached when primitive blood vessels begin to form in the embryonic mesoderm. The complex process of angiogenesis, the formation of new blood vessels from pre-existing vessels, begins to play an important role at this time [67].

The blood supply to the skull bones is mainly provided by branches from the internal and external carotid arteries. The internal carotid artery serves the anterior part of the brain, while the external carotid artery branches off gracefully to serve the scalp and facial regions.

As development progresses, these arterial networks undergo extensive branching and weave a complex vasculature that penetrates the bones of the skull and supplies the surrounding tissues. Critical anastomoses, or connections between different blood vessels, are meticulously created to ensure redundancy and uninterrupted blood flow and serve as a lifeline to these newly developing regions.

Ensuring effective venous drainage is at least as important as arterial supply. The dural venous sinuses, located between the layers of the meninges, emerge as vital channels that collect venous blood passing through the bones of the skull and scalp. Eventually, this venous blood is directed to the internal jugular vein, providing a harmonized circulation [67].

Nerve Function in the Scalp and Bones of the Skull: The complex journey of nerve development in the cranial region involves neural crest cells, specialized entities that arise from the embryonic ectoderm. These remarkable cells serve as the architects behind various components of the nervous system, including sensory neurons that hold the key to cranial sensation.

Numerous cranial nerves play important roles in the sensory innervation of the scalp and skull bones. Among these, the trigeminal nerve (CN V) stands out as illuminating. Its branches, such as the ophthalmic (V1), maxillary (V2), and mandibular (V3) divisions, emerge as the main sensory contributors to different areas of this complex landscape [68].

The sensory innervation of the scalp depends on a dermatomal pattern in which separate spinal nerves serve specific areas of the skin. For example, the ophthalmic division of the trigeminal nerve expertly supervises the sensory areas of the forehead and scalp [69].

Free nerve endings and sensory receptors, including specialized structures such as Meissner's corpuscles and Pacinian corpuscles, are distributed throughout the scalp and skull bones. These complex receptors play the role of vigilant sentinels, always ready to detect a range of sensory stimuli, from gentle touches and pressures to temperature changes and pain signals.

Sensory information gathered from the scalp and skull bones makes the journey to the brain, where it is meticulously processed and integrated. This information contributes significantly to various functions, including somatosensory perception, motor responses, and finely tuned mechanisms responsible for maintaining homeostasis [70].

During fetal development, the establishment of blood flow and nerve function in the scalp and skull bones unfolds as a symphony of orchestrated processes. The sensitivity of the vasculature ensures the delivery of vital nutrients and oxygen, while the sensory innervation network allows for the keen perception of various sensory cues. Understanding the intricacies of these developmental aspects is instrumental in understanding the conditions associated with craniofacial anomalies and neurological disorders that can affect these vital regions.

2. Childhood Development

Continued Cranial Bone Growth: In early childhood, cranial bone growth remains a prominent developmental process. The expansion of the braincase and the cranial vault continues to accommodate the growing brain [71]. As a child matures, fontanelles, the soft spots on the skull, gradually close. This closure results from the progressive fusion of cranial bones, particularly at the sutures. By around the age of two, fontanelles typically complete their closure.

There are several basic processes in the development of the skull bones that contribute to their growth and adaptation:

Sutural growth: The flat skull bones are enclosed in connective tissue membranes, with one side adjacent to the brain and the other to the skin. As the brain grows, the skull bones are pulled outwards, partly due to the expanding meninges, which have osteogenic properties. This outward displacement stimulates the osteogenic sutural membranes to produce membranous bone in proportion to the degree of displacement. This process increases the circumference of each bone and stabilizes the articulation between them.

Remodeling: Remodelling is an ongoing process that involves the deposition and reabsorption of bone tissue in specific areas of a bone. This dynamic process reshapes and resizes bones as they continue to grow.

Displacement Movements: Displacement movements occur in all skull bones and contribute to their separation at the points of connection between them. Primary displacement occurs with the natural growth of a bone, while secondary displacement is influenced by the expansion of neighboring or distant bones or soft tissues. During primary displacement, the moving bone and other skeletal parts grow simultaneously, while secondary displacement is not directly related to the growth of the bone itself.

These growth processes cause changes in the size and thickness of the skull bones. Deposits along the edges of the sutures and the outer surface of the bones, combined with bone removal from the inner surface, lead to bone growth while maintaining the size of the skull cavity.

Notably, the growing brain does not physically push the bones outwards. Instead, each flat bone is suspended in a network of collagen fibers of the inner (meningeal) and outer (cutaneous) periosteal layers. These membranes grow outwards in front of the expanding brain, causing the bones to shift with them. This separation creates tensile forces that stimulate bone production.

The stimulus for this bone-producing response comes primarily from the expanding brain, which sends signals through the dura mater. As the brain expands and the synchondroses (cartilaginous growth plates) at the skull base lengthen, the sutures respond by adding intramembranous (IM) bone at their edges. This allows the cranial vault to accommodate the expanding brain while maintaining the width of the sutures.

At birth, the skull bones are widely separated by sutures, facilitating the flexibility needed for the relatively large fetal head to pass through the birth canal. Later, bone deposition along the edges of the fontanelles eliminates these gaps. However, a thin line of periosteum keeps the bones apart for many years before they fuse in adulthood [65].

Advancements in Scalp and Hair Growth: The development of the scalp continues throughout childhood. The epidermis, dermis, and subcutaneous tissue layers mature, influencing the texture and resilience of the skin. Hair growth becomes more apparent, and changes in hair thickness and texture may be observed.

3. Adult Changes

   Ongoing Cranial Bone Remodelling: In adulthood, the cranial bones undergo a lifelong process of remodeling. This involves a delicate balance between bone resorption (destruction) and bone formation. Remodeling helps maintain bone strength and adaptability in response to mechanical stresses and functional requirements.

   Maintenance of Sutures: While fontanelles close during childhood, cranial sutures persist into adulthood. These sutures provide a degree of flexibility and allow minimal movement between the cranial bones. They also contribute to the even distribution of stress across the cranial vault.

Scalp and Hair Ageing: As individuals age, various changes can occur in the scalp. These changes may include decreased blood flow to the scalp, thinning of the epidermis, and changes in hair texture and pigmentation. Conditions such as alopecia, characterized by hair loss, may become more common with age.

Understanding the complex developmental changes in the scalp and calvarium is essential for health professionals across a range of specialties, including pediatricians, neurologists, dermatologists, and orthopedic surgeons. It informs the assessment of normal development, helps to identify developmental abnormalities or disorders, and facilitates the diagnosis and treatment of conditions affecting these regions at different life stages. It also provides a basis for research efforts aimed at unraveling the complexity of craniofacial development and aging processes, ultimately contributing to advances in medical science and healthcare [65, 72, 73].

3.6.2 Clinical Relevance of Developmental Changes (Cranial Sutures and Craniosynostosis, Fontanelle Closure, Age-Related Changes in the Scalp)

Developmental changes occurring in the scalp and calvarium have profound clinical significance spanning a variety of medical specialties. These changes not only serve as diagnostic indicators but also guide treatment approaches, influencing patient care across the lifespan. Let us comprehensively examine the clinical significance of these developmental changes:

Cranial Sutures and Craniosynostosis: Clinical Significance: Cranial sutures, fibrous joints between the cranial bones, play a crucial role in cranial development and growth. Their proper function is critical to accommodate the growth of the brain and maintain the shape of the skull. When one or more cranial sutures fuse prematurely, it leads to craniosynostosis, which can cause craniofacial deformities and increased intracranial pressure. Early diagnosis and intervention are very important [74]. Healthcare providers, including pediatricians and craniofacial surgeons, rely on an understanding of cranial suture development for timely diagnosis and surgical correction of craniosynostosis. Surgical release of fused sutures is often necessary to allow for normal cranial growth.

Fontanelle Closure: Fontanelles, the soft, membranous spaces between the skull bones in infants, serve as windows to intracranial health. The timing and pattern of their closure are vital clinical indicators. Pediatricians and neonatologists use the status of fontanelles (open, closing, or closed) as part of routine infant assessments. Deviations from the expected closure timeline may indicate underlying problems such as dehydration, hydrocephalus, or genetic syndromes. Fontanelle assessment helps diagnose and monitor conditions related to intracranial pressure and cranial development. It guides further evaluation and treatment decisions [75].

Age-related changes in the scalp: The scalp undergoes significant histological and functional changes throughout a person's lifetime, affecting skin health, hair conditions, and dermatological assessments. Dermatologists and plastic surgeons consider age-related scalp changes when diagnosing and treating various conditions. Decreased blood flow and thinning of the epidermis in older individuals can affect wound healing, skin health, and response to cosmetic procedures [76].

Alopecia and Hair Loss: Age-related hair thinning and conditions such as androgenetic alopecia are common concerns. Scalp specialists use their knowledge of these changes to develop customized treatment plans that may include topical medications, hair transplantation, or other interventions.

A comprehensive understanding of the clinical significance of developmental changes in the scalp and calvarium is essential for multi-disciplinary healthcare providers. It enables them to recognize developmental anomalies, address health problems promptly, and deliver patient-centered care across the entire lifespan. Furthermore, this knowledge fuels ongoing research on craniofacial development, bone disorders, dermatological conditions, and innovative treatment modalities, promoting advances in medical science and improving patient outcomes [77].

3.7 Conclusion

3.7.1 Summary of Key Points in Developmental Anatomy and Histology of the Scalp and Calvarium

Our literature research on the developmental anatomy and histology of the scalp and calvarium revealed a wealth of vital information. Here is a detailed summary of the key points discussed:

1. Embryonic Origins: The scalp and calvarium originate from the ectodermal and mesodermal layers during embryonic development.

   Neural crest cells, a specialized group of cells, play an important role in the formation of cranial bones, the development of cranial nerves, and the production of melanin by melanocytes.
2. Histology of the Scalp: The scalp is composed of different layers with unique histological features, including the epidermis, which consists of stratified squamous epithelium containing melanocytes responsible for skin and hair pigmentation. The dermis harbors hair follicles, sebaceous glands, blood vessels, and sensory nerves. The subcutaneous tissue, rich in adipose (fat) cells, provides insulation and cushioning. Several layers of connective tissue, including the galea aponeurotica and pericranium, offer structural support.

   Blood vessels and nerves traverse these layers, providing nutrients, oxygen, and sensation to the scalp.
3. Histology of Cranial Bones: The cranial bones exhibit a unique histological composition characterized by the following: The outer layer of compact bone is composed of osteons with concentric lamellae around Haversian canals. Spongy bone in the inner layer, composed of trabeculae and containing red bone marrow. Diploic cavities in some cranial bones, containing cancellous bone and marrow. The periosteum is a connective tissue membrane that covers the bones of the skull and promotes growth and repair.
4. Developmental changes over time: The scalp and calvarium undergo dynamic changes throughout developmental stages, including fetal development, childhood, and adulthood:

   Fetal development includes cranial bone formation, brain growth, and initial development of the scalp layers. During childhood, the growth of the cranial bones, the closure of the fontanelle, and the progression of epidermal and hair development of the scalp continue. In adulthood, the skull bones remodel throughout life, skull sutures continue, and age-related changes affect scalp health and hair conditions.
5. Clinical Significance: Developmental changes in the scalp and calvarium are of great clinical significance: Cranial sutures and fontanelles are crucial for the diagnosis and management of conditions such as craniosynostosis, where premature closure of sutures can lead to craniofacial deformities. Age-related scalp changes, including reduced blood flow and changes in skin and hair texture, affect dermatological assessments, hair loss treatments, and surgical interventions.

Understanding the intricacies of developmental anatomy and histology in the scalp and calvarium is imperative for healthcare professionals in a variety of specialties, from pediatricians and neurosurgeons to dermatologists and plastic surgeons. This knowledge forms the basis for accurate diagnosis, effective treatment strategies, and optimal patient care. It also fuels ongoing research into craniofacial development, bone disorders, and skin diseases, contributing to advancing medical science and improving patient outcomes.

3.7.2 Importance of This Knowledge in Clinical Practice

Understanding the developmental anatomy and histology of the scalp and calvarium is the cornerstone of clinical practice across a diverse range of medical disciplines. This knowledge underpins accurate diagnosis, effective treatment strategies, and improved patient care. Let us explore in more depth the profound importance of this knowledge and its transformative impact on clinical practice:

1. Precision in Diagnosis and Assessment:

   An in-depth understanding of skull bone development and the complex histological structure of the scalp enables healthcare professionals to make precise diagnoses in clinical settings.

   Pediatricians use this knowledge to assess the condition of fontanelles, detect anomalies, and monitor intracranial pressure in infants. Neurosurgeons use their expertise in cranial suture development to meticulously plan and execute surgical interventions, especially in craniosynostosis and other cranial anomalies. Dermatologists utilize knowledge of scalp histology to diagnose and effectively treat a wide range of skin diseases and hair disorders [78, 79].
2. Tailored Treatment Strategies:

   Insights gained from developmental changes across the lifespan enable the creation of tailored treatment plans, optimizing patient outcomes. Pediatric surgeons proactively intervene in cases of craniosynostosis, initiating surgical procedures to release fused cranial sutures and ensure optimal craniofacial development. Armed with a deep understanding of cranial bone growth dynamics, plastic, and reconstructive surgeons create precise and individualized corrective procedures to address complex craniofacial anomalies. Guided by their knowledge of age-related scalp changes, dermatologists design bespoke treatment regimens for patients, effectively managing wound healing, hair restoration, and overall skin health [80, 81].
3. Improving Patient Care:

   Proficiency in the developmental anatomy and histology of the scalp and calvarium raises the standard of patient care by improving diagnostic accuracy and treatment efficacy. Rapid diagnosis and intervention in pediatric cases involving cranial anomalies ensure superior craniofacial development and overall well-being. Dermatological care for scalp conditions, expertly informed by scalp histology, improves patients' quality of life and self-confidence. The ability to address the subtleties of age-related scalp changes empowers healthcare providers to effectively address concerns associated with the natural aging process [82, 83].
4. Catalyst for Research Advances:

   This fundamental knowledge catalyzes pioneering research efforts in craniofacial development, bone disorders, and dermatological conditions. The knowledge gained from such research contributes to the development of innovative treatments, cutting-edge therapies, and transformative medical breakthroughs. The advancement of medical science depends on a deep understanding of the nuances specific to the anatomy and histology of the scalp and calvarium [84].
5. Promoting Multidisciplinary Collaboration:

   Collaborative healthcare guided by multidisciplinary expertise is a cornerstone in addressing complex conditions involving the scalp and skull bones. A culture of information sharing and interdisciplinary collaboration ensures the delivery of comprehensive, holistic patient care, emphasizing the overall health and well-being of the individual [85].

In summary, an in-depth understanding of the developmental anatomy and histology of the scalp and calvarium goes beyond academic enrichment and plays a central role in clinical practice. It equips healthcare providers with the tools needed to make well-informed decisions, provides highly personalized patient care, and advances the frontiers of medical science. The ripple effect of this knowledge extends far beyond the confines of textbooks and ultimately promotes better health and enriched lives for patients at all stages of life.

References

1. Eid S, Iwanaga J, Oskouian RJ, Loukas M, Jerry Oakes W, Tubbs RS. Ventriculosubgaleal shunting-a comprehensive review and over two-decade surgical experience. Childs Nerv Syst. 2018;34(9):1639–42.
2. Troupis TG, Dimitroulis D, Paraschos A, Michalinos A, Protogerou V, Vlasis K, Troupis G, Skandalakis P. Lingual and facial arteries arising from the external carotid artery in a common trunk. Am Surg. 2011;77(2):151–4.
3. Kemp WJ 3rd, Tubbs RS, Cohen-Gadol AA. The innervation of the scalp: a comprehensive review including anatomy, pathology, and neurosurgical correlates. Surg Neurol Int. 2011;2:178.
4. Lin SJ, Hanasono MM, Skoracki RJ. Scalp and calvarial reconstruction. Semin Plast Surg. 2008;22(4):281–93.
5. Chen H, Jin R, Yu M, Weng T. Clinical decision model for the reconstruction of 175 cases of scalp avulsion/defect. Am J Otolaryngol. 2021;42(1):102752.
6. Kawaguchi M, Kato H, Matsuo M. CT and MRI features of scalp lesions. Radiol Med. 2019;124(10):1049–61.
7. Barranco R, Tettamanti C, Bonsignore A, Ventura F. Otorrhagia in strangulations: an important but often underestimated finding in forensic pathology. J Forensic Sci. 2022;67(4):1739–42.
8. Yang L, Yang MC, Qu PR, Zhang D, Ge M, Li DP. A retrospective study comprising 228 cases of pediatric scalp and skull lesions. BMC Pediatr. 2023;23(1):478.
9. White HE, Goswami A, Tucker AS. The intertwined evolution and development of sutures and cranial morphology. Front Cell Dev Biol. 2021;9:653579.
10. Luo J, Qian Q, Zheng W, Gripkauskaite I, Wu S, Zhang M, Li J, Fu B, Bhogal R, Murray P, Rowson M, Li B, Xue X, Gu X, Yang Y, Jin L, Gunn DA, Wang S. Scalp hair loss is not random across follicular units: a new insight into human hair ageing. Int J Cosmet Sci. 2023;45(4):548–55.
11. Koontz A, Urrutia HA, Bronner ME. Making a head: neural crest and ectodermal placodes in cranial sensory development. Semin Cell Dev Biol. 2023;138:15–27.
12. Cui CY, Kunisada M, Esibizione D, Douglass EG, Schlessinger D. Analysis of the temporal requirement for eda in hair and sweat gland development. J Invest Dermatol. 2009;129(4):984–93.
13. Streit A. Early development of the cranial sensory nervous system: from a common field to individual placodes. Dev Biol. 2004;276(1):1–15.
14. Tajran J, Gosman AA. Anatomy, head and neck, scalp. 2023 Jul 24. In: StatPearls [Internet]. Treasure Island (FL): StatPearls Publishing.
15. Suh DC. Where did the dura mater come from? Neurointervention. 2020;15(1):2–3.
16. Celik S, Tomruk C, Tanriover DE, Uyanikgil Y, Bilge O, Turgut M. Embryological and histological features of the cranial sutures. In: The sutures of the skull: anatomy, embryology, imaging, and surgery. Cham: Springer International Publishing; 2021. p. 19–42.
17. Mishina Y, Snider TN. Neural crest cell signaling pathways critical to cranial bone development and pathology. Exp Cell Res. 2014;325(2):138–47.
18. Opperman LA. Cranial sutures as intramembranous bone growth sites. Dev Dyn. 2000;219(4):472–85.
19. Santagati F, Rijli FM. Cranial neural crest and the building of the vertebrate head. Nat Rev Neurosci. 2003;4(10):806–18.
20. Sommer L. Generation of melanocytes from neural crest cells. Pigment Cell Melanoma Res. 2011;24(3):411–21.
21. Kim J. Treatment of scalp scars. Facial Plast Surg Clin North Am. 2017;25(1):83–8.
22. Shevel E. A method for determining when the superficial scalp arteries are the source of migraine pain. S Afr Med J. 2017;107(8):691–3.
23. Seery GE. Surgical anatomy of the scalp. Dermatologic Surg. 2002;28(7):581–7.
24. Germann AM, Jamal Z, Al Khalili Y. Anatomy, head and neck, scalp veins. [Updated 2023 Jan 13]. In: StatPearls [Internet]. Treasure Island (FL): StatPearls Publishing; 2023 Jan-.
25. American Academy of Dermatology. Alopecia areata: self-care. 2019.
26. Piérard-Franchimont C, Piérard GE. Alterations in hair follicle dynamics in women. Biomed Res Int. 2013;2013:957432.
27. Torkamani N, Rufaut NW, Jones L, Sinclair RD. Beyond goosebumps: does the arrector pili muscle have a role in hair loss? Int J Trichology. 2014;6(3):88–94.
28. Glover JD, Wells KL, Matthäus F, Painter KJ, Ho W, Riddell J, Johansson JA, Ford MJ, Jahoda CAB, Klika V, Mort RL, Headon DJ. Hierarchical patterning modes orchestrate hair follicle morphogenesis. PLoS Biol. 2017;15(7):e2002117.
29. Wortsman X, Carreño L, Ferreira-Wortsman C, Poniachik R, Pizarro K, Morales C, Calderon P, Castro A. Ultrasound characteristics of the hair follicles and tracts, sebaceous glands, montgomery glands, apocrine glands, and Arrector pili muscles. J Ultrasound Med. 2019;38(8):1995–2004.
30. Miranda BH, Charlesworth MR, Tobin DJ, Sharpe DT, Randall VA. Androgens trigger different growth responses in genetically identical human hair follicles in organ culture that reflect their epigenetic diversity in life. FASEB J. 2018;32(2):795–806.
31. Harvard Medical School. Telogen effluvium. 2019.
32. Cui CY, Schlessinger D. Eccrine sweat gland development and sweat secretion. Exp Dermatol. 2015;24(9):644–50.
33. Curtin HD, Gupta R, Bergeron RT. Embryology, anatomy, and imaging of the temporal bone. In: Som PM, Curtin HD, editors. Head and neck imaging. 5th ed; 2011.
34. Kiesler J, Ricer R. The abnormal fontanel. Am Fam Physician. 2003;67(12):2547–52.

35. Chemke J, Robinson A. The third Fontanelle. J Pediatr. 1969;75(4):617–22.
36. Lachkar S, Dols MM, Ishak B, Iwanaga J, Tubbs RS. The diploic veins: a comprehensive review with clinical applications. Cureus. 2019;11(4):e4422.
37. Goldberg AN, Oroszlan G, Anderson TD. Complications of frontal sinusitis and their management. Otolaryngol Clin N Am. 2001;34(1):211–25.
38. Konan LM, Reddy V, Mesfin FB. Neuroanatomy, cerebral blood supply. 2023 Jul 24. In: StatPearls [Internet]. Treasure Island (FL): StatPearls Publishing; 2023 Jan–.
39. Thomas JL, Jacob L, Boisserand L. Système lymphatique et cerveau [Lymphatic system in central nervous system]. Med Sci (Paris). 2019;35(1):55–61. French
40. Turner GA, Hoptroff M, Harding CR. Stratum corneum dysfunction in dandruff. Int J Cosmet Sci. 2012;34(4):298–306.
41. Rassman WR, Pak JP, Kim J, Estrin NF. Scalp micropigmentation: a concealer for hair and scalp deformities. J Clin Aesthet Dermatol. 2015;8(3):35–42.
42. De Rosa G, Mignogna C. The histopathology of psoriasis. Rheumatism. 2007;59(Suppl 1):46–8.
43. Rolfe P, Burton PJ, Crowe JA, Basarab-Horwath I, Goddard PJ, Woolfson J, Slevin P, Johnson P. Foetal scalp mass spectrometer blood-gas transducer. Med Biol Eng Comput. 1982;20(3):375–82.
44. Singh A, Prieto VG, Czelusta A, McClain KL, Duvic M. Adult Langerhans cell histiocytosis limited to the skin. Dermatology. 2003;207(2):157–61.
45. Kwack MH, Yang JM, Won GH, Kim MK, Kim JC, Sung YK. Establishment and characterization of five immortalized human scalp dermal papilla cell lines. Biochem Biophys Res Commun. 2018;496(2):346–51. https://doi.org/10.1016/j.bbrc.2018.01.058.
46. Paus R, Cotsarelis G. The biology of hair follicles. N Engl J Med. 1999;341(7):491–7.
47. Ro BI, Dawson TL. The role of sebaceous gland activity and scalp microfloral metabolism in the etiology of seborrheic dermatitis and dandruff. J Investig Dermatol Symp Proc. 2005;10(3):194–7.
48. Roshani RR, Sachin SV, Vinita AP, Amresh SB. Sweat gland tumor (Eccrine Porocarcinoma) of the scalp: a rare tumor. Indian J Plastic Surg. 2005;38(01):51–3.
49. Jung D, Kim YB, Lee JB, Muhamed AMC, Lee JY. Sweating distribution and active sweat glands on the scalp of young males in hot-dry and hot-humid environments. Eur J Appl Physiol. 2018;118(12):2655–67.
50. Suihko V. Modelling the response of scalp sensory receptors to transcranial electrical stimulation. Med Biol Eng Comput. 2002 Jul;40(4):395–401.
51. Mehrara BJ, Disa JJ, Pusic A. Scalp reconstruction. J Surg Oncol. 2006;94(6):504–8.
52. Williams R, Pawlus AD, Thornton MJ. Getting under the skin of hair aging: the impact of the hair follicle environment. Exp Dermatol. 2020;29(7):588–97.
53. Muszynski CA, Robertson DP, Goodman JC, Baskin DS. Scalp hibernoma: case report and literature review. Surg Neurol. 1994;42(4):343–5.
54. Sharman AM, Kirmi O, Anslow P. Imaging of the skin, subcutis, and galea aponeurotica. Semin Ultrasound CT MR. 2009;30(6):452–64.
55. Barty G. Die Galea aponeurotica als Fasziale Struktur. DO-Deutsche Zeitschrift für Osteopathie. 2014;12(01):34–8.
56. Nahian A, Chauhan PR. Histology, periosteum and endosteum. [Updated 2023 May 1]. In: StatPearls [Internet]. Treasure Island (FL): StatPearls Publishing; 2023 Jan-.
57. Jizong Z. The study of bone histology in the human skeleton. Acta Anthropologica Sinica. 2008;27(04):325.
58. Bohnert M. Burns and scalds. Encyclopedia of forensic sciences. 2nd ed. Academic Press; 2013. p. 11–4.
59. Huang AH, Sun HH, Skolnick GB, Woo AS. Thickness of calvarium and diploic space in children ages 0 to 17 as assessed by computed tomography. Eur J Plast Surg. 2015;38:193–8.
60. Dwek JR. The periosteum: what is it, where is it, and what mimics it in its absence? Skeletal Radiol. 2010;39(4):319–23.
61. Kolabas ZI, Kuemmerle LB, Perneczky R, Förstera B, Ulukaya S, Ali M, Kapoor S, Bartos LM, Büttner M, Caliskan OS, Rong Z, Mai H, Höher L, Jeridi D, Molbay M, Khalin I, Deligiannis IK, Negwer M, Roberts K, Simats A, Carofiglio O, Todorov MI, Horvath I, Ozturk F, Hummel S, Biechele G, Zatcepin A, Unterrainer M, Gnörich J, Roodselaar J, Shrouder J, Khosravani P, Tast B, Richter L, Díaz-Marugán L, Kaltenecker D, Lux L, Chen Y, Zhao S, Rauchmann BS, Sterr M, Kunze I, Stanic K, Kan VWY, Besson-Girard S, Katzdobler S, Palleis C, Schädler J, Paetzold JC, Liebscher S, Hauser AE, Gokce O, Lickert H, Steinke H, Benakis C, Braun C, Martinez-Jimenez CP, Buerger K, Albert NL, Höglinger G, Levin J, Haass C, Kopczak A, Dichgans M, Havla J, Kümpfel T, Kerschensteiner M, Schifferer M, Simons M, Liesz A, Krahmer N, Bayraktar OA, Franzmeier N, Plesnila N, Erener S, Puelles VG, Delbridge C, Bhatia HS, Hellal F, Elsner M, Bechmann I, Ondruschka B, Brendel M, Theis FJ, Erturk A. Distinct molecular profiles of skull bone marrow in health and neurological disorders. Cell. 2023;186(17):3706–3725.e29.
62. Pan A, Chang L, Nguyen A, James AW. A review of hedgehog signaling in cranial bone development. Front Physiol. 2013;4:61.
63. Takagi K, Urist MR. The reaction of the dura to bone morphogenetic protein (BMP) in repair of skull defects. Ann Surg. 1982 Jul;196(1):100–9.
64. Weickenmeier J, Fischer C, Carter D, Kuhl E, Goriely A. Dimensional, geometrical, and physical constraints in skull growth. Phys Rev Lett. 2017;118(24):248101.
65. Jin SW, Sim KB, Kim SD. Development and growth of the normal cranial vault : an embryologic review. J Korean Neurosurg Soc. 2016;59(3):192–6.

66. Smith DW, Gong BT. Scalp-hair patterning: its origin and significance relative to early brain and upper facial development. Teratology. 1974;9(1):17–34.
67. Rehman B, Muzio MR. Embryology, Week 2–3. [Updated 2023 May 1]. In: StatPearls [Internet]. Treasure Island (FL): StatPearls Publishing; 2023 Jan-.
68. Geoffrey HS, Steven MS. Embryology and development of the facial skeleton. Aesthetic surgery of the facial skeleton. Elsevier; 2022. p. 117–24.
69. Anderson BC, McLoon LK. Cranial nerves and autonomic innervation in the orbit. Encyclopedia of the eye. Academic Press; 2010. p. 537–48.
70. Broekhuizen R, De Rydt T, Lutters E, Klooster RT, De Bruyne G. Head sensitivity for designing bicycle helmets with improved physical comfort. In: Rebelo F, Soares M, editors. Advances in ergonomics in design. AHFE 2018. Advances in intelligent systems and computing, vol. 777. Cham: Springer; 2019. p. 14–9.
71. Garn SM, Rohmann CG, Wagner B, Ascoli W. Continuing bone growth throughout life: a general phenomenon. Am J Phys Anthropol. 1967;26(3):313–7.
72. Taylor PJ. Big head? Bald head! Skull expansion: alternative model for the primary mechanism of AGA. Med Hypotheses. 2009;72(1):23–8.
73. Semalty M, Semalty A, Joshi GP, Rawat MS. Hair growth and rejuvenation: an overview. J Dermatolog Treat. 2011;22(3):123–32.
74. Katsianou MA, Adamopoulos C, Vastardis H, Basdra EK. Signaling mechanisms implicated in cranial sutures pathophysiology: craniosynostosis. BBA Clin. 2016;6:165–76.
75. D'Antoni AV, Donaldson OI, Schmidt C, Macchi V, De Caro R, Oskouian RJ, Loukas M, Shane TR. A comprehensive review of the anterior fontanelle: embryology, anatomy, and clinical considerations. Childs Nerv Syst. 2017;33(6):909–14.
76. Friedman D, Kazmerski V, Fabiani M. An overview of age-related changes in the scalp distribution of P3b. Electroencephalogr Clin Neurophysiol. 1997;104(6):498–513.
77. Hadshiew IM, Foitzik K, Arck PC, Paus R. Burden of hair loss: stress and the underestimated psychosocial impact of telogen effluvium and androgenetic alopecia. J Invest Dermatol. 2004;123(3):455–7.
78. Rabiner JE, Friedman LM, Khine H, Avner JR, Tsung JW. Accuracy of point-of-care ultrasound for diagnosis of skull fractures in children. Pediatrics. 2013;131(6):e1757–64.
79. Cummins DM, Chaudhry IH, Harries M. Scarring alopecias: pathology and an update on digital developments. Biomedicines. 2021;9(12):1755.
80. Marijon P, Bertolus C, Foy JP, Marechal G, Caruhel JB, Benassarou M, Carpentier A, Degos V, Amelot A, Mathon B. Custom surgical management of invasive malignant tumors of the scalp. Acta Neurochir. 2020;162(12):2991–9.
81. Shay T, Mitchell KA, Belzberg M, Zelko I, Mahapatra S, Qian J, Mendoza L, Huang J, Brem H, Gordon C. Translucent customized cranial implants made of clear polymethylmethacrylate: an early outcome analysis of 55 consecutive cranioplasty cases. Ann Plast Surg. 2020;85(6):e27–36.
82. Chao AH, Yu P, Skoracki RJ, Demonte F, Hanasono MM. Microsurgical reconstruction of composite scalp and calvarial defects in patients with cancer: a 10-year experience. Head Neck. 2012;34(12):1759–64.
83. Cormier NS, Lin SJ. Trends and outcomes of cranioplasty alone versus single-stage composite scalp and calvarial reconstruction. J Craniofac Surg. 2022;33(5):1271–5.
84. Woeppel KM, Cui XT. Nanoparticle and biomolecule surface modification synergistically increases neural electrode recording yield and minimizes inflammatory host response. Adv Healthc Mater. 2021;10(16):e2002150.
85. Kyriakou A, Neufeld E, Werner B, Paulides MM, Szekely G, Kuster N. A review of numerical and experimental compensation techniques for skull-induced phase aberrations in transcranial focused ultrasound. Int J Hyperth. 2014;30(1):36–46.

Regeneration of the Scalp and Cranium

4

Pengfei Guo and Fuyou Guo

4.1 Introduction

Severe cranial damage or extirpation of tumors requires reconstructive surgeries to protect the underlying brain and to restore cranial contour and scalp integrity, as well as avoid complications such as neurocognitive decline. Various advanced substitutes, including biological and synthetic materials, have been developed for this purpose. Biological materials can be further subdivided into autologous grafts, allografts, and xenografts [1, 2]. On the other hand, the wide utilization of preoperative methods, such as computed tomography (CT), magnetic resonance imaging (MRI) or 3D printer (3D-Printer), also fundamentally plays a critical role in perfect regeneration of major defects of the scalp and cranium [3]. The advantage of current preoperative evaluation is that it provides not only an optimal definition for defects and the adjacent structures status but also effective guidance for subsequent successful reconstruction. The present chapter highlights plastic surgical concepts and techniques applied to regeneration of major scalp and cranium defects.

4.2 Development of Cranium

The cranial bones develop in the mesenchymal tissue surrounding the head end of the notochord. This developmental process consists of condensation (beginning at the end of the first month) and thickening of the mesenchyme into masses, which are the first distinguishable cranial elements. A portion of the forming cranial bones are shaped into cartilage, while the others form directly from membranous tissue. Most of the cranial vault and a portion of the base of the skull are composed of membranous bone [4, 5].

4.3 Anatomy of the Scalp and Cranium

The scalp is composed of five segments as follows: skin, subcutaneous connective tissue, rigid galea aponeurosis, underlying areolar tissue, and skull pericranium in the frontal-parietal-occipital area. However, in the temple section, there are six unique layers composed of skin, subcutaneous connective tissue, superficial temporal fascia,

P. Guo
Department of Burn and Reconstruction, The First Affiliated Hospital of Zhengzhou University, Zhengzhou, Henan, China

F. Guo (✉)
Department of Neurosurgery, The First Affiliated Hospital of Zhengzhou University, Zhengzhou, Henan, China

International Joint Laboratory of Nervous System Malformation, Zhengzhou, Henan, China
e-mail: chyou666@hotmail.com

M. Turgut et al. (eds.), *Lesions of the Scalp and Cranial Vault*,
https://doi.org/10.1007/978-3-031-88244-9_4

deep temporal fascia, temporal muscle, and skull pericranium.

The scalp has an abundant blood supply with a thick network of collateral vessels. There are six principal arteries on each side, which include the supratrochlear artery, supraorbital artery, superficial temporal artery, posterior artery, posterior auricular artery, and occipital artery [6]. The arteries feeding on the scalp originated from the internal carotid artery and external carotid artery.

The cranium is the part of the skull that encloses the brain and is divided into the cranial base and calvaria. The calvaria has three distinct layers in adults: the hard internal and external laminae and the cancellous middle layer, or the diploe. The etiology of cranium defects is commonly traumatic cranium fracture and neoplasm invasion of the skull (benign or malignant lesion), as well as congenital defects such as encephaloceles or meningoencephaloceles.

4.4 Regeneration of the Scalp and Cranium Regions

4.4.1 Regeneration of Scalp

4.4.1.1 Defect Assessment of the Scalp and Management Choices

Skin grafting was carried out for pure scalp defects if the defect contained viable periostem, and the defect could be closed quickly with a retroauricular full-thickness skin graft or a split-thickness skin graft regardless of the size of the scalp defect. However, surgical repair of complex scalp deficiency is commonly regarded as the repair of scalp defects with exposed bone or simultaneous deficiency of the scalp and skull bone. Wound repair is performed by skin flap transplantation, which involves the use of either rotation flaps or free skin flaps.

According to the degree of deficiency, diverse management strategies should be administered individually. When $10\ cm^2 < \text{defect area} < 20\ cm^2$, a free skin flap is the best choice for management. A high height on the lateral thigh is the ideal donor site because the cutting scar is easily concealed with clothing; if wounds surpass $20\ cm^2$, when conditions are suitable, the initial defect can be closed with either rotation flaps or bipedicle flaps, and the donor sites will require skin grafting. When defects exceed 50%, regeneration with free omentum was described successfully by Mclean and Buncke in 1972 [7], which has been proven to be an attractive alternative for extensive scalp defects [8, 9].

4.4.1.2 Surgical Techniques for the Scalp

When employing free skin grafts for direct wound repair or applying skin grafting for defect closure, surgical techniques, including the following steps, play an important role in successful operation: ① The ideal choice of donor site is usually harvesting from the lateral thigh (Fig. 4.1) or the posterior trunk. ② It is necessary to maintain drainage for several days through graft transplantation perforations. ③ Skin graft fixation should be reliable with appropriate pressure, and surgical failure can easily occur after tissue damage from excessive pressure on the graft.

The fundamental principles of flap coverage are as follows: (1) To move available tissue with intact circulation from an area of relative excess to the zone of deficiency. (2) To optimize the vascularity of the flap [6]. Hence, the superficial temporal artery and its accompanying vein are first chosen for reconstructing scalp defects through free flap transplantation. Second, the superficial temporal vein and its concomitant vein via a longer subcutaneous tunnel may be considered for microvascular anastomosis. Of course, flap regeneration should be conducted after effective inflammation control for infected wounds or necrotic bone resection. In addition, aesthetic outcomes are achieved by multilobed flap transplantation or the combined use of omental flaps and skin grafts for large scalp defect reconstruction. For the repair of large scalp defects with exposed bones, the outer layer of cranium was drilled at 1 cm intervals to facilitate vascularization between the flap and wound bed.

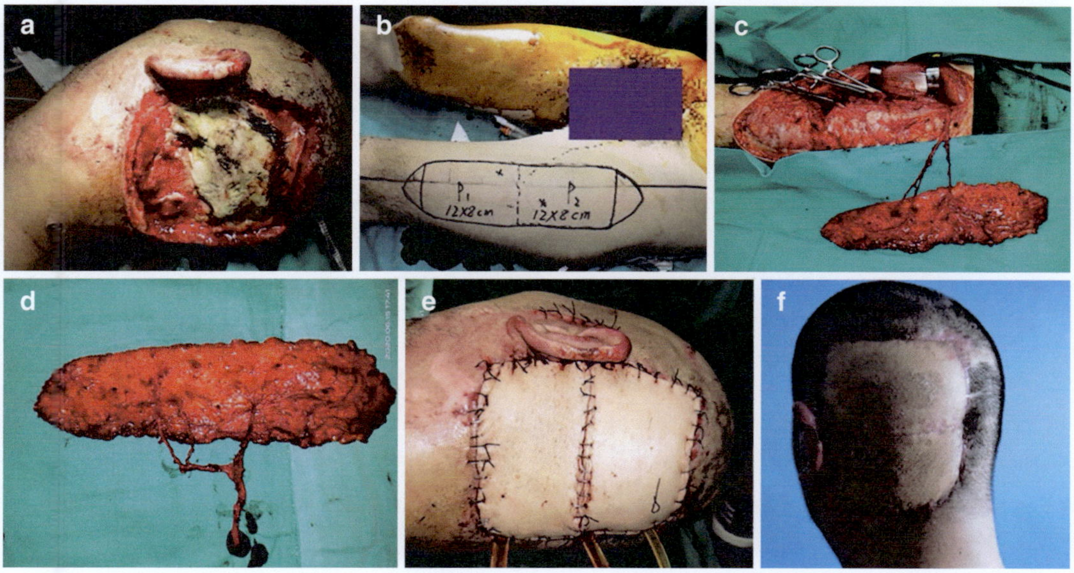

Fig. 4.1 Extensive electric burn scalp defect with exposed bone (**a**), preoperative design for anterolateral thigh flap on the right leg (**b**), and left anterolateral femoral skin flap obtained for reconstruction (**c** and **d**). Successful repair was achieved by anterolateral femoral skin flap graft (**e**), and favorable outcomes were observed after three months of follow-up (**f**)

4.4.1.3 Surgical Complications Associated with Scalp Repair

Distal tip necrosis and delayed healing due to a narrow pedicle base have been reported for flap grafts [10]. Artificial skin substitute templates have been shown to be a reliable solution for the reconstruction of large scalp defects with exposed skull bones. Complications such as template necrosis (4%), infections (4%), ulcerations (3%), and autograft necrosis (2%) were also found in a series of 68 patients [11].

4.4.2 Regeneration of Cranium

4.4.2.1 Surgical Indication

① Large cranium decompression, such as bone deficiency surpassing 3 cm and lack of protection for brain tissue; ② severe headache, dizziness, and other symptoms of syndrome of the trephine, vague discomfort at the site of the cranium defect; ③ epilepsy caused by bone defect and scar formation; and ④ unsuccessful deterioration for the expected cosmetic appearance.

4.4.2.2 Cranioplasty Materials and Surgical Timing

Autologous bone grafts are usually considered the ideal option for cranioplasty procedures due to their lower incidence of complications [12, 13]. However, increasing evidence has demonstrated that an increased reoperation rate is more common in patients who underwent autologous bone repair than in those who underwent alloplastic cranioplasty, which indicates that autologous bone grafts are inferior to synthetic materials [14–17]. In our clinical center, cranioplasty can be performed with titanium mesh and a PEEK overlay via custom-assisted design and manufacturing customization (Fig. 4.2). In addition, it is not appropriate if the patient's bone has infection or resorption. Hence, a variety of alloplastic biomaterials, including hydroxyapatite and polymethylmethacrylate, have been similarly developed for use in cranioplasty. With advances in alloplastic materials and custom manufacturing of implants, additional new and effective substances will be adopted in the future.

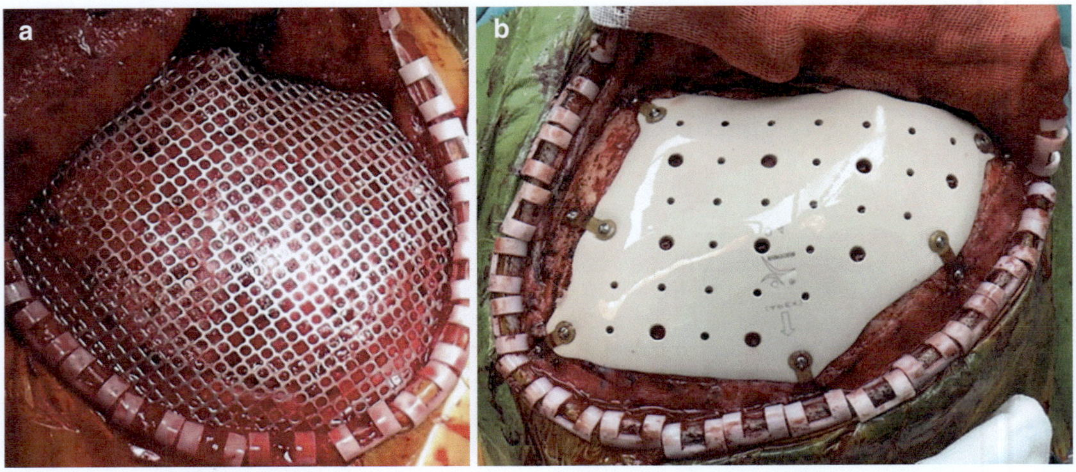

Fig. 4.2 Intraoperative photographs showing cranioplasty with titanium mesh and PEEK material (**a** and **b**)

There is no consensus regarding the optimal timing of cranioplasty based on the previous literature. The timing of cranioplasty varies and ranges from 6 weeks to more than 12 months after traumatic decompression [18]. The following factors, including the cerebral swelling state, clinical recovery, resolution of any infection, and evaluation of soft tissues at the defect site, will predominantly contribute to the surgical results of bone grafting. Consequently, the optimal timing for performing cranioplasty should be tailored for patients with minimal complications. Satisfactory outcomes are usually obtained for cranioplasty (Fig. 4.3). Single-stage cranioplasty with a template is usually recommended for benign skull tumors since surgical resection is potentially curative (Fig. 4.4). However, bone regeneration should be performed carefully if the tumor is highly malignant and requires further radiation therapy. Last, it is not suitable for pediatric cranioplasty with alloplastic material in children younger than 7–8 years because the cranium continues to develop significantly until that age.

4.4.2.3 Surgical Techniques for Cranium Repair

Cranioplasty surgery techniques play important roles in restoring neurological function and in ensuring a good cosmetic appearance. The skull flap was removed gently from the underlying dura and brain. In view of the potential adhesion between the dura and brain tissue, intraparenchymal hemorrhage may occur if the skull flap is dissected roughly. In addition, dural tears should be repaired in a timely manner to avoid cerebrospinal fluid collection and fever. It is wise to suspend the dura at the core of a large bone defect to prevent epidural hematoma. Separation of the scalp flap and temporalis muscle from the underlying dura or dura substitute is critical for a good outcome. At the end of the procedure, wound sur-

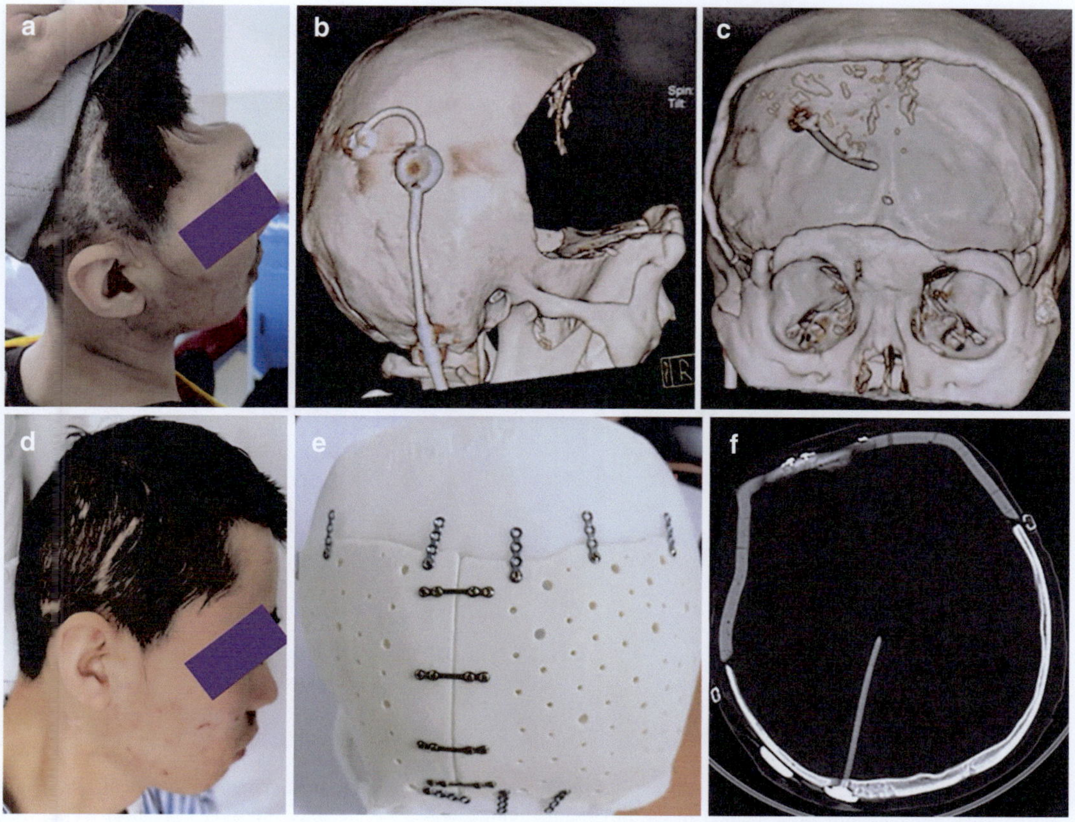

Fig. 4.3 A male patient aged 27 years underwent bifrontal decompressive craniectomy (DC) due to severe traumatic brain injury and subsequent ventriculoperitoneal shunt resulting from hydrocephalus. An obvious brain tissue collapse was observed at 8 months after DC (**a**), 3D reconstructions of the CT scan demonstrating a large bone defect before cranioplasty (**b** and **c**), a satisfactory cosmetic appearance was achieved after bone repair (**d**), the PEEK material adopted in this case (**e**) and postoperative CT showing bifrontal reconstruction with PEEK (**f**)

face irrigation with hydrogen peroxide and saline with gentamicin as well as drainage tube placement contributed to reducing infection.

4.4.2.4 Complications of Cranium Repair

Cranioplasty, although a routine neurosurgical procedure, can lead to significant morbidity, with rates of total major complications ranging between 10.9% and 40.4%, as described in the previous literature [19]. Andrabi SM [20] reported that wound infection/dehiscence was the most common complication encountered after skull repair, and postoperative hematoma was also a significant complication following cranioplasty. Other complications, including seizures, bone resorption, and sunken bone plates, were observed in 236 patients. Notably, there was no statistically significant difference in the infection rate between autologous and synthetic cranial grafts of acrylic for cranioplasty based on the report of Klinger DR [21]. Additionally, unilateral or bilateral subdural fluid collections may form if there has been intrinsic loss of brain parenchyma so that the brain does not fully rebuild to fill the skull. Despite the reported high rate of these complications, serious complications such as meningitis, air embolism, and death are rare during cranioplasty [22].

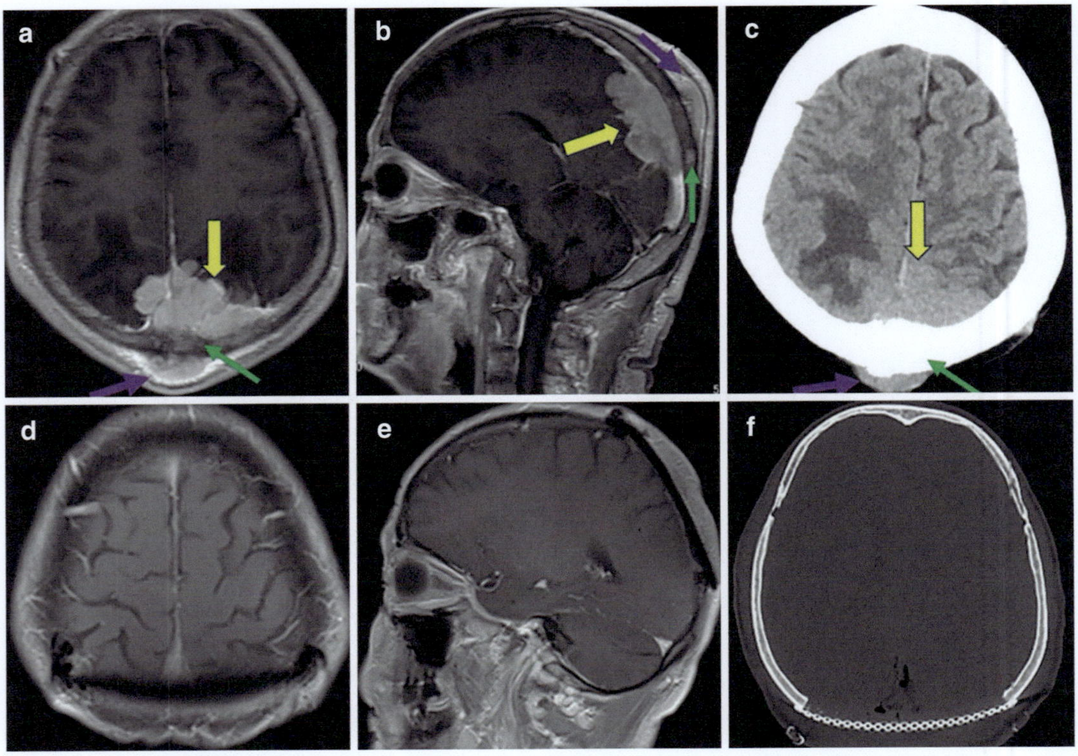

Fig. 4.4 Preoperative enhanced axial and sagittal MR images illustrating meningioma located in the biparietal lobe and sagittal sinus. The yellow arrow shows the tumor, the green arrow and the purple arrow demonstrate involvement in the cranium and subcutaneous connective tissue, respectively (**a** and **b**), and the CT scan shows the tumor marked by the yellow arrow, green arrow, and purple arrow demonstrating involvement in the cranium and subcutaneous connective tissue, respectively (**c**). Postoperative enhanced axial and sagittal MR images illustrating that the tumor was completely removed and that one-stage cranioplasty was performed with titanium mesh (**d** and **e**); postoperative CT image showing cranium reconstruction with titanium mesh (**f**)

4.5 Conclusion

Regeneration of the scalp and cranium restores the normal architecture of the skull, which not only provides significant psychosocial benefits to the patient by reestablishing the protective barrier of the skull but also effectively solves the cosmetic problem. However, the optimal surgical timing and ideal material choice for cranioplasty are currently disputed. In addition, regeneration of the scalp and cranium is a well-practiced and utilized neurosurgical procedure aiding in skull reconstruction, and postoperative complications such as wound infection and hematoma should be considered. The relationship between cranioplasty and long-term neurological outcomes should be extensively investigated in the future.

References

1. Alkhaibary A, Alharbi A, Alnefaie N, Oqalaa Almubarak A, Aloraidi A, Khairy S. Cranioplasty: a comprehensive review of the history, materials, surgical aspects, and complications. World Neurosurg. 2020;139:445–52.
2. Mee H, Anwar F, Timofeev I, Owens N, Grieve K, Whiting G, Alexander K, Kendrick K, Helmy A, Hutchinson P, Kolias A. Cranioplasty: a multidisciplinary approach. Front Surg. 2022;9:864385.
3. Thimukonda Jegadeesan J, Baldia M, Basu B. Next-generation personalized cranioplasty treatment. Acta Biomater. 2022;154:63–82.
4. Retzlaff Ernest W, Mitchell FL. The cranium and its sutures. Berlin: Springer; 1987.
5. Carlson BM. Human embryology and developmental biology. 5th ed. Elsevier Saunders; 2014.
6. Schmidek & Sweet. Operative neurosurgical techniques: indications, methods and results, vol. 1. 4th ed. Elsevier Science; 2002.

7. McLean DH, Buncke HJ Jr. Autotransplant of omentum to a large scalp defect, with microsurgical revascularization. Plast Reconstr Surg. 1972;49(3):268–74.
8. Losken A, Carlson GW, Culbertson JH, Scott Hultman C, Kumar AV, Jones GE, Bostwick J 3rd, Jurkiewicz MJ. Omental free flap reconstruction in complex head and neck deformities. Head Neck. 2002;24(4):326–31.
9. Kim JW, Woo SH, Jang SY, Kim WS, Bae TH, Kim HK. Facial artery as a recipient vessel for extensive scalp reconstruction with free omental flap without vein graft. J Craniofac Surg. 2018;29(3):e271–3.
10. Krishna D, Khan MM, Dubepuria R, Chaturvedi G, Cheruvu VPR. Reconstruction of scalp and forehead defects: options and strategies. Cureus. 2023;15(7):e41479.
11. Benecke J, Koenen W, Mager L, Weina K, Klemke CD, Felcht M, Faulhaber J. Reconstruction of full thickness defects on the scalp with artificial dermal regeneration template: analysis of long-term results in 68 cases. Dermatologic Surg. 2021;47(1):e1–4.
12. Fan MC, Wang QL, Sun P, Zhan SH, Guo P, Deng WS, Dong Q. Cryopreservation of autologous cranial bone flaps for cranioplasty: a large sample retrospective study. World Neurosurg. 2018;109:e853–9.
13. Oberoi MK, Mirzaie S, Huang KX, Caprini RM, Hu VJ, Dejam D, Ge S, Cronin BJ, Pfaff MJ, Lee JC. Meta-analysis and meta-regression of complications and failures of autologous heterotopic cranial bone versus alloplastic cranioplasties. Plast Reconstr Surg. 2023;154:757e. https://doi.org/10.1097/PRS.0000000000011093.
14. Piitulainen JM, Kauko T, Aitasalo KM, Vuorinen V, Vallittu PK, Posti JP. Outcomes of cranioplasty with synthetic materials and autologous bone grafts. World Neurosurg. 2015;83(5):708–14.
15. Malcolm JG, Mahmooth Z, Rindler RS, Allen JW, Grossberg JA, Pradilla G, Ahmad FU. Autologous cranioplasty is associated with increased reoperation rate: a systematic review and meta-analysis. World Neurosurg. 2018;116:60–8.
16. van de Vijfeijken SECM, TJAG M, Spijker R, LHE K, Vandertop WP, Becking AG, Ubbink DT, CranioSafe Group. Autologous bone is inferior to alloplastic cranioplasties: safety of autograft and allograft materials for cranioplasties, a systematic review. World Neurosurg. 2018;117:443–452.e8.
17. Rosinski CL, Patel S, Geever B, Chiu RG, Chaker AN, Zakrzewski J, Rosenberg DM, Parola R, Shah K, Behbahani M, Mehta AI. A retrospective comparative analysis of titanium mesh and custom implants for cranioplasty. Neurosurgery. 2020;86(1):E15–22.
18. Baumeister S, Peek A, Friedman A, et al. Management of postneurosurgical bone flap loss caused by infection. Plast Reconstr Surg. 2008;122(6):195e–208e.
19. Piazza M, Grady MS. Cranioplasty. Neurosurg Clin N Am. 2017;28(2):257–65.
20. Andrabi SM, Sarmast AH, Kirmani AR, Bhat AR. Cranioplasty: indications, procedures, and outcome - an institutional experience. Surg Neurol Int. 2017;8:91.
21. Klinger DR, Madden C, Beshay J, White J, Gambrell K, Rickert K. Autologous and acrylic cranioplasty: a review of 10 years and 258 cases. World Neurosurg. 2014;82(3–4):e525–30.
22. Sahoo NK, Tomar K, Thakral A, Rangan NM. Complications of Cranioplasty. J Craniofac Surg. 2018;29(5):1344–8.

5 Clinical Presentations of Lesions of the Scalp and Calvarium

Hatim Belfquih and Ali Akhaddar

Abbreviations

CSF Cerebrospinal fluid
CT Computed tomography
MRI Magnetic resonance imaging

5.1 Introduction

Scalp and calvarial lesions occur in the region ranging from the external occipital protuberance to the supraorbital margin and between two ears lateraly; they may comprise skin, subcutaneous connective tissue, epicranial aponeurosis, loose areolar connective tissue, the pericranium, and the skull that consists of an inner table, bone marrow space, and an outer table. Too often more than one layer of the scalp and skull is involved [1].

The lesions can be asymptomatic and discovered fortuitously or are detected as palpable, painful, or painless mass during physical examination. Their pathological nature is multivarious and may be neoplastic (benign and malignant neoplasia), congenital, inflammatory, traumatic, vascular, infectious lesions, or even idiopathic [1, 2].

The medical history and clinical features including the age of patient are a principal factor in the diagnostic process. However, identifying the type of the lesion is still a clinical challenge in some cases and the diagnosis was confirmed by radiologic and histological examination [2].

In this chapter, the clinical presentations of lesions of the scalp and calvarium will be described according to the pathology nature of the lesions (Table 5.1). This chapter is focalized essentialy on the pathologies which seen in neurosurgical practice.

H. Belfquih (✉)
Department of Neurosurgery, Avicenne Military Hospital of Marrakech, Cady Ayyad University, Marrakech, Morocco
e-mail: hatimbelfquih@gmail.com

A. Akhaddar
Department of Neurosurgery, Avicenne Military Hospital of Marrakech, Mohammed V University in Rabat, Rabat, Morocco

M. Turgut et al. (eds.), *Lesions of the Scalp and Cranial Vault*,
https://doi.org/10.1007/978-3-031-88244-9_5

Table 5.1 The different lesions of the scalp and calvarium described clinically in the text according to their pathology nature

Lesions Location	Neoplastic lesions		Congenital and developmental lesions	Traumatic lesions	Vascular and pseudovascular lesions	Infectious lesions	Miscellaneous lesions (inflammatory, heamatologic, metabolic, iatrogenic and others)
	Benign	Malign					
Scalp	Trichilemmal cysts Pilomatricoma Seborrhoeic keratosis Acquired melanocytic naevus Blue naevus Sebaceoma Hidrocystoma Syringomas Dermatofibroma Neurofibroma Leiomyoma	Cutaneous squamous cell carcinoma Intraepidermal squamous cell carcinoma Basal cell carcinoma Malignant melanoma Malignant proliferating trichilemmal tumour Pilomatrix carcinoma Sebaceous carcinoma Porocarcinoma Leiomyosarcoma Dermatofibrosarcoma protuberans Fibrosarcoma Merkel cell carcinoma	Congenital melanocytic naevus	Scalp injury Cephalohematoma deformans Keloid scar Hypertrophic scar Scalp pressure ulcers	Infantile haemangiomas Venous malformation Arteriovenous malformation Lymphangioma Cutaneous angiosarcoma	Scalp folliculitis Folliculitis decalvans Tufted hair folliculitis Acne keloidalis nuchae Impetigo Tinea Syphilitic alopecia Pediculosis capitis Scalp abscesses	Rosai-Dorfman disease Scalp necrosis Juvenile xanthogranuloma

Scalp and Calvarium	Lipomas Meningiomas Intracranial neoplasms with involvement of the scalp and calvarium	Liposarcoma Metastatic tumors Malign meningiomas Intracranial neoplasms with involvement of the scalp and calvarium	Epidermal cysts Dermoid cyst Congenital midline scalp and skull defects Dermal sinus tracts Sinus pericranii Heterotopic brain tissue Encephaloceles, meningoceles and meningoencephaloceles Aplasia cutis congenita	Scalp and calvarial injury Leptomeningeal Iatrogenic Lesions: (Surgical and Nonsurgical): burr holes, bone flaps, Mayfield (head-holders), stereotactic frame, cervical traction, radionecrosis cysts	Venous lakes Intraossous hemangiomas Aneurysmal bone cyst	Pott puffy tumour Calvarial hydatid cysts	Lymphoma Eosinophilic granuloma
Calvarium	Osteomas Giant cell tumor Juvenile psammomatoid ossifying fibroma	Osteosarcomas Chondrosarcomas Ewing sarcoma	Congenital depression of the skull Craniosynostosis	Calvarial injury	Hemangiosarcoma	Osteomyelitis Calvarial tuberculosis	Fibrous dysplasia Paget's sarcoma Multiple myeloma Calvarial sarcoidosis Hyperparathyroidism, Renal osteodystrophy acromegaly Amyloidosis Chronic anemia Osteopenia Thalassemia Osteopetrosis

5.2 Neoplastic Lesions of the Scalp and Calvarium

5.2.1 Benign Neoplastic Lesions of the Scalp and Calvarium

5.2.1.1 Trichilemmal Cysts "Pilar Cyst"

Trichilemmal cysts are common in middle-aged women, keratin filled nodules derived from the outer hair root sheath and lacking a central punctum. They present as firm, mobile, subcutaneous nodules measuring 0.5–5 cm in diameter. There is no central punctum, unlike an epidermoid cyst. The cyst wall is thick and not prone to rupture. They can be painful if inflamed (Fig. 5.1) [3].

5.2.1.2 Pilomatrixomas

Pilomatrixomas are hair follicle tumors that arise in childhood derived from hair matrix cells. They present as a single skin-colored or purplish lesion. They are rock-hard and lobulated. Most pilomatrixomas are 5–10 mm in diameter [4].

5.2.1.3 Seborrhoeic Keratosis

Seborrhoeic keratosis are commonly seen in adults over 60 years of age, flat or raised papule or plaque, 1 mm to several cm in diameter in size. Skin colored, yellow, grey, light brown, dark brown, black or mixed colors. Smooth, waxy or warty surface. Solitary or grouped in certain areas, such as within the scalp [5].

5.2.1.4 Acquired Melanocytic Naevus

Acquired melanocytic naevus are a flat or raised localized proliferation of melanocytes, follow sun exposure. They may be flat or protruding. Pink or flesh tones to dark brown, steel blue, or black in color. Mostly round or oval in shape, moles are sometimes unusual shapes. They range in size from a couple of millimeters to several centimeters in diameter [6].

5.2.1.5 Blue Naevus

Blue naevus is usually 0.5–1 cm in diameter. The cellular blue naevus is more nodular and is at least 1 cm in diameter. Usually blue to grey hues, but sometimes brown or yellowish [7].

5.2.1.6 Sebaceoma and Sebaceous Adenoma

Sebaceoma and Sebaceous adenoma are Sebaceous cell proliferations that manifest as

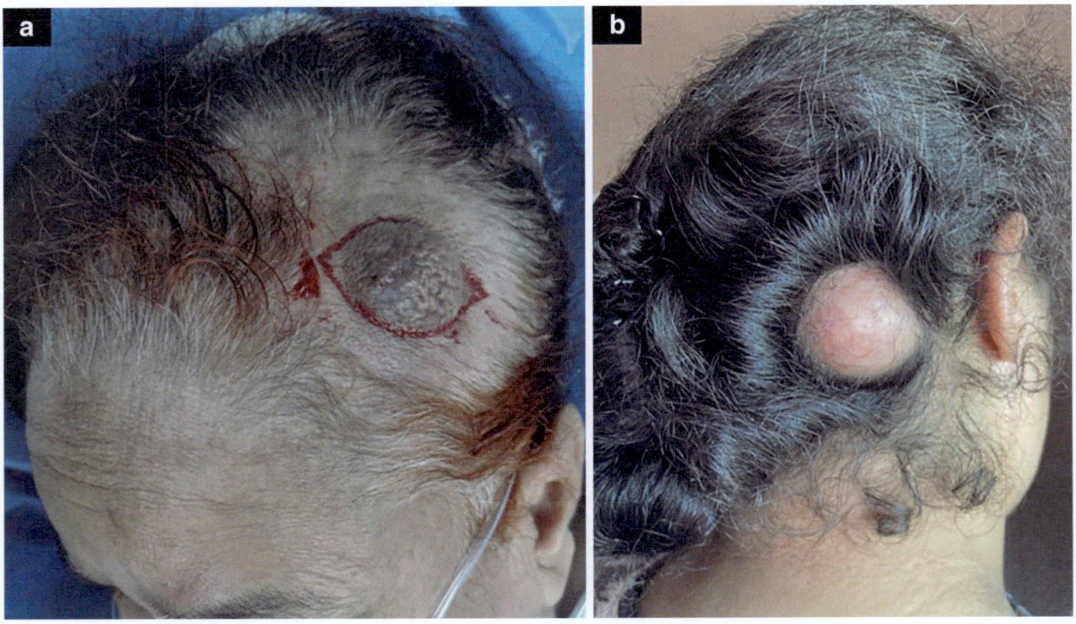

Fig. 5.1 Trichilemmal cyst. Firm, mobile, subcutaneous nodule of the scalp with coexisted hair loss on the left frontal area (**a**) and on the right occipital area (**b**)

skin colored or yellow nodules originating from deeper in the skin (sebaceoma) or superficially (sebaceous adenoma) [8].

5.2.1.7 Hidrocystomas

Hidrocystomas is apocrine or eccrine derived skin colored or blue cysts which may arise as solitary or multiple lesions [9].

5.2.1.8 Syringomas

Syringomas are harmless sweat duct tumors. They start to appear in adolescence and are more common in women than men. Firm skin colored or yellow papules millimeters in diameter and commonly occurring in clusters on the eyelids [10].

5.2.1.9 Dermatofibromas

Dermatofibromas are solitary, firm papules or nodules of variable coloration that may dimple on pinching [11].

5.2.1.10 Neurofibromas

Neurofibromas are derived from Schwann cells, fibroblasts, mast cells, and vascular components of underlying nerves. They are well circumscribed, superficial, soft button-like brown-, pink-, or skin-colored superficial nodules with soft or firm consistency. Occurs in association with café-au-lait macules in Neurofibromatosis 1 (NF1) (Fig. 5.2) [12].

5.2.1.11 Lipomas

Lipomas are the most common benign tumor of the scalp in adults. They are common in men between the ages of 30 and 50 years. Growth slowly over several years. A dome-shaped or egg-shaped lump about 2–10 cm in diameter (some may grow even larger). They feel soft and smooth and are easily moved under the skin with the fingers. They may have a rubbery or doughy consistency. Most lipomas are symptomless, but some are painful when applying pressure. A lipoma

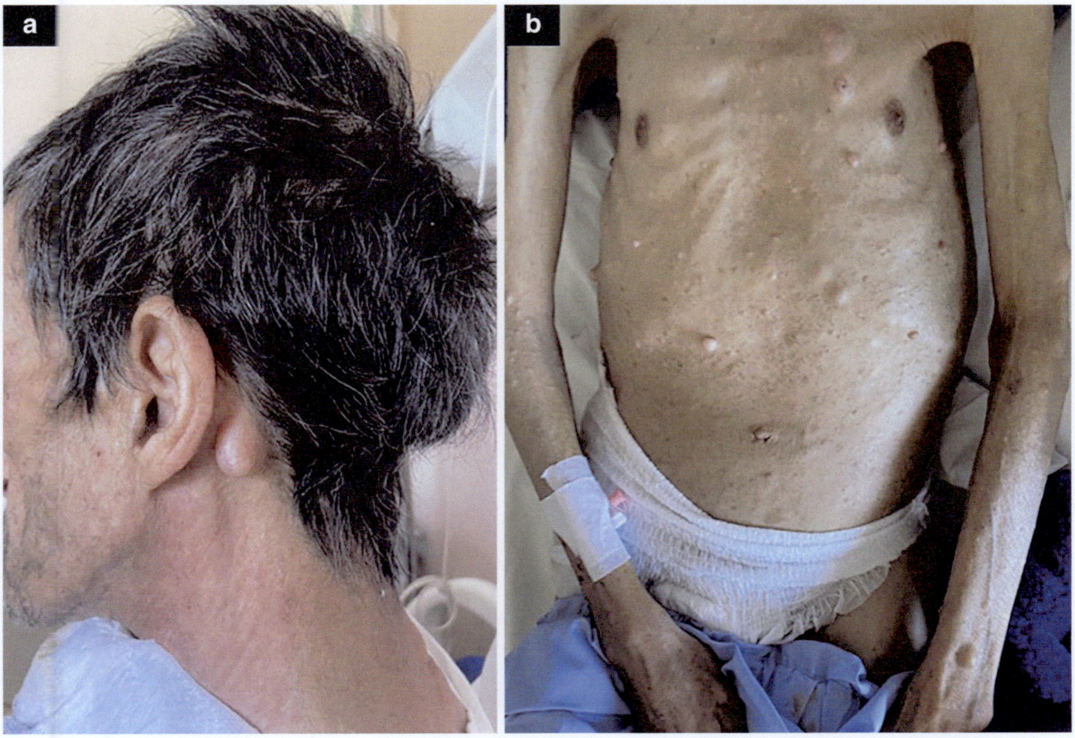

Fig. 5.2 Neurofibroma. Well circumscribed, superficial, soft button-like skin colored nodule with soft consistency on the left side of occipital area (**a**), mosaic cafe-au-lait macules and neurofibromas characterize neurocutaneous disorder (**b**) "Neurofibromatosis type 1"

that is tender or painful is usually an angiolipoma. There are four types: soft tissue lipoma which pressures the outer table; periosteal lipoma that causes hyperostosis and bone erosion; intraosseous lipoma originating from the bone marrow, with a tendency to expand and distort the bone; liposarcoma (Fig. 5.3a) [13].

5.2.1.12 Leiomyomas

Leiomyomas are the proliferations of myocytes which can develop from both smooth and skeletal muscle. Typically present as firm, smooth, and tender hyperpigmented or red-brown nodules [14].

5.2.1.13 Meningiomas

The most common presentation of meningiomas is the extra-axial dural based tumor with reactive hyperostosis of the adjacent calvarium. Occasionally, they can produce marked bone thickening with outward growth of the outer table of the skull. Primary extradural meningioma or intraosseous meningiomas are a rare subtype of meningioma (<2% of all meningiomas), classified as extracalvarial, purely calvarial or calvarial with extracalvarial extension. When they are palpable, meningiomas are immobile, occasionally painful [15].

5.2.1.14 Osteomas

Osteomas are the most common benign lesions that arise from the outer table of the skull and grow slowly. They usually occur before 30 years of age. They are firm, immobile, non-tender, and broad-based. The parasagittal frontal bone is the most location. Sometimes, multiple lesions are associated with Gardner syndrome. The complaints are cosmetically disturbing swelling and diplopia if they are localized at the orbit (Fig. 5.3b) [16].

5.2.1.15 Giant Cell Tumors "Brown Tumors"

Giant cell tumors are the benign osseous lesions associated mainly with hyperparathyroidism. They can be multifocal or solitary. Brown tumor is a localized accumulation of fibrous tissue and giant cells which can replace bone and cause bone expansion. Brown tumors are generally well-defined unilocular or multilocular pure lytic lesions, which stimulate little reactive bone formation [17].

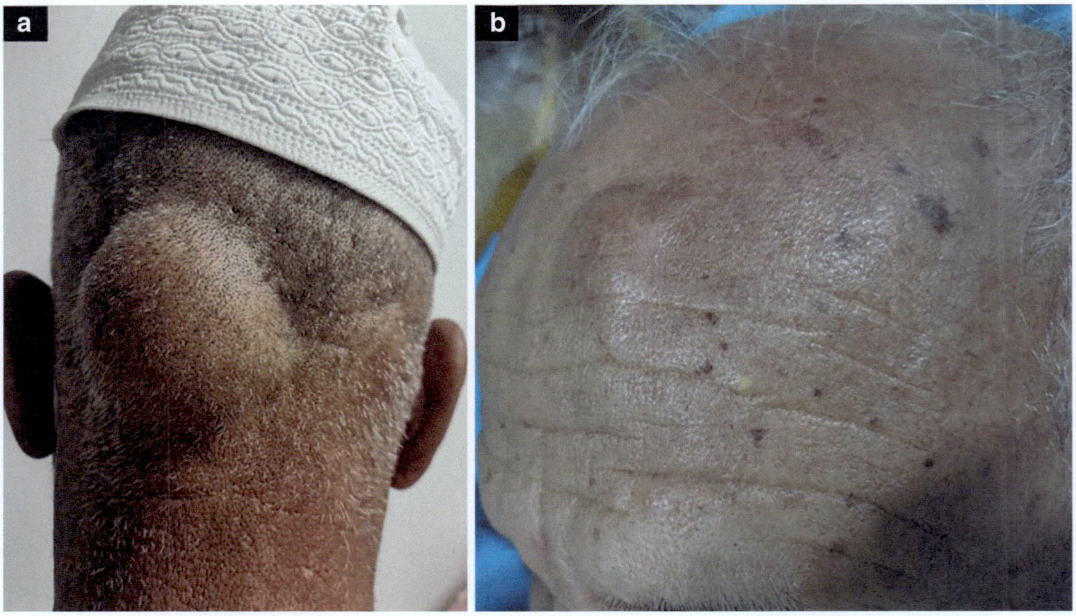

Fig. 5.3 (**a**) Lipoma. Dome-shaped lump with rubbery consistency on the left occipital area. (**b**) Osteoma. Firm, immobile, nontender swelling on the parasagittal frontal bone

5.2.1.16 Juvenile Psammomatoid Ossifying Fibroma

Juvenile psammomatoid ossifying fibroma is a rare, most commune benign form of ossifying fibromas. Mean age ranges from 16 to 33 years. Sometimes past history of trauma may be associated with the affected region. The tumor presented with an enlarging mass noted incidentally on imaging or while grooming their hair [18].

5.2.2 Malign Neoplastic Lesions of the Scalp and Calvarium

5.2.2.1 Cutaneous Squamous Cell Carcinomas

Cutaneous squamous cell carcinoma are a malignant proliferation of keratin producing cells extending beyond the epidermis. Particularly prevalent in elderly males. However, they also affect females and younger adults. They grow over weeks to months. They are often tender or painful, may ulcerate. Size varies from a few millimeters to several centimeters in diameter [19].

5.2.2.2 Intraepidermal Squamous Cell Carcinoma

Intraepidermal squamous cell carcinoma are also known as Bowen's disease. A malignant proliferation of keratin producing cells localized within the epidermis (Fig. 5.4a) [20].

5.2.2.3 Basal Cell Carcinomas

Basal cell carcinoma are a malignant proliferation of keratin producing cells extending beyond the epidermis, locally invasive skin tumor. The main characteristics are slowly growing plaque or nodule, skin colored, pink or pigmented, varies in size from a few millimeters to several centimeters in diameter, spontaneous bleeding or ulceration and have a higher propensity for recurrence (Fig. 5.4b) [21].

5.2.2.4 Malignant Melanomas

Malignant melanomas are potentially very serious skin cancer in which there is an uncontrolled growth of melanocytes (pigment cells). Scalp melanomas are more commonly seen in older men and are associated with alopecia. Compared

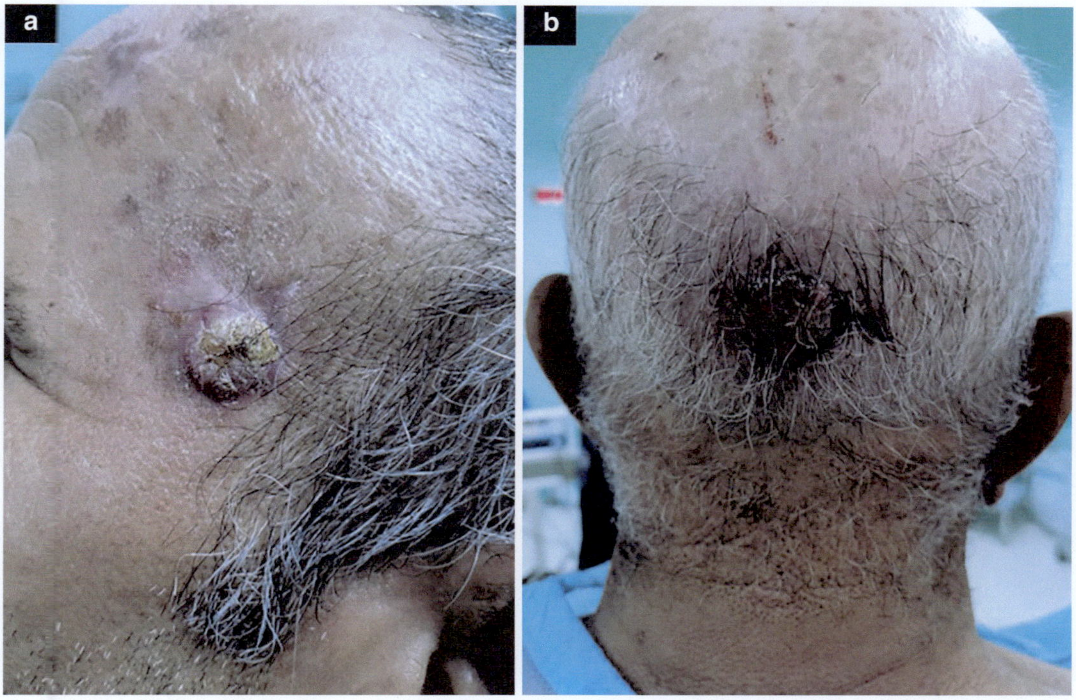

Fig. 5.4 (**a**) Intraepidermal squamous cell carcinoma. Irregular scaly plaque, pink-yellow colored on the left temporal scalp. (**b**) Basal cell carcinoma. Irregular, pink, pigmented, ulcerated nodule on the occipital area

to other body areas, there may be a higher propensity to present as recurrent desmoplastic or amelanotic melanoma. The lesions are also more likely to develop ulceration (Fig. 5.5a) [22].

5.2.2.5 Malignant Proliferating Trichilemmal Tumors

Malignant proliferating trichilemmal tumors are the keratinized nodules or cysts derived from outer hair root sheath cells with low potential for metastasis. They may develop from trichilemmal cysts in most cases, the sign of malignancy is the rapid growth. The malignant cyst may be a recurrence of a previously diagnosed and excised proliferating trichilemmal cyst. Most lesions have been found in women aged between 50 and 75 years of age. Most lesions are greater than 5 cm, these may cause pressure and necrosis on underlying tissues [23].

5.2.2.6 Pilomatrix Carcinomas

Pilomatrix carcinomas are a low-grade adnexal carcinoma derived from hair matrix cells that may manifest as skin colored or purplish irregular papules [24].

5.2.2.7 Sebaceous Carcinomas

Sebaceous carcinomas are a form of adnexal carcinoma where the cells demonstrate a differentiation into sebaceous cells. Lesions lack distinguishing features but may appear as yellow nodules or plaques with ulceration or crusting [25].

5.2.2.8 Apocrine Carcinoma and Poro Carcinoma

Apocrine carcinoma and Poro carcinoma originate from sweat gland. Clinically, these lesions present as rapidly growing nodules within a long-standing, previously stable lesion. They have a nondescript appearance and may manifest as ulcerating or bleeding nodules (Fig. 5.5b) [26].

5.2.2.9 Liposarcomas

Liposarcoma are a malignant proliferation of adipocytes that can resemble an enlarging lipoma. Differentiated from lipoma on the basis of histology findings [27].

5.2.2.10 Leiomyosarcomas

Leiomyosarcomas are a malignant proliferation of smooth muscle cells that may also develop in the dermis or subcutaneous tissue [28].

5.2.2.11 Dermatofibrosarcoma Protuberans

Dermatofibrosarcoma protuberans are usually presents as a painless thickened area of skin (plaque and/or nodule) that feels rubbery or firm to touch and is fixed to the underlying skin. They may be red-brown or skin colored. It usually

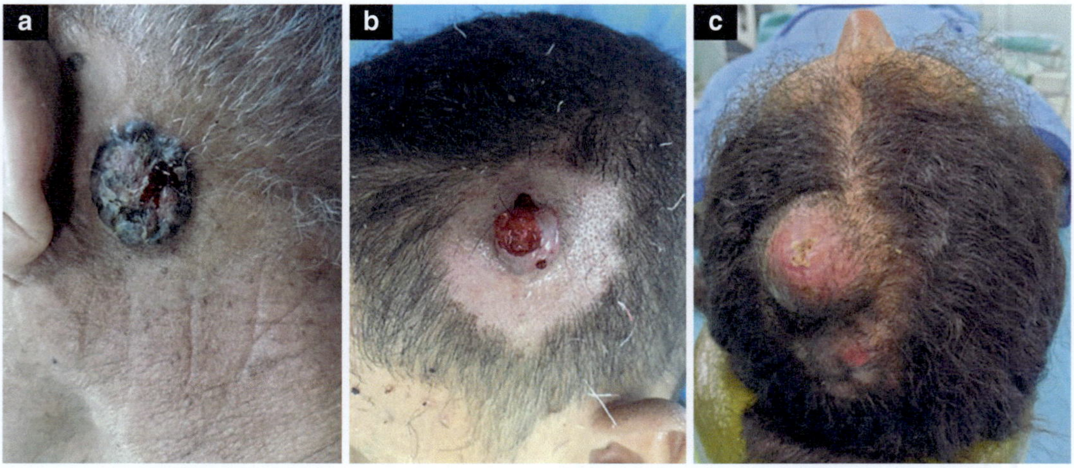

Fig. 5.5 (**a**) Malignant melanoma. Retroauricular papule, dark-brown colored with bleeding and ulcerating. (**b**) Porocarcinoma. Ulcerating and bleeding nodule on the left fronto-parietal scalp. (**c**) Dermatofibrosarcoma. Two painless lichenified nodules, red-brown colored, rubbery and firm to touch, fixed to underlying skin on the left parasagittal parietal area

grows very slowly over months to years (Fig. 5.5c) [29].

5.2.2.12 Fibrosarcomas

Fibrosarcomas are a malignant proliferation of spindled fibroblasts or myofibroblasts which are typically firm and spherical but otherwise nondescript in appearance [30].

5.2.2.13 Merkel Cell Carcinomas

Merkel cell carcinomas are aggressive tumors with high metastatic potential, thought to be derived from pressure receptors (Merkel cells) in the skin. They are typically larger and present as a rapidly enlarging, solitary, irregular red nodule. They spread through the lymphatic system and multiple metastases can develop around the main tumor (local recurrence). They may also spread to lymph nodes in the neck, axillae, and groin [31].

5.2.2.14 Osteosarcomas

Osteosarcomas are the most common malignant calvarial tumor, rapidly growing, painful, or asymptomatic [32].

5.2.2.15 Chondrosarcomas

Chondrosarcomas are slow growing malignant lesions accounting. They arise from remnants of embryonal cartilage, endochondral bone, or primitive mesenchymal cells. The typical location of these tumors is off-midline, centered at the petro-occipital fissure/synchondrosis [33].

5.2.2.16 Ewing Sarcomas

Ewing sarcomas are a highly malignant bone tumor, shows varying degrees of neuroectodermal differentiation. They are more prevalent in young adults and in children. They are more prevalent in frontal and parietal convexities. They are present as a gradually progressive fungating swelling band aching pain in midline occipital region [34].

5.2.2.17 Metastatic Tumors

The metastatic tumors of the scalp and calvaria are arisine from various malignancies, mostly seen from breast, lung, prostate, kidney, pelvis, and thyroid primaries. The most common calvarial metastasis in adults is breast cancer. In children, the most common calvarial metastases are neuroblastoma. Clinically are usually an incidental finding. However, metastatic lesions, when symptomatizing, were presented with various manifestations, scalp swelling, non-tender masse, dome-shaped, may be boggy, rubbery, or rock-hard, painful when the periost is infiltrated and headaches. Intracranial growth can result in neurological symptoms including headaches, neurological deficits, and seizures [35].

5.2.3 Intracranial Neoplasms with Involvement of the Scalp and Calvarium

The tumors may be intra or extra-axial associated with increased intracranial pressure and focal neurologic disturbance. They may rupture the outer table of the skull and involve the scalp inducing prominence on the head and skull deformity (meningioma, hemangiopericytoma, oligodendroglioma, astrocytoma, glioblastoma, intracranial metastatic tumors, ….)

5.3 Congenital and Developmental Lesions of the Scalp and Calvarium

5.3.1 Epidermal Cysts

Epidermal cysts are the benign cysts derived from the infundibulum or upper portion of a hair follicle. They are common in young to middle-aged adults and are rare in children. The clinical features include Firm, flesh-colored or yellow papules/nodules which may have a central punctum that exudes foul smelling debris, cyst wall is delicate and prone to rupture. The lesions are usually solitary or multiple in Gardner's syndrome and basal cell nevus syndrome (Fig. 5.6) [36].

5.3.2 Dermoid Cysts

Dermoid cysts consist of an ectodermal inclusion and occur in the midline or other embryonic fusion lines. They appear in early childhood, with about 40% present at birth. They are made up of

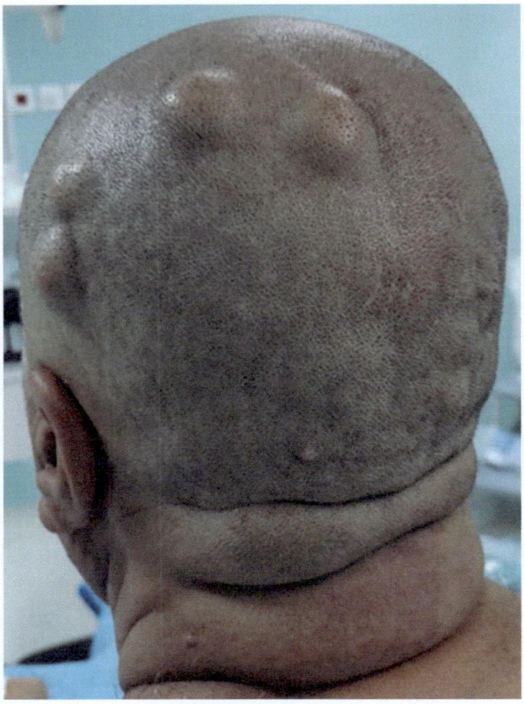

Fig. 5.6 Scalp epidermoid cyst. Multiple firm, flesh-colored nodules which have a central punctum

epidermal and dermal components: keratinocytes, hair follicles and hair, and sweat glands. The cyst is usually a solitary, firm, dough-like lump and ranges in size from 0.5 to 6 cm in diameter. It can be associated with a nearby pit and/or sinus tract to underlying tissues (cause for infectious meningitis). They may produce an intracranial mass by extending through a defect in the cranium. The cyst may broadcast the keratinous and sebaceous material into the cerebrospinal fluid (CSF), resulting in chemical meningitis (Fig. 5.7) [37].

5.3.3 Congenital Melanocytic Naevus (American Spelling Nevus)

Congenital melanocytic naevus are the proliferation of benign melanocytes that are present at birth or develop shortly after birth. Present as single or multi-shaded, round or oval-shaped pigmented patches, they may have increased hair growth (hypertrichosis). They may become darker, raised, bumpier and hairier, particularly around the time of puberty. They are usually asymptomatic, some may be itchy, particularly larger lesions. The overlying skin may become fragile and erode or ulcerate [38].

5.3.4 Congenital Midline Scalp and Skull Defects

Congenital midline scalp and skull defects are usually parieto-occipital and most commonly affect females, due to congenital deficiencies in the process of embryological development. Meningitis, ulceration, and hemorrhage may occur [39].

5.3.5 Congenital Depression of the Skull

Congenital depression of the skull is related to trauma during difficult labor, by obstetric maneuvers or pressure from forceps. Skull depressions may occur with or without fractures and can be classified as linear, depressed, or "ping-pong" fractures and occipital osteodiastasis. They most frequently occur in the temporal and parietal bones. In the majority of cases, deficits are a rare association, often secondary to intra- or extra-axial hematomas [40].

5.3.6 Dermal Sinus Tracts

Dermal sinus tracts appear in childhood as dimples overlying a midline occipital scalp. Intracranially, these tracts may end in the fourth ventricle as a dermoid tumor. Recurrent meningitis is often aseptic and results from chemical irritation from cholesterol crystals [41].

5.3.7 Encephaloceles, Meningoceles, and Meningoencephaloceles

Encephaloceles, meningoceles, and meningoencephaloceles are the developmental lesions present at birth that result from faulty closure of the cephalic end of the neural tube. Encephalocele is

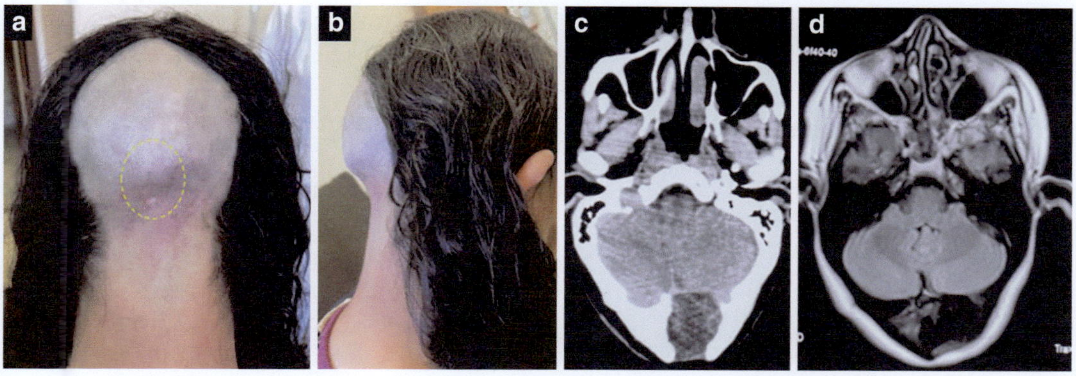

Fig. 5.7 Intradiploic dermoid cyst. (**a**, **b**): Posterior and lateral view; occipital bony protrusion (yellow dotted circle). (**c**): Axial CT scan demonstrating a hypodense multiloculated cystic lesion located in the occipital region associated with osteolysis of the inner and outer table of the occipital bone. (**d**): On T1-weighted image the lesion appears slightly inhomogeneous, mostly hypointense

the herniation of intracranial tissue through a defect in the skull. They are called meningoceles when they contain only meninges, or meningoencephaloceles if brain tissue is included. They are usually midline or Para midline and occur most commonly in the occipital scalp. They can be either sessile or pedunculated, there is a marked variation in size. Cephaloceles have a bluish tinge; tense, cystic, compressible; and may pulsate. Transillumination may indicate the presence of CSF [42].

5.3.8 Sinus Pericranii

Sinus pericranii is a developmental abnormality of childhood that can also be secondary to trauma. It consists of abnormal communications between the intracranial and extracranial venous circulation through a small ostium. Most commonly it occurs in the frontal midline scalp and generally communicate with the large sagittal sinus. It is well-circumscribed, soft, fixed to bone, respect to the skin, compressible and increases in size when the patient strains or reclines as a result of Valsalva maneuver, crying, coughing, and from jugular vein compression [43].

5.3.9 Heterotopic Brain Tissue

Heterotopic brain tissue is a glial tissue and meninges with intracranial connection. It most often occurred in the occipital or parietal areas. The cystic or solid mass has a blue-red hue, fixed to the overlying skin, mobile below (the underlying bone is usually intact). The hair overlying the lesions is usually absent or located just at the periphery "hair collar sign" [44].

5.3.10 Aplasia Cutis Congenita

Aplasia cutis congenital is a congenital absence of the skin, and it presents with a focal ulcer over the vertex of the skull in the midline. The surface is usually shiny, flat, hairless plaque, rarely pulsatile when the underlying bone may be absent. The defect may involve the calvaria and the dura mater, with 20–30% of cases presenting with associated anomalies. Larger defects revealing the dura and sagittal sinus require treatment at birth to avoid complications such as meningeal infection and hemorrhage (Fig. 5.8) [45].

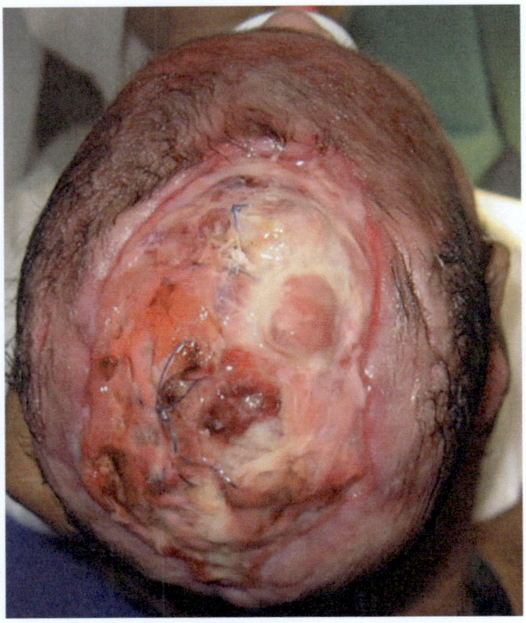

Fig. 5.8 Aplasia cutis congenital. Large defect in the midline of the skin with the underlying bone revealing the dura and sagittal sinus

5.3.11 Craniosynostosis

Craniosynostosis are a major congenital craniofacial disorder characterized by the premature closure of a cranial suture(s) which causes abnormal calvarial growth. They consist of a restriction of skull growth perpendicular to the affected suture and leading to an abnormal cranial contour. The four main sutures implicated in craniosynostosis are the sagittal, coronal, metopic, and lambdoid sutures. Defects in each of these sutures present with distinct clinical manifestations. Craniosynostosis can occur either as part of a recognized genetic syndrome or as an isolated pathology. Severe craniosynostosis often have impairments in hearing, vision, intracranial pressure, and/or neurocognitive functions. Syndromic craniosynostosis may present with other deformities or symptoms including respiratory problems [46].

5.4 Traumatic Lesions of the Scalp and Calvarium

5.4.1 Scalp and Calvaria Injury

Scalp and calvaria injury must be evaluated according to the mechanism of head injury (closed, penetrating, high or low velocity, gunshot wounds…), the characteristics of the scalp wound (location, size, and depth, involving pericranium, calvarium, dura, etc.), associated subgaleal hematoma, the calvarial fractures (simple or compound, linear or communited, depressed or elevated, diasthestic fractures, widening of sutures in children) (Figs. 5.9a–c, 5.10a, b, and 5.11a–d).

5.4.2 Leptomeningeal Cysts

Leptomeningeal cysts are an uncommon late complication of a calvaria fracture in infants and young children. The cyst is formed by the arachnoidal membranes that are trapped through a traumatic dural tear and grows by the pulsations of the CSF. So much pressure will cause bone erosion and widening of the fracture. A history of headache is frequent. The mass is soft, pulsatile, typically elongated, occurring along the fracture line, compressible and becomes more apparent when the patient reclines. Parietal and parieto occipital scalp are the most common locations for these cysts [47].

5.4.3 Cephalohematoma Deformans

Cephalohematoma deformans is defined as a sequela of subperiosteal hemorrhage confined by cranial sutures (Cephalohematoma), after perinatal trauma. Subperiosteal hematoma may calcify, and new bone formation then circumscribes the area under the raised periosteum [48].

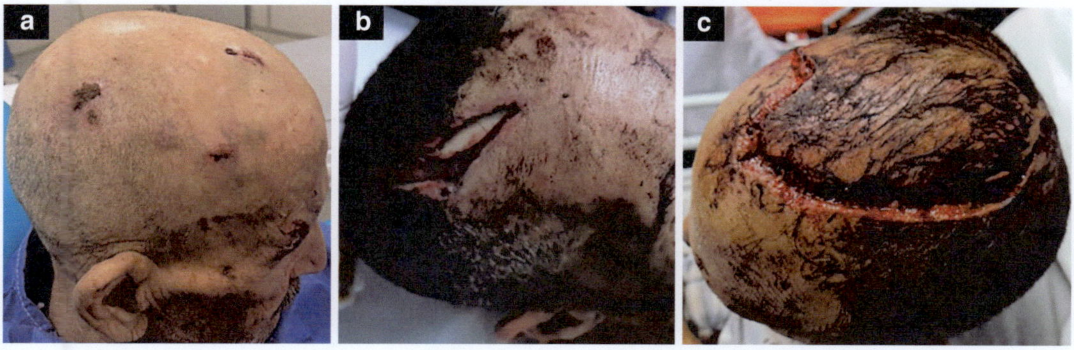

Fig. 5.9 Scalp wounds: (a) Small wound, (b) medium wound with bone fracture and (c) large wound

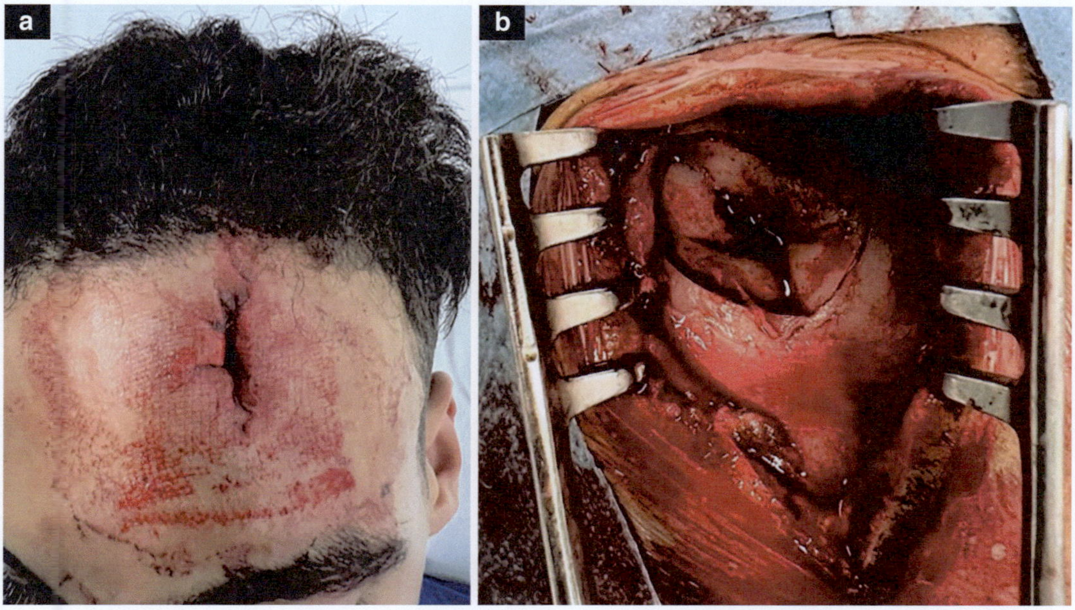

Fig. 5.10 (a) Frontal scalp wound. (b) Bone fracture depressed visualized after exposure

5.4.4 Keloid Scar

Keloid scar is a firm, smooth fibrous tissue that occurs as a result of excessive scar formation after skin injury. Keloids are usually purplish red, can be uncomfortable and itchy, and can occur years after injury and extend beyond the site of the precipitating injury (Fig. 5.12a) [49].

5.4.5 Hypertrophic Scar

Hypertrophic scar is a growth of fibrous tissue that develops as part of wound healing processes. Typically, it begins as red and prominent before becoming flat and pale. It is usually pink to red, slightly raised or flat, and can be uncomfortable and itchy. Usually occurs within weeks of injury. Limited to the confines of the initiating wound [49].

5.4.6 Scalp Pressure Ulcers

Scalp pressure ulcers are the skin or soft tissue injuries following prolonged pressure exerted over specific areas of the scalp most frequently occipital area. The pressure causes lesions with different stages: tissue ischemia, necrosis, tissue loss, and possible involvement of the bone (Fig. 5.12b) [50].

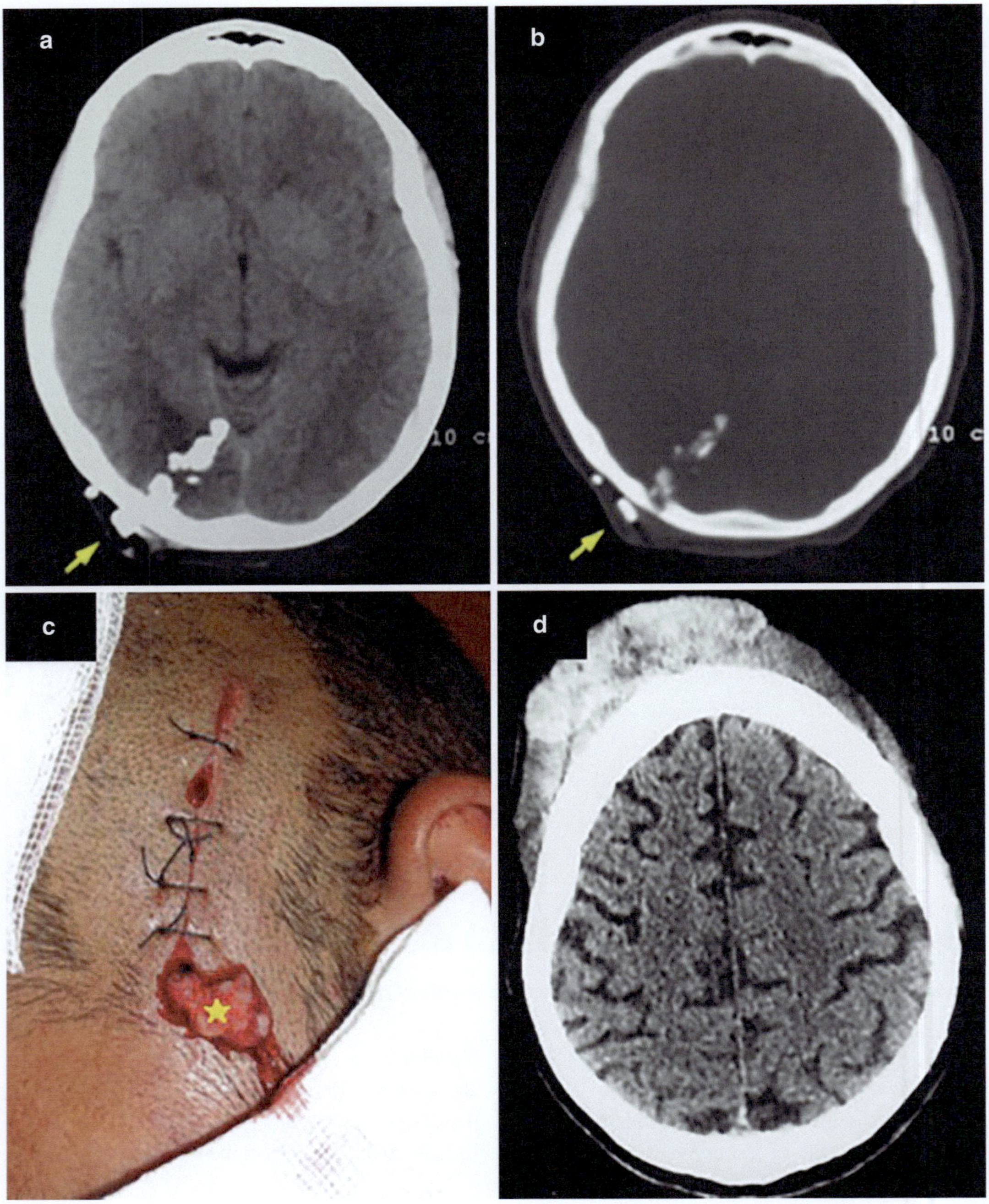

Fig. 5.11 (**a**, **b**): CT, right parieto-occipital penetrating craniocerebral wound. (**c**): left temporal penetrating craniocerebral wound with extravasation of tissue parenchyma (asterix). (**d**): CT, right frontal subgaleal hematoma

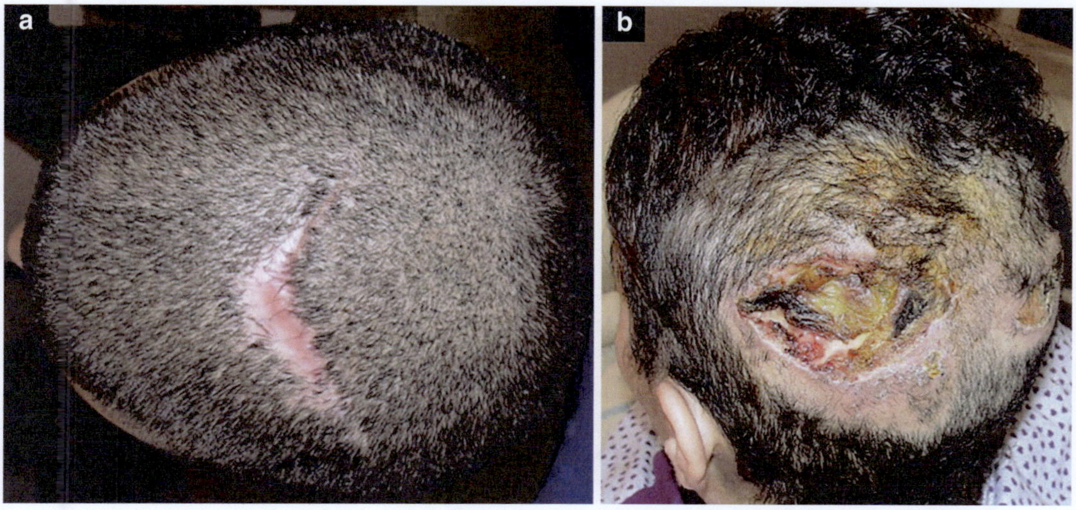

Fig. 5.12 (**a**) Frontoparietal keloid scar. (**b**) Occipital scalp pressure ulcers

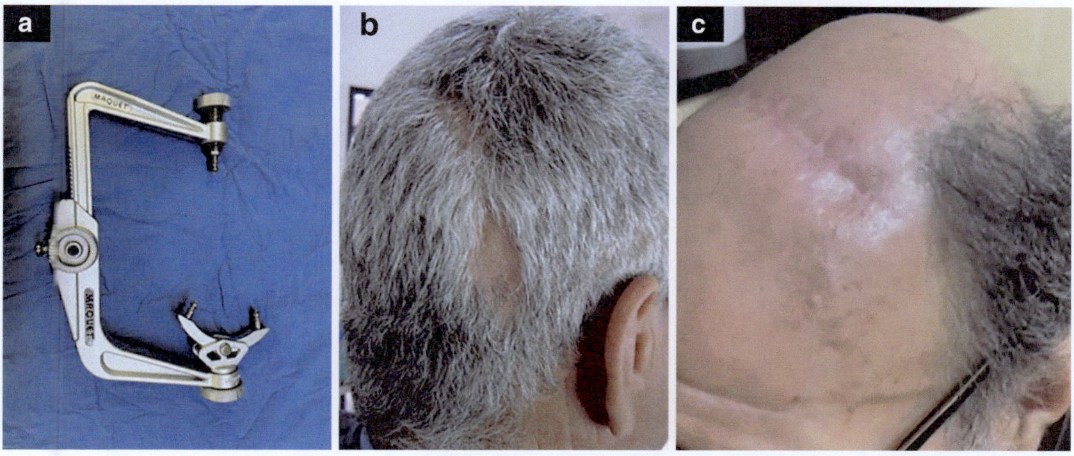

Fig. 5.13 Iatrogenic lesions. (**a**) Mayfield (head-holders), (**b**) Alopecia in the site of the spikes of the mayfield, (**c**) Burr hole and de bone flap scar

5.4.7 Iatrogenic Lesions

(Surgical and Nonsurgical): burr holes, bone flaps, Mayfield (head-holders), Stereotactic frame, cervical traction, radionecrosis, scalp necrosis, shunted hydrocephalus (Fig. 5.13).

5.5 Vascular Lesions of the Scalp and Calvarium

5.5.1 Infantile Hemangiomas

Infantile hemangiomas represent a vascular malformation in the dermis or subcutaneous tissue. Typically, they are solitary, maybe segmental or multiple. The clinical features are determined by the depth of the lesion, distribution pattern, and phase of growth. Bright red, blue or flesh-colored, non-tender and non-pulsatile papules/plaques. Involvement of internal organs is usually indicated by multiple cutaneous lesions [51].

5.5.2 Venous Malformations

Venous malformations are a type of vascular naevus or birthmark. They consist of a congenital malformed dilated vein which appears as a soft and non-pulsatile blue or purple swelling of variable size. These are sometimes associated with other abnormalities in various vascular syndromes (Maffucci syndrome, Bean syndrome) [52].

5.5.3 Arteriovenous Malformations

Arteriovenous malformations refer to communication between an artery and a vein. The affected skin feels warmer than the surrounding skin. It may be possible to feel a "thrill" due to the high flow of blood through the arteriovenous malformation. These are sometimes associated with other abnormalities in various vascular syndromes (Fig. 5.14) [53].

5.5.4 Lymphangioma

Lymphatic malformation is a type of vascular naevus or birthmark due to malformed and dilated lymphatic vessels. They are always present at birth, more obviously during infancy and childhood. Variable in size, often appear red or blue because of the involvement of adjacent blood vessels [54].

5.5.5 Venous Lakes

Transcalvarial venous channels consist of holes in the calvarium through which emissary veins

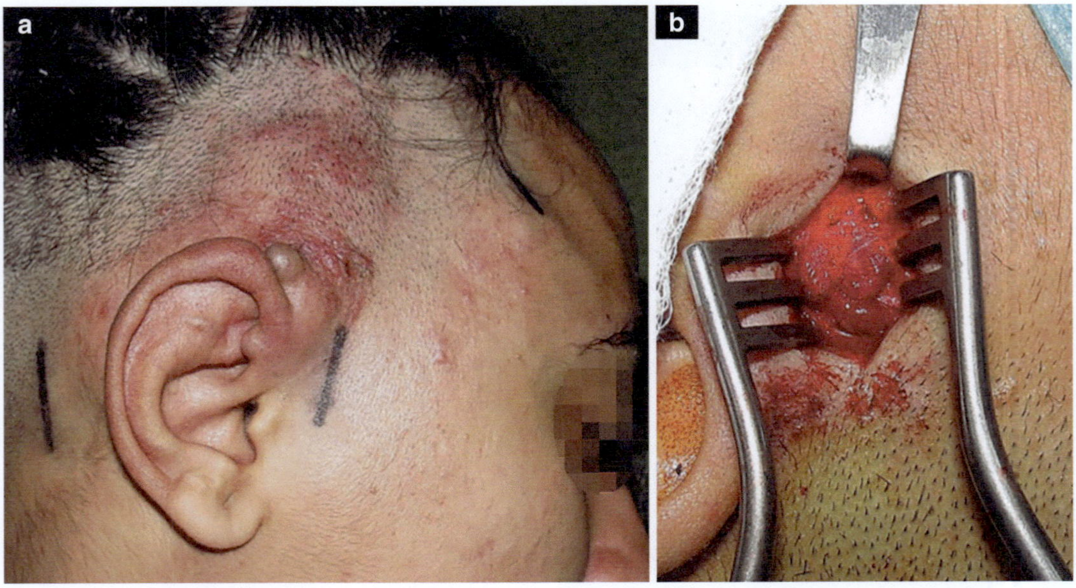

Fig. 5.14 (**a**, **b**): Right temporal arteriovenous malformation of the scalp

pass, connecting the dural venous sinuses with veins external to the skull. They usually present as serpiginous or linear lucencies with sclerotic borders through the skull and are sometimes confounded with fractures or sutures. When these veins are enlarged, they are known as venous lakes [55].

5.5.6 Cutaneous Angiosarcoma

Cutaneous angiosarcoma is presented either as a nodular or diffuse lesion of the scalp. It often presents insidiously as a bruise like lesion or a purplish papule that may be mistaken for a benign lesion such as hemangioma. It may manifest as painful rapidly growing bruises, blue–black nodules, or persistent ulcers [56].

5.5.7 Intraosseous Hemangiomas

Intraosseous hemangiomas are benign vascular neoplasms originate in the skull diploic vessels. Classified as either infantile or congenital hemangiomas. In adult, they are more common in middle aged females and are located in the parietal less in the frontal area. The tumors are boggy or doughy and compressible. They are often asymptomatic; further growth can cause painful swelling, tender or soft masse, fluctuating, and pulsating masse, overlying skin may contain telangiectasis. The lesions undergo periods of rapid growth followed by gradual resolution. Some congenital hemangiomas may never involute [57].

5.5.8 Aneurysmal Bone Cyst

Aneurysmal bone cyst is a benign, cystic lesion composed of multiple blood-filled cavities divided by connective tissue septa, rarely affecting the skull (2–6% of all cases). Local swelling and tenderness represent the most common clinical findings. Pulsation can be observed if the lesion breaks through the inner table of the cranium [58, 59].

5.6 Infectious Lesions of the Scalp and Calvarium

5.6.1 Infections of the Scalp

Infections of the scalp are one of the most seen reasons for admission to dermatology clinics. The most seen are bacterial: Folliculitis, folliculitis decalvans, tufted hair folliculitis and acne keloidalis nuchae. Fungal: Tinea capitis, favus and kerion celsi. Protozoal: Syphilitic alopecia. Pediculosis capitis is the most common worldwide infestation of the scalp. They may present the predisposing factors for more serious infectious complications (scalp abscesses, osteomyelitis, post-neurosurgical decompensations) [60–67].

5.6.2 Scalp Abscesses

Scalp abscesses are the purulent infectious collections involving principally the subgaleal space. Subgaleal abscesses may be spontaneous, owing to contiguous spread (from a paranasal sinus infection), acquired or iatrogenic, following trauma or surgery. The main signs are tender, fluctuant swelling, erythema, and local heat. Sometimes, pus formation, purulent fistula, and discharge with a foul odor can be seen. Tenderness out of proportion to soft tissue findings suggests osteomyelitis of the skull rather than scalp abscess. General and/or regional signs of infection may also be encountered, such as fever, chills, fatigue, irritability, headache, and lymphadenopathy. Clinical symptoms may be more serious (meningitis and neurologic complications) if the infection progresses into deep anatomic structures such as the cranial bone and intracranial space (Fig. 5.15) [68].

5.6.3 Subperiosteal Abscess "Pott Puffy Tumor"

Pott puffy tumor refers to the edema and swelling of the forehead and scalp caused by a subperiosteal abscess overlying frontal bone osteomyelitis.

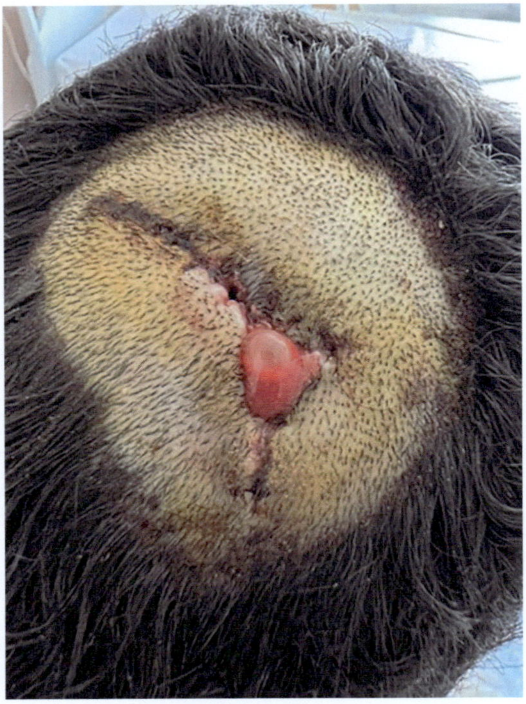

Fig. 5.15 Scalp abscesses following post-traumatic wound

The infection can spread directly through the thin bone wall of the sinus or through the small veins that drain its mucosa. Frontal sinusitis and trauma are the most common causes of this condition. The most common causal organisms are streptococci, staphylococci, and anaerobic bacteria. Intracranial complications are more common in adult males in the fourth decade of their lives, the most common of which are epidural abscesses or empyemas [69].

5.6.4 Osteomyelitis

Osteomyelitis is an inflammatory condition of the bone (osteitis) and bone marrow (myelitis), caused by pyogenic bacteria, fungal infection in both immunosuppressed and immunocompetent patients. Three main sources of infection: direct extension from a contiguous site of infection, postsurgical or posttraumatic direct inoculation, hematogenous dissemination from a source of infection. Local signs of infection are swelling, pus formation, purulent fistula, and discharge with a foul odor. The cranial bone may be exposed. General signs of infection are represented by fever, chills, fatigue, lethargy, irritability, headache, and lymphadenopathy. Meningitis and neurologic syndromes should alert for intracranial complications [70].

5.6.5 Calvarial Tuberculosis

Calvarial tuberculosis is a rare manifestation of extrapulmonary tuberculosis, and it constitutes 0.1–3.7% of all skeletal tuberculosis cases. Most cases are secondary to pulmonary tuberculosis. Patients are mostly between the age of 11 and 20 years. Trauma is a predisposing factor. The patient had painless fluctuant scalp swelling [71].

5.6.6 Calvarial Hydatid Cysts

Calvarial hydatid cysts are predominantly seen in young adult males. Its symptomatology varies according to the cyst location and growth direction. Frequently, the inner table ruptured, and the vesicular larva passes into the epidural space allowing symptoms of increased intracranial pressure and focal neurologic disturbance. Less frequently, cysts may rupture the outer table of the skull and involve the scalp inducing prominence on the head and skull deformity [72].

5.7 Miscellaneous Lesions of the Scalp and Calvarium (Inflammatory, Hematologic, Metabolic, Iatrogenic and Others)

5.7.1 Fibrous Dysplasia

Fibrous dysplasia is a benign condition characterized by replacement of normal bone by proliferative immature fibro osseous. Most frequently seen in childhood and adolescence. The skull is involved in both the monostotic and polyostotic form of the disease. Generally, it is asymptomatic and painless, symptoms in increased mass, asym-

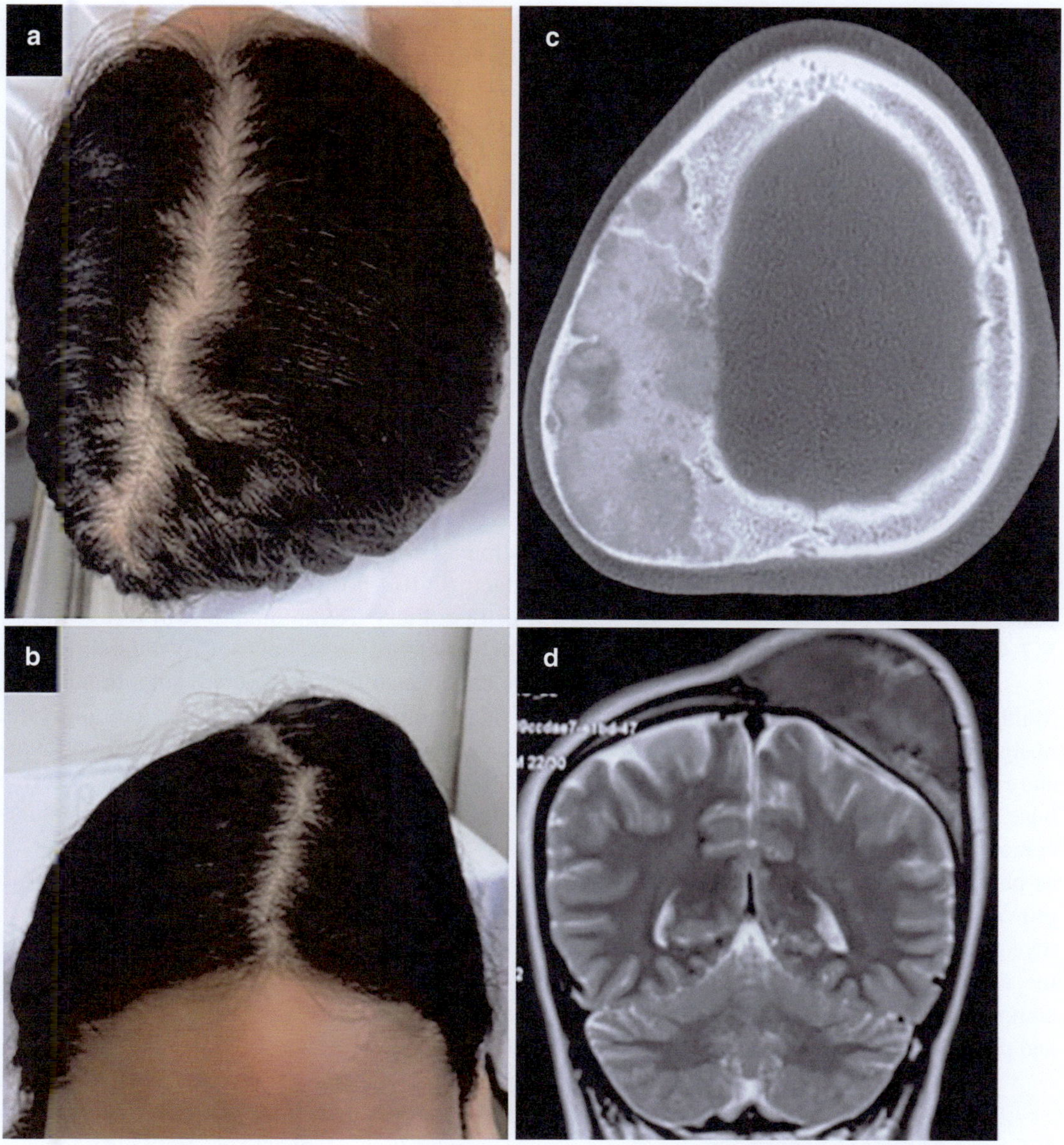

Fig. 5.16 Fibrous dysplasia. (**a**, **b**): Left parietal bone swelling causing asymmetry of the head. (**c**): axial CT head image showing an expansible lesion with internal ground-glass opacity emerging from left parietal bone. (**d**): On coronal T2-weighted image, the lesion shows iso signal intensity

metry of skull and facial bone, majorly found in frontal and temporal bones (Fig. 5.16) [73].

5.7.2 Paget's Disease "Osteitis Deformans"

Paget's disease is a chronic disorder characterized by focal or multifocal excessive remodelling and disorganized bone structure. Paget's disease may be divided into three phases: initial (active), middle (intermediate), and late (inactive). Each phase is associated with distinctive pathologic, radiologic, and clinical features. The vast majority of patients are asymptomatic in all stages and most of the symptoms are related to weakened and thickened bones. Patients frequently complain of pain. The most common complications comprise arthropathy, fractures, neurologic dysfunction, hypercalcemia, and hypercalciuria in immobilized patients and the tumor transformation commonly into osteosarcoma [74].

5.7.3 Lymphoma

Lymphoma is a malignant proliferation of lymphocytes. The most commonly occurring variants on the scalp include primary cutaneous follicle center and/or marginal zone lymphomas. Osseous lymphoma belongs to the non-Hodgkin lymphoma classification, specifically a diffuse large cell lymphoma. The usual clinical presentation is the presence of scalp swelling, without neurological deficits. If intraparenchymal infiltration is present, neurological deficits may become the most important clinical manifestation of disease [75].

5.7.4 Multiple Myeloma

Multiple myeloma is the most common primary malignant bone lesion occurring between the fourth and eighth decades. It is a malignant disorder of the bone marrow in which there is monoclonal proliferation of plasma cells. Solitary lesions are known as plasmacytomas. They are asymptomatic rapid growing masses or have bone pain. Multiple myeloma lesions are usually disseminated through the axial skeleton, affecting the vertebrae most commonly, as well as the ribs, skull, pelvic girdle, and proximal appendicular skeleton [76].

5.7.5 Calvarial Sarcoidosis

Sarcoidosis is an inflammatory disorder of unknown cause characterized by the presence of non-caseating granulomas in tissues. Skull involvement in sarcoidosis is very rare with few cases reported. Clinically calvarial sarcoidosis may manifest with headaches and skull tenderness [77].

5.7.6 Eosinophilic Granuloma

Eosinophilic granuloma is the local benign form of langerhans cell histiocytosis that develops after the abnormal proliferation of the histiocyte and has an unknown etiology. The parietal bone is the most common location of skull bones. At clinical presentation, patients can be asymptomatic or have a palpable soft-tissue mass, immobile, doughy, and pulsatile if associated with underlying bone destruction. Tenderness and local swelling are usually the presenting symptoms [78].

5.7.7 Juvenile Xanthogranuloma

Juvenile xanthogranuloma is a type of non--Langerhans cell histiocytosis usually limited to the skin in very young children. It is a polyclonal proliferation of cholesterol-containing factor XIIIa-positive histiocytes. It can occur with solitary asymptomatic skin lesion (80%) or with multiple lesions and systemic involvement. It manifests as domed, smooth and firm papules/nodules, large lesions can ulcerate. Lesion color progresses from red through yellow to brown before fading. Atypical forms include giant, generalized, clustered, subcutaneous [79].

5.7.8 Rosai–Dorfman Disease

Rosai–Dorfman disease is called sinus histiocytosis with massive lymphadenopathy, is a non--Langerhans histiocytic disease. The skin is the most common extra nodal site. Cutaneous Rosai–Dorfman disease typically occurs in older females and presents in various forms, ranging from single papules to multiple nodules and plaques of red, red-brown, or yellow coloration [80].

5.7.9 Acromegaly

Growth hormone hypersecretion associated with bony abnormalities including thinning of the cranial vault, prominence and enlargement of frontal and maxillary sinuses, prominence of the occipital protuberance, enlargement, and elongation of the mandible [81].

5.7.10 Chronic Hemolytic Anemia

Patients with hemolytic anemia have a widening of the diploic space caused by marrow hyperplasia [82].

5.7.11 Others Metabolic Disorders of the Scalp and Calvarium

There are a large spectrum of systemic conditions that can affect the calvaria and can be identified as palpable masses or as incidental findings on radiologic studies (Hyperparathyroidism, renal osteodystrophy, amyloidosis, phenytoin-induced hyperostosis, osteopenia, thalassemia, osteopetrosis…).

5.7.12 Normal Variants Mimicking Pathology (Pseudolesions)

Calvarial pseudolesions include arachnoid granulations, prominent venous lakes, hyperostosis frontalis, thinning of the parietal bones. Knowing these entities is important to not mistake them for true pathology.

5.8 Suggestive Signs: Historic and Clinical Features

The clinical examination is an interesting step in diagnosis and therapeutic strategy of the scalp and calvarial lesions. It must specify the location, size, number, mobility, tenderness, local pain, color, pulsation, bruit, ulceration, consistency, aspect, and invasion of the underlying structures. All these findings can be helpful to assist the diagnosis; moreover there are some suggestive signs allowing the recognition some lesions; however they are still no specific and the confirmation is provided by the radiologic and anatomopathological studies (Table 5.2).

Table 5.2 The table summarizing some example of suggestive signs

Highly suggestive conditions and findings	Differential diagnosis
Trauma (Surgical and Nonsurgical)	Cephalohematoma deformans Osteoma Hemangioma Meningioma Lipoma Leptomeningeal cyst Scalp and calvaria injury Iatrogenic Lesions Hypertrophic scar, keloid scar
Family history	Cephalocele Developmental neural anomalies Metabolic disorders Craniosynostosis Neurofibromas
Neurologic symptoms: increased intracranial pressure, focal neurologic disturbance, seizures	Intracranial Neoplasms with Involvement of the Scalp and Calvarium: meningioma, hemangiopericytoma, oligodendroglioma, intracranial metastatic tumors Midline lesions
History of meningitis: indicative of a connection from the skin to the intracranial space	Dermoid tumor Dermal sinus Encephaloceles, meningoceles and meningoencephaloceles

(continued)

Table 5.2 (continued)

Highly suggestive conditions and findings		Differential diagnosis
Pulsatile masses: Any lesion that is continuous with the CSF or cerebral or cranial vasculature will pulsate		Arteriovenous malformations Sinus pericranii and other vascular tumors Encephaloceles, meningoceles and meningoencephaloceles Leptomeningeal cysts Extending intracranial neoplasms Aplasia cutis congenita
Bruits and trills		Vascular tumors Arteriovenous malformations
Turgor alterations: Lesions filled with CSF or bloodwill also change sizeor turgor when the patient changes position or cries		Leptomeningeal cysts Encephaloceles, meningoceles and meningoencephaloceles Vascular lesions Arteriovenous malformations
Transillumination: Presence of CSF or any fluid can mimic CSF		Encephaloceles, meningoceles and meningoencephaloceles Gliomas Leptomeningeal cysts Dermoid tumors
Consistency	Rock-hard	Osteomas Intracranial hemangiomas Cephalhematoma deformans Eosinophilic granulomas Pilomatricomas Ossifying fibroma Fibrous dysplasia
	Soft and compressible	Vascular lesions Encephaloceles, meningoceles, meningoencephaloceles, Heterotopic brain tissue, leptomeningeal cysts
	Rubbery, firm	Dermoid and epidermoid tumors
	Doughy	Lipomas
Discharge from a central pore: Leakage of fluid from a central pore, can be indicative of CSF, sweat, or sebaceous material		Epidermal cysts Complex dermoid tumors
Immobility/fixed		Deep fixation: Lesions with intracranial extension. Intraosseous tumors with outward extension Intramuscular or subgaleal lesions Skin fixation: Lesions located within the dermis Tumors with sinus tracts to the external surface
Tenderness		Eosinophilic granulomas Hemangiomas Meningiomas Osteogenic sarcomas
Associated anomalies: Abnormal hair growth on and around the tumor, Associated hemangiomas…		Developmental anomaly Vascular malformations
Midline location		Sinus pericranii Cephalocele Aplasia cutis congenita Dermoid and epidermal tumors Dermal sinus tumors
Malign signs: Irregular borders, rapid growth, bleeding, ulceration, painful mass…		Malign lesions, Metastatic tumors
General and systemic signs		Inflammatory Hematologic Metabolic Metastatic tumors
Infectious signs		Scalp abscesses Pott puffy tumor Osteomyelitis

5.9 Conclusion

Summarizing, there are some semiotics that can help the practitioner in the differential diagnosis and there are highly suggestive findings in the evaluation of scalp and calvarial lesions. Clinical information and extensive knowledge of possible differential diagnoses are useful in differentiating benign from malignant lesions. In difficult cases, the evaluation of the lesions may be aided by the association of different imaging techniques, especially computed tomography and magnetic resonance imaging particularly in the intracranial extension.

References

1. Yang L, Yang MC, Qu PR, Zhang D, Ge M, Li DP. A retrospective study comprising 228 cases of pediatric scalp and skull lesions. BMC Pediatr. 2023;23(1):478.
2. Gomez CK, Schiffman SR, Bhatt AA. Radiological review of skull lesions. Insights Imaging. 2018;9(5):857–82.
3. Abreu Velez AM, Brown VM, Howard MS. An inflamed trichilemmal (pilar) cyst: not so simple? N Am J Med Sci. 2011;3(9):431–4.
4. Waydadi O, Bijou W, Laachoubi M, Oukessou Y, Roubal M, Mahtar M. Huge pilomatrixomas of the scalp: a case report. Int J Surg Case Rep. 2021;84:106048.
5. Wollina U. Seborrheic keratoses - the most common benign skin tumor of humans. Clinical presentation and an update on pathogenesis and treatment options. Open Access Maced J Med Sci. 2018;6(11):2270–5.
6. Sah K-Y, Bolognia JL. Signature nevi. J Am Acad Dermatol. 2009;60(3):508–14.
7. Borgenvik TL, Karlsvik TM, Ray S, Fawzy M, James N. Blue nevus-like and blue nevus-associated melanoma: a comprehensive review of the literature. ANZ J Surg. 2017;87(5):345–9.
8. Takayama K, Usui Y, Ito M, Goto H, Takeuchi M. A case of sebaceous adenoma of the eyelid showing excessively rapid growth. Clin Ophthalmol. 2013;7:667–70.
9. Tejaswi C, Rangaraj M, Karthikeyan K. Apocrine hidrocystoma arising from nevus sebaceous on the scalp. Indian Dermatol Online J. 2016;7(2):111–3.
10. Choi J, Tschen J, Cohen PR. Incidental clear cell syringoma of the scalp in a patient with lichen planopilaris. Cureus. 2021;13(6):e16064.
11. Jialiandri J, Wang XY, Liu ZJ, Zhang JW, Xu Y. Dermoscopic patterns of dermatofibroma in 72 Chinese patients. Chin Med J. 2019;132(17):2121–2.
12. Hom GL, Moodley S, Rothner AD, Moodley M. The clinical spectrum of mosaic neurofibromatosis in children and adolescents. J Child Neurol. 2020;35(3):242–6.
13. Vlad MM, Dupont M, Kayser F. Subgaleal lipoma: imaging findings. J Belg Soc Radiol. 2021;105(1):23.
14. Holst VA, Junkins-Hopkins JM, Elenitsas R. Cutaneous smooth muscle neoplasms: clinical features, histologic findings, and treatment options. J Am Acad Dermatol. 2002;46(4):477–90.
15. Tokgoz N, Oner YA, Kaymaz M, Ucar M, Yilmaz G, Tali TE. Primary intraosseous meningioma: CT and MRI appearance. AJNR Am J Neuroradiol. 2005;26(8):2053–6.
16. Farah RA, Poletti A, Han A, Navarro R. Giant frontal sinus osteoma and its potential consequences: illustrative case. J Neurosurg Case Lessons. 2021;1(21):CASE21105. Published 2021 May 24
17. Xie C, Tsakok M, Taylor N, Partington K. Imaging of brown tumours: a pictorial review. Insights Imaging. 2019;10(1):75.
18. Chung RT, Montejo JD, Kerr DA, Hong J. Juvenile psammomatoid ossifying fibroma of the parietal bone and review of calvarial presentations: illustrative case. J Neurosurg Case Lessons. 2021;2(10):CASE21361.
19. Fania L, Didona D, Di Pietro FR, Verkhovskaia S, Morese R, Paolino G, Donati M, Ricci F, Coco V, Ricci F, Candi E, Abeni D, Dellambra E. Cutaneous squamous cell carcinoma: from pathophysiology to novel therapeutic approaches. Biomedicines. 2021;9(2):171.
20. British Association of Dermatologists' guidelines for the management of squamous cell carcinoma in situ (Bowen's disease) 2022 — British Association of Dermatologist.
21. Kim JY, Kozlow JH, Mittal B, Moyer J, Olencki T, Rodgers P. Guidelines of care for the management of basal cell carcinoma. J Am Acad Dermatol. 2018;78(3):540–59.
22. Elder DE, Bastian BC, Cree IA, Massi D, Scolyer RA. The 2018 World Health Organization classification of cutaneous, mucosal, and uveal melanoma: detailed analysis of 9 distinct subtypes defined by their evolutionary pathway. Arch Pathol Lab Med. 2020;144(4):500–22.
23. Goyal S, Jain BB, Jana S, Bhattacharya SK. Malignant proliferating trichilemmal tumor. Indian J Dermatol. 2012;57(1):50–2.
24. Jones C, Twoon M, Ho W, Portelli M, Robertson BF, Anderson W. Pilomatrix carcinoma: 12-year experience and review of the literature. J Cutan Pathol. 2018;45(1):33–8.
25. Kibbi N, Worley B, Owen JL, et al. Sebaceous carcinoma: controversies and their evidence for clinical practice. Arch Dermatol Res. 2020;312(1):25–31.
26. Storm CA, Seykora JT. Cutaneous adnexal neoplasms. Am J Clin Pathol. 2002;118(Suppl 1):S33–49.
27. Kessler A, Berenholz L, Eviatar E, Segal S. Liposarcoma of the scalp: a case report and review

of the literature. Otolaryngology–Head Neck Surg. 1997;117(4):412–4.
28. Kamian S, Ebrahimi A, Zadeh KE, Behzadi B. Primary intracranial leiomyosarcoma presenting with frontal bone mass: a case report. Radiat Oncol J. 2020;38(4):282–6.
29. David MP, Funderburg A, Selig JP, et al. Perspectives of patients with dermatofibrosarcoma protuberans on diagnostic delays, surgical outcomes, and nonprotuberance. JAMA Netw Open. 2019;2(8):e1910413.
30. Kumar R, Jagdewan A, Sharma MC. Congenital infantile fibrosarcoma of scalp. Is adjuvant therapy essential? Indian J Surg Oncol. 2014;5(4):297–9.
31. Heath M, Jaimes N, Lemos B, et al. Clinical characteristics of Merkel cell carcinoma at diagnosis in 195 patients: the AEIOU features. J Am Acad Dermatol. 2008;58(3):375–81.
32. Huvos AG. Clinicopathologic spectrum of osteogenic sarcoma. Recent observations. Pathol Annu. 1979;14(Pt 1):123–44.
33. Konovalov A, Shekhtman O, Shekhtman AP, Bezborodova T. Chondrosarcoma of the skull base: a case study and literature review. Cureus. 2020;12(12):e12412.
34. Hadfield MG, Luo VY, Williams RL, et al. Ewing's sarcoma of the skull in an infant. A case report and review. Pediatr Neurosurg. 1996;25:100–4.
35. Gupta S, Sharma G, Sajeevan S, et al. Varied clinical presentation and management of calvarial metastases. Asian J Neurosurg. 2022;17(4):631–4.
36. Liu M, Liu X, Wang Y, et al. Epidermal cyst on the scalp induced by forceps injury during delivery: a case report and epidemiological analysis of 3949 patients. Clin Cosmet Investig Dermatol. 2023;16:593–601.
37. Splendiani A, Bruno F, Mariani S, et al. A rare localization of pure dermoid cyst in the frontal bone. Neuroradiol J. 2016;29(2):130–3.
38. Takaya K, Kato T, Ishii T, Sakai S, Okabe K, Aramaki-Hattori N, Asou T, Kishi K. Clinical analysis of cultured epidermal autograft (JACE) transplantation for giant congenital melanocytic nevus. Plast Reconstr Surg Glob Open. 2021;9(1):e3380.
39. Lassman LP, Sims DG. Congenital midline scalp and skull defect. Arch Dis Child. 1975;50(12):958–60.
40. Vidal Mico S, Lopez Navarro M, Téllez de Meneses M, et al. Spontaneous resolution of a congenital depressed skull fracture. An Esp Pediatr. 2004;54:78–80.
41. Hong S, Maruyama K, Hatanaka R, et al. Frontotemporal dermoid cyst with incomplete dermal sinus tract in an adult: a case report. Surg Neurol Int. 2020;11:429.
42. Alberts A, Lucke-Wold B. Craniofacial Encephalocele: updates on management. J Integr Neurosci. 2023;22(3):79.
43. Fujino S, Enokizono M, Ihara S, Kono T, Miyama S. Sinus pericranii associated with syntelencephaly: a case report. BMC Neurol. 2022;22(1):316.
44. Commens C, RogersM KA. Heterotropic brain tissue presenting as bald cysts with a collar of hypertrophic hair. Arch Dermatol. 1989;125:1253–6.
45. Abbott R, Cutting CB, Wisoff JI-I, et al. Aplasia cutis congenita of the scalp: issues in its management. Pediatr Neurosurg. 1991–1992;17:182–84.
46. Stanton E, Urata M, Chen JF, Chai Y. The clinical manifestations, molecular mechanisms and treatment of craniosynostosis. Dis Model Mech. 2022;15(4):dmm049390.
47. Kim H, Jo KW. Treatment of a traumatic leptomeningeal cyst in an adult with fibrinogen-based collagen. J Korean Neurosurg Soc. 2013;53(5):300–2.
48. Goodwin MD, Persing JA, Duncan CC, Shin JH. Spontaneously infected cephalohematoma: case report and review of the literature. J Craniofac Surg. 2000;11:371–5.
49. Ogawa R, Dohi T, Tosa M, Aoki M, Akaishi S. The latest strategy for keloid and hypertrophic scar prevention and treatment: the Nippon medical school (NMS) protocol. J Nippon Med Sch. 2021;88(1):2–9.
50. Kottner J, Cuddigan J, Carville K, Balzer K, Berlowitz D, Law S, Litchford M, Mitchell P, Moore Z, Pittman J, Sigaudo-Roussel D, Yee CY, Haesler E. Pressure ulcer/injury classification today: an international perspective. J Tissue Viability. 2020;29(3):197–203.
51. Endicott AA, Chamlin SL, Drolet BA, et al. Mapping of segmental and partial segmental infantile hemangiomas of the face and scalp. JAMA Dermatol. 2021;157(11):1328–34.
52. Dubois J, Garel L. Imaging and therapeutic approach of hemangiomas and vascular malformations in the pediatric age group. Pediatr Radiol. 1999;29:879–93.
53. Kaul A, Kanuparthi SP, Erkmen K. A vascular quartet : scalp arteriovenous malformation, Sinus Pericranii, dural arteriovenous fistula, and arteriovenous brain malformation in a single patient. Cureus. 2023;15(4):e37140.
54. Cheng J, Liu B, Lee HJ. 30-Day outcomes analysis of NSQIP-pediatric for surgical management of head and neck lymphatic malformations in children. Int J Pediatr Otorhinolaryngol. 2019;118:21–4.
55. Kiritsi O, Noussios G, Tsitas K, et al. Anatomical variants of the emissary veins: unilateral aplasia of both, the sigmoid sinus and the internal jugular vein and development of the petrosquamosal sinus. A rare case report. Folia Morfol. 2011;70:305–8.
56. Albores-Saavedra J, Schwartz AM, Henson DE, et al. Cutaneous angiosarcoma: analysis of 434 cases from the surveillance, epidemiology, and end results program, 1973-2007. Ann Diagn Pathol. 2011;15(2):93–7.
57. Politi M, Romeike BF, Papanagiotou P, Nabhan A, Struffert T, Feiden W, Reith W. Intraosseous hemangioma of the skull with dural tail sign: radiologic features with pathologic correlation. AJNR Am J Neuroradiol. 2005;26(8):2049–52.
58. Hermann AL, Polivka M, Loit MP, Guichard JP, Bousson V. Aneurysmal bone cyst of the frontal bone - a radiologic-pathologic correlation. J Radiol Case Rep. 2018;12(7):16–24.
59. Strohm JA, Strohm PC, Kühle J, Schmal H, Zwingmann J. Management of juvenile and aneu-

rysmal bone cysts: a systematic literature review with meta-analysis. Eur J Trauma Emerg Surg. 2023;49(1):361–72.
60. Lin HS, Lin PT, Tsai YS, Wang SH, Chi CC. Interventions for bacterial folliculitis and boils (furuncles and carbuncles). Cochrane Database Syst Rev. 2021;2(2):CD013099.
61. Breshtilova V, Bardarov E, Kazandjieva J, Marina S. Tufted hair folliculitis: a case report and literature review. Acta Dermatovenerol Alp Pannonica Adriat. 2011;20:27–9.
62. Umar S, Lee DJ, Lullo JJ. A retrospective cohort study and clinical classification system of acne Keloidalis Nuchae. J Clin Aesthet Dermatol. 2021;14(4):E61–7.
63. Hartman-adams H, Banvard C, Juckett G. Impetigo: diagnosis and treatment. Am Fam Physician. 2014;90(4):229–35.
64. Zaraa I, Hawilo A, Trojjet S, El Euch D, Mokni M, Ben OA. Letter: tinea capitis in infants in their first 2 years of life: a 12-year study and a review of the literature. Dermatol Online J. 2012;18:16.
65. Liu ZH, Zhang Y, Zhu J, Dai YQ, Shen H. Successful treatment of severe kerion celsi in an immunocompromised girl with evacuation of pus, terbinafine and short course glucocorticosteroids. J Mycol Med. 2016;26:42–5.
66. Hernández-Bel P, Unamuno B, Sánchez-Carazo JL, Febrer I, Alegre V. Syphilitic alopecia: a report of 5 cases and a review of the literature. Actas Dermosifiliogr. 2013;104:512–7.
67. Feldmeier H. Treatment of pediculosis capitis: a critical appraisal of the current literature. Am J Clin Dermatol. 2014;15:401–12.
68. Goodman SJ, Cahan L, Chow AW. Subgaleal abscess: a preventable complication of scalp trauma. West J Med. 1977;127(2):169–72.
69. Sideris G, Davoutis E, Panagoulis E, Maragkoudakis P, Nikolopoulos T, Delides A. A systematic review of intracranial complications in adults with pott puffy tumor over four decades. Brain Sci. 2023;13(4):587.
70. Khan MA, Quadri SAQ, Kazmi AS, et al. A comprehensive review of skull base osteomyelitis: diagnostic and therapeutic challenges among various presentations. Asian J Neurosurg. 2018;13(4):959–70.
71. Rengarajan S, Krishnasamy L. Calvarial tuberculosis - a report of seven cases from a tertiary care hospital. J Neurosci Rural Pract. 2023;14(1):123–6.
72. Demir MK, Yapıcıer O, Hasanov T, Yılmaz B, Kılıç T. Hydatid disease: MR imaging of calvarium and superior sagittal sinus involvement. Neuroradiol J. 2018;31(3):320–3.
73. Mierzwiński J, Kosowska J, Tyra J, et al. Different clinical presentation and management of temporal bone fibrous dysplasia in children. World J Surg Oncol. 2018;16(1):5.
74. Shankar YU, Misra SR, Vineet DA, Baskaran P. Paget disease of bone: a classic case report. Contemp Clin Dent. 2013;4(2):227–30.
75. Nitta N, Moritani S, Fukami T, Nozaki K. Characteristics of cranial vault lymphoma from a systematic review of the literature. Surg Neurol Int. 2022;13:231.
76. Michels TC, Petersen KE. Multiple myeloma: diagnosis and treatment. Am Fam Phzecian. 2017;95(6):373–83.
77. Nessrine A, Zahra AF, Taoufik H. Musculoskeletal involvement in sarcoidosis. J Bras Pneumol. 2014;40(2):175–82.
78. Dukmak ON, Abualia SMS, Meqbil YJI, Emar M, Basal SI, Itaidek S. Eosinophilic granuloma affecting the parietal bone of the skull: a case report and literature review.
79. Höck M, Zelger B, Schweigmann G, et al. The various clinical spectra of juvenile xanthogranuloma: imaging for two case reports and review of the literature. BMC Pediatr. 2019;19(1):128.
80. Sampaio R, Silva L, Catorze G, Viana I. Cutaneous Rosai-Dorfman disease: a challenging diagnosis. BMJ Case Rep. 2021;14(2):e239244.
81. Baptista LC, Martins MM, Marcos VN. Radiographic findings in acromegaly: pictorial essay. Radiol Bras. 2023;56(2):110–5.
82. Ogwang E, Odongo CN, Namusisi J, Okello PA, Acan M. Hair-on-end sign in a 9-year-old girl presenting with acute stroke in sickle cell disease. Int Med Case Rep J. 2022;15:69–73.

Imaging of Scalp and Calvarial Lesions

6

Ersen Ertekin, Srinivas Dwarakanath, and Ahmet T. Turgut

6.1 Introduction

Scalp and calvarial lesions are mostly detected incidentally on central nervous system imaging studies. In addition to these lesions which are associated with any clinical symptom, systemic diseases, infectious processes, and tumoral processes can also have scalp or skull involvement. While radiological imaging is not usually required, it may be necessary to resort to radiological imaging procedures, especially in the characterization of systemic/metabolic diseases and tumoral lesions. While ultrasound (US)/Doppler US is accepted as the initial imaging tool for the diagnosis of scalp lesions, magnetic resonance imaging (MRI) is more useful in differential diagnosis thanks to its superior soft tissue resolution. Although X-ray and computed tomography (CT) are considered as the first imaging tool for bone lesions, though the inherent radiation exposure poses a significant disadvantage. MRI would be more appropriate in evaluating the medullary bone marrow as it shows better the spread of skull base lesions [1, 2]. In this chapter, common scalp and skull lesions, their imaging findings and differential diagnoses will be discussed.

E. Ertekin (✉)
Department of Radiology, Hitit University Faculty of Medicine, Çorum, Türkiye
e-mail: drersen@hotmail.com

S. Dwarakanath
Department of Neurosurgery, National Instiute of Mental Health and Neurosciences, Bengaluru, Karnataka, India

A. T. Turgut
Department of Radiology, Ankara Medipol University Faculty of Medicine, Ankara, Türkiye

6.2 Scalp Lesions

Scalp is the part of skin that surrounds the skull and is covered with hair. In addition to general skin lesions, lesions originating from hair follicles are more frequently seen on the scalp. Lesions covered by hair are less visible and usually present with symptoms such as skin thickening or swelling. Examples of common lesions will be presented here.

6.2.1 Trichilemmal Cyst

Trichilemmal cysts are keratin accumulations that mostly appear on the scalp. Lesions, also known as pilarkysts, can be seen along the intracutaneous extension of the outer hair follicle sheath (tricylemma). These lesions, which are mostly detected incidentally, are found in 2.5% of adult patients who undergo head imaging. Most incidental ones are asymptomatic and have no clinical significance [3]. They are hard cystic structures containing largely white semi-solid

M. Turgut et al. (eds.), *Lesions of the Scalp and Cranial Vault*,
https://doi.org/10.1007/978-3-031-88244-9_6

material. They often contain areas of dystrophic calcification. Rarely, they may show neoplastic transformation into locally aggressive "proliferating trichilemmal cysts."

In radiological imaging, they appear as small round or oval, well-circumscribed nodules under the skin. There is no involvement of adjacent skin or bone [4]. Lesions that are mostly hypoechoic on US have a heterogeneous internal structure. While most lesions show posterior acoustic enhancement, they do not show blood supply on Doppler US due to their avascular nature [1, 5]. While it appears as well-circumscribed lesion with soft tissue density on CT, it may contain mottled calcifications and high-density areas due to the cholesterol crystals and keratin it contains. Lesions that are iso-hyperintense on T1-weighted images due to dense content on MRI may have linear or reticular hypointensities on T2-weighted images due to the calcifications they contain. They do not show internal enhancement in CT or MRI contrast-enhanced series [3].

If the lesion is larger than 5 cm, has grown rapidly, is heterogeneously hyperintense on T2-weighted images, or shows contrast enhancement, neoplastic transformation into proliferating trichilemmal cysts should be suspected. Epidermal inclusion cysts, also known as epidermoid or sebaceous cysts, which are included in the differential diagnosis, are rare on the scalp and often have high or mixed signal intensities on both T1- and T2-weighted images [3].

6.2.2 Proliferative Trichilemmal Cyst

Proliferative trichilemmal cysts, also known as proliferative trichilemmal tumors, are dermal or subcutaneous tumors with squamoid cytological features and trichilemmal-type keratinization that usually occur on the scalp. Proliferative trichilemmal cysts have a female predominance [6, 7]. Cases associated with Cowden syndrome have been reported. Proliferative trichilemmal cysts appear in the scalp as lobulated masses ranging in size from a few millimeters to centimeters in size. Histopathologically, it shows intense epithelial proliferation, mild cytological nuclear atypia and mitotic activity. Despite being benign, it is locally invasive in nature. Rarely, it may present with a clinical picture of infection or malignant transformation [6].

Proliferative trichilemmal cysts usually appear as multiple complex subcutaneous solid or cystic masses. On US, they appear as heterogeneous hypoechoic lesions with posterior acoustic enhancement. Cystic components sometimes contain layers of high-density proteinaceous material. Sometimes a ring-like mineralization pattern is also encountered. On CT, benign lesions appear as well-circumscribed, non-contrast-enhancing masses, while areas with dense content may show mild hyperdensity [4, 5]. On MRI, they generally appear as well-circumscribed lesions that are hypo/isointense on T1- and heterogeneous hyperintense on T2-weighted images. Areas with dense content can be selected as hyperintense on T1-, and areas of calcification can be selected as hypointense on T2-weighted images. The fact that the lesion borders are irregular and contain areas with contrast enhancement areas implies the infiltrative nature of the lesion [8].

While epidermal inclusion cysts primarily come to mind in the differential diagnosis of benign lesions, other soft tissue tumors should also be considered in locally invasive/malignant lesions.

6.2.3 Epidermal Inclusion Cyst

Epidermal inclusion cyst or epidermal cysts are frequently encountered lesions that occur in the dermis or subdermis as a result of the proliferation of squamous epithelium. It is also considered a type of dermoid cyst or called as an epidermoid cyst by some authors. Although the term sebaceous cyst is sometimes used incorrectly, this naming is incorrect because it does not originate from the sebaceous glands [9]. While most lesions are detected incidentally, the most common symptom is a palpable, painless, hard mass. If they rupture, inflammatory changes may be observed around the lesion. Scalp, face, and nape are the most common locations. Rarely, they can also be seen within bones. Rarely, they may transform into squamous cell carcinoma. Etiologically, trauma or surgical implantations, congenital cell residues, or human papillomaviruses are blamed [10, 11].

Epidermal inclusion cysts appear on US as hypoechoic, well-circumscribed, round masses compared to the subcutaneous fatty tissue. Sometimes they may have a lobulated contour, less often a tubular shape. Small lesions may be anechoic, while large lesions may have heterogeneous echoes due to fat, calcification, or mucoid matter. When they become infected, the internal density increases due to purulent material. When they rupture, their contours may show lobulation, their borders become irregular, and they may show vascularity [10, 11].

They appear as water-dense lesions on CT. They generally have a thin hyperdense wall. On MRI like central nervous system epidermoid cysts, they are observed as hypointense or intermediate signal intensity on T1-weighted images and hyperintense on T2-weighted images. While a T2 flare effect is seen in diffusion-weighted imaging (DWI), hypointensity due to diffusion restriction can be observed on the ADC map in some lesions. While no central contrast enhancement is observed in contrast-enhanced series, they may show peripheral thin-wall contrast enhancement. Ruptured lesions may be accompanied by thick and irregular peripheral enhancement and heterogeneous enhancement in the adjacent subcutaneous fatty tissue [10, 11].

Pilomatrichoma, neurogenic tumors, nodular fasciitis, and myxoid tumors can be considered in the differential diagnosis.

6.2.4 Pilomatricoma

Pilomatricoma is a rare, benign tumor thought to arise from hair cortex cells. They constitute 0.1% of cutaneous tumors and 20% of hair follicle tumors. It is more common in women (F:M = 3:2). There are two peaks in the first and sixth decades. Overall, 40% of cases occur before age of 10 and 60% before the third decade of the life. Sarcoidosis can be seen together with pathologies such as Gardner and Turner syndrome [1, 5]. In total, approximately 50% of cases occur in the head and neck region. They generally appear as painless, hard, mobile masses ranging from 0.5 to 5 cm in diameter. It is located superficially and a bluish-red discoloration may be detected on the skin. Their growth rate is low [12].

Pilomatricomas are superficial lesions observed at the junction of the skin and subcutaneous fatty tissue. They mostly appear as well-circumscribed oval or round lesions showing calcification. The skin over the lesion is generally thinned. On US, they appear as target lesions containing hyperechoic epithelial cells surrounded by a capsule of hypoechoic connective tissue [13]. Subcutaneous nodular lesions containing well-circumscribed microcalcifications are seen on CT. On MRI, on T1-weighted images, they are seen as low, medium or high signal lesions depending on their content, while on T2-weighted images they are observed as intermediate or high signal with homogeneous or heterogeneous intensity. Contrast-enhanced images may show variable peripheral contrast enhancement in some lesions [1, 14].

Epidermal inclusion cyst, calcified hematoma, dermoid cyst, and foreign body reaction should be kept in mind in the differential diagnosis of pilomatricoma.

6.2.5 Dermatofibrosarcoma Protuberans

Dermatofibrosarcoma protuberans (DFSP) is a low-grade malignant neoplasm arising from the skin and (sub)cutaneous tissues. Although they are generally rare, they are the most common cutaneous sarcoma. Although it generally shows positive results, local recurrence rates are high. Although it is more common between the ages of 20–50, it can be encountered at any age of the life. It is slightly more common in men. Lesions begin as multi-nodular masses on the skin and spread to subcutaneous tissues [15]. It is most commonly found on the trunk and proximal extremities, followed by the head and neck area of the body. These tumors, which are neglected due to their slow growth, can reach large sizes.

Lesions ranging in size from 1 cm to very large sizes have been described in the literature [16].

They appear as non-mineralized, round or oval soft tissue masses within the skin and subcutaneous fatty tissue. They are generally well-circumscribed and have slightly lobulated contours [1]. On US, they generally appear as heterogeneous hypoechoic lesions. Focal hypoechoic areas separated by linear or ovoid hypoechoicities may be seen. They may contain small echogenic foci that do not show comet artifact. Posterior acoustic enhancement is common. They show moderate blood flow, mostly peripheral, on Doppler US [16]. On CT, they generally appear as subcutaneous masses with homogeneous soft tissue density. They often show homogeneous contrast enhancement in contrast-enhanced examination. In large tumors, low-density areas due to intratumoral necrosis or cystic degeneration may be seen [17]. On MRI, they are hypointense on T1-weighted images and are isointense or hyperintense with the subcutaneous fatty tissue on T2-weighted images. They maintain high signal in fat-suppressed T2-weighted images. They show significant enhancement in postcontrast sequences [16, 17].

6.2.6 Dermoid/Epidermoid Cysts

Dermoid/epidermoid cysts, which are generally seen in the intracranial region, spine, bone and genital organs, are inclusion cysts originating from the ectoderm. Rarely, they are also seen under the skin on the scalp. Dermoid cysts also have skin appendages, including hair, sebaceous and sweat glands, while epidermoid cysts are lined only by squamous epithelium. Although mature cystic teratoma and dermoid cyst are used interchangeably, teratomas must contain tissues from at least two embryological layers [1, 18].

They appear as well-circumscribed oval or round subcutaneous cystic lesions. Epidermoid cysts appear hypodense on CT, whereas on MRI they appear mild hyperintense in contrast to cerebrospinal fluid (CSF) on T1-weighted and iso/hyperintense on T2-weighted images. Sometimes linear or leveling hypointensity can be detected on T2-weighted images due to debris content. Hyperintensity due to diffusion restriction is characteristic in diffusion-weighted images. Dermoid cysts, on the other hand, appear significantly hypodense (in fat density) on CT due to their fat content, while they are observed as hyperintense on T1-weighted MRIs. Signal loss in fat-suppressed sequences aids diagnosis. Unlike lipomas, they have variable T2-weighted signal rangingfrom hypo- to hyperintensity [18, 19]. Both lesions retain contrast in the form of a thin peripheral rim in contrast-enhanced examinations, but cystic component contrast enhancement is not detected. When infected or ruptured, thick wall and septa enhancement may be observed [1, 19].

6.2.7 Lipoma

They are benign tumors originating from mature adipocytes. Scalp is not a frequent location for lipomas, which are quite common. These tumors, which are often located superficially under the skin on the trunk and extremities, can rarely be seen in deep localization in the muscle, bone, retroperitoneum in the thorax. They usually present as painless soft masses [1].

Lipomas are well-circumscribed masses with a thin capsule, and sometimes very thin compartments that have homogeneous fat imaging properties. Their sonographic appearance is variable and they are mostly iso/hyperechoic with subcutaneous fatty tissue. In encapsulated lesions, it is very difficult to detect the capsule on US. They do not show blood flow on Doppler US. Large size with internal heterogeneity and increased blood supply on Doppler US may be indicative for in terms of liposarcoma [1]. On CT, they typically appear as hypodense lesions with homogeneous fat density. The presence of areas of internal soft tissue density, especially in larger lesions with deeper location, should bring liposarcoma to mind. The presence of calcification is also more commonly associated with liposarcoma [1]. MRI is more sensitive than either examination for the differential diagnosis of liposarcoma. While lipomas are observed as hyperintense on both T1- and

T2-weighted images, they are suppressed on fat-suppressed sequences. Non-suppressed areas in fat-suppressed T2-weighted images should suggest liposarcoma. In contrast studies lipomas do not show any enhancement. The presence of enhanced areas and irregular margins may imply liposarcoma [20].

6.2.8 Infantile Hemangioma

Infantile hemangiomas, a benign vascular neoplasm, are among the most common head and neck tumors of infancy. These tumors, which are frequently seen in the orbital and parotid regions, are less common on the scalp. Lesions, which are typically not observed at birth, appear in the first year of life and grow rapidly. After a subsequent stable period, it starts to regress and 50% disappears by the age of 5 and 70% by the age of 7. Lesions that show red or blue discoloration depending on the depth of the skin are sometimes seen as lumps on the skin [21].

Lesions that appear radiologically as a well-circumscribed hyperechoic subcutaneous mass on US may show high-flow arterial and low-resistance venous flow patterns on Doppler US. On CT, they appear as lobulated masses that are isodense with adjacent muscle tissues and show intense homogeneous contrast enhancement. On MRI, they have intermediate signal intensity on T1-weighted and are hyperintense with signal void areas on T2-weighted images and maintain homogeneous contrast [22].

6.2.9 Basal Cell Carcinoma

Basal cell carcinoma is one of the most frequent types of non-melanocytic cancer of the skin. It is encountered in men and light-skinned people. It originates from the basal layer of the epidermis. It is generally locally aggressive and has high local recurrence rates. Distant metastasis rates are quite rare [23].

Sonographically, they appear as well-circumscribed skin lesions, being hypoechoic or having heterogeneous echotexture. The presence of hyperechoic areas within the lesions that do not cause posterior acoustic shadowing is useful in distinguishing them from other skin cancers. They may extend into deeper skin layers or muscle tissues with local invasion [24]. On MRI, they are iso/hyperintense compared to muscle tissue on T1-weighted images, while they are significantly hyperintense on T2-weighted images. They show contrast enhancement in contrast-enhanced T1-weighted images [24].

6.2.10 Keloid Scar

They are extreme fibrotic skin reactions secondary to injury or inflammation. Histopathologically, there is type I and type III collagen proliferation in the hypodermis. Its limits may extend beyond the original injury site. Clinically, they present as hard nodules that may be accompanied by pain and itching. While hypertrophic scars are limited to the injury site, keloids generally tend to exceed these boundaries [25].

Sonographically, keloids are hypoechoic lesions located in the dermis-hypodermis. Calcification may be observed. Doppler US is useful in demonstrating vascularity in the proliferative phase [26]. On MRI, lesions have low signal on both T1- and T2-weighted images due to the fibrous reaction. Moderate to severe contrast enhancement can be observed in the proliferation phase in postcontrast series. In the presence of necrosis, the lesion may acquire a heterogeneous appearance due to cystic areas [1]. Dermatofibrosarcoma protuberans, hypertrophic scar, and scleroderma should be kept in mind in the differential diagnosis.

6.2.11 Melanocytic Nevus (Mole)

Nevus, which form as a result of benign proliferation of melanocytic cells, can be seen at epidermal junctions, called “junctional nevi,” in the dermis (intradermal nevi), or in both compartments, called “compound nevi.” Melanocytic nevi, also called moles, are most common in the fourth to fifth decades. Women are more affected.

There is a linear relationship between lesion size and the risk of malignant transformation. Nevus that increases in size should be followed closely in this regard. Congenital forms on the scalp tend to regress over time [27].

Melanocytic nevi appear as flat patch lesions on the skin. Although they are generally limited to the skin, subcutaneous tissue invasions can rarely be observed in large-sized ones. Due to the melanin content, the lesions are observed as hyperdense on CT. Due to the paramagnetic effect of melanin, they are selected as hyperintense on T1-weighted and hypontense on T2-weighted MRI [1].

6.2.12 Primary Cutaneous Melanoma

It is a very aggressive tumor originating from pigment-producing melanocytes. Since melanocytes are located in the basal layer of the skin, they are generally seen on the skin, but they can appear in any part of the body. They are more common in the sixth decade and in men. They are the skin cancer that most frequently causes death due to high metastasis rates, although they are less common than other skin cancers [28]. Etiologically, the most common causes are excessive sun and therefore ultraviolet ray exposure, having light-colored skin, radiation or solvent exposure, CDKN2A mutation and xeroderma pigmentosum. Due to pigment production, the lesions have a distinctly pigmented appearance on inspection, but no color change is observed on the skin in amelanocytic forms. Lesions may spread superficially throughout the basal layer, or they may spread deeply, as in nodular melanoma. There is a direct correlation between lesion size and distant metastasis and lymph node involvement. Lesions located on the scalp tend to be larger than other regions [28, 29].

Due to the paramagnetic effect of melanin, lesions appear hyperintense on T1-weighted images and hypointense on T2-weighted images on MRI. These lesions appear hyperdense on CT. Amelanotic melanomas are iso-hypointense on T1W and hyper-isointense on T2W. Lesion signal becomes heterogeneous in the presence of intratumoral hemorrhage and necrosis [29, 30].

6.2.13 Squamous Cell Carcinoma

Squamous cell cancer (SCC), one of the most common skin cancers, is less common on the scalp. It usually occurs in the sixth to seventh decades. SCCs located on the scalp are diagnosed at an advanced stage because they are diagnosed later and are an indicator of poor prognosis. Tumor size greater than 10 mm, poor margins, and history of radiation are indicators of high risk [31].

They generally appear as flat skin lesions like BCCs. Tumors that appear nonspecifically hypointense on T1-weighted images and iso-hyperintense on T2-weighted images on MRI can not be distinguished from BCC. They show enhancement on contrast-enhanced T1-weighted images. In large lesions, they may show ulcerations and heterogeneity. Due to their tendency to be more invasive than BCC, invasion into deep soft tissues is detected more frequently [30, 32].

6.3 Calvarial Lesions

The bone structure that protects the brain tissue from the external environment is called calvarium. It consists of frontal, parietal, occipital, temporal, sphenoid, and ethmoid bones, which hold each other tightly with immovable joints called sutures. Calvarial lesions may arise directly from the calvarium or may occur secondary to invasion from the skin or intracranial lesions. The medullary bone that fills the gap between the cortical bone tissue, called the inner and outer tabula, is called the diploe distance [2]. Congenital, infective/inflammatory, tumoral, or traumatic events can affect the calvarium, and benign/malignant focal lesions will be mentioned here.

6.3.1 Eosinophilic Granuloma

It is a component of the spectrum of Langerhans Cell Histiocytosis, which occurs as a result of monoclonal uncontrolled proliferation of Langerhans cells and is characterized by "granuloma." Eosinophilic granuloma is a form characterized by single organ involvement and a single lesion, and the calvarium is the most commonly affected tissue. The clinic varies depending on the organ involved. It is more common in the pediatric population and in males [33].

On CT, they are seen as solitary lytic lesions, mostly in the parietal bone. Generally, sclerotic rim is not observed. Bone tissue residue can be seen within the lesion, which is called "button sequestrum." On MRI, the lesions appear nonspecifically hypointense on T1-weighted and hyperintense on T2-weighted images, while they show contrast enhancement in contrast-enhanced series [2, 33]. Epidermoid cyst, intradiploic hemangioma, and osteoblastoma should be considered in the differential diagnosis (Fig. 6.1a–d).

6.3.2 Intradiploic Epidermoid/Dermoid Cyst

Epidermoid and dermoid cysts can rarely be located in the diploe distance. They generally appear as slowly growing swellings. Parietal and temporal bones are more commonly involved. While epidermoid cysts are generally seen in people between the ages of 20 and 50, dermoid cysts occur mostly in the first 3 years of life [2].

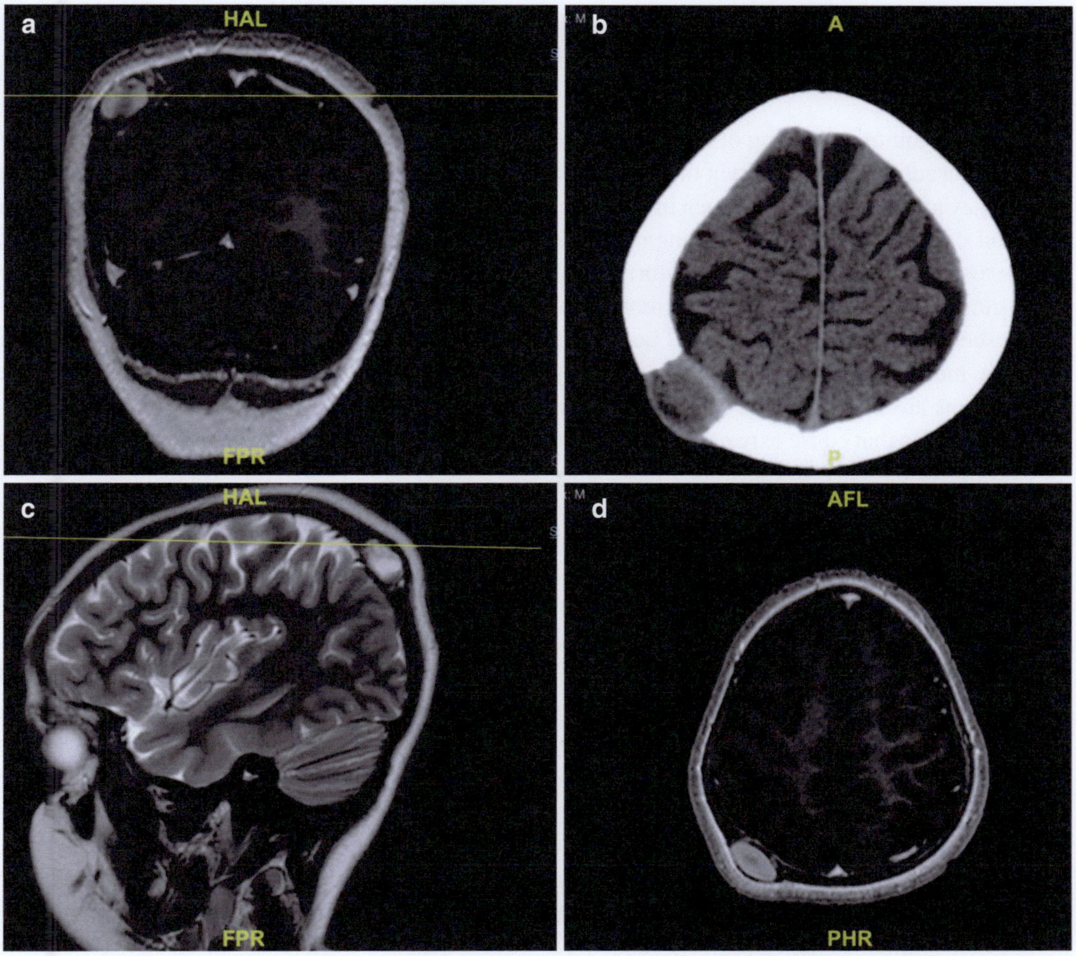

Fig. 6.1 (**a**–**d**) T1 coronal contrast enhanced, T2 sagittal and axial postcontrast MRIs (**a**–**c**) and Plain CT axial images (**d**) showing a T2 hetero-intense lesion enhancing on contrast in the parietal region. Biopsy: Hematoma with xanthogranulomatous reaction and dense inflammation

The lesions appear as lytic lesions with well-defined borders and sclerotic edges on plain radiography and CT. As a result of expansion in the bone structure, they cause thinning and springing in the tables, especially in the inner tables. On MRI, epidermoid cysts are mild hyperintense on T1-weighted images and iso or hyperintense on T2-weighted images in contrast to CSF, and they do not show contrast enhancement. Diffusion restriction is characteristic in diffusion-weighted images. Dermoid cysts are observed as hyperintense on T1-weighted images due to their fatty content [34, 35]. In the differential diagnosis, eosinophilic granuloma and hemangioma should be considered.

6.3.3 Primary Intraosseous Hemangioma

It is a benign tumor consisting of small and large diameter vascular channels seen in the diploe distance. They are most commonly seen in the vertebrae and calvarium. Calvarial hemangiomas are called "osseous venous vascular malformation" in the current nomenclature. They are most commonly seen in the frontal and parietal bones and they are more common in older women [33]. Most lesions are asymptomatic due to their slow growth. Lesions that cause expansion can present as swelling in the calvarium. Sometimes pathological fractures or high flow rates may cause shunt-related symptoms. Among cavernous, capillary and venous histopathological types, the cavernous form is most frequent one [36].

On CT, they appear as slightly expanded, lytic lesions with sclerotic edges. The "sunburst pattern" caused by thickened trabeculae radiating from the central part is characteristic. Thinning due to expansion can be detected in the inner and outer tables. The lesion signal on MRI may vary depending on the amount of fat it contains. While a typical hemangioma appears hyperintense on T1- and T2-weighted images, it shows significant homogeneous enhancement on contrast-enhanced T1-weighted images [36, 37]. In the differential diagnosis, epidermoid/dermoid cyst and eosinophilic granuloma can be considered.

6.3.4 Intraosseous Lipoma

Intraosseous lipomas, which constitute 1–2% of all bone lesions, are benign tumors consisting of mature fat clusters in the medullary space. It is most commonly seen in men in fourth and fifth decades. Lipomas, which are mostly seen in the lower extremities, are found in the calvarium at a rate of 7%. It is most commonly observed in the frontal, parietal and temporal bones. Their average size is around 3–5 cm. Areas of necrosis or calcifications may develop within the lesions. While lipomas are mostly asymptomatic clinically, the presenting complaint is usually pain [38].

In lipomas, which generally appear as well-circumscribed lytic lesions on radiography, calcification may be observed within the lesion (cockade sign). On CT, lipomas appear as medullary mass lesions with fat density. On MRI, they are observed as hyperintense on T1- and T2-weighted images due to their fat content. In the presence of necrosis within the lesion, hypointense and hyperintense areas can be detected on T1 and T2-weighted images, respectively. If calcification is present, hypointense foci can be detected on the aforementioned MR sequences [38, 39].

6.3.5 Intraosseous Meningioma

Intraosseous meningiomas, the most common form of extradural meningiomas, constitute less than 1% of osseous tumors. Although embryologically it is thought to arise from arachnoid meningothelial valve cell remnants extending to the sutures, most lesions have no relation with the sutures. It is often confused with the most plaque meningiomas, which are accompanied by a significant intracranial mass. Hyperostosis or bone invasions can be observed in the most plaque meningiomas. In meningiomas, which are more common in women, the clinical picture results mostly from mass effect. A palpable mass is also among the frequent findings (Fig. 6.2a–d) [40, 41].

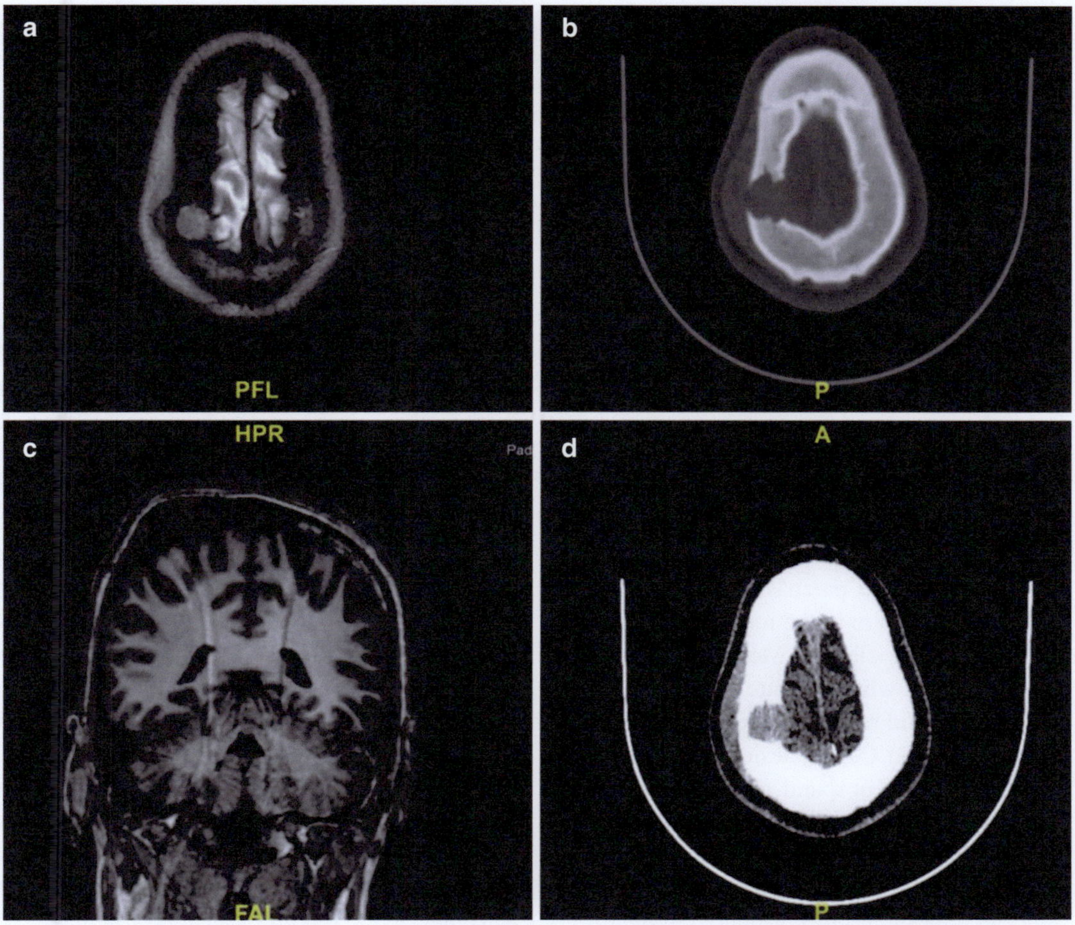

Fig. 6.2 (**a–d**) MRI Brain T2 axial and T1 coronal and CT brain plain axial—Bone window and postcontrast axial showing a lesion in the right parietal region. Biopsy: Langerhans cell Histiocytosis

The appearance of the lesions varies depending on whether they are osteoblastic or osteolytic. Most lesions are osteoblastic and are observed on CT with sclerosis causing expansion of the bone structure. Osteolytic lesions are observed as lesions with hypodense soft tissue density on non-contrast CT. On MRI, hypointensity on T1- and iso/hyperintensity on T2-weighted iamges are detected along with expansion of the bone structure. They show significant enhancement on contrast-enhanced images, similar to dural meningiomas [40, 41]. In the differential diagnosis, Paget's disease (no contrast enhancement), fibrous dysplasia (more expansile), and osteosarcoma (irregular contour and heterogeneous contrast enhancement) should be kept in mind.

6.3.6 Calvarial Donut Lesions

They are radiolucent skull defects with a peripheral sclerotic halo. Irregular bone nidus can be observed within the lesion, which consists of mesenchymal and fibrous tissue elements. Lesions of unknown etiology are mostly detected in middle-advanced ages. It is usually solitary. Most cases are asymptomatic and are detected incidentally [42].

On radiography, the lesions appear as lucent areas with peripheral sclerotic lines anywhere in the calvarium. In large lesions, sclerotic edges may become irregular. Irregularly shaped sclerotic densities can be detected in the lucency center of the lesion. The appearance is similar on CT. Sometimes lesions may cause expansion in the external table. On MRI, lesions appear hypointense on T1- and especially T2-weighted sequences due to fibrous elements. A hypointense sclerotic ring surrounds the lesion. Since the central nidus is also hypointense on MRI, CT is superior for nidus imaging [42, 43]. Eosinophilic granuloma, epidermoid cyst, and hemangioma can be considered in the differential diagnosis.

6.3.7 Osteoma

They are benign bone tumors consisting of lamellar/cortical type bone. They are often observed in the calvarium. The female/male ratio is equal. Most lesions are asymptomatic and are detected incidentally. They are usually found in the bone cortex, often in the paranasal sinuses and skull base. When they are in the medullary bone, they are called “bone islands.” Most of the time they are solitary, but when they are multiple, Gardner syndrome should be considered [44].

On X-ray and CT, the lesions appear as cotically located, oval or round, distinct dense formations. On MRI, they are observed as significantly hypointense on both T1- and T2-weighted images [44, 45]. Exocytosis, fibrous dysplasia, and osteosarcoma should be considered in the differential diagnosis.

6.3.8 Hyperostosis Frontalis Interna

Hyperostosis frontalis interna, defined by Morgagni in 1719 as a pathology accompanying virilism and obesity, is characterized by excessive growth of the internal table of the frontal bone. Sometimes it may be continuous with the parietal bones. The inner tabula can be smooth and nodular in character. Its etiology is unknown and it has no clinical significance. Most cases are detected incidentally [2, 46].

In radiological examinations, it is observed as a diffuse widening of the diploe distance in the frontal bones. The inner tabula may be well-circumscribed or nodular. Sometimes parietal bones are also involved, which is defined as hyperostosis fronto-parietalis. The affected bones maintain normal signal structure [46, 47]. Fibrous dysplasia is at the forefront in the differential diagnosis.

6.3.9 Craniofacial Fibrous Dysplasia

Fibrous dysplasia is a benign bone tumor that occurs as a result of disruption in mature lamellar bone formation and intramedullary fibro-osseous proliferation. One of the most common sites of involvement is cranial and facial bones. Although it is mostly seen in young adults and children, it can be detected at any age. There are monostotic forms involving a single bone or polyostotic forms involving more than one bone. While most cases are asymptomatic, the most common findings are bone pain, visual and hearing disorders secondary to expansion and compression. Anterior bones such as frontal, sphenoid, and maxillary bones are more frequently affected (Fig. 6.3a, b) [48].

Expansion of the affected bone structure and loss of cortico-medullary distinction are essential. While a homogeneous ground-glass density appearance is generally dominant on CT, sometimes a mixed pattern with lucent and sclerotic areas can be observed. Preservation of the inner and outer tabulae (cortex) is an important finding in distinguishing Paget’s disease. Generally, the border of the lesion with normal bone is unclear, but it can also be seen with sharp boundaries [49, 50]. On MRI, heterogeneous intermediate signal intensity on T1- and heterogeneous hypointensity on T2-weighted images are the dominant findings in the expanded bone medulla. Sometimes it may be accompanied by hyperintense areas on T2-weighted images. It has been reported that a heterogeneous enhancement is seen in contrast-enhanced T1-weighted MRIs [49, 50]. Paget’s disease, metastases, and intraosseous meningioma should be kept in mind in the differential diagnosis.

6.3.10 Metastasis

Distant organ metastasis of an existing tumoral lesion via hematogenous route occurs frequently to the bones, despite being less common than

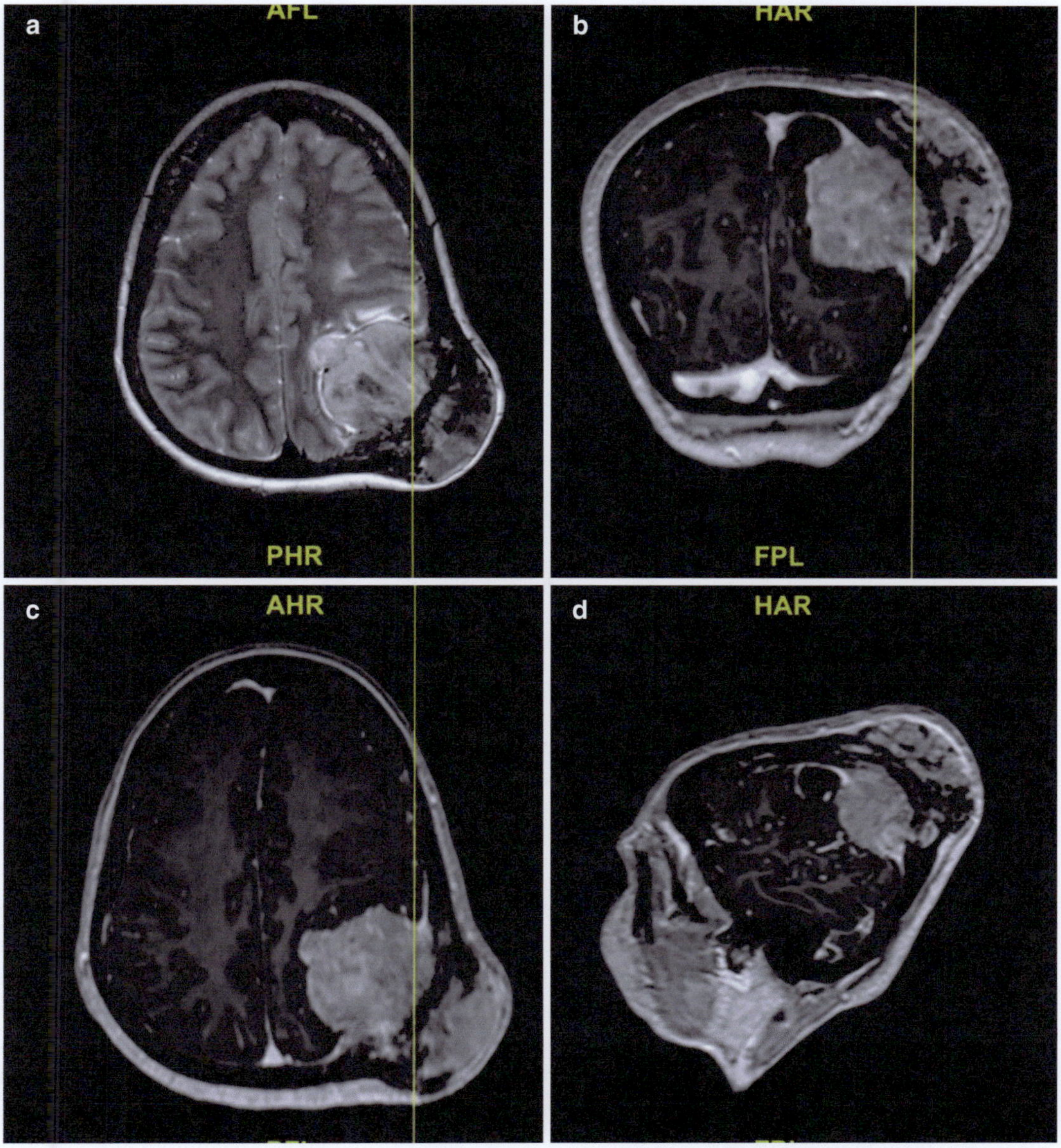

Fig. 6.3 (**a–d**) MRIs (axial T2, postcontrast coronal, axial and sagittal T1). Preoperative appearance of the meningioma with trans-dural extension and bony hyperostosis

lung and liver. Although bone metastases are mostly to the vertebrae and pelvic bones where the red bone marrow is located, calvarium metastases are also seen at a significant rate. The most common metastases to the calvarium are from lung, breast, and prostate cancers and renal cell carcinoma. Metastases usually present with local bone pain and a palpable mass, though the patients are mostly asymptomatic. They can be lytic, sclerotic (osteoblastic) or mixed types. Lung, kidney, and thyroid cancers are more likely to cause lytic metastases, while prostate and breast cancers are more prone to cause sclerotic metastases (Fig. 6.4a–c) [51–55].

The radiological appearance of bone metastases varies depending on whether they are lytic, sclerotic, or mixed. The sensitivity of plain radiographs in detecting metastasis is relatively low.

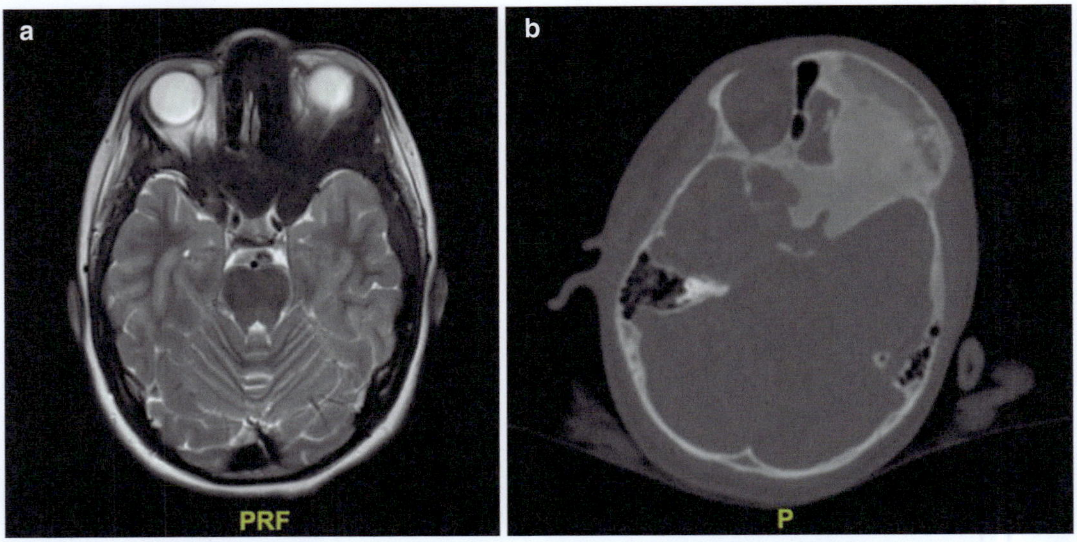

Fig. 6.4 (**a**, **b**) T2 MRI (**a**) and Plain CT scan (**b**) axial slices show diffuse enlargement of the fronto-orbital region with compression of the optic nerve foramina secondary to fibrous dysplasia

Scanning the whole body with CT is not preferred because it will cause high radiation exposure. Although MRI is very sensitive in bone marrow evaluation, whole body MRI is not widely used. In this regard, bone scintigraphy is generally preferred in screening for bone metastasis in the presence of a known malignancy [2].

Osteolytic bone metastases appear as poorly circumscribed lucent lesions on radiographs. Bone metastases often occur in the medullary bone, and cortical involvement generally occurs with the spread of the medullary lesion. For a medullary metastasis to be visible on direct radiograph, at least 50% loss of bone trabeculae is required. In this regard, plain radiographs have low sensitivity in detecting bone metastasis. Additionally, lesion detection becomes more difficult in patients with osteoporosis. On CT, osteolytic metastases are observed as lucent lesions in soft tissue density. The destruction of the cortex and periosteal reaction can be easily demonstrated in cortical and periosteal lesions, respectively. In particular, cortex destruction and periosteal reactions in periosteal lesions in cases with cortical lesions can be easily demonstrated. MRI is quite reliable in detecting medullary lesions and differentiating osteolytic/osteoblastic metastases due to its high soft tissue resolution. Osteolytic lesions are observed as hypointense on T1- and hyperintense on T2-weighted images. Fat-suppressed T2-weighted sequences and diffusion-weighted imaging (DWI) are more sensitive sequences in detecting metastasis. Although their appearance varies on contrast-enhanced images, most osteolytic metastases show enhancement [51–55].

Osteoblastic bone metastases are observed as well-defined radio-opacities on radiography. On CT, osteoblastic metastases appear as distinct hyperdense, oval or round lesions. MRI is very sensitive in detecting osteoblastic metastases located in the bone marrow. On T1- and T2-weighted images, the lesions are hypointense and easily differentiated from normal bone marrow. However, MRI is disadvantageous for cortical lesions and osteoblastic metastases in bones with small diploe distance [51–55].

Mixed type metastases have the characteristics of both types of metastases in varying proportions. In the differential diagnosis, multiple myeloma, lymphoma, and non-ossifying fibroma should be considered primarily in lytic lesions, while bone islands, osteoma, or a treated lytic metastasis may come to mind in sclerotic lesions. In mixed type metastases, non-ossifying fibroma, fibrous dysplasia, and Paget's disease should be considered.

6.3.11 Multiple Myeloma/Plasmocytoma

These tumors, which are formed as a result of monoclonal proliferation of plasma cells in the bone marrow, are called plasmocytoma when they are solitary, and are called "multiple myeloma" in case they are multiple. Its incidence increases in men over the age of 50. It is one of the most common bone malignancies in adults. Clinically, it most commonly presents with intermittent bone pain. In time, the pain becomes permanent. Anemia, hyperkalemia, proteinuria, and renal failure are other findings. Bone lesions may cause compression fractures, more commonly in the vertebrae or long bones. Although it is most commonly seen in the vertebrae, skull involvement is also quite frequent [56–58].

Imaging is useful in diagnosing disease as well as demonstrating complications and monitoring disease progression. They usually appear as multiple sharply circumscribed lytic lesions. Punched out lucencies are the most important finding on plain radiographs. This appearance, caused by numerous lesions, is called "raindrop skull." Lesions adjacent to the cortex may cause endosteal scalloping. It can rarely be seen in sclerotic lesions. CT has higher sensitivity and specificity, and lytic soft tissue lesions can be easily visualized, similar to X-ray [56, 58].

MRI is more sensitive than these two examinations in showing bone marrow lesions. Lesions are generally hypointense on T1- and hyperintense on T2-weighted images, with significant contrast. In the presence of diffuse involvement, they may appear isointense with normal bone marrow on T1-weighted images. On diffusion MRI, lesions show significant diffusion restriction. MRI enhancement patterns can be focal, diffuse, or mixed [56–58]. In the differential diagnosis, metastatic disease should first be kept in mind.

6.3.12 Chordoma

Chordomas, which are rare malignant tumors, originate from the embryological remains of the primitive notochord. It can be seen in bones at any level from Rathke's pouch to the coccyx. The most common region after the sacrococcygeal region is the clivus. They are locally aggressive tumors. They are most commonly seen in men aged 20–40. Due to their slow growth, they generally do not cause symptoms, or radiological findings related with pressure on adjacent structures may be observed [54, 59].

Although MRI, which has superior soft tissue resolution, is quite helpful for the diagnosis of the lesion, CT is more useful in determining the calcification pattern within the lesion and evaluating osteolysis. Lesions are observed on CT as well-circumscribed, destructive and expansile soft tissue masses. Sclerosis may be seen at the lesion borders. Irregular calcifications due to sequestrum, hypodense areas due to necrosis and hemorrhage may be observed within the lesion. Moderate to severe contrast enhancement may be observed [54, 59].

On MRI, the lesions have low or intermediate signal intensity on T1-weighted images, while hyperintense on T2-weighted images. Heterogeneous contrast enhancement is observed in contrast-enhanced series, and non-enhancing calcification areas may cause a "honeycomb" appearance. Significant diffusion restriction indicates poor prognosis [54, 59, 60]. Chondrosarcoma and plasmacytoma should be considered in the differential diagnosis.

6.3.13 Chondrosarcoma

Chondrosarcomas, which are cartilage-derived malignant tumors, are the third most common malignant bone tumor, but calvarial involvement is less than 2%. Involvement of the petro-occipital synchondrosis, sphenoethmoidal junction, and sella turcica is observed in the calvarium, respectively. Most lesions present with findings due to mass effect on adjacent tissues. They are usually sporadic. Unlike chordomas, they are generally observed outside the midline. With local spread, they spread to the cavernous sinuses, paranasal sinuses and skull base [54, 61].

Chondrosarcomas are usually larger than 4 cm at the time of diagnosis. Lesions are generally seen as lytic lesions on plain radiography and CT. There is a high rate of matrix calcifications (annular and arc-shaped calcifications are characteristic) within the lesion. Endosteal scalloping is a common finding. On MRI, low-signal calcifications can be observed within lesions with low signals on T1- and high signals on T2-weighted images. Chondrosarcomas show heterogeneous contrast enhancement on CT and MRI. Since diffusion restrictions are greater than chordoma, they show lower apparent diffusion coefficient (ADC) values [54, 60, 61].

Chordoma and metastases should be considered first in the differential diagnosis.

6.4 Conclusion

Scalp and calvarium are the anatomical sites where lesions associated with numerous pathologies can be seen, and patient age, clinical history, as well as radiological findings are important for differential diagnosis. There are many other lesions which are rarer and need to be kept in mind for the differential diagnosis (Figs. 6.5, 6.6, 6.7, 6.8 and 6.9). Familiarity with the typical localization of the lesions and radiological imaging features signals will help narrow the differential diagnosis.

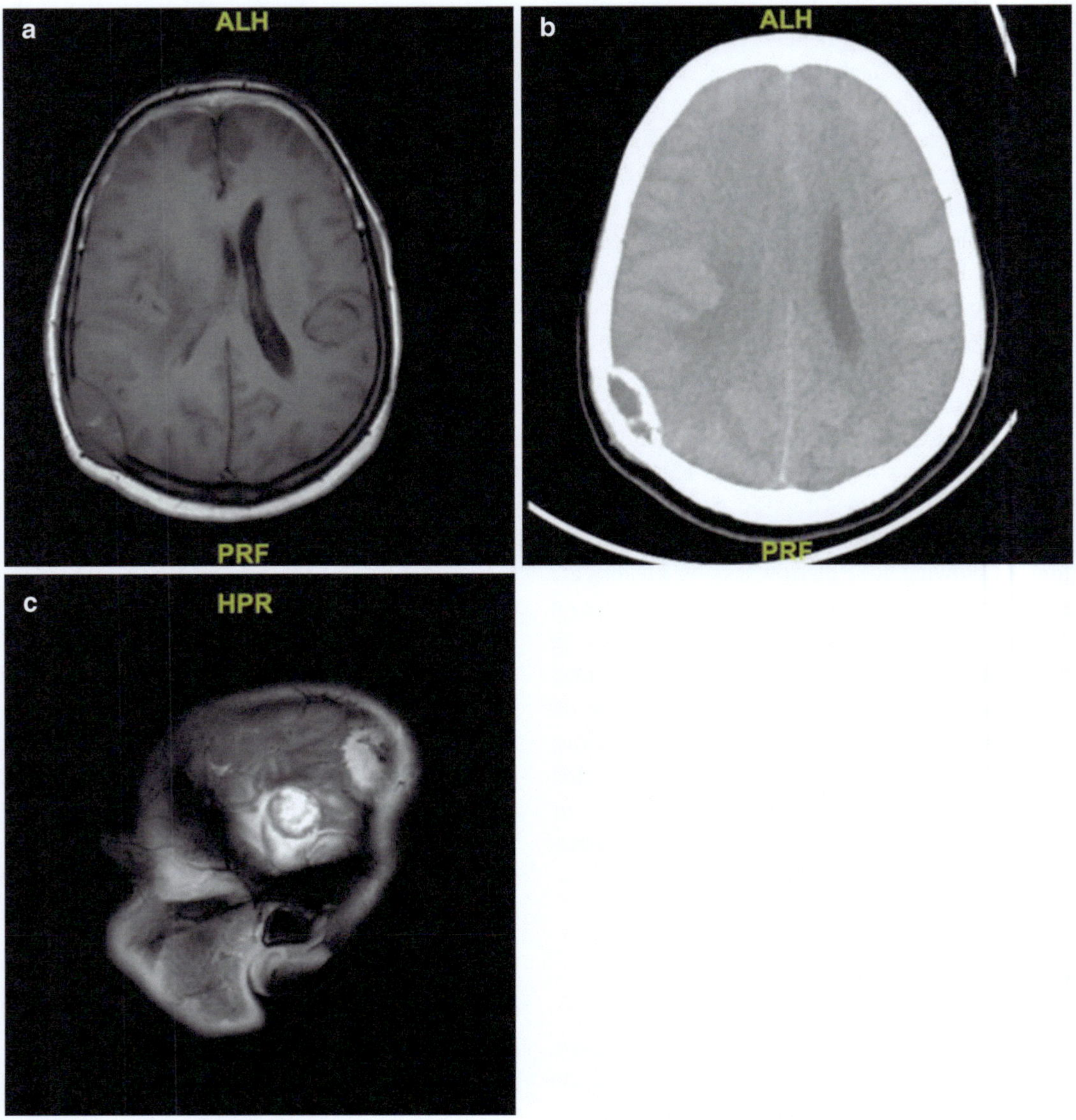

Fig. 6.5 (**a–c**) Axial slices of MRI T1 plain and T2 sagittal (**a**, **b**) and axial plain CT (**c**) a calvarial lesion of the right parietal region. Biopsy: Metastatic papillary adenocarcinoma

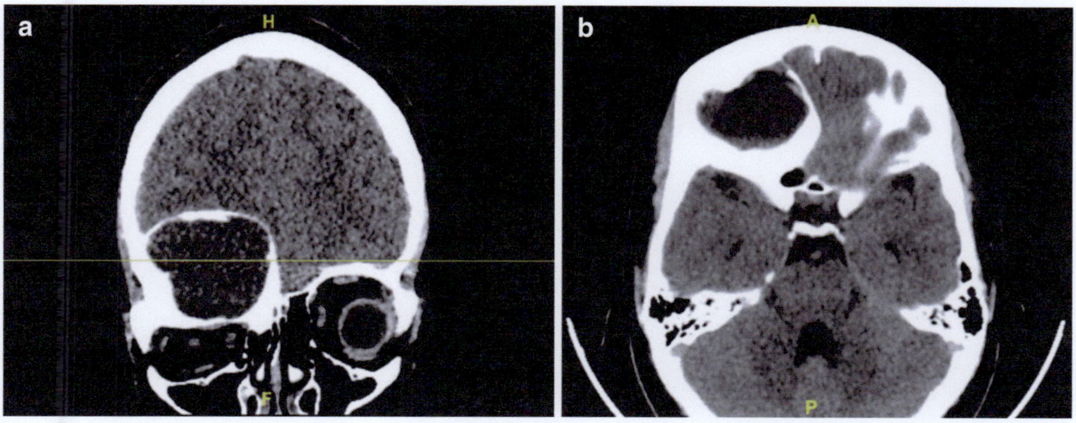

Fig. 6.6 (**a**, **b**) Plain CT scan axial images showing a cystic bony interosseus lesion of the orbit. Biopsy: Psammomatoid juvenile ossifying fibroma

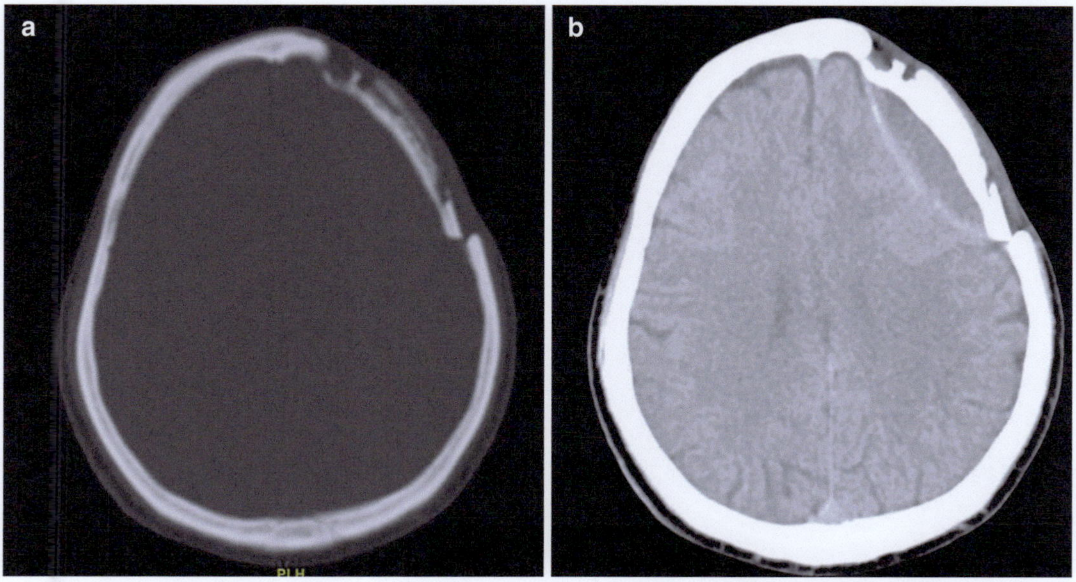

Fig. 6.7 (**a**, **b**) Computed tomography axial bone window and axial postcontrast showing destruction of the bone of the left frontal region with islands of normal bone in between along with subdural pus suggestive of osteomyelitis of the skull

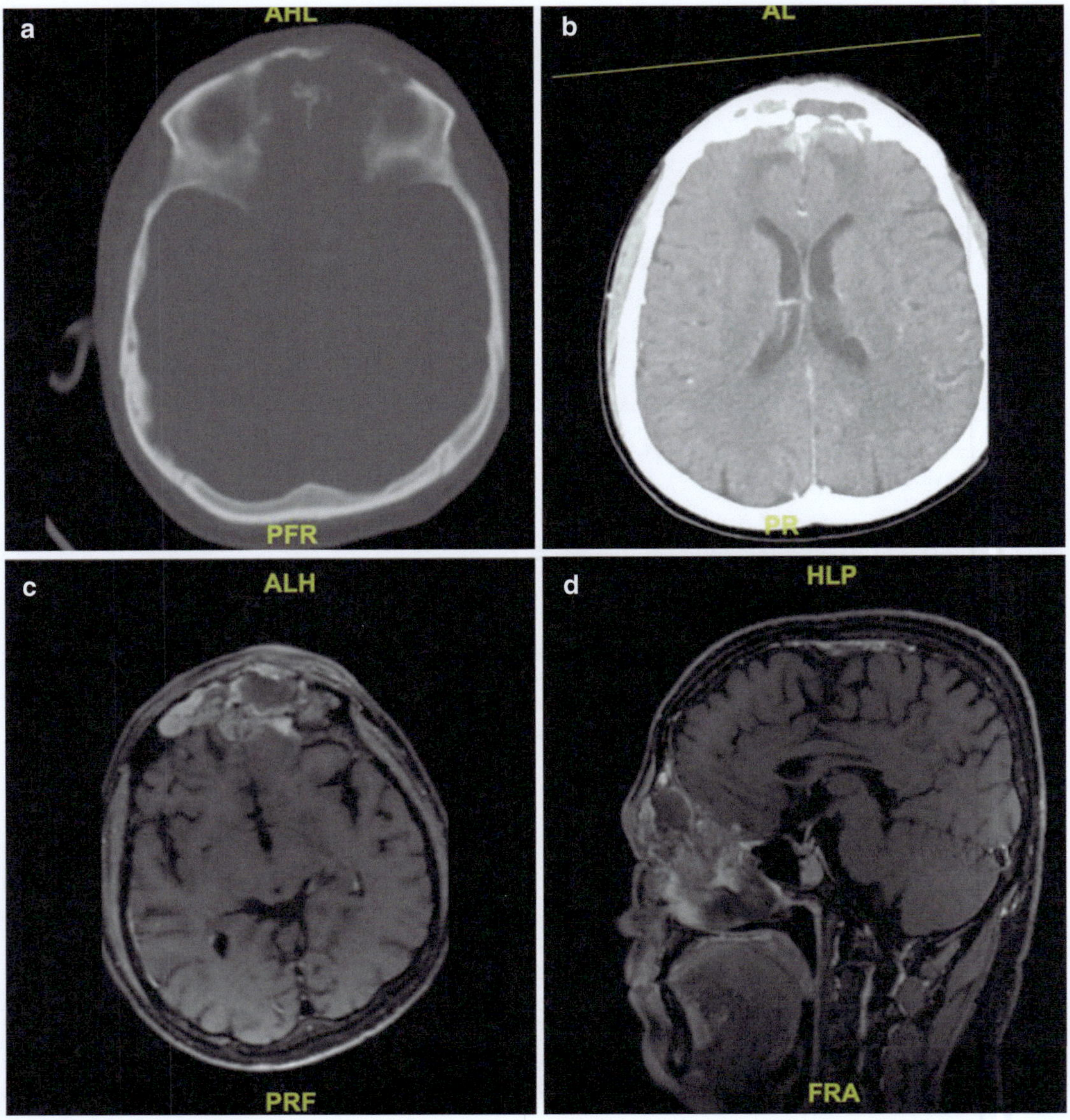

Fig. 6.8 (**a**–**d**) CT Brain plain axial–Bone window and postcontrast axial and MRIs (postcontrast T1 axial and sagittal) showing a lesion in the frontal bone and orbita. Biopsy: Recurrent Ewing's Sarcoma)

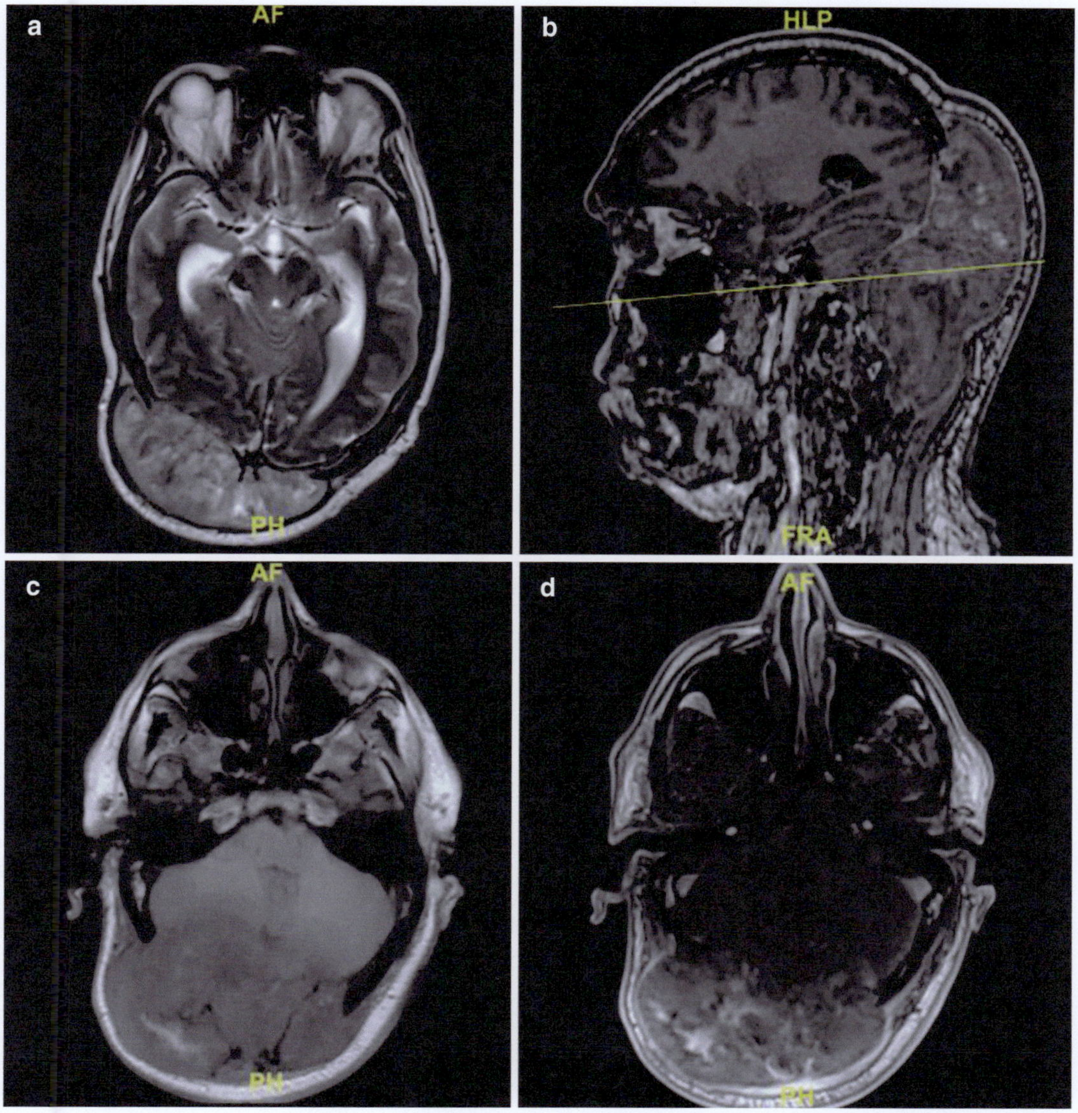

Fig. 6.9 (**a**–**d**) MRI Brain T2 axial and T1 axial plain T1 sagittal and axial–post contrast showing a lesion in the right parieto occipital region. Biopsy: Spindle cell sarcoma; occcipitocalvarial

References

1. Kawaguchi M, Kato H, Matsuo M. CT and MRI features of scalp lesions. Radiol Med. 2019;124(10):1049–61.
2. Yalçin O, Yildirim T, Kizilkiliç O, Hürcan CE, Koç Z, Aydin V, Sen O, Kayaselçuk F. CT and MRI findings in calvarial non-infectious lesions. Diagn Interv Radiol. 2007;13(2):68–74.
3. Gossner J, Larsen J. Incidental subcutaneous nodules on the scalp in patients undergoing CT of the brain; frequency, appearance, and differential diagnosis. Clin Radiol. 2010;65(5):427–8.
4. Kawaguchi M, Kato H, Suzui N, Miyazaki T, Tomita H, Hara A, Matsuyama K, Seishima M, Matsuo M. Imaging findings of trichilemmal cyst and proliferating trichilemmal tumour. Neuroradiol J. 2021;34(6):615–21.
5. He P, Chen W, Zhang Q, Cui L, Zhang Q. Distinguishing a trichilemmal cyst from a pilomatricoma with ultrasound. J Ultrasound Med. 2020;39(10):1939–45.
6. Chang SJ, Sims J, Murtagh FR, McCaffrey JC, Messina JL. Proliferating trichilemmal cysts of the scalp on CT. AJNR Am J Neuroradiol. 2006;27(3):712–4.
7. Sau P, Graham JH, Helwig EB. Proliferating epithelial cysts. Clinicopathological analysis of 96 cases. J Cutan Pathol. 1995;22(5):394–406.

8. Kim HJ, Kim TS, Lee KH, Kim YM, Suh CH. Proliferating trichilemmal tumors: CT and MR imaging findings in two cases, one with malignant transformation. AJNR Am J Neuroradiol. 2001;22(1):180–3.
9. Ranabhat S, Tiwari M, Maharjan S. Teratoid cyst of the postauricular region: the first ever case report. Case Rep Pathol. 2017;2017:9235925.
10. Hong SH, Chung HW, Choi JY, Koh YH, Choi JA, Kang HS. MRI findings of subcutaneous epidermal cysts: emphasis on the presence of rupture. AJR Am J Roentgenol. 2006;186(4):961–6.
11. Kim HK, Kim SM, Lee SH, Racadio JM, Shin MJ. Subcutaneous epidermal inclusion cysts: ultrasound (US) and MR imaging findings. Skeletal Radiol. 2011;40(11):1415–9.
12. Van der Horn G, Rutten MJ. Pilomatrixoma. JBR-BTR. 2011;94(3):142–3.
13. Garioni E, Danesino GM, Madonia L. Pilomatricoma: sonographic features. J Ultrasound. 2008;11(2):76–8.
14. De Beuckeleer LH, De Schepper AM, Neetens I. Magnetic resonance imaging of pilomatricoma. Eur Radiol. 1996;6(1):72–5.
15. Allen A, Ahn C, Sangüeza OP. Dermatofibrosarcoma protuberans. Dermatol Clin. 2019;37(4):483–8.
16. Hao X, Billings SD, Wu F, Stultz TW, Procop GW, Mirkin G, Vidimos AT. Dermatofibrosarcoma protuberans: update on the diagnosis and treatment. J Clin Med. 2020;9(6):1752.
17. Ren Q, Li J, Shangguan J, Feng X, Ma X. Imaging features of dermatofibrosarcoma protuberans. J Cancer Res Ther. 2022;18(2):476–81.
18. Al-Khateeb TH, Al-Masri NM, Al-Zoubi F. Cutaneous cysts of the head and neck. J Oral Maxillofac Surg. 2009;67(1):52–7.
19. Prior A, Anania P, Pacetti M, Secci F, Ravegnani M, Pavanello M, Piatelli G, Cama A, Consales A. Dermoid and epidermoid cysts of scalp: case series of 234 consecutive patients. World Neurosurg. 2018;120:119–24.
20. Einarsdottir H, Söderlund V, Larson O, Jenner G, Bauer HC. MR imaging of lipoma and liposarcoma. Acta Radiol. 1999;40(1):64–8.
21. Bertino F, Trofimova AV, Gilyard SN, Hawkins CM. Vascular anomalies of the head and neck: diagnosis and treatment. Pediatr Radiol. 2021;51(7):1162–84.
22. Abdel Razek AAK, Elmokadem AH, Soliman M, Mukherji SK. MR imaging of vascular malformations and tumors of head and neck. Magn Reson Imaging Clin N Am. 2022;30(1):199–213.
23. Baheti AD, Tirumani SH, Giardino A, Rosenthal MH, Tirumani H, Krajewski K, Ramaiya NH. Basal cell carcinoma: a comprehensive review for the radiologist. AJR Am J Roentgenol. 2015;204(2):W132–40.
24. Catalano O, Corvino A. Ultrasound of skin cancer: what we need to know. Semin Ultrasound CT MR. 2023:S0887-2171(23)00094-X.
25. Lee JY, Yang CC, Chao SC, Wong TW. Histopathological differential diagnosis of keloid and hypertrophic scar. Am J Dermatopathol. 2004;26(5):379–84.
26. Lobos N, Wortsman X, Valenzuela F, Alonso F. Color Doppler ultrasound assessment of activity in keloids. Dermatol Surg. 2017;43(6):817–25.
27. Hauschild A, Egberts F, Garbe C, Bauer J, Grabbe S, Hamm H, Kerl H, Reusch M, Rompel R, Schlaeger M, expert group "Melanocytic nevi". Melanocytic nevi. J Dtsch Dermatol Ges. 2011;9(9):723–34.
28. Long GV, Swetter SM, Menzies AM, Gershenwald JE, Scolyer RA. Cutaneous melanoma. Lancet. 2023;402(10400):485–502.
29. Pathak P, Wondimu B, Jalilianhasanpour R, Pooyan A, Matesan MC, Mansoori B. Skin malignancies: imaging review with radiologic-histopathologic correlation. Radiographics. 2023;43(12):e230093.
30. Kawaguchi M, Kato H, Tomita H, Hara A, Suzui N, Miyazaki T, Matsuyama K, Seishima M, Matsuo M. MR imaging findings for differentiating cutaneous malignant melanoma from squamous cell carcinoma. Eur J Radiol. 2020;132:109212.
31. Prodinger CM, Koller J, Laimer M. Scalp tumors. J Dtsch Dermatol Ges. 2018;16(6):730–53.
32. Kim JH, Kim JY, Chun KA, Jee WH, Sung MS. MR imaging manifestations of skin tumors. Eur Radiol. 2008;18(11):2652–61.
33. Gomez CK, Schiffman SR, Bhatt AA. Radiological review of skull lesions. Insights Imaging. 2018;9(5):857–82.
34. Demir MK, Yapıcıer O, Onat E, Toktaş ZO, Akakın A, Urgun K, Kılıç T. Rare and challenging extra-axial brain lesions: CT and MRI findings with clinico-radiological differential diagnosis and pathological correlation. Diagn Interv Radiol. 2014;20(5):448–52.
35. Splendiani A, Bruno F, Mariani S, La Marra A, Capretti I, Di Cesare E, Masciocchi C. A rare localization of pure dermoid cyst in the frontal bone. Neuroradiol J. 2016;29(2):130–3.
36. Yang Y, Guan J, Ma W, Li Y, Xing B, Ren Z, Su C, Wang R. Primary intraosseous cavernous hemangioma in the skull. Medicine (Baltimore). 2016;95(11):e3069.
37. Brandner JS, Rawal YB, Kim LJ, Dillon JK. Intraosseous Hemangioma of the frontal bone. Report of a case and review of the literature. J Oral Maxillofac Surg. 2018;76(4):799–805.
38. Han Z, Liu Y, Hao X, Li C, Tian Y. Large intraosseous lipoma of the skull: a case report and review of the literature. World Neurosurg. 2018;120:525–9.
39. Pekcevik Y, Arslan IB, Arslan Y. CT and MRI findings of the incidental intraosseous lipomatous lesions of the sphenoid bone. Head Neck. 2016;38(2):E41–4.
40. Gao L, Chen P, Yang L, Li Y, Han F, Liu H, Zhang J. Imaging features of primary intraosseous meningiomas. J Comput Assist Tomogr. 2023;47(6):934–9.
41. Omofoye OA, Huynh T, Jhun R, Ashfaque H, Cronk K. Primary intraosseous meningioma of the calvarium: a systematic review. Clin Neurol Neurosurg. 2020;199:106283.

42. Baumgartner D, Gassner I, Sperl W, Salzer-Kuntschik M, Judmaier W, Steinmann B. Calvarial "doughnut lesions": clinical spectrum of the syndrome, report on a case, and review of the literature. Am J Med Genet. 2001;99(3):238–43.
43. Som PM, Anderson PJ, Wolf BS. A malignant calvarial doughnut lesion ("button sequestrum?"). Mt Sinai J Med. 1978;45(3):390–3.
44. Tarsitano A, Ricotta F, Spinnato P, Chiesa AM, Di Carlo M, Parmeggiani A, Miceli M, Facchini G. Craniofacial osteomas: from diagnosis to therapy. J Clin Med. 2021;10(23):5584.
45. Langlie JA, Hullfish H, Jabori SK, Thaller SR. Diagnosis and management of craniofacial osteomas. J Craniofac Surg. 2023;34(5):1515–21.
46. Raikos A, Paraskevas GK, Yusuf F, Kordali P, Meditskou S, Al-Haj A, Brand-Saberi B. Etiopathogenesis of hyperostosis frontalis interna: a mystery still. Ann Anat. 2011;193(5):453–8.
47. Bracanovic D, Djuric M, Sopta J, Bracanovic M, Djonic D. Radiological evaluation of Hyperostosis frontalis interna: is it of clinical importance? Homo. 2020;71(2):155–60.
48. DiCaprio MR, Enneking WF. Fibrous dysplasia. Pathophysiology, evaluation, and treatment. J Bone Joint Surg Am. 2005;87(8):1848–64.
49. Kushchayeva YS, Kushchayev SV, Glushko TY, Tella SH, Teytelboym OM, Collins MT, Boyce AM. Fibrous dysplasia for radiologists: beyond ground glass bone matrix. Insights Imaging. 2018;9(6):1035–56.
50. Lisle DA, Monsour PA, Maskiell CD. Imaging of craniofacial fibrous dysplasia. J Med Imaging Radiat Oncol. 2008;52(4):325–32.
51. Harrison RA, Nam JY, Weathers SP, DeMonte F. Intracranial dural, calvarial, and skull base metastases. Handb Clin Neurol. 2018;149:205–25.
52. Mitsuya K, Nakasu Y, Horiguchi S, Harada H, Nishimura T, Yuen S, Asakura K, Endo M. Metastatic skull tumors: MRI features and a new conventional classification. J Neurooncol. 2011;104(1):239–45.
53. Isaac A, Dalili D, Dalili D, Weber MA. State-of-the-art imaging for diagnosis of metastatic bone disease. Radiologe. 2020;60(Suppl 1):1–16.
54. Pons Escoda A, Naval Baudin P, Mora P, Cos M, Hernandez Gañan J, Narváez JA, Aguilera C, Majós C. Imaging of skull vault tumors in adults. Insights Imaging. 2020;11(1):23.
55. Poon D, Tang C, Vijayanathan S, Mak D. The use of MRI for the imaging of metastatic bone lesions. Q J Nucl Med Mol Imaging. 2023;67(4):271–9.
56. Kosmala A, Bley T, Petritsch B. Imaging of multiple myeloma. Rofo. 2019;191(9):805–16.
57. Baffour FI, Glazebrook KN, Kumar SK, Broski SM. Role of imaging in multiple myeloma. Am J Hematol. 2020;95(8):966–77.
58. Solis F, Gonzalez C. Raindrop skull. N Engl J Med. 2018;378(20):1930.
59. Soule E, Baig S, Fiester P, Holtzman A, Rutenberg M, Tavanaiepour D, Rao D. Current management and image review of skull base chordoma: what the radiologist needs to know. J Clin Imaging Sci. 2021;11:46.
60. Oh HC, Hong CK, Lee KS, Cha YJ, Ahn SJ, Suh SH, Park HH. Apparent diffusion coefficient as a prognostic factor in clival chordoma. Sci Rep. 2021;11(1):486.
61. Hasegawa H, Shin M, Niwa R, Koizumi S, Yoshimoto S, Shono N, Shinya Y, Takami H, Tanaka S, Umekawa M, Amemiya S, Kin T, Saito N. Revisitation of imaging features of skull base chondrosarcoma in comparison to chordoma. J Neurooncol. 2022;159(3):581–90.

Part II

Congenital and Anatomic Variants of the Scalp and Calvarium

Editor's Summary

In this "Part II: Congenital and Anatomic Variants of the Scalp and Calvarium," there are three chapters that address the common normal anatomic variations that involve the scalp and calvarium and are seen in different age groups. 7 describes normal anatomical structures such as arachnoid granulations, dilated venous channels and lakes, and sinus pericranii found in various age groups as well as enlarged parietal foramina and meningeal herniations found in the young and hyperostosis frontalis interna that is seen primarily in the elderly. Surgical burr holes are iatrogenic in nature and are presented in this chapter. A topic of significant importance that primarily involves the calvarium and warrants its own thorough discussion in Chap. 8 is craniosynostosis. An uncommon occurrence that involves both the scalp and the calvarium in two conjoined twins is craniopagus which is covered in Chap. 9.

Congenital and Anatomic Variants of Lesions of the Scalp and Calvarium

7

Muhammad S. Jalal and Walter A. Hall

7.1 Prominent Venous Channels and Lakes

Prominent venous channels are common benign findings, often identified incidentally in pediatric patients. Prominent vascular channels typically appear as dilated blood vessels located within the skull on imaging. Venous lakes or lacunae are large venous spaces within the skull that can often communicate with the dural venous sinuses [1, 2]. Venous lakes usually occur near to the location of the superior sagittal sinus and can have direct connections to the sinus via emissary veins [2]. Diploic veins are extracranial venous channels that are found within the cancellous bone in the skull. These diploic veins often drain into emissary veins and venous lakes. These emissary veins and venous lakes subsequently drain into the dural venous sinuses, thus allowing for a direct connection between the extracranial and intracranial vasculature. In some ways, venous lakes simply represent enlarged emissary veins. There are several suggested physiologic functions of emissary veins. It has been suggested that these veins are important in brain temperature regulation, primarily cooling. The valveless nature of these veins allows for bi-directional blood flow between the extracranial and intracranial venous systems that in turn regulates temperature [3]. Changes in the rate of venous outflow via these emissary veins can also serve as a compensatory mechanism in times of elevated intracranial pressure [4]. Prominent venous channels and venous lakes can appear both as lytic lesions on computed tomography (CT) imaging and on occasion, may be mistaken for other pathological processes.

M. S. Jalal · W. A. Hall (✉)
Department of Neurosurgery, State University of New York (SUNY) Upstate Medical University, Syracuse, NY, USA
e-mail: hallw@upstate.edu

7.1.1 Operative Considerations

It is important to recognize the risks associated with bleeding from venous lacunae intraoperatively. Preoperative planning in pediatric patients should include careful identification of lacunae prior to planning a craniotomy. Additionally, injury to venous lakes and emissary veins can also result in life threatening venous thromboembolic events [5]. Furthermore, these venous structures can also serve as pathways for extracranial infections to migrate intracranially. All of these factors must be taken into careful consideration preoperatively.

7.2 Sinus Pericranii

Sinus pericranii refers to calvarial lesions that represent an abnormal connection between the intracranial and extracranial venous systems [6].

M. Turgut et al. (eds.), *Lesions of the Scalp and Cranial Vault*,
https://doi.org/10.1007/978-3-031-88244-9_7

We have previously discussed the nature of the diploic veins and emissary veins. Sinus pericranii develop as an abnormal venous network located between these venous structures and are typically found near the superior sagittal sinus. In contrast to arteriovenous malformations, these vascular channels are often very low-flow venous lesions [7]. Their origin may be congenital, or they can be acquired after trauma. In many cases, they will appear as a soft, parasagittal scalp mass. This abnormal venous connection typically exits the skull via a parasagittal foramina and a skull defect is often visible on plain radiographs [8]. A soft tissue mass with a small skull defect may also be visualized on CT imaging. In addition, given the valveless nature of the diploic veins, these lesions can often increase in size with the valsalva maneuver and when in the supine position.

7.2.1 Indications for Treatment

While sinus pericranii is a benign entity, there are a variety of different indications for their treatment. Prior bleeding episodes from sinus pericranii often represent an indication for treatment. Some patients also prefer treatment for cosmesis [9–11]. Due to the potential risk of scalp bleeding from these lesions, many of them are typically treated early in childhood. The gold standard for treatment of sinus pericranii involves surgical resection and obliteration. Some neurosurgeons prefer to obtain venous imaging in the form of a preoperative magnetic resonance (MR) venogram. Many neurosurgeons, however, choose to resect these lesions en bloc, while tracing and obliterating any draining veins, intraoperatively. Because this lesion typically presents as a prominent, localized, scalp mass, preoperative venous mapping is often not necessary to allow for an adequate resection. In any case, if an MR venogram with appropriate 3D venous mapping is available, complete obliteration of the sinus pericranii is often successful. Surgical resection typically involves circumferentially dissecting around the lesion and ligating any penetrating veins as they are identified [12, 13]. After the lesion has been circumferentially isolated, it is then possible to trace the draining emissary vein to the skull defect. This draining vein is then ligated at the site of the skull defect to ensure complete obliteration. Surgical resection, however, is not without its inherent risks. There is a risk for significant intraoperative hemorrhage if the involved veins are not successfully ligated. There is a risk of incomplete obliteration if the major draining vein is not identified or if the lesion cannot be traced to the skull defect. Additionally, not all sinus pericranii are similar. Some lesions may contain larger draining veins or can simply involve many veins. All these factors must be considered preoperatively when selecting appropriate candidates for surgical resection. As we will discuss later, there are alternative emerging treatment modalities that may also be of use in certain more complex situations.

7.2.2 Additional Treatment Modalities and Recurrence

The role of endovascular embolization (Fig. 7.1) and ultrasound-guided sclerotherapy has also been described for the treatment of sinus pericranii. Ultrasound-guided sclerotherapy has been

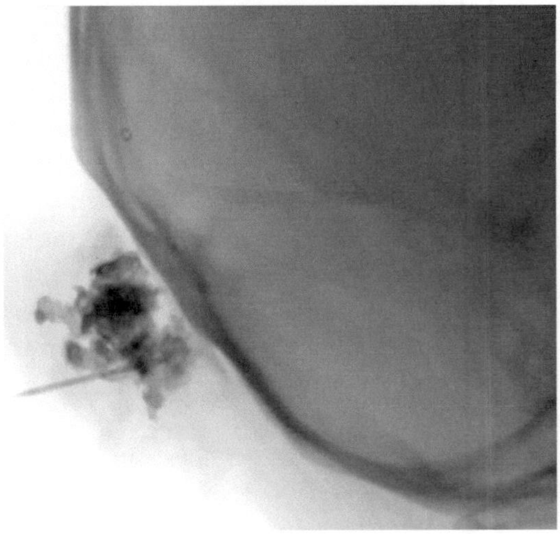

Fig. 7.1 Direct percutaneous embolization of sinus pericranii using fluoroscopy

reported in younger pediatric patients and can occasionally be used in conjunction with surgical resection to aid in the complete obliteration of the lesion [14]. Direct or percutaneous endovascular embolization of the lesion has also been reported but has not been well studied. Endovascular embolization by a transvenous approach can be limited by the access to the draining emissary vein. This technique may be more common in infants and younger pediatric patients. Recurrence rates after surgical resection are typically very low, although they have not been well studied [15]. While surgical resection remains the gold standard for treatment, further studies must be performed to evaluate the role of ultrasound-guided sclerotherapy and endovascular embolization in the treatment of sinus pericranii.

7.3 Bony Deformities

There are a variety of congenital and acquired bony deformities of the calvarium. In this section, we will discuss a few more common abnormalities and their clinical relevance.

7.3.1 Bilateral Thinning of the Parietal Bones

Bilateral thinning of the parietal bones or biparietal osteodystrophy involves a symmetric decrease in the thickness of the bilateral parietal cortical and cancellous bony layers [16–18]. This process has a prevalence of 0.25–0.8% and has a female predominance. While it may be congenital, it is typically a slowly progressive, acquired condition that often affects individuals in the fifth or sixth decade of life [18, 19]. This entity is often an incidental finding, and most patients are asymptomatic at presentation. In rare cases, scalp depressions may be visibly apparent [16, 20]. There are a variety of theories addressing the development of bilateral thinning of the parietal bones. Histological studies in this patient population demonstrate an absence of osteoclasts which may suggest an osteoporotic process [18]. Some reports suggest that devascularization of the scalp may contribute to thinning of the parietal bone [16]. In any case, bilateral thinning of the parietal bone is a largely asymptomatic process that is often found incidentally.

7.3.2 Enlarged Parietal Foramina

Enlarged parietal foramina represent paired, symmetric, parasagittal calvarial foramina [21]. These foramina are congenital and are typically located at the junction of the lambdoidal and sagittal suture lines and are thought to be secondary to variations in the embryological development of the skull [22, 23]. The ossification of the parietal bone begins around the eighth week of life. The parietal notch is a bony landmark that forms during this process. Incomplete ossification during gestation can lead to the delayed closure of the parietal notch, resulting in enlarged parietal foramina (Fig. 7.2). On exam, one may feel a pal-

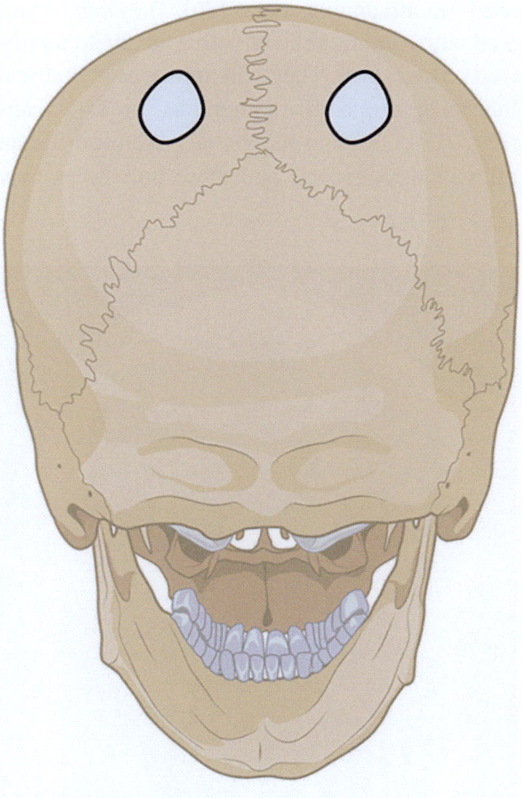

Fig. 7.2 Enlarged parietal foramina. Imaging created using Biorender software

pable parietal defect. Skull radiography will demonstrate a pair of symmetric parietal lytic lucencies. While enlarged parietal foramina represent well studied calvarial defects, incomplete ossification at other centers can lead to a variety of congenital foramina. Some have suggested that carriers of the ALX4 or MSX2 genes are more prone to developing enlarged parietal foramina, in addition to other craniofacial abnormalities [24]. Enlarged parietal and other congenital foramina are typically benign incidental findings, that may contain other vascular structures.

In some cases, parietal emissary veins and branches of the occipital artery may pass through the parietal foramina bilaterally [25]. This information is important to know preoperatively when considering surgery near these structures.

7.4 Surgical Burr Holes

Surgical burr holes are iatrogenic skull lesions used for intracranial access [26]. They can be created with a craniotome or with a handheld motorized or twist drill. They will appear as cylindrical lucencies on skull radiographs or CT scans (Fig. 7.3). Different individuals exhibit different rates of osteogenesis and these burr holes may

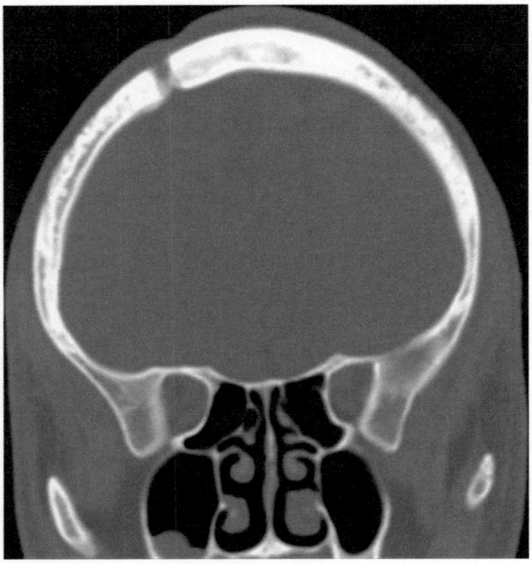

Fig. 7.3 Prior surgical burr hole

persist as partial lucencies on imaging for many years. In some cases, large burr holes may need to be covered with metal plates [27]. In any case, burr holes are regarded as benign entities.

7.5 Arachnoid Granulations

7.5.1 Pathophysiology

Arachnoid granulations (Fig. 7.4) or pacchionian granulations are outpouchings of the arachnoid membrane that are connected to the dural-based venous sinuses. In this manner, they serve as a direct communication between the cerebrospinal fluid (CSF) space and the cerebral venous system. The pathophysiology behind the development of arachnoid granulations is not well understood. These structures are thought to develop early in life and can vary greatly in size and location [28]. In some cases, these CSF-filled arachnoid outpouchings may also communicate directly with the inner table of the skull. Arachnoid granulations can be associated with any dural based venous sinus but typically occur near the location of the superior sagittal sinus and often communicate directly with the sinus or with surrounding lacunae [29]. This direct connection allows for continuous resorption and re-distribution of CSF. Certain pathological processes result in variations in the size of the arachnoid granulations. Arachnoid granulations have been noted to be prominent and enlarged in patients with idiopathic intracranial hypertension [30].

7.5.2 Imaging Characteristics

It is important to note that arachnoid granulations, while benign in nature, can mimic other types of pathology. Given that these granulations are largely filled with CSF, on MRI, they do not exhibit internal diffusion restriction [31, 32]. Arachnoid granulations have a propensity to appear near venous sinuses and within skull defects on imaging. In short, arachnoid granulations are benign CSF-filled outpouchings that can extend into the dural venous sinuses or the inner

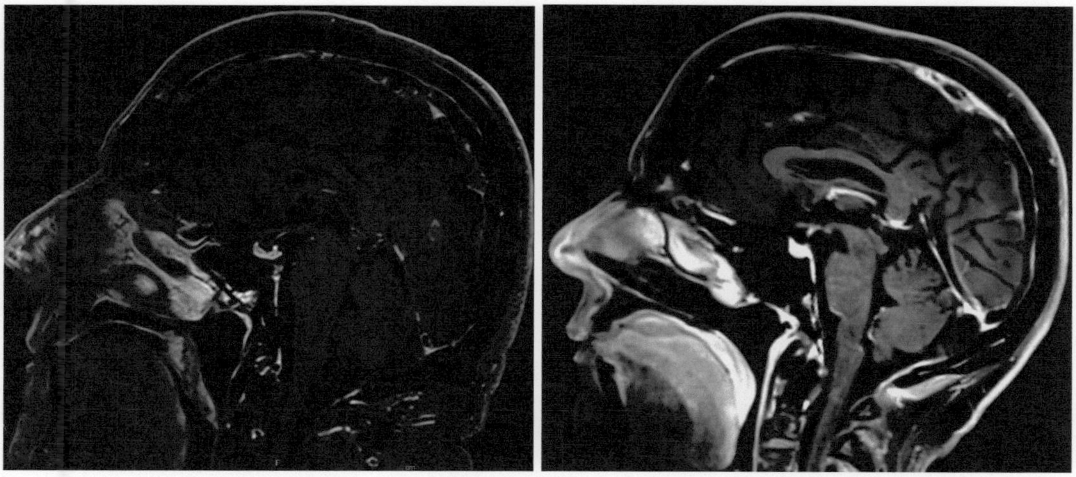

Fig. 7.4 Arachnoid granulations near the superior sagittal sinus

table of the skull and must be carefully discriminated from other pathological processes on imaging.

7.6 Conclusion

There are a variety of lesions of the scalp and calvarium. Many of these lesions are often incidentally found when obtaining routine imaging. It is important to understand that many of these lesions are benign congenital and anatomic variants. This chapter provided a brief overview of these lesions and how to distinguish them from the pathologic processes they may mimic.

References

1. Gomez CK, Schiffman SR, Bhatt AA. Radiological review of skull lesions. Insights Imaging. 2018;9(5):857–82.
2. Benson JC, Hamilton-Cave M, Carr CM, Lane JI. Prevalence of intra-osseous veins and venous lakes in the posterior skull base on 3T MRI. Neuroradiol J. 2023;36:19714009231187350.
3. Gulmez Cakmak P, Ufuk F, Yagci AB, Sagtas E, Arslan M. Emissary veins prevalence and evaluation of the relationship between dural venous sinus anatomic variations with posterior fossa emissary veins: MR study. Radiol Med. 2019;124(7):620–7.
4. Mortazavi MM, Tubbs RS, Riech S, Verma K, Shoja MM, Zurada A, et al. Anatomy and pathology of the cranial emissary veins: a review with surgical implications. Neurosurgery. 2012;70(5):1312–8. discussion 8-9.
5. Klein BM, Bordoni B. Anatomy, head and neck, emissary veins. Treasure Island (FL): StatPearls; 2023.
6. Vinas FC, Valenzuela S, Zuleta A. Literature review: sinus pericranii. Neurol Res. 1994;16(6):471–4.
7. Ota T, Waga S, Handa H, Nishimura S, Mitani T. Sinus pericranii. J Neurosurg. 1975;42(6):704–12.
8. Sinus Pericranii. In: Jallo GI, Kothbauer KF, Recinos VMR, editors. Handbook of pediatric neurosurgery. 1st ed: Thieme Medical Publishers, Inc.; 2018.
9. Sinus Pericranii. In: Albright AL, Pollack IF, Adelson PD, editors. Principles and practice of pediatric neurosurgery. 3rd ed: Thieme Medical Publishers, Inc.; 2014.
10. Sheu M, Fauteux G, Chang H, Taylor W, Stopa E, Robinson-Bostom L. Sinus pericranii: dermatologic considerations and literature review. J Am Acad Dermatol. 2002;46(6):934–41.
11. Ruge JR, Tomita T, Naidich TP, Hahn YS, McLone DG. Scalp and calvarial masses of infants and children. Neurosurgery. 1988;22(6 Pt 1):1037–42.
12. Pavanello M, Melloni I, Antichi E, Severino M, Ravegnani M, Piatelli G, et al. Sinus pericranii: diagnosis and management in 21 pediatric patients. J Neurosurg Pediatr. 2015;15(1):60–70.
13. Gandolfo C, Krings T, Alvarez H, Ozanne A, Schaaf M, Baccin CE, et al. Sinus pericranii: diagnostic and therapeutic considerations in 15 patients. Neuroradiology. 2007;49(6):505–14.
14. Ryu JY, Lee JH, Lee JS, Lee JW, Lee SJ, Lee JM, et al. Combined treatment of surgery and sclerotherapy for sinus pericranii. Arch Craniofac Surg. 2020;21(2):109–13.
15. Tamura G, Ogiwara H, Morota N. Characteristics of recurrent congenital sinus Pericranii: case report and review of the literature. Pediatr Neurosurg. 2019;54(4):265–9.

16. Yiu Luk S, Fai Shum JS, Wai Chan JK, San Khoo JL. Bilateral thinning of the parietal bones: a case report and review of radiological features. Pan Afr Med J. 2010;4:7.
17. Lloret I, Server A, Taksdal I. Calvarial lesions: a radiological approach to diagnosis. Acta Radiol. 2009;50(5):531–42.
18. Lim ST, Sohn MH. Bilateral symmetric photon defects in the parietal bones on Tc-99m MDP bone scintigraphy: bilateral parietal thinning. Clin Nucl Med. 2001;26(6):570–1.
19. Cederlund CG, Andren L, Olivecrona H. Progressive bilateral thinning of the parietal bones. Skeletal Radiol. 1982;8(1):29–33.
20. Khodarahmi I, Alizai H, Chalian M, Alaia EF, Burke CJ, Slasky SE, et al. Imaging spectrum of calvarial abnormalities. Radiographics. 2021;41(4):1144–63.
21. Fink AM, Maixner W. Enlarged parietal foramina: MR imaging features in the fetus and neonate. Am J Neuroradiol. 2006;27(6):1379–81.
22. Reddy AT, Hedlund GL, Percy AK. Enlarged parietal foramina. Assoc Cerebral Venous Cortical Anomalies. 2000;54(5):1175–8.
23. Mavrogiannis LA, Wilkie AOM. Enlarged parietal foramina. In: Adam MP, Mirzaa GM, Pagon RA, Wallace SE, Bean LJH, Gripp KW, et al., editors. GeneReviews((R)). Seattle (WA); 1993.
24. Griessenauer CJ, Veith P, Mortazavi MM, Stewart C, Grochowsky A, Loukas M, et al. Enlarged parietal foramina: a review of genetics, prognosis, radiology, and treatment. Childs Nerv Syst. 2013;29(4):543–7.
25. Reddy AT, Hedlund GL, Percy AK. Enlarged parietal foramina: association with cerebral venous and cortical anomalies. Neurology. 2000;54(5):1175–8.
26. Easwer HV, Rajeev A, Varma HK, Vijayan S, Bhattacharya RN. Cosmetic and radiological outcome following the use of synthetic hydroxyapatite porous-dense bilayer burr-hole buttons. Acta Neurochir 2007;149(5):481–5; discussion 5–6.
27. Izci Y, Seçer HI, Ilica AT, Karaçalioglu O, Onguru O, Timuçin M, et al. The efficacy of bioceramics for the closure of burr-holes in craniotomy: case studies on 14 patients. J Appl Biomater Funct Mater. 2013;11(3):e187–96.
28. Haroun AA, Mahafza WS, Al Najar MS. Arachnoid granulations in the cerebral dural sinuses as demonstrated by contrast-enhanced 3D magnetic resonance venography. Surg Radiol Anat. 2007;29(4):323–8.
29. Leach JL, Meyer K, Jones BV, Tomsick TA. Large arachnoid granulations involving the dorsal superior sagittal sinus: findings on MR imaging and MR venography. AJNR Am J Neuroradiol. 2008;29(7):1335–9.
30. Watane GV, Patel B, Brown D, Taheri MR. The significance of arachnoid granulation in patients with idiopathic intracranial hypertension. J Comput Assist Tomogr. 2018;42(2):282–5.
31. Trimble CR, Harnsberger HR, Castillo M, Brant-Zawadzki M, Osborn AG. "Giant" arachnoid granulations just like CSF?: NOT!! AJNR Am J Neuroradiol. 2010;31(9):1724–8.
32. Lu CX, Du Y, Xu XX, Li Y, Yang HF, Deng SQ, et al. Multiple occipital defects caused by arachnoid granulations: emphasis on T2 mapping. World J Radiol. 2012;4(7):341–4.

Craniosynostosis

8

George W. Koutsouras, Satish Krishnamurthy, and Walter A. Hall

8.1 Introduction

Craniosynostosis is a major congenital craniofacial disorder characterized by premature fusion of at least one cranial suture [1]. The sagittal suture located between both parietal bones is the most affected suture, followed by the coronal and metopic sutures. Craniosynostosis can result from mutations, chromosomal abnormalities, or adverse environmental effects and can occur in isolation or in association with numerous syndromes [1]. Over 80% of craniosynostosis cases are attributed to genetic alterations [2]. The only method of treatment is surgical, and these surgeries are major procedures performed on an infant that have significant risks. There are no other methods of treatment for craniosynostosis.

The skull (or cranium) is a composite structure made up of neurocranium, which surrounds and protects the brain, and the viscerocranium which forms the skeleton of the face. The neurocranium can be subdivided into the cartilaginous part which forms the base of the skull (chondrocranium) and the membranous part which forms the cranial vault or calvarium. [1] The cranial vault consists mainly of the flat bones: paired frontal and parietal bones, the squamous parts of the temporal bone, and the interparietal part of the occipital bone. All these bones are formed by intramembranous ossification (IM), as opposed to the development of long bones which are formed by endochondral ossification [3].

Prenatal development and growth of the human cranial vault involves two phases. The first phase is the embryonic phase which occurs in the first 8 weeks of pregnancy. In this phase, formation of the cranial vault is preceded by the formation of mesenchymal cells by epithelial-mesenchymal transformation via the mesenchymatous or precondensation cells. Simultaneously, development of the cranial bones begins with condensation of mesenchymal cells [3]. Viscerocranium forms the facial skeleton and is derived from the neural crest. The neural crest provides the mesenchyme forming the frontal, sphenoid, squamous temporal bones as well as the facial bones. Paraxial mesoderm plays a direct role in the skeletogenesis of the parietal, petrous temporal, and occipital bones, which forms the neurocranium. A small line of the neural crest is derived from mesenchyme and remains between the two parietal bones and contributes to the signaling system that governs the growth of the cranial vault at the sutures and the development of the underlying meninges. During the fifth week of gestation, the mesenchyme that gives rise to the membranous neurocranium is first arranged as a capsular membrane around the

G. W. Koutsouras (✉) · S. Krishnamurthy · W. A. Hall
Department of Neurosurgery, State University of New York (SUNY) Upstate Medical University, Syracuse, NY, USA
e-mail: koutsoug@upstate.edu

M. Turgut et al. (eds.), *Lesions of the Scalp and Cranial Vault*,
https://doi.org/10.1007/978-3-031-88244-9_8

developing brain [4]. This membrane which is called *meninx primitiva* is the first sign of the cranial vault which appears around the 30th day of gestation [3]. The meninx primitiva can be subdivided into two layers: the endomeninx which contributes to the formation of the pia and arachnoid and the ectomeninx which contributes to the formation of the inner dura mater and an outer periosteal layer with osteogenic and chondrogenic properties.

Cranial sutures of the skull vault including the metopic, coronal, lambdoid, and sagittal sutures are fibrous joints that connect the skull bones, coordinate growth and development of the skull and brain, enable minor movements, and serve as shock absorbers [1]. Most calvarial sutures lie at neural crest-mesoderm boundaries, with two exceptions: the metopic suture which lies between the two neural crest-derived frontal bones, and the lambdoid suture, which lies between the two mesoderm derived parietal and occipital bones [1, 5, 6].

Craniosynostosis is seldom diagnosed prenatally and is most often identified through physical examination in the early months after birth. Normally the metopic suture closes between 3 and 8 months of life and is the only suture that completely fuses with bone, unlike the other sutures that fuse with fibrous tissue in between. In fact, other sutures, including the facial bone sutures, may not fuse until adulthood. The patency of the cranial sutures is critical for cranial and brain growth. As described by Virchow in 1851, cranial growth is parallel to that of a fused suture, where if a suture is fused, growth occurs along the suture line that is not fused [7].

8.2 Pathophysiology

Syndromes associated with craniosynostosis include Pfeiffer, Apert, Crouzon, and others [2]. These syndromes have a large phenotypic variation and are more likely to have multiple suture involvement, such as in bicoronal craniosynostosis. Patients with these syndromes may have other craniofacial anomalies such as cleft palate or lip, proptosis, and peripheral connective tissue findings such as syndactyly that is seen in Apert syndrome or broad-based thumbs and great toes as seen in Pfeiffer syndrome [8, 9].

The identification of pathogenic mutations in syndromic craniosynostosis patients has provided tremendous benefits for genetic consulting, diagnostic testing, risk assessment, reproductive advice, prognostic guidance, treatment planning, and disease mechanism studies. Overall, the genetic basis for craniosynostosis can be identified in only 20–30% of patients, whereas 86% of these identifiable genetic causes consist of single-gene mutations and the remainder are associated with chromosomal abnormalities [10]. The inheritance patterns of causative mutations are typically autosomal dominant. They are also less commonly X-linked or recessive [11]. Craniosynostosis is associated with over 180 syndromes. Mutations associated with familial craniosynostosis, including those in Fibroblast Growth Factor Receptor (FGFR) pathway genes, *TWIST1* and *EFNB1*, among others, often occur in genes with critical functions in craniofacial and/or skeletal morphogenesis and are thus highly penetrant or cause severe clinical abnormalities in patients [1]. FGFR mutations are well known in commonly described in craniofacial syndromes, including Crouzon, Apert, Muenke, and Pfeiffer syndromes. These are autosomal dominant, with variable penetrance, and are FGFR1-3 gain-of-function mutations. Other genetic mutations, such as TWIST1 gene, are seen in Saethre-Chotzen syndrome [9].

8.3 Environmental Risk Factors in Craniosynostosis

The etiology of non-syndromic craniosynostosis in most infants is unknown and most cases occur in families with no history of the disease [9, 12]. Overall, 70–80% of all craniosynostosis cases manifest with no described genetic cause, which indicates that new disease-causing mutations remain to be identified, as do potential environmental factors or gene–environment interactions [11, 13]. The idea that environmental risk factors contribute to the etiology of craniosynostosis is also consistent with clinical variability, such as asymmetric suture fusions and variable phenotypic penetrance. Even in syndromic craniosynostosis with defined genetic mutations, there is substantial variation in clinical manifestations, suggesting the potential involvement of environmental risk factors [1].

Diabetes: Mothers of infants with craniosynostosis have a significantly higher rate of gestational diabetes than mothers of non-affected infants [13]. Studies have demonstrated that 11.6–13.5% of mothers of children with craniosynostosis were diagnosed with gestational diabetes which is significantly higher than in mothers with normal children (2.9%) [13]. Furthermore a case control study found diabetes to be a significant risk factor for having a craniosynostotic child [14].

Smoking: Maternal smoking appears to be the greatest risk factor [odds ratio (OR) 1.6] to the developing fetus after the first trimester, and the risk increases with the number of cigarettes smoked per day [14]. A large retrospective study of 173,687 children born with malformations and 11.7 million controls found that craniosynostosis is 33% more likely to occur in children whose mothers smoked during pregnancy than in those whose mothers did not smoke [OR 1.33; 95% confidence interval (CI) 1.03–1.73] [15]. In mothers who smoked more than one pack per day during pregnancy, the likelihood of having a child with craniosynostosis rose to 3.5 times that of non-smokers [16].

Clomiphene citrate: Clomiphene citrate, a fertility drug used in early pregnancy, has been associated with craniosynostosis. [14, 17, 18] One case-control study on risk factors associated with both syndromic and non-syndromic craniosynostosis identified clomiphene citrate as one of the strongest independent risk factors (OR 12.71; 95% CI 1.42–113.6) [14]. A study using data from the National Birth Defects Prevention Study (1997–2005) found that the use of clomiphene citrate increased the odds of craniosynostosis development by 1.9 times (95% CI 1.2–3.0) after adjusting for potential confounders [17].

For a detailed description of the molecular mechanisms and insights gained from animal models of craniosynostosis, the reader is referred to several articles published recently [1, 3, 4, 13].

8.4 Diagnosis

In neonates, the skull may appear abnormal as it travels through the birth canal and may appear asymmetrical after birth. The confirmation of the skull shape will take form under standard circumstances, in which the deposition of premineralized bone matrix will occur along the suture line. Early closure as seen in craniosynostosis will be identified by visible skull distortion, abnormal closure of the posterior and anterior fontanelles, and hypotelorism.

Additionally, cephalometric indices, such as the horizontal cephalic index, AP diameter, and vertical cranial index, are objective measures that the clinician can use to identify synostosis. Upon identification, obtaining a CT image, with 3D skull reconstruction, allows further characterization and a definitive diagnosis. Many have also advocated for the early screening and use of photography and machine learning algorithms to characterize synostosis [19–23].

Outside of an abnormal appearing head, there are key manifestations that can develop from untreated synostosis [24]. Neurocognitive delays with increased intellectual disability and behavioral difficulties may occur at higher rates than in the general population. This has been thought to be due to elevated intracranial pressure along with focal compression and deformity of the underlying brain parenchyma. Elevated ICP may occur in up to 40% of children with single suture synostosis and up to 70% in multisutural synostosis, and elevated ICP that is longstanding has correlated well with neurocognitive disturbances. Furthermore, syndromic craniosynostosis may develop with elevated ICP at a greater rate than in non-syndromic patients, given the rapidity of the synostosis development.

8.5 Craniosynostosis Types and Potential Management

Sagittal suture synostosis (scaphocephaly or dolicocephaly) is the most common form of synostosis comprising up to 60% of all synostosis. The hyperostosis of the sagittal suture is rather prominent yielding a pronounced anterior-posterior diameter of the skull (Fig. 8.1). In these cases, the sagittal suture may have pronounced hyperostosis. Additionally, there are secondary causes of non-syndrome scaphocephaly as depicted in Fig. 8.2, in a patient with hydrocephalus who developed premature fusion of the sagittal suture.

Anterior plagiocephaly (unilateral coronal synostosis, Fig. 8.3) or bilateral synostosis (brachycephaly) is the early fusion of one or both coronal sutures as seen in Fig. 8.4. Anterior plagiocephaly may result in various phenotypes. The Harlequin deformity may either be unilateral or bilateral and is described as ipsilateral elongation of the lesser wing of the sphenoid bone and the lower face, as well as elevation of the ipsilateral orbit (Fig. 8.3). The type of synostosis is the second most common form in up to 30% of patients with craniosynostosis.

The metopic suture is the first suture to close and if premature closure ensues may yield the presence of a keel-like deformity of the frontal bone. About 70% of metopic premature fusion is idiopathic, while syndromes that include Jacobsen or Baller–Gerold have been associated with isolated metopic synostosis. Typically, the brain lengthens longitudinally and horizontally given the presence of functional coronal and sagittal sutures (Fig. 8.5). The frontal lobes are not able to advance forward, yielding a greater than usual posterior longitudinal growth of the brain. Hypotelorism is often visualized. Suturectomy may either be offered minimally invasively or with a bicoronal craniotomy approach. A small bicoronal incision 2 cm on either side of midline at the level of the coronal suture allows exposure to the anterior fontanelle and coronal suture, and the ability to resect the synostosed metopic suture that extends to the frontonasal suture. Factors such as the timing of diagnosis and surgery as well as the desire to correct hypotelorism may require a larger bicoronal incision to complete a fronto-orbital advancement. This may occur if there is coexistent frontoethmoidal suture synostosis, which requires completion of a bandeau osteotomy with the fronto-orbital advancement.

Lambdoid synostosis: Commonly, described to be the least common single suture (Fig. 8.6) pathology and if bilateral will yield a flattened occipital bone. It is critical for the clinician to differentiate unilateral posterior lambdoid plagiocephaly from positional plagiocephaly. CT imaging in addition to a skull X-ray may be the diagnostic option of choice as lambdoid sutures may not be visible on a plain radiograph alone. It is key to identify premature suture fusion to avoid improper diagnosis as non-surgical management

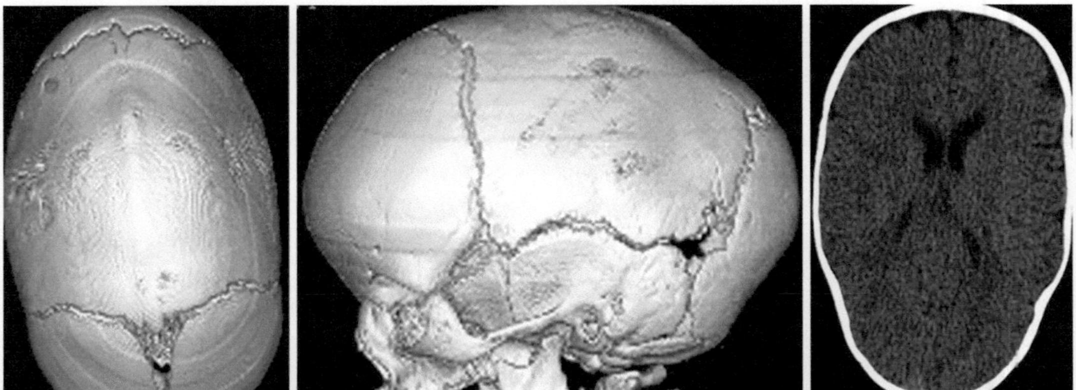

Fig. 8.1 Nonsyndromic scaphocephaly with elongated anterior-posterior diameter of the cranial vault on CT head and 3D reconstruction

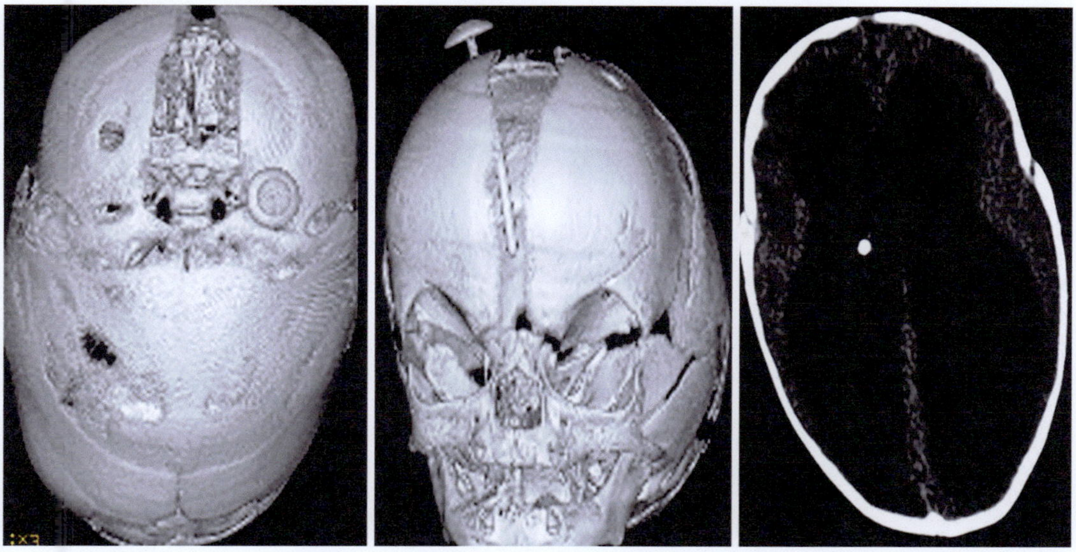

Fig. 8.2 Latrogenic sagittal synostosis in premature patient with ommaya reservoir placement with post-hemorrhagic hydrocephalus

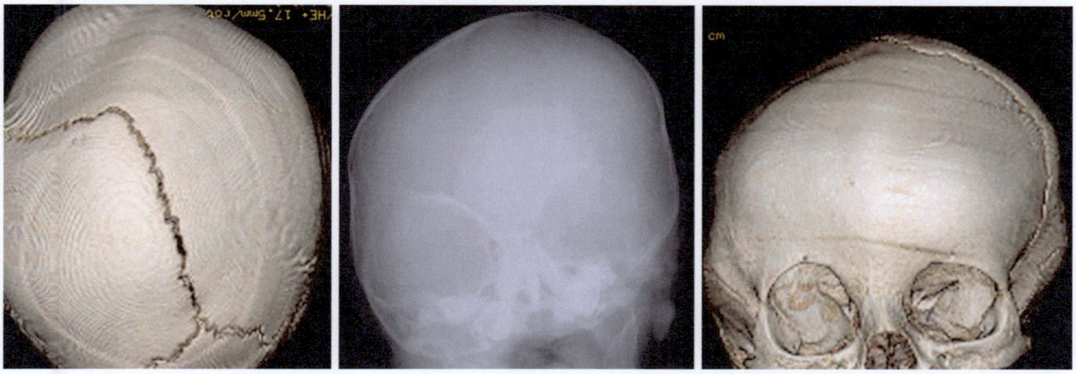

Fig. 8.3 Unilateral right-sided coronal synostosis with elevation of ipsilateral orbit

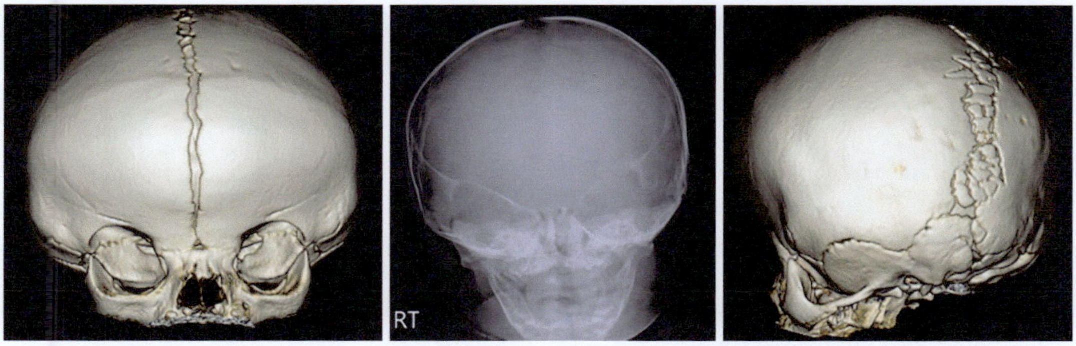

Fig. 8.4 Brachycephaly with harlequin deformity in non-syndromic synostosis

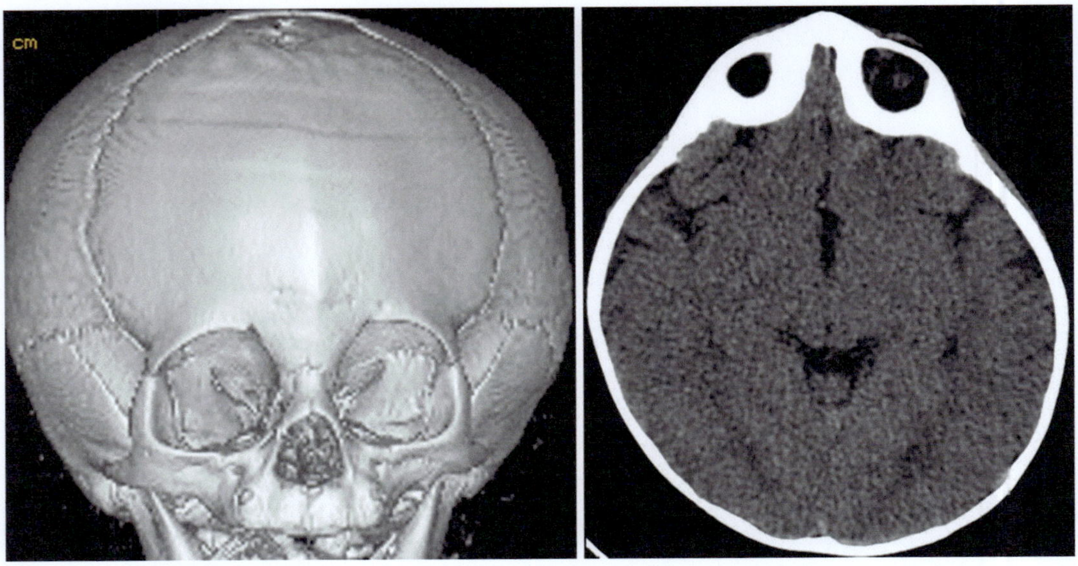

Fig. 8.5 Non-syndrome metopic craniosynostosis with trigoncephaly seen on CT with 3D reconstruction

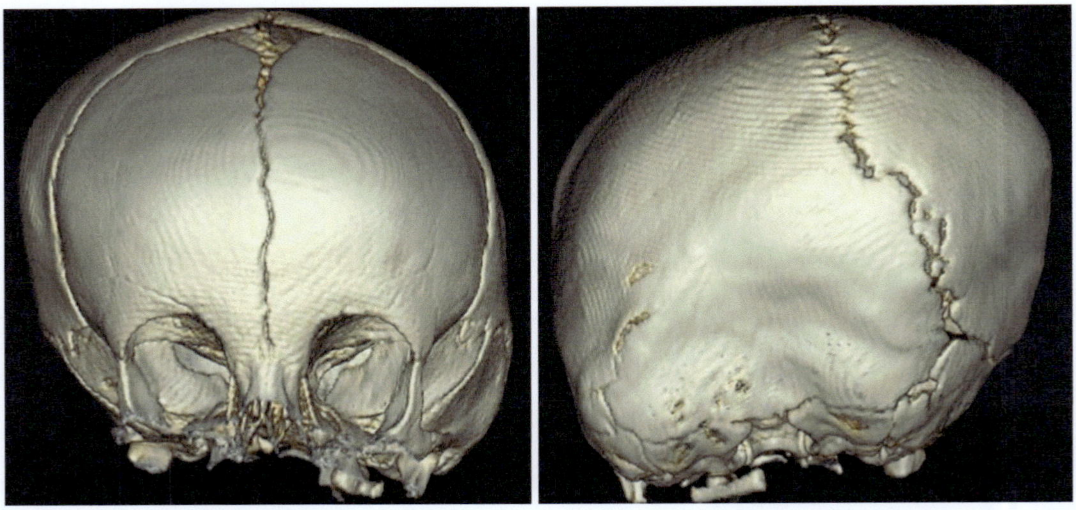

Fig. 8.6 Unilateral lambdoid synostosis on CT-3D reconstruction

is the standard advisable care for positional plagiocephaly.

Multiple suture synostosis (Figs. 8.7, 8.8 and 8.9) occurs in less than 5% of patients and is associated with elevated intracranial pressure with cranial imaging demonstrating other findings that include Chiari I malformation. This synostosis may be seen in brachycephaly or bilateral lambdoid synostosis, but also in other types of synostosis involving more than one suture (Fig. 8.10). These types may be more associated with genetic alterations, or cases of pansynostosis or Cloveleaf skull (Kleeblattschadel) deformity. Nonetheless, the surgical correction is often more challenging and requires an open cranial vault reconstruction.

Surgical indications and management: An in-depth description of the surgical correction of the more complex and less common forms of craniosynostosis such as Apert, Crouzon, Pfeiffer, and

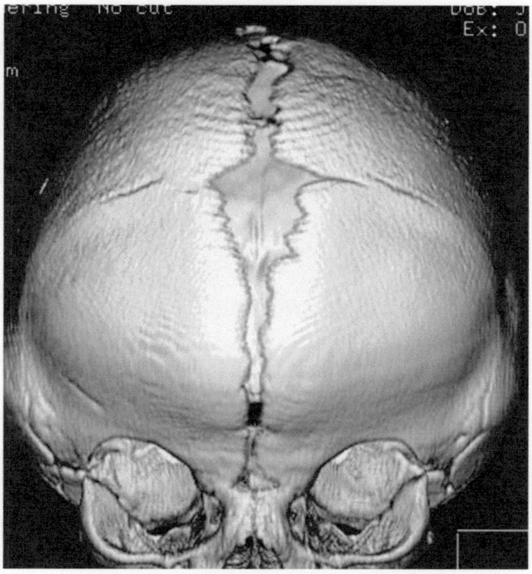

Fig. 8.7 Turribrachycephaly (flat forehead with bilateral craniosynostosis) in Pfeiffer syndrome

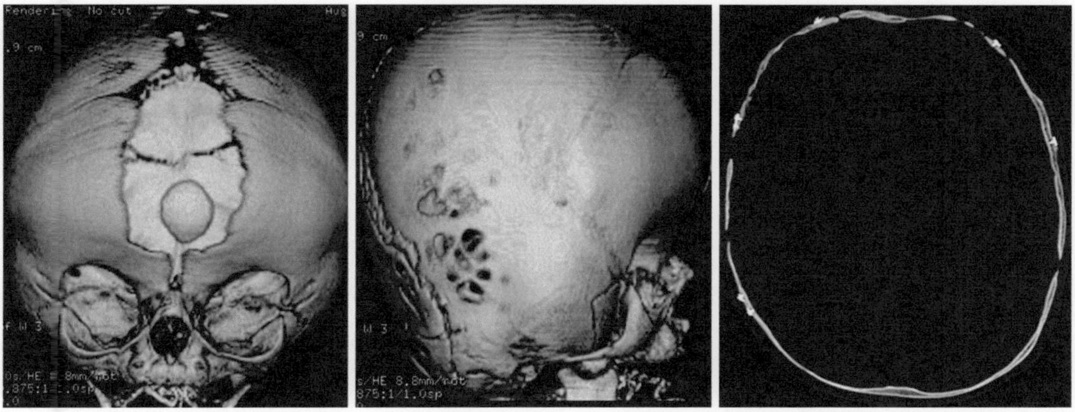

Fig. 8.8 Acrocephalosyndactlyly as seen in Apert syndrome with bilateral coronal synostosis and an expanded, bulging anterior fontanelle concerning for elevated intracranial pressure on initial reconstruction with normal AP diameter seen after 13 year follow-up CT imaging

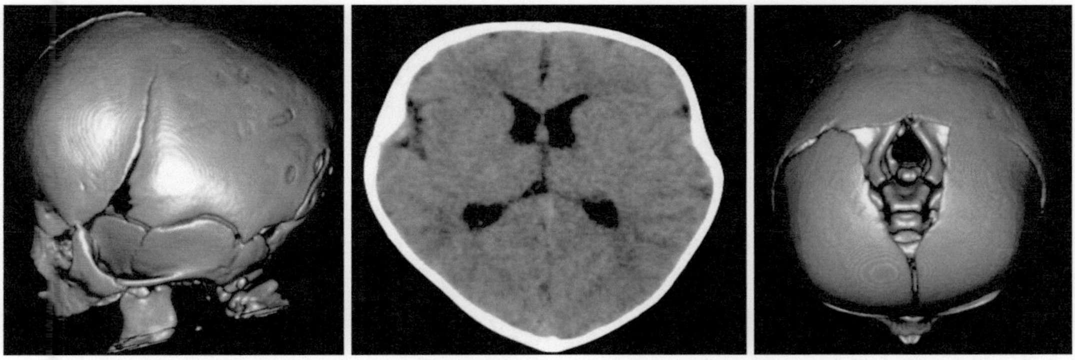

Fig. 8.9 A 1-year-old prior to open cranial vault reconstruction with bilateral lambdoid synostosis, and unilateral coronal synostosis

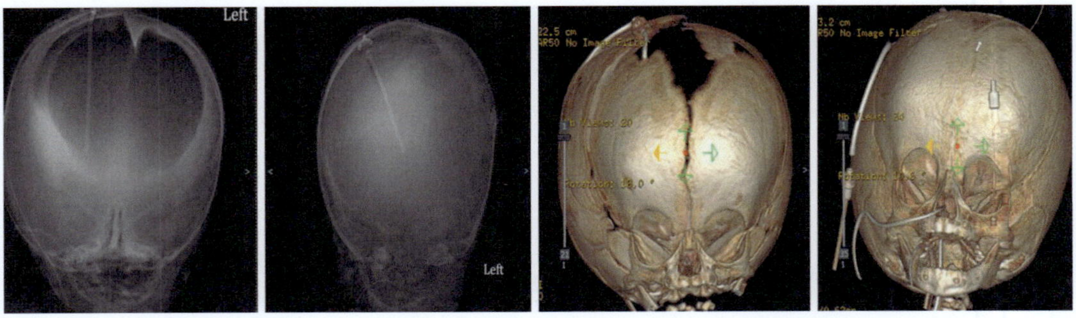

Fig. 8.10 Shunted ventriculomegaly leading to iatrogenic craniosynostosis with bilateral brachycephaly

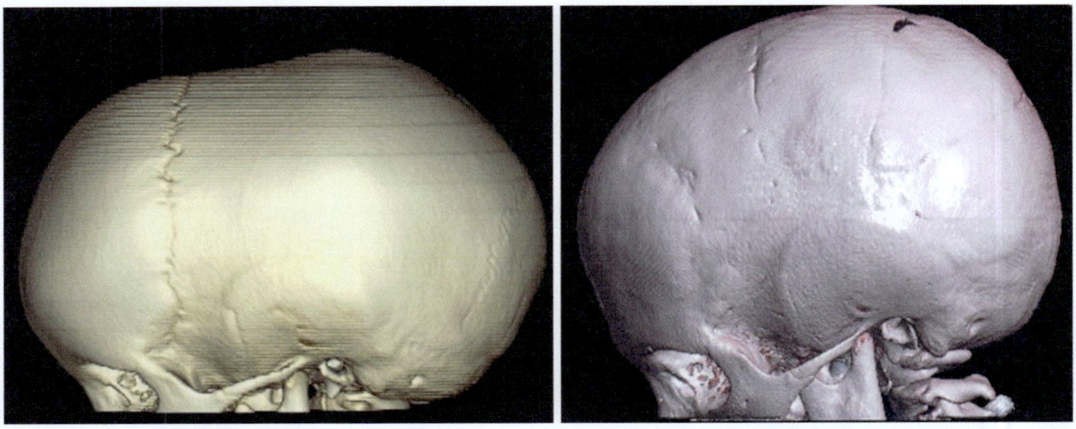

Fig. 8.11 Twenty-two-month-old with scaphocephaly (Image Left) and papilledema on physical examination and 3 years following open cranial vault reconstruction with resolution of scaphocephaly (Image Right)

Kleeblatschadel is outside the scope of this chapter; however, it is critical to understand that craniosynostosis is a surgical pathology, treated by trained craniofacial surgeons and neurological surgeons [1, 24]. Early diagnosis of synostosis allows for early deformity correction, including minimally invasive endoscopic suturectomy and osteotomy, combined with distraction maneuvers. Suturectomy deals with the excision of the hyperostotic bone that occurs along the course of the prematurely fused suture. The bony excision, or osteotomy, will extend beyond the region of the normal suture line, allowing for deformity correction. Suturectomy is best accomplished prior to 7 months of life if possible and diminishes the risk of permanent skull deformity and deformation of the brain. As synostosis is prolonged over time, open cranial vault reconstruction may be the only option available for the child, which will require a larger operation with an extended recovery phase. Figure 8.11 describes a child with scaphocephaly that underwent open cranial vault reconstruction.

8.6 Conclusion

The premature fusion of cranial sutures may be associated with both environmental and genetic risk factors, much of which are related to FGFR mutations. Surgery remains the gold standard management for these lesions, and earlier identification provides the potential for expedited correction of these deformities, which may yield improved aesthetic and neurodevelopmental results for the child.

References

1. Stanton E, Urata M, Chen JF, Chai Y. The clinical manifestations, molecular mechanisms and treatment of craniosynostosis. Dis Model Mech. 2022;15(4)
2. Ko JM. Genetic syndromes associated with craniosynostosis. J Korean Neurosurg Soc. 2016;59(3):187–91.
3. Jin SW, Sim KB, Kim SD. Development and growth of the normal cranial vault : an embryologic review. J Korean Neurosurg Soc. 2016;59(3):192–6.
4. Ang PS, Matrongolo MJ, Zietowski ML, Nathan SL, Reid RR, Tischfield MA. Cranium growth, patterning and homeostasis. Development. 2022;149(22)
5. Balczerski B, Zakaria S, Tucker AS, Borycki AG, Koyama E, Pacifici M, et al. Distinct spatiotemporal roles of hedgehog signalling during chick and mouse cranial base and axial skeleton development. Dev Biol. 2012;371(2):203–14.
6. Di Ieva A, Bruner E, Davidson J, Pisano P, Haider T, Stone SS, et al. Cranial sutures: a multidisciplinary review. Childs Nerv Syst. 2013;29(6):893–905.
7. Delashaw JB, Persing JA, Broaddus WC, Jane JA. Cranial vault growth in craniosynostosis. J Neurosurg. 1989;70(2):159–65.
8. Ciurea AV, Toader C. Genetics of craniosynostosis: review of the literature. J Med Life. 2009;2(1):5–17.
9. Wilkie AO. Craniosynostosis: genes and mechanisms. Hum Mol Genet. 1997;6(10):1647–56.
10. Johnson D, Wilkie AO. Craniosynostosis. Eur J Hum Genet. 2011;19(4):369–76.
11. Durham EL, Howie RN, Cray JJ. Gene/environment interactions in craniosynostosis: a brief review. Orthod Craniofac Res. 2017;20 Suppl 1(Suppl 1):8–11.
12. Lajeunie E, Crimmins DW, Arnaud E, Renier D. Genetic considerations in nonsyndromic midline craniosynostoses: a study of twins and their families. J Neurosurg. 2005;103(4 Suppl):353–6.
13. Sergesketter AR, Elsamadicy AA, Lubkin DT, Krucoff KB, Krucoff MO, Muh CR. Characterization of perinatal risk factors and complications associated with nonsyndromic craniosynostosis. J Craniofac Surg. 2019;30(2):334–8.
14. Ardalan M, Rafati A, Nejat F, Farazmand B, Majed M, El Khashab M. Risk factors associated with craniosynostosis: a case control study. Pediatr Neurosurg. 2012;48(3):152–6.
15. Hackshaw A, Rodeck C, Boniface S. Maternal smoking in pregnancy and birth defects: a systematic review based on 173 687 malformed cases and 11.7 million controls. Hum Reprod Update. 2011;17(5):589–604.
16. Alderman BW, Bradley CM, Greene C, Fernbach SK, Baron AE. Increased risk of craniosynostosis with maternal cigarette smoking during pregnancy. Teratology. 1994;50(1):13–8.
17. Reefhuis J, Honein MA, Schieve LA, Rasmussen SA. National Birth Defects Prevention S. Use of clomiphene citrate and birth defects, National Birth Defects Prevention Study, 1997-2005. Hum Reprod. 2011;26(2):451–7.
18. Reefhuis J, Honein MA, Shaw GM, Romitti PA. Fertility treatments and craniosynostosis: California, Georgia, and Iowa, 1993-1997. Pediatrics. 2003;111(5 Pt 2):1163–6.
19. Blessing M, Gallagher ER. Epidemiology, genetics, and pathophysiology of craniosynostosis. Oral Maxillofac Surg Clin North Am. 2022;34(3):341–52.
20. Bookland MJ, Ahn ES, Stoltz P, Martin JE. Image processing and machine learning for telehealth craniosynostosis screening in newborns. J Neurosurg Pediatr. 2021;27(5):581–8.
21. Callejas Pastor CA, Jung IY, Seo S, Kwon SB, Ku Y, Choi J. Two-dimensional image-based screening tool for infants with positional cranial deformities: a machine learning approach. Diagnostics (Basel). 2020;10(7)
22. Visse HS, Meyer U, Runte C, Maas H, Dirksen D. Assessment of facial and cranial symmetry in infants with deformational plagiocephaly undergoing molding helmet therapy. J Craniomaxillofac Surg. 2020;48(6):548–54.
23. Wilbrand JF, Wilbrand M, Pons-Kuehnemann J, Blecher JC, Christophis P, Howaldt HP, et al. Value and reliability of anthropometric measurements of cranial deformity in early childhood. J Craniomaxillofac Surg. 2011;39(1):24–9.
24. Dias MS, Samson T, Rizk EB, Governale LS, Richtsmeier JT, Section On Neurologic Surgery SOP, et al. Identifying the misshapen head: craniosynostosis and related disorders. Pediatrics. 2020;146(3)

Craniopagus Conjoined Twins

9

Ali Çağlar Turgut, Kubilay Doğan Kılıç, Sahar Ebrahem Orif, Emine Meliknur Kılıç, Fedi Ercan, and Farideh Nejat

Abbreviations

2D	Two-dimensional
3D	Three-dimensional
BGB	Bürgerliches Gesetzbuch (German Civil law book)
CP	Craniopagus
CPT	Craniopagus twins
CT	Conjoined twins
CTS	Computed tomography scanning
CSF	Cerebrospinal fluid
CVS	Peripheral venous sinus
DWI	Fast imaging techniques
EPI	Single-shot Fast Spin Echo (SSFSE), Echo Planar Imaging
HASTE	Half-Fourier Acquisition Single-shot Turbo spin Echo
MRI	Magntic resonance imaging
RP	Rapid prototyping
SDVS	Shared dural venous sinuses
TA	Total angular
TV	Total vertical
UN	United Nations
UNCRC	United Nations Committee on the Rights of the Child
US	Ultrasonofraphy

A. Ç. Turgut
Department of Histology and Emryology, Aydın Adnan Menderes University Institute of Health Sciences, Aydın, Türkiye

Department of Radiology, Ege University Faculty of Medicine, İzmir, Türkiye

K. D. Kılıç (✉)
Department of Histology and Embryology, Ege University Faculty of Medicine, İzmir, Türkiye

Leibniz Institute for Evolution and Biodiversity Science, Museum für Naturkunde, Berlin, Germany
e-mail: kubilay.dogan.kilic@ege.edu.tr

S. E. Orif
Department of Anatomy and Embryology, Mansoura University Faculty of Veterinary Medicine, Mansoura, Egypt

Department of Stem Cell, Ege University Institute of Health Sciences, İzmir, Türkiye

E. M. Kılıç
Department of Civil Law, İzmir Bakırçay University Faculty of Law, İzmir, Türkiye

Program of Private Law Doctorate, Dokuz Eylül University Institute of Social Sciences, İzmir, Türkiye

Department of Civil Law, Trier University Faculty of Law, Trier, Germany

F. Ercan
Department of Gynecology and Obstetrics, Aydın Adnan Menderes University Faculty of Medicine, Aydın, Türkiye

F. Nejat
Department of Neurosurgery, Children's Hospital Medical Center, Tehran University of Medical Science, Tehran, Iran

M. Turgut et al. (eds.), *Lesions of the Scalp and Cranial Vault*,
https://doi.org/10.1007/978-3-031-88244-9_9

9.1 Introduction

9.1.1 Overview of Conjoined Twins

Conjoined twins (CT) are individuals who are physically connected to each other from pregnancy to birth. This phenomenon was first detected in the Neolithic era. The reason for this situation is thought to be due to the fission or fusion process in monozygotic twin pregnancies that split after the 13th day. These twins typically share a single placenta (monochorionic) and amniotic sac (monoamniotic). CT, which are more common in women with a ratio of 1 male to 3 females, occur in approximately 1 in every 50,000–200,000 births. The incidence of stillbirths is around 60%, which is quite high. Managing this complex condition requires a collaborative approach of various medical disciplines [1].

Theoretically, a "parasitic twin" has unidentical development. A parasitic fetus can fully develop and link to the body of its spouse. Depending on the degree of the pathology, just a mass of viable tissue may be left [2, 3]. CT, on the other hand, is extremely unusual, and the rachipagus is even rarer (Fig. 9.1) [4, 5]. An ectopicorauxiliary limb linked to the back is a very rare and unusual disorder, with only a few recorded occurrences in the global literature [6, 7].

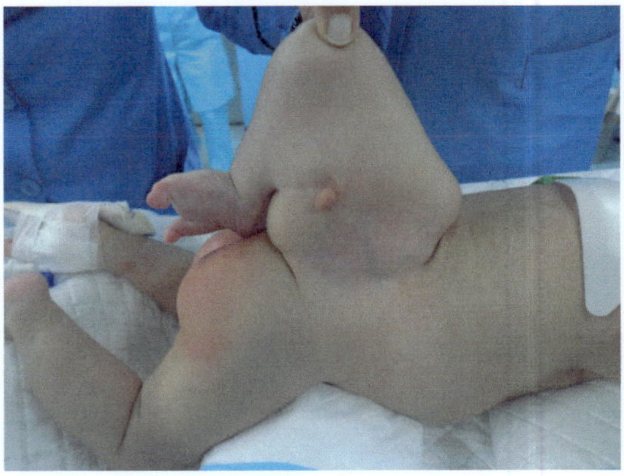

Fig. 9.1 A representative figure of rachiaphagus case, among all types rachiphagus is one of the rarest, reported by Navaei et al. (2015) [5]

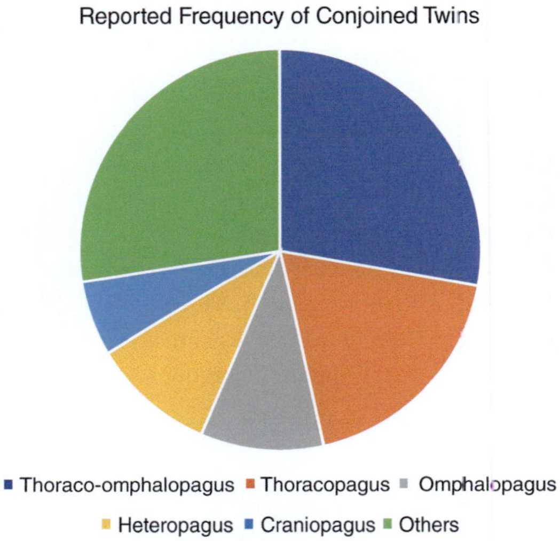

Fig. 9.2 Piechart of the conjoined twins frequency rates

Types of CT and Their Frequency

CT can be classified according to their point of attachment; The most common types are "Thoraco-omfalopagus" (joined at the chest and abdomen) with 28%, "Thoracopagus" (joined at the chest) with 18.5%, and "Omphalopagus" with 18.5%. "(joined at the abdominal part) is 10%, "Heteropagus" (parasitic twins) is 10%, and "Craniopagus" (joined at the skull level) is 6%. Less common types include "Pyopagus" (joined at the sacrum and perineum region), "Rachipagus" (joins at the spine), "Ischiopagus" (joins at the lower abdomen and pelvis), and "Cephalopagus" (joins at the head to the umbilical region). Typically, about 25% of live births survive long enough to be considered candidates for surgical intervention (Fig. 9.2) [8].

CT is attributed to "incomplete fission" or "secondary fusion"; Both processes may explain the embryological and anatomical features observed in CT. However, these theories focusing on fission and fusion do not cover all conceivable conjunctions and cannot be universally applied to a variety of observations in CT. There are two main categories of CT: "dorsally non-CT" and "dorsally CT," which include ventral, lateral, and caudal conjunctions.

Non-dorsal unions can occur in various ways; the most common involves sharing a common umbilical cord and organs. In contrast, dorsal junctions are characterized by two umbilical cords and primarily distinct internal organs. The proposition suggests that non-dorsal association results from duplication of axial primordia, leading to a shift in axial orientation and/or interaction aplasia. Dorsal union, on the other hand, may result from the secondary fusion of initially separate monozygotic twins [9].

9.1.2 Definition and Classification of Craniopagus Conjoined Twins

"Craniopagus twins" (CPT) represent a rare congenital anomaly characterized by twins conjoined at the head. This condition accounts for only 2–6% of CT and occurs in approximately 1 in 2.5 million live births. While intracranial coupling typically occurs in homologous positions, both vertically and angularly, in each twin, the face and foramen magnum is usually unaffected [10].

In contrast, "Craniopagus parasiticus" refers to CPT in which one of the twins is significantly underdeveloped [11]. The origin of this condition is believed to be due to the loss of cord blood flow to one of the craniopagus-conjoined twins or the intrauterine death of one of the twins [12]. This syndrome is extremely rare, as evidenced by an American study in which 81 CT were detected out of seven million births, and only eight of them were parasitic. Female pregnancies tend to predominate in this subgroup [13–15].

Today, effective separation has grown increasingly common as neuroimaging, neuroanesthesia, and neurosurgery procedures have advanced, although craniopagus twins have a high prenatal and postnatal mortality rate. Surgery is technically complex because of joined brain tissue, shared arteries and veins, and abnormalities in the skull and dura, and neuroimaging plays an essential part in preoperative planning [16]. The classification system of CPT is as follows (Fig. 9.3):

Various classification schemes have been proposed for CPT. The first classification developed by O'Connell [17] distinguishes between total and partial CPT. Total CPT has a large surface area and involves widely interconnected cranial cavities, whereas partial CPT affects a smaller, superficial surface area. O'Connell also classified partial CPT by the degree to which one head turned towards the other. This classification includes "Type I" vertical CPT where both heads face the same direction (less than 40 degrees of rotation), "Type II" CPT where heads face opposite sides (140 to 180 degrees of rotation), and "Type III" twins each has a moderate angle of rotation (40 to less than 140 degrees) which occurs with various brain abnormalities and abnormal circulation.

Stone and Goodrich [18] presented another classification that emphasizes the presence or absence of major common dural venous sinuses. Partial CPT, according to their classification, lacks major shared dural venous sinuses; total CPT shares a significant portion of these sinuses, leading to significant brain compression and cranial distortion. Stone and Goodrich divided twins into "angular" and "vertical" groups based on their long axis angle. In their system, vertical CPTs have a continuous longitudinal skull that is further differentiated by intertwin axial facial rotation. Angular CPT twins, on the other hand, have an intertwin longitudinal angle of less than 140 degrees, regardless of axial rotation. Stone and Goodrich's classification is widely accepted in this field.

9.1.3 Historical Perspective on CPT

The earliest recorded instance of CPTs dates back to 1491 in Bavaria, Germany, and is documented as a terrifying phenomenon interpreted as "Ein MONSTERUM," or a divine warning. These frontal CPT, born near Worms, Germany, lived for about 10 years [19]. Craniopagus parasiticus, also called épicome or epicomus, involves a parasitic twin head with an underdeveloped or undeveloped body attached to the head of the developed twin, as seen in the "two-headed child of Bengal" born in 1783 [15, 20].

Historical publications on CPT include works by Ambroise Paré in the sixteenth century, Sir Everard Home in the eighteenth century, and August Förster in the nineteenth century. The

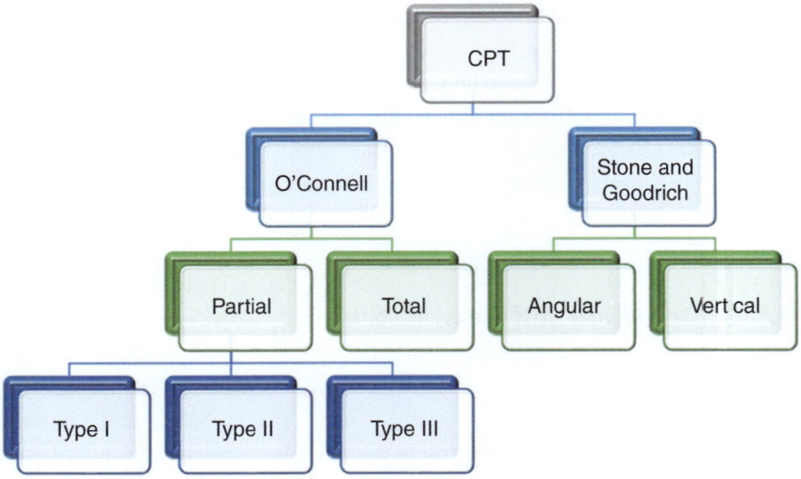

Fig. 9.3 Diagram of the CPT classification

concept of Siamese twins gained popularity through traveling "side shows" exemplified by Chang and Eng, who became public figures in the nineteenth and twentieth centuries [21]. From the 1950s to the 1980s, exhibitions of "freaks of nature" such as Yvonne and Yvette McCarther in Los Angeles were sometimes used to defray their medical expenses [19].

Dr. Before Goodrich's contributions, CPT separation involved single, prolonged operations; This led to challenges such as the development of collateral circulation and high morbidity and mortality rates. Cameron [22] published the first report on craniopagus detachment in 1928 in The Lancet. Grossman and colleagues [23] performed the first instance of a successful CPT twin separation involving 14-month-old twin boys in JAMA in 1953. Dr. Oscar Sugar [24] performed the complex procedure, which required extensive blood transfusion, in five stages. Unfortunately, neither twin survived long after surgery.

Voris et al. [25] reported twin sisters, ages 7 months, being split apart in 1957, which was indicative of long-term survival. The surgical approach evolved from the 1960s to the 1970s; Dr. Oscar Sugar pioneered the use of polyethylene sheets for gradual cutting, ligation, and separation of the venous vasculature. The earliest application of the operating microscope was in craniopagus surgery in 1974 [26]. Dr. from Salt Lake City, Utah, in the 1980s, Ted Roberts successfully staged the separation of type I and II total vertical (TV) CPT and they had a long survival [27, 28]. Drummond et al. [29] described in 1991 the use of a screw clamp to gradually separate the CPT for progressively closing the connecting vessel, but prolonged survival remained unclear.

9.2 Embryonic Development and Etiology

9.2.1 Embryonic Origins of CT

CT, also called "conjoined siblings" or "Siamese twins," is a fascinating and extremely rare phenomenon in the field of human reproduction. Their existence is a testament to the extraordinary complexity and occasional aberrations that can occur during the intricate process of embryonic development. Understanding the embryonic origins of CT requires a journey into the fascinating world of monozygotic twinning and the precise timing of the division of the fertilized egg [30]. These exceptional individuals are the result of a highly unusual event in early embryogenesis. It is important to emphasize that the formation of CT is an extremely rare and complex biological event. Typically, CT arise when a single fertilized egg, scientifically known as a zygote, encounters unique challenges during its division into two distinct individuals. This crucial moment in embryonic development occurs within the first 2 weeks following fertilization [9].

Investigating the origin of CT involves examining various theories that attempt to elucidate how this incomplete separation of the zygote occurs:

1. "Late Cleavage": One intriguing theory proposes that the zygote begins the process of splitting into two separate embryos but, for reasons that are not fully understood, fails to complete the division sufficiently. As a result, CT share certain organs or body parts. This incomplete division can occur due to genetic anomalies or environmental factors [31].
2. "Fusion of Early Embryos": In some cases, two initially separate embryos may fuse spontaneously in the early stages of development. This fusion process can occur at various points in embryonic development and can result in varying degrees of physical connection between twins. It's crucial to keep in mind that these twins are genetically identical because they originate from two separate embryos that fuse [32].
3. "Abnormalities in Cell Division": Errors or abnormalities in the complex process of cell division in the early stages of embryonic development can lead to CT. These developmental irregularities can affect the migration of cells and the subsequent formation of different parts of the body. Genetic mutations or environmental factors can contribute to these anomalies [33].

It is very important to recognize that the exact causes and mechanisms underlying the occurrence of CT are still the subject of ongoing research and discovery. The occurrence of CT is extremely rare, estimated to be around 1 in every 200,000 live births, and the exact factors leading to this phenomenon are still not understood. Moreover, the outcomes of CT can vary considerably depending on the specific stage during embryonic development at which incomplete separation or fusion occurs. The degree of physical connection between CT also varies greatly; some twins are united at the chest, abdomen, pelvis, and even the head. As a result, the medical challenges and considerations are unique to each case [34–36].

CT may share certain organs, have duplicated organs, or encounter other distinct anatomical complexities. Considering the potential for surgical separation, if deemed medically appropriate, involves complex and delicate procedures. These surgeries require meticulous planning, as CT often have different and complex vascular (blood vessel) and neural connections, making the separation process extremely complex [37].

In summary, the study of CT provides profound insights into the extraordinary complexity of human embryonic development. These rare individuals not only fascinate our scientific curiosity but also challenge the medical community to develop innovative solutions to improve their quality of life. Despite their rarity, CT stand as a testament to the mysteries of biology and continually inspire medical professionals and researchers worldwide to unravel the complexities surrounding their formation and care.

9.2.2 Factors Contributing to CT Formation

CT represent an extraordinary and extremely rare phenomenon in the field of human reproduction. Their unique existence is a testament to the complex interplay of genetic factors, environmental influences, and the intricate processes governing embryonic development. To comprehensively explore the factors that contribute to CT formation, we must embark on a detailed journey into the multifaceted dynamics of monozygotic twinning and the complex mechanisms that can lead to this extraordinary phenomenon.

1. Genetic Factors: Genetic influences have a crucial role in the formation of CT. These twins arise from a single fertilized egg, scientifically termed a monozygotic zygote, and typically result in the development of two genetically identical individuals. CT, however, deviate from this norm due to unique genetic conditions [38].

2. Genetic Mutations: Mutations or changes in certain genes involved in embryonic development can disrupt the normal process of separation of the monozygotic zygote. These genetic abnormalities can affect the precise division and differentiation of cells, leading to the formation of CT [39].
3. Chromosomal Aberrations: Abnormalities in chromosomal structure or number can affect embryonic development and contribute to the formation of CT. Such chromosomal abnormalities can disrupt the complex genetic instructions that guide the division of cells during early development [32].
4. Epigenetic Changes: Epigenetic factors, which involve changes in gene expression without altering the underlying DNA sequence, can influence the development of CT. These changes can affect critical genes responsible for the differentiation of body parts and organ formation [40].
5. Environmental Factors: Environmental factors encompass a wide range of external influences that can affect embryonic development. While the genetic blueprint is critical, environmental factors can interact with genetic predispositions to influence the formation of CT [41].
6. Maternal Health and Lifestyle: Maternal health and lifestyle choices during pregnancy can influence the development of CT. Factors such as maternal nutrition, exposure to toxins, and maternal age may contribute to anomalies in embryonic development [42].
7. Exposure to Teratogens: Teratogens are substances such as drugs, chemicals, or radiation that can cause birth defects when a developing embryo is exposed to them. If a developing embryo undergoes incomplete separation due to teratogenic exposure, it can result in the formation of CT. Teratogens represent a subset of environmental factors that deserve special attention in the context of CT formation. Some chemicals, such as thalidomide and retinoids, have been associated with the formation of CT when exposed at critical stages of embryogenesis. These substances can disrupt precise cellular processes that lead to the proper separation of the monozygotic zygote [43].
8. Radiation: Prenatal exposure to ionizing radiation is a known teratogen that can interfere with cell division and differentiation. When radiation exposure affects the early stages of embryonic development, it can lead to the formation of CT [44].

In conclusion, the formation of CT is a complex biological phenomenon influenced by a complex interaction of genetic factors, environmental influences, and the potential for exposure to teratogens. While monozygotic twinning normally results in two genetically identical individuals, deviations from this course due to genetic mutations, chromosomal abnormalities, epigenetic modifications, and various environmental factors can lead to CT. Understanding the multifaceted factors that contribute to CT formation is important not only for scientific research but also for the medical community. CT present unique medical challenges and their care requires an in-depth comprehension of the fundamental reasons and potential complications associated with their condition. Further investigation of the genetic and environmental factors influencing CT formation is crucial to advance our knowledge of embryonic development and improve the care and outcomes of these exceptional individuals.

9.2.3 Theories on the Development of CPT

The development of CPT, a rare and complex medical phenomenon, has been a subject of curiosity and scientific research for many years. These twins are connected through the cranium (skull) and often share complex anatomical structures, including brain tissue. Although the mechanisms leading to the formation of CPT are not fully understood, several specific theories have been proposed to shed light on this unique phenomenon, as follows [30]:

1. Incomplete Embryonic Division: The prevailing theory suggests that CPT are primarily caused by the incomplete division of a single fertilized egg during early embryonic devel-

opment. Usually in monozygotic (identical) twins with CP, the zygote begins to divide but does not fully separate. This partial division results in twins that are linked at the skull level, sharing not only the bones of the skull but often parts of the brain as well. The theory of incomplete embryonic division is consistent with the fact that CPT are almost always monozygotic and originate from a single embryo [45].
2. Disruptions in Signalling Pathways: One particular theory suggests that disruptions in specific molecular signaling pathways, or molecules critical for cellular differentiation and development, have a central role in the formation of CPT. During embryogenesis, various signaling processes direct the growth and differentiation of cells, particularly in the head region. Anomalies in these signaling pathways can potentially lead to misdirected cellular growth, causing embryos to fuse at the level of the skull. This theory highlights the importance of molecular signaling in skull development and separation [39].
3. Vascular Disorders: Another specialized theory explores the possibility that vascular complications during early embryonic development contribute to CPT formation. Irregularities in blood flow or the development of blood vessels in the head region may prevent the separation of embryos, leading to fusion at the cranial level. This theory underlines the critical role of vascular dynamics in cranial embryogenesis [46].
4. Random Chance and Unpredictable Outcomes: Finally, it is important to recognize that the development of CPT can be an extremely rare and random event. In some cases, this condition can occur without identifiable genetic or environmental factors, underlining the unpredictable nature of conjoined twinning in the CP region. This particular theory emphasizes the inherent complexity and variability of human embryonic development.

CPT represent an incredibly complex and rare medical phenomenon. Due to the rarity and complexity of these cases, specialized research into the exact causes of their development remains challenging. As genetic research and embryology continue to advance, there may be opportunities for more profound comprehension of the specific factors that contribute to CPT formation. For now, however, these theories provide a specialized perspective on the fascinating and puzzling phenomenon of CPTs.

9.3 Incidence and Demographics

9.3.1 Global Incidence of CPT

CPT are an extremely rare birth condition, with an incidence of only 0.6 per million births. In these cases, twins may be partially or completely fused; This condition can involve not only the skin and skull, but also the dura and even deeper structures such as brain tissue and blood vessels [47].

A very important factor in this case is the shared superior sagittal sinus, a vital venous brain structure. Its involvement is an important consideration in surgical planning and successful weaning, as any compromise can lead to serious consequences such as venous infarction or life-threatening bleeding during surgery [48].

9.3.2 Geography, Demographic Variations, Ethnic Factors, and Gender Distribution

In the literature, there is a most comprehensive one. For this title sorted data of this study is used [49]. In Mutchnick's review [49] of 383 CT, 21 cases of CP constituted 5.5% of the total cases. The distribution of these cases according to regions is illustrated in the following map (Fig. 9.4). In the same study, we observed that 13 cases were female and 6 cases were male. In two cases, gender could not be determined. In this very limited data, it can be tentatively concluded that the incidence in females is twice that of males. In the same study, CT were also classified into four categories according to ethnicity:

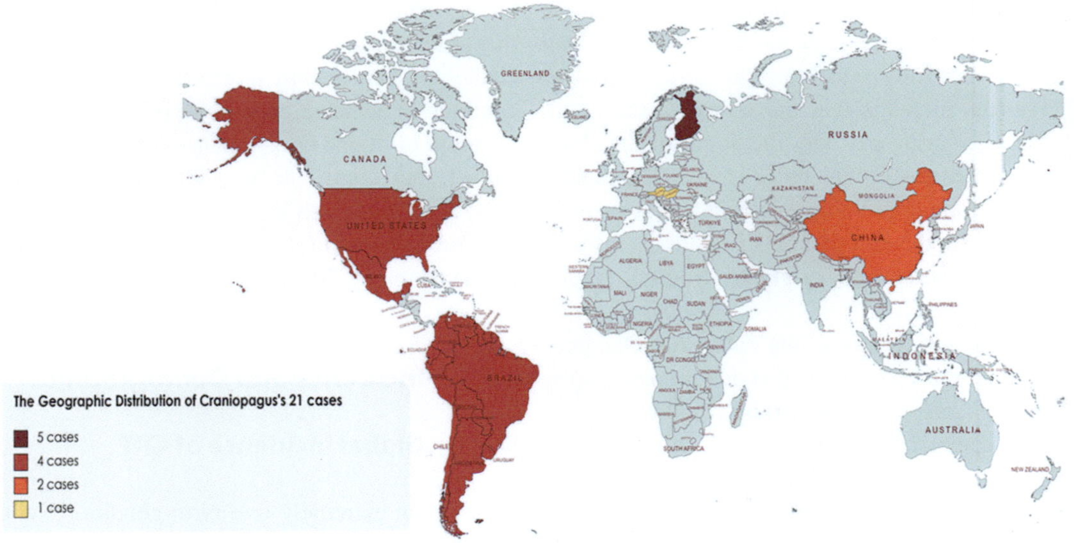

Fig. 9.4 The geographical distribution of 21 cases of craniopagus is given in the map according to regions (Produced from data of study of Mutchinick et al., 2011) [49]

Anglo-Saxon/Caucasian, Chinese, Latin American, and Latin European. The ethnic group of Latin Americans had a higher predominance. There were statistically significant variations when compared with the Anglo-Saxon/Caucasian, Chinese, and Latin-European ethnic groups. Statistical point of view, other comparisons were insignificant. For Cranophagius, the results were demographically consistent with the general values.

9.4 Clinical Presentation

9.4.1 Physical Characteristics of CPT

CPT depend solely on the calvaria, excluding the attachment of the face, vertebrae, skull base, or foramen magnum. In contrast, the cephalopagus includes the brain, face, ribcage, and upper abdomen, the parapagus diprosopus has two faces in a single-bodied head, and the rachipagus connects dorsally along the spine and sometimes extends to the occiput. The accompanying figure shows a cephalophagus case showing the combination of brain, face, upper ribcage, and abdomen. Postmortem images of the same case show two vertebralis and medulla spinalis columns (Fig. 9.5). In cases of CPT, the connection is rarely symmetrical and can affect any part of the head, comprising underlying tissues as the meninges, venous sinuses, and cortex. The architectural complexity of separation varies based on the attachment position, degree of rotation, and angle between the twins [50].

In "partial CPT," cranial junctions typically occur anteriorly, with occipital or vertical biparietal junctions occurring less frequently. In partial CPT, the diameter of the junction is usually smaller than in other forms, and a missing layer of bone could exist in between the twins. In partial CPT, individual calvarial convexities are found in each child, and cerebral abnormalities and compression are localized and small [51]. Each twin's dura can either be intact or damaged, and the cortical gyri may entwine. The presence of interdigitate gyri makes surgical separation difficult, and while leptomeninges can sometimes be separated if accompanied by leptomeningeal vascular transmission, division can cause postoperative morbidity. Shared dural venous sinuses (SDVS) are either absent or negligible. Successful separation in partial CPT occurs at a younger age than in total CPT, and both children

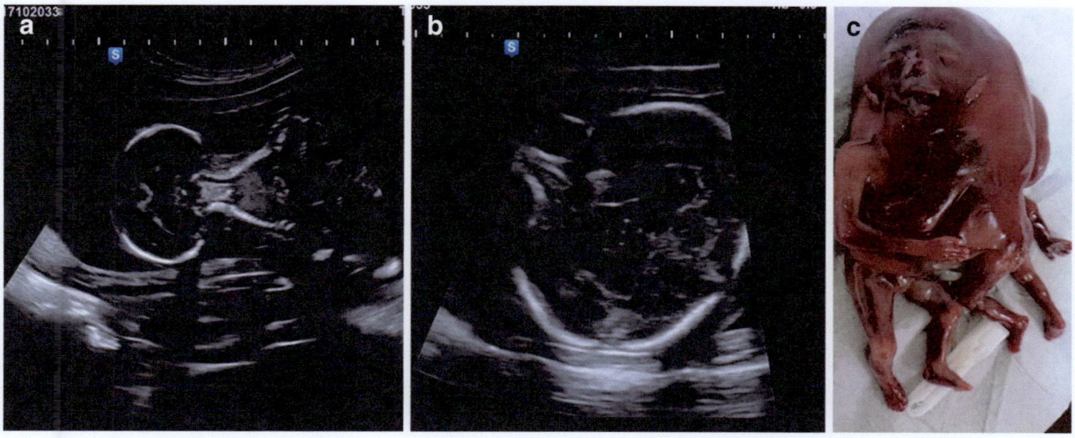

Fig. 9.5 Intrauterine (**a**, **b**) and postmortem (**c**) images of a cephalophagus case are shown. In (**a**), two separate columna vertebralis structures are observed, and in (**b**), a single calvarium is observed. In (**c**), it is observed that the postmortem cranium, thorax, and upper abdomen are common

are more likely to survive without serious damage [52].

In contrast, the TV CPT type is characterized by a longitudinal arrangement with a common continuous skull residing the four cerebral hemispheres. The minimum longitudinal inclination or "stovepiping" between twins is usual, with the longitudinal intertwin axis or angle varying from 140° to 180°. The single-layer transverse dural septum, whether defective or complete, often divides the cerebral hemispheres deeply within the adherent zone. Falx cerebri is typically absent or abnormal [17]. Primary cerebral arterial supply is frequently limited to every twin. Along with tiny interconnected leptomeningeal vessels, adherent brain tissue may comprise a bigger artery that requires detachment during surgery, for example the shared circulation of middle cerebral artery, making safe division difficult and potentially impeding [53].

Given that the entire CPT lacks two complete dural wrappers, a "peripheral venous sinus" (CVS) is surrounded by the peripheral dural shelf in the combined cerebral hemispheric region. CVS in TV CPT often extends at least half the circumference of the adherent area, replacing the superior sagittal sinus that is missing in both twins. By the lateral hemispheric division plane, CVS adopts an increasingly oblique orientation with increasing interaxial rotation between TV CPT [17].

Each twin's homolateral superior cerebral hemisphere is drained by CVS, drains into a common or asymmetrically shared posterior sinus junction, and might join one twin's lateral sinus to the other's lateral sinus. Examples of shared venous drainage comprise venous sinus "lakes," a single shared superior sagittal sinus, or separate superior sagittal sinuses with various connections. Due to the potential for considerable blood loss and disastrous outcomes for one or both kids during separation difficulties, the structure of the cerebral venous system becomes a critical predictor of an effective separation [54].

In "TV type I CPT," the cerebral hemispheres generally exhibit symmetrical superior biparietal or compactive apex flattening. The anterior and middle fossa are large, and the posterior fossa are minor. Facial asymmetry is caused by slight bending or telescoped axial rotation. Intertwin orientation and limited singular twin movement constrained by the weight and position of the other twin contribute to diffuse positional plagiocephaly later in life [55].

Conversely, in "TV types II and III," increased twins axial rotation during growth leads to a more pronounced obliquity of the conjoined junction. As a result, cerebral hemispheric oblique compression, craniofacial abnormalities, and deformities in the middle and posterior fossa occur. Significant bony, dural, and cerebral asymmetries in TV type II and III CPT make surgical differentiation difficult. Along with condensed cerebral tissue, TV CPT exhibits a united cerebral cortex and underlying white matter [17].

"Total angular (TA) CPT" is characterized by more acute intertwin longitudinal angulation and SDVS, associated with intricate, interconnected venous channels (or CVS) and severely deformed cerebral hemispheres. Surgical separation is further complicated by the presence of the brain of one twin within the calvaria of the other twin [56]. Skull base deformity may occur due to cerebral compression, distortion, and displacement. The majority of CPT TA forms are associated asymmetrically with intertwin axial rotation; however some are essentially symmetrical. TA twins are extra difficult to disperse because TA CPT reveals more adherent brain tissue, counting cerebellum and cerebral arterial cross-filling, compared to TV CPT [57].

9.4.2 Associated Medical Conditions and Complications

The advancement of recent medicine, particularly in radio imaging, surgery, and anesthesia, has enabled several CT to get surgical separation and have a complete life. Few surgeries are as difficult as surgically separating a CT [58, 59]. During the perioperative stage, significant preparation and multidisciplinary collaboration are required, as there are many associated medical conditions and complications related to CT in general and here for CP cases especially [60].

Depending on the case report discussed by Goodrich and Staffenberg [61], here some of the complications that the CP cases can suffer from are reviewed. In that report, because of the CPT vertex joining, those children slept on their backs all the time. This position resulted in recurring aspiration pneumonia in both children who were fed orally. Both children were roughly 60% of their usual body weight when they arrived, a weight reduction that was caused by chronic aspirations and illness. Both twins developed aspiration pneumonia, as well as chest X-rays that revealed diffuse infiltrates. Both children developed modest but distinct hemipareses as a result of continuous positioning on one side. Both children had developmental delays as a result of social isolation and a lack of speech development. Also, one of the children required four cardiac drugs to manage the blood pressure, even though some degree of hypertension is essential for both brain perfusion. Surprisingly, medication provided to one child did not affect the other.

The case study published by Rutka, et al. [53] demonstrates the health issues that the twins may face if the choice to have surgery is delayed. At the time of referral, the twins were 3 years old and had vertex CP. Although they appeared to be in good health, twin A developed cardiomegaly while awaiting surgery as a result of her cardiac output being diverted to twin B. Moreover, twin B's blood urea nitrogen and creatinine levels were rising, indicating acute renal failure. As a result, the operation team must work fast and efficiently before one or both twins are pronounced incapable medically to undertake surgery.

The "dominant twin" will thrive and have a stronger clinical presentation, whereas the non-dominant twin may suffer from the effects of hypotension and poor cardiac output, such as oliguria, low weight, aspiration pneumonia, and failure to get better. The dominant twin will receive most midline structures, including the circumferential venous sinus, with the division plane on the side of the non-dominant twin [16].

9.5 Diagnosis and Prenatal Evaluation

9.5.1 Prenatal Diagnosis of CPT

CPT pregnancy has symptoms similar to normal twin pregnancies and is characterized by the size of the uterus being larger than expected for gestational age. Improvements in imaging technology have facilitated early diagnosis through prenatal imaging in most cases [11]. The most effective method for diagnosis at early pregnancy is still "first-trimester ultrasonography (US)." Prenatal magnetic resonance imaging (MRI) has proven valuable in assisting with embryological abnormalities, tissue characterization, and determination of union type. Postnatal MRI should be guided by prenatal imaging, and when necessary, modern techniques such as three-dimensional (3D) printing can assist in surgical pre-planning and subsequent differentiation [62].

Prenatal Imaging Modalities

CPT can be detected in utero using prenatal US and fetal MRI. Both modalities are good for prenatal imaging due to their lack of ionizing radiation. The US can be used to provide an antenatal diagnosis of CT as early as "12 weeks gestation," which is critical for effective obstetric care [63].

If a single gestational sac does not reveal distinct fetuses, prenatal suspicion may arise and be confirmed later. Diagnostic support comes from sonographic observations such as the split appearance of the early fetal pole, more than three vessels in the umbilical cord, stable level and plane of the heads, and relative lack of movement between fetuses over time [64]. 3D US can provide more precise information than two-dimensional (2D) US, especially in determining shared skull space and orientation of faces [65].

On the other hand, fetal MRI provides a superior evaluation of intracranial tissues, comprising the fetal brain, vascular structures, and other soft tissue components, making it widely used in prenatal measurement of CPT [66]. Fast imaging techniques (DWI), including Half-Fourier Acquisition Single-shot Turbo spin Echo (HASTE), Single-shot Fast Spin Echo (SSFSE), Echo Planar Imaging (EPI), steady-state precession true-speed imaging, and Diffusion Weighted Imaging, are used to study the anatomical details of the moving fetal brain, bleeding and diffusion limitations [67].

9.5.2 Challenges in Prenatal Counseling

Pregnancy with CT is complicated and increases the chance of major problems significantly. Twins with CP or a single cardiac mass have the worst prognosis, and just a fraction of twins who undergo separation surgery survive [68]. CPT babies must be delivered surgically via cesarean section; they are also more likely to be born early 2–3 weeks before the due date, and one or both may be stillborn or die immediately after birth. Severe health difficulties for twins, such as difficulty breathing or cardiac problems, can emerge immediately. Scoliosis, cerebral palsy, and learning difficulties may develop later in life [69]. Accurate early diagnosis using the US is critical in counseling parents so that they can make an informed decision. Fetal echocardiography, Doppler tests, and MRI are effective adjuncts in the prenatal period for additional anatomical evaluation and prognosis. Early referral to a tertiary care facility composed of maternal-fetal medicine specialists, neonatologists, and pediatric surgeons will provide counseling and offer parents the choice of terminating the pregnancy, appropriate pregnancy management, and a successful separation surgery [70]. Many parents choose to terminate pregnancy due to prognosis and quality-of-life concerns because therapy for CT varies widely. If the couple decides to keep the pregnancy going, the mother and babies will be continuously observed [16]. Complications are possible depending on where the twins are united, the organs or other areas of the body they share, and the healthcare team's expertise and experience. When twins are predictable, the family and the healthcare team must thoroughly explore the potential complications and how to prepare for them [18].

9.5.3 Ethical Considerations in Decision-Making

CPT, which occur at a rate of four to six per ten million births, present complex ethical and technical challenges and require the involvement of a multidisciplinary medical team for separation planning [71]. Because of the high risks of death or brain damage, the decision to separate becomes especially complex when twins share vital organs such as the brain or heart. The success and prognosis of separation surgery largely depends on the degree of organ sharing. Similar to intrauterine twin-to-twin transfusion, vascular shunts and cross-circulation between twins can lead to serious consequences if not managed appropriately [72]. It is important to weigh the benefits of integrated multidisciplinary consultation against the risk of overwhelming parents. Offering consistent, clear communication and support is crucial. Parents are encouraged to seek out support groups and therapists to cope with psychological stressors during such a challenging time. Discussions about media exposure and the possibility of relocating for comprehensive prenatal and postnatal care are also critical [74].

9.6 Treatment Options

9.6.1 Multidisciplinary Care Team for Management of Patients with CT

There are essentially three indications for deciding on CPT surgery. The first option is to leave the twins together and let nature take its course or to separate them immediately if one of the twins gets extremely ill or dies. The third option is to perform an elected separation [75]. Computed tomography scanning (CTS) and MRI remain the cornerstones of neurosurgical investigation and should be the first neurosurgical investigations conducted after delivery, coupled with a skull X-ray. The CT scan best shows the bone join, whereas the MRI scan (containing the MR venogram) best shows the relationship between the adjacent brains and shared venous sinuses [76].

Anaesthesia Concerns

In the case of CT, several anesthesia difficulties must be addressed. Even though they are CT, each twin has his or her circulation and sensitivity to drugs. Medication given to one twin does not always affect the other. When one child receives intravenous fluids, the other twin may urinate [77]. Several authors have documented significant blood loss while trying separation, which frequently results in cardiac arrest. With this in mind, the anesthetist may be called upon to manage the hemodynamically unstable patient, and as such, the anesthetic team's role in integrating with the surgical team is critical [78].

The involvement of the plastic surgeon is as important as that of the neurosurgeon in preventing postoperative complications such as wound rupture, cerebrospinal fluid (CSF) leak, and meningitis. Preoperative tissue expanders and flap rotations may be necessary to ensure adequate closure of large junctional defects. In cases where full coverage is not possible, split-thickness skin grafts can be used as an alternative. Ideally, both twins should equally share available scalp tissue, but if one twin is weaker or facing imminent death, it may be acceptable to allocate the majority of the scalp to the healthier twin [75].

Fascia lata graft stands out as the most suitable material for dural covering. Difficulties arise when a large surface area of the exposed brain must be covered. In many countries, lyophilized dura is not a viable option due to the risk of Jacob-Creutzfeldt disease. Although other artificial dural materials are available, they have a high risk of infection and are not guaranteed to prevent CSF leaks. An alternative approach involves filling the defect with surgery or a similar agent and placing a drain that remains until the wound heals (usually 4–5 days) to prevent CSF leak [79].

In summary, preoperative discussions regarding the management of CT should include parents, neurosurgeons, neonatologists, general pediatric surgeons, and plastic and reconstructive surgeons [80].

9.6.2 Surgical Separation of CPT

Separation of CPT requires a multidisciplinary team that includes parental involvement and significant financial and administrative support. Success rates are higher in vertical CPT, with factors such as early surgery (before 12 months) and a staged approach being beneficial [54, 81]. The nature of shared venous sinus drainage is also an important determinant. Detailed classification and comprehensive case report documentation are crucial for effective case discrimination [54]. Imaging techniques for newborns and older babies differ; the former often uses the "feed and wrap" method without sedation, while the latter may require general anesthesia [82]. Specialist neuroanesthesia teams play a critical role, with closed-loop communication and meticulous labeling required to prevent errors [83, 84]. Drug pharmacokinetics may be complicated by circulatory interference between twins. Difficulties in mask ventilation and intubation are noted due to the angle between the twins' heads [77, 85]. For better surgical planning, it is recommended that twins be positioned for surgery so that they are visible on the operating table during imaging [86].

Intraoperative Techniques

Plastic surgery arranges the skin incision to produce the best skin reconstructive results possible, while the neurosurgery team performs the underlying tissue dissection guided by neuromonitoring. The absence of muscle relaxants may be recommended by the neurosurgical team to avoid monitoring fallacies and further complications during intubation. The neurosurgery team also requests pediatric surgery to attend and ensure the absence of any visceral abnormalities that may interfere with the separation operation [87].

The Single-Stage Technique

In the one-stage technique, one twin receives the implanted circumferential venous sinus, while the other twin develops a deep venous drainage system through successive closure of the draining veins over several months [16]. However, this weaning strategy has demonstrated minimal effectiveness, with procedures often exceeding 20–30 h. The complexity of this technique, combined with the abrupt changes in hemodynamic forces and stresses that occur when attempting to bypass the entire cerebral venous outflow, results in these efforts rarely being successful. Given the complexity of these cases and the difficulties in predicting the adequacy of individual venous outflow that must operate immediately after separation, the preferred approach is a multistage surgical strategy [88].

As procedures have improved, the one-stage approach has become the standard for separating complete CPT. In this approach, the surviving twin usually removes the majority of the upper dural venous sinuses, often causing significant damage, and operations can take up to 22–100 h. Although surgical outcomes for total craniopagus twins have steadily improved over the years, single-stage results are likely no better than previously developed multistage separation methods [18, 56, 75, 78].

The Multi-stage Procedures

Despite numerous earlier unsuccessful attempts, the first successful separation of CPT occurred in 1953, when a multistaged technique was adopted. "Partial CPT" frequently does not necessitate multi-stage procedures [27]. In "complete CPT," multi-stage surgical separation is the favored current management [54]. In the non-dominant twin, who does not receive the superior sagittal sinus, gradually splitting bridging veins stimulates collateral development and dilatation of shared or connecting veins. This increases venous drainage, lowering the risk of cerebral edema and cerebrospinal fluid leak. Furthermore, by the end of the third stage, the cardiac and renal difficulties, as well as the quantity of drugs required, improve [16].

9.6.3 Long-Term Physical and Neurological Outcome and Quality of Life, Psychosocial Considerations

As a general rule, the outcome is determined by a variety of factors, because there are numerous types of CPT and each pair's connection might differ. The doctors can analyze the situations in great depth using several diagnostic tests and develop a treatment plan focused on improving the children's health and quality of life [58].

CT have a poor prognosis in general. The overall success rate is 7.5%. Only 60% of cases that have been surgically separated survive. As a result, the decision to split the twins depends on their chances of survival and the quality of life for each infant. There is no doubt that staying connected is the only option when separation surgery is impossible and some CT live happy, healthy, and full lives [89].

Complications of separation surgery include organ failure, skin abnormalities, surgical infection, bleeding, harm to internal organs and/or vasculature, and inability to complete the procedure [90]. Moreover, CT pose a significant psychological and social problem. Surgical separation is fraught with ethical quandaries, particularly in circumstances of unequal separation. Furthermore, CT struggle to establish uniqueness and may exhibit a twinning reaction [91].

9.6.4 Rehabilitation and Support

The CPT should first be admitted to a pediatric rehabilitation hospital for healthcare, weight gain, and motor and intellectual development. In retrospect, this turned out to be a crucial decision in the care of the children [92]. The eating problems can be resolved by the use of feeding tubes in close coordination with the rehabilitation team. Also, if there is aspiration, pneumonia can be nearly completely resolved once the children are repositioned during feeding. Both twins can gain enough weight over time [61]. The presence of social workers is critical in the care of CT. Patient education about the difficulties of CT and the poor prognosis can assist the family in caring for the CT [73].

9.7 Medicolegal Aspects of Management of CPT

Under this headline, consent to the treatment to be applied to CT will be discussed from a legal perspective. To ensure the integrity of the subject, the principles of informed consent, the person authorized to give consent on behalf of the child, and the best interest of the child will be briefly discussed, considering international regulations.

9.7.1 Informed Consent

salus et voluntasaegrotisupremalex

9.7.1.1 Generally Informed Consent

By Article 5 of the 1997 Convention for the Protection of Human Rights and Dignity of the Human Being about the Application of Biology and Medicine: Convention on Human Rights and Biomedicine, medical intervention can be carried out by the informed consent of the person regarding the treatment and its risks. How information should be provided has been developed and revealed by case law throughout history [93–97]. Therefore, the nature of information may vary depending on countries, legal systems, and jurisprudence.

Informed consent aims to respect the individual's right to autonomy by making the person adopt the relevant perspective to eliminate the information asymmetry. It aims to protect the person against manipulations in a relationship that involves information asymmetry and interference with bodily integrity, which is part of personal rights [96, 98, 99]. As a rule, a valid informed consent includes a total of five basic elements: voluntarism, capacity, disclosure, understanding, and decision [93, 96, 100, 101]. In order not to disrupt the integrity of the subject, these five elements can be briefly defined: "Voluntarism" refers to the patient's own free will, free from any kind of pressure or coercion [102]. A patient's ability to make health care decisions can be pointed out as "capacity" [96, 103]. The concept of disclosure, providing the patient with the information needed to understand the treatment procedure and potential risks associated with not seeking or seeking treatment [95, 104]. Disclosure aims to the occurrence of "understanding" which requires the patient to comprehend the information given and appreciate its relevance to their situation [104, 105]. "Decision" refers to authorization given by the patient to the physician to execute the proposed treatment [94, 104].

In this context, general information should be provided by the physician who will perform the procedure or a person (BGB § 630/e 1-2) with technical knowledge about the intervention. It should include the diagnosis and diagnosis of the disease, the complications with their possibilities, and the consequences of not applying or applying the treatment [95]. The physician must inform the person who will give consent most simply and unambiguously, by the patient's age, and social and cultural level [94, 95, 106]. However, minors who are mature enough to understand the nature, purpose, and result of medical intervention should also be informed [99]. This situation is also set out in Article 6 of the Convention on Human Rights and Biomedicine. If the procedure is not urgent, information should be given to the patient within a reasonable period for him/her to consider and evaluate [98]. In this way, the patient can make a more rational decision.

9.7.1.2 Person Authorized to Give Consent

Consent does not constitute a legal transaction due to its legal nature, and the validity rules governing legal transactions are not fully applicable in terms of consent to medical intervention [98, 107]. Due to the absence of specialized regulations within legal systems about competence in providing consent for medical interventions, rules governing capacity for legal transactions may be considered as a point of reference. Anyone who has reached the age of majority and is in full sanity is authorized to consent unless the contrary is proved [98]. The person who will consent to medical intervention must be competent in this regard [94, 96]. Individuals who are incapable of understanding the significance and value of the legal interest to which the intervention is directed, foreseeing the consequences and risks of their consent, or evaluating which option would be more advantageous in terms of the outcome toward which the consent is directed, are deemed legally incompetent to give consent to medical intervention [107, 108].

As a rule, competent adults possess the authority to provide consent for medical interventions directed towards themselves. In the case of minors, consent for medical interventions is typically granted by their parents or legal guardians. It is a generally accepted view in the doctrine that minors who possess the cognitive capacity to comprehend the purpose, outcome, and process of a medical intervention may, in principle, provide consent for such interventions [109, 110]. A physician who determines that the minor lacks the maturity required for the specific procedure should seek consent for the intervention from the child's parents or legal guardian if one exists. If parental custody rights are intact, parents should jointly make decisions regarding the medical intervention to be administered to their child [109, 111]. In other words, for informed consent, information is provided to both parents, and the outcome of the medical intervention to be administered is determined according to the overlapping will of both parents.

9.7.2 The Best Interest of the Child as the Limit of Custody Rights

The supremacy of the best interests of the child has been established by the United Nations Committee on the Rights of the Child (UNCRC) as one of the four general principles of the 1989 United Nations (UN) Convention, and therefore all rights of children should be interpreted and implemented under the guidance of this principle [112]. The Committee has further emphasized that the best interests of the child constitute a tripartite concept, encompassing a substantive right, a procedural rule, and a fundamental interpretive legal principle [113].

The Convention places an obligation on States to make every effort to protect the child's right to life and development. By Article 6 of the UNCRC, States are obligated to respect the decisions regarding the upbringing and care of the child made by parents, legal guardians, or those legally responsible for the child. In this regard, States have committed to taking 'all appropriate measures' (Article 19) for the protection of children against all forms of abuse and maltreatment, including physical or mental violence, neglect or negligent treatment, and sexual abuse, among others. These measures encompass legal, administrative, social, and educational aspects. The limitation imposed on parental rights by the principle of the best interests of the child under the UNCRC is also reflected in the domestic laws of countries. In these regulations, the "best interests of the child" principle emerges as a significant factor in restricting parental rights, to safeguard the rights of the child [111, 114, 115]. In other words, the custodian of parental rights is obliged to consider the best interests of the child while exercising the authority granted to them. Examples of such regulations can be found in Article 346 of the Turkish Civil Code, Article 307 of the Swiss Civil Code, and Section 1697a of the German BGB, which are all drafted in a similar vein. In this context, it should be noted that parental rights are neither unlimited nor irrevocable. If the child's welfare and development are at risk, and if the custodian of parental rights proves to be inadequate, the court will take the necessary measures [109, 111, 114]. In this context, it is crucial to emphasize that the state's intervention should not be about challenging every decision made by parents, but rather, it should be focused on upholding a fundamental right with high importance, such as the child's right to life. When balancing the interests for intervention, the parent's right to respect their private and family life stands in opposition to the child's rights. The aim here is to keep the interests in balance and not to intervene in the private family life of the parents unless it is in the best interest of the child [116–118].

The principle of the best interests of the child and the rights of parents in custody can be better illustrated with a sensational example like the CT' case of Mary and Jody [119]. In this case, state intervention is aimed at protecting the child's right to life.

The twins born at St. Mary's Hospital in Manchester were connected at the pelvis with four legs and united spinal cords [120, 121]. Each had their brain, arms, legs, and other vital organs. However, one of the CT (Jodie) was biologically and neurologically stronger. The weaker one (Mary) had a non-functioning heart and lungs; the oxygenated blood her body needed was supplied by the stronger twin [122, 123]. The twins shared a common artery. The family expressed that the twins' condition was God's will, and they did not want the surgery. However, doctors determined that separation surgery was inevitable to keep Jody alive. The possibilities were as follows: both twins would die if Jody's heart failed in the months following, and in the case of Mary, who had lower life functions, and passed away earlier, Jody could be saved by immediate surgery, but her chances of survival would be low. Without immediate separation surgery, it appeared inevitable that both children would die [124].

The case was heard by the Court of Appeal to decide the best interest of the child. The court concluded that the only proper legal path when there is a conflict of interest between CT is "to choose the lesser of two evils." Considering that Mary's organs were not fully developed and her chances of surviving independently were lower, a decision was made in favor of Jody's right to life, prioritizing it over Mary's right to life, which was practically parasitic on Jody's body [120–122].

9.7.3 CPT

Considering the above discussion, the concept of medical intervention will be evaluated in the context of the separation surgery for CPT. By the medical explanations provided above, it is assumed that consent for the medical intervention will be provided by the child's parents when the surgery is to be performed during a period when the child's skull bone development has not yet been completed. Therefore, information concerning the risks, complications, alternative methods, and the expected outcome if the surgery is not performed should be provided to the parents. The physician should be attentive to the elements of informed consent as outlined in the earlier section (Sect. 9.7.1.1 Generally Informed Consent).

Regarding the medical interventions to be performed, parents are obligated to consider the child's best interests when making decisions. The twins' best interest will be determined in each specific case, considering medical indications and risks. If available, the family is free to choose alternative treatment methods that they believe would cause less agitation for the child [109]. Throughout the process, the physician performing a public duty and the hospital administration are monitored by the State to ensure that the child's best interests are considered. If it is noticed from a medical perspective that the child's best interests are not being considered or that the child is being severely neglected (which often results in the child's life being at risk or in the loss of limbs), the State may intervene by petitioning the court for the judge's intervention. The judicial intervention can be made on a case-by-case basis, or in some situations, it may involve appointing a representative deputyship to make decisions regarding the child's medical interventions [109, 125, 126]. Consequently, when a representative deputyship is appointed for the child, the parent's authority to make decisions on behalf of the child regarding medical interventions will be restricted.

9.8 Case Studies and Notable Cases

9.8.1 Examination of Historic and Contemporary CPT Cases

Chang and Eng Bunker (1811–1874) Chang and Eng Bunker, born in Siam (now Thailand), were the world's most famous CT in the nineteenth century. Their thoracic-omphalopagus (joined at the chest and partly at the liver) condition fascinated audiences worldwide. They coined the term "Siamese Twins," which later became synonymous with CT. Chang and Eng lived relatively normal lives despite their physical connection. They traveled extensively, married two sisters, and had a total of 21 children. Their entrepreneurial spirit led them to financial success. Their legacy extends to cultural idioms and legal precedents, particularly in the context of marriage and legal guardianship of CT [127].

Jadon and Anias McDonald (2015) Born in 2015, Jadon and Anias McDonald underwent groundbreaking separation surgery at Montefiore Medical Centre in New York. They were CPT, their heads joined together. Their case attracted international attention and highlighted the latest medical techniques and the collaborative efforts of medical professionals. The successful separation of Jadon and Anias exemplified significant advances in neurosurgery, imaging technology, and perioperative care. It also raised ethical questions regarding informed consent and the best interests of the twins [21].

Ronnie and Donnie Galyon (1951–2020) Ronnie and Donnie Galyon are the longest-surviving CT in history, living to the age of 68. They were joined at the lower chest and shared organs. Their lives shed light on the challenges and triumphs of CT, including societal attitudes, access to healthcare, and disability advocacy [128].

Abby and Brittany Hensel (1990) Abby and Brittany Hensel are dicephalic parapagus twins, meaning they have two heads on one body. They have overcome the complexities of everyday life, including education, driving, and career choices while challenging societal perceptions of CT [129].

Masha and Dasha Krivoshlyapova (1950–2003) Masha and Dasha are CPT living in Russia. Their lives were shaped by medical experiments during their first years under Soviet rule, followed by years of isolation and medical neglect. Their story highlights the ethical concerns surrounding the treatment of CT [130].

Ladan and Laleh Bijani (1974–2003) Ladan and Laleh Bijani were Iranian CPT who sought separation surgery as adults. Their case highlighted the complexity and risks of such procedures which resulted in their unfortunate deaths during surgery [131].

These historical and contemporary CP and other twin cases provide a multifaceted perspective on the challenges, triumphs, medical advances, and ethical dilemmas associated with CT. They also serve as a reminder of the need for medical innovation, community support, and ethical considerations in the care and treatment of individuals with unique medical conditions.

9.8.2 Examination of Notable Case

In the case report, the urgent separation of CPT, a rare congenital anomaly in which twins are joined at the head, is discussed. CPT are typically operated on electively after extensive preoperative evaluations, but in cases where one twin dies, immediate separation is necessary due to the risk of life-threatening complications for the surviving twin. The presented case involved twins born prematurely at 28 weeks, and one of the twins died suddenly. Surgical separation performed at 32 weeks was successful, making it the youngest and mildest case of successful separation reported. The surviving twin developed a pseudo meningocele, requiring a second surgery and placement of a cystoperitonealshunt. Despite this, the twin's good condition at the last follow-up highlights the difficulties and complexities involved in separating CPT, especially in emergencies. The report underscores the importance of a multidisciplinary team and comprehensive preoperative evaluations for optimal outcomes in CPT separations [132].

9.9 Future Directions and Research

9.9.1 Advances in Surgical Techniques and Technologies

Rapid prototyping (RP), also called advanced digital manufacturing, involves creating 3D objects from computer designs using technologies that add layers rather than traditional subtraction methods. Technologies such as stereolithography and 3D printing are examples of RP methods [133]. RP models, in craniopagus, are invaluable in aiding decision-making, informed consent, surgical planning, and postoperative care at all stages of twin separation, improving both knowledge and quality of care [134]. Advocates the use of open source software in 3D reconstruction and virtual navigation to manage costs. This approach was applied to a case involving CPT using a variety of imaging techniques for evaluation and open source software for cost-effective surgical planning. The study highlights the importance of interdisciplinary collaboration and the potential of open-source solutions in addressing complex medical cases such as CPT, improving surgical outcomes through advanced 3D modelling.

9.10 Conclusions

The results of this chapter regarding CPT will be summarized and grouped under the following subheading:

1. *Medical Advances in CPT Separation: CPT* pose an exceptional medical challenge that requires innovative solutions. Surgeons, together with interdisciplinary medical teams, are constantly pushing the boundaries of medical knowledge and technology to improve separation procedures. The importance of this lies not only in the successful separation of these twins but also in the knowledge gained during the process. These medical advances often have far-reaching implications affecting neurosurgery, pediatric medicine, and surgical techniques.
2. *Ethical Considerations Surrounding CPT:* The ethical dimensions of CPT separation are multifaceted. They involve complex questions about autonomy, consent, and the best interests of the twins. Social norms and ethical principles play a critical role in guiding medical decisions. The ethical debate extends to the role of parents, medical professionals, and society in making choices that profoundly affect the lives of twins.
3. *Public Awareness and Understanding*: Cases of CPT often capture the public imagination. Extensive media coverage and documentaries serve as educational tools to help the public

understand the challenges faced by these twins and their families. Increased awareness fosters empathy, reduces stigma, and promotes inclusion for individuals with unique medical conditions. It also encourages support for research and health initiatives aimed at improving the lives of CT.

4. *Psychosocial Impact on CPT*: CT, including those with CP, navigate a complex psychosocial environment. Their experiences may include issues related to self-identity, body image, social acceptance, and personal privacy. Societal attitudes and support systems significantly influence their psychological well-being. Sociological research examines how societal perceptions and interactions affect the mental and emotional health of these individuals.
5. *Disability Advocacy and Inspirational Role Models*: CPT who have undergone separation surgery often become advocates for people with disabilities. Their life stories and resilience inspire others and contribute to changing societal attitudes towards disability. They leave a lasting impact on disability advocacy movements by emphasizing the importance of inclusion, accessibility, and equal opportunities for individuals of all abilities.
6. *Contributions to Research, Education, and Medical Knowledge*: The study of CPT provides valuable insights into embryonic development, genetics, and rare medical anomalies. Their unique condition serves as a valuable resource for medical researchers and educators. By improving our understanding of these twins, researchers can make discoveries that will benefit a wider range of patients and potentially influence medical practices and treatments.
7. *Cultural and Religious Perspectives on CT*: Cultural and religious beliefs shape how societies view CPT and their families. Sociological studies investigate various cultural and religious perspectives on CT and examine the impact of these beliefs on social perceptions, medical decisions, and social support systems. These studies help to promote cross-cultural understanding and respect for different opinions.
8. *Legal Frameworks and Guardianship Challenges*: CPT may face complex legal challenges, particularly regarding their legal status, rights, and guardianship. Societal views on individual autonomy, informed consent, and the legal framework for making medical decisions on their behalf are important aspects of sociological analysis. These legal aspects emphasize the need for legal and ethical frameworks that take into account the unique circumstances of CT.

In summary, each aspect of the sociological significance of CPT provides a nuanced understanding of their impact on medicine and society. These twins serve as a lens through which we examine ethics, public awareness, psychosocial dynamics, disability advocacy, research, cultural influences, legal frameworks, and more. Their presence challenges societal norms and encourages critical reflection on our values and responsibilities as a compassionate and inclusive society.

References

1. Mian A, Gabra NI, Sharma T, Topale N, Gielecki J, Tubbs RS, Loukas M. Conjoined twins: from conception to separation, a review. Clin Anat. 2017;30(3):385–96.
2. Chadha R, Lal P, Singh D, Sharma A, Choudhury SR. Lumbosacral parasitic rachipagus twin. J Pediatr Surg. 2006;41(1):e45–8.
3. Ratan SK, Rattan KN, Magu S, Rohilla S, Purwar P, Mathur SK. Thoracolumbar rachipagus parasite. Pediatr Surg Int. 2004;20(4):298–300.
4. Chadha R, Bagga D, Malhotra CJ, Dhar A, Kumar A. Accessory limb attached to the back. J Pediatr Surg. 1993;28(12):1615–7.
5. Navaei AA, Habibi Z, Moradi E, Nejat F. Parasitic rachipagus twins; report of two cases. Childs Nerv Syst. 2015;31(6):1001–3.
6. Debnath B, Biswas SK. Heteropagus twinning on back – a case report. J Indian Med Assoc. 2011;109(7):514–5.
7. Zhang J, Duan H, Zhang Y, Yi Z, Bao S. Parasitic rachipagus conjoined twins with spina bifida, diplomyelia, scoliosis, tethered cord syndrome, and ven-

tricular septal defect – case report. Neurol Med Chir (Tokyo). 2011;51(10):736–9.
8. Baken L, Rousian M, Kompanje EJ, Koning AH, van der Spek PJ, Steegers EA, Exalto N. Diagnostic techniques and criteria for first-trimester conjoined twin documentation: a review of the literature illustrated by three recent cases. Obstet Gynecol Surv. 2013;68(11):743–52.
9. Boer LL, Schepens-Franke AN, Oostra RJ. Two is a crowd: two is a crowd: on the enigmatic etiopathogenesis of conjoined twinning. Clin Anat. 2019;32(5):722–41.
10. Spitz L, Kiely EM. Conjoined twins. JAMA. 2003;289(10):1307–10. https://doi.org/10.1001/jama.289.10.1307.
11. Caceres A, Segura-Masis JL, Caceres-Alan A, Gutierrez-Duran F, Zamora-Chaves J, Segura-Valverde JL. Craniopagus parasiticus: successful separation of a 28-week preterm newborn from parasite sibling twin bearing lethal congenital anomalies associated to Cantrell's pentad and sirenomelia-case-based review of the literature. Childs Nerv Syst. 2021;37(7):2139–46.
12. Bondeson J, Allen E. Craniopagus parasiticus. Everard Home's two-headed boy of Bengal and some other cases. Surg Neurol. 1989;31(6):426–34.
13. Edmonds LD, Layde PM. Conjoined twins in the United States, 1970-1977. Teratology. 1982;25(3):301–8.
14. Stephens TD, Siebert JR, Graham JM Jr, Beckwith JB. Parasitic conjoined twins, two cases, and their relation to limb morphogenesis. Teratology. 1982;26(2):115–21.
15. Bosmia AN, Smelser LB, Griessenauer CJ. An apocryphal case of craniopagus parasiticus: the legend of Edward Mordake. Childs Nerv Syst. 2015;31(12):2211–2.
16. Goldman-Yassen AE, Goodrich JT, Miller TS, Farinhas JM. Preoperative evaluation of craniopagus twins: anatomy, imaging techniques, and surgical management. AJNR Am J Neuroradiol. 2020;41(6):951–9.
17. O'Connell JE. Craniopagus twins: surgical anatomy and embryology and their implications. J Neurol Neurosurg Psychiatry. 1976;39(1):1–22.
18. Stone JL, Goodrich JT. The craniopagus malformation: classification and implications for surgical separation. Brain. 2006;129(Pt 5):1084–95.
19. Browd SR, Goodrich JT, Walker ML. Craniopagus twins. J Neurosurg Pediatr. 2008;1(1):1–20.
20. Machado LE, Bonilla-Musoles F, Osborne N, Skeletal anomalies. The fetus in three dimensions: imaging, embryology, and fetoscopy. In: Kurjak A, Azumendi G, editors. Informa Healthcare. London; 2007. p. 341–60.
21. Lehrich BM, Brown NJ, Shahrestani S, Sahyouni R, Hsu FPK. James T. Goodrich, MD, PhD, 1946-2020: a historical perspective and his contributions to craniopagus separation. J Neurosurg Pediatr. 2020;26(4):454–60.
22. Todorov AB, Cohen KL, Spilotro V, Landau E. Craniopagus twins. J Neurol Neurosurg Psychiatry. 1974;37(12):1291–8.
23. Grossman HJ, Sugar O, Greeley PW, Sadove MS. Surgical separation in craniopagus. JAMA J Am Med Assoc. 1953;153(3):201–7.
24. Sugar O, Grossman H, Greeley P, Destro V. The Brodie craniopagus twins. Trans Am Neurol Assoc. 1953;3(78th Meeting):198–9.
25. Voris HC, Slaughter WB, Christian JR, Cayia ER. Successful separation of craniopagus twins. J Neurosurg. 1957;14(5):548–60. https://doi.org/10.3171/jns.1957.14.5.0548.
26. Duhamel B. La séparation des jumelles craniopages [Letter: The separation of craniopagic twins]. Nouv Press Med. 1975;4(24):1811.
27. Roberts TS. Cerebral venous abnormalities in craniopagus twins. In: Kapp JP, Schmidek HH, editors. The cerebral venous system and its disorders. Grune & Stratton; 1984. p. 355–71.
28. Roberts TS. Craniopagus twins. In: Wilkins RH, Rengachary SS, editors. Neurosurgery, vol. 3. McGraw-Hill; 1985. p. 2091–6.
29. Drummond G, Scott P, Mackay D, Lipschitz R. Separation of the Baragwanath craniopagus twins. Br J Plast Surg. 1991;44(1):49–52.
30. Kaufman MH. The embryology of conjoined twins. Childs Nerv Syst. 2004;20(8–9):508–25.
31. Vandenberg LN, Levin M. Consistent left-right asymmetry cannot be established by late organizers in Xenopus unless the late organizer is a conjoined twin. Development. 2010;137(7):1095–105.
32. Spencer R. Parasitic conjoined twins: external, internal (fetuses in fetu and teratomas), and detached (acardiacs). Clin Anat. 2001;14(6):428–44.
33. Nowosad J, Kucharczyk D. First report of the occurrence and different types of conjoined twins in common whitefish Coregonus maraena larvae originating from the Baltic Sea. Dis Aquat Org. 2019;132(3):163–70.
34. Spencer R. Conjoined twins: theoretical embryologic basis. Teratology. 1992;45(6):591–602.
35. Spencer R. Anatomic description of conjoined twins: a plea for standardized terminology. J Pediatr Surg. 1996;31(7):941–4.
36. Hockley AD, Gornall P, Walsh R, Nishikawa H, Lam H, MacPherson L, Bissenden J, Downey G, Spitz L. Management of pyopagus conjoined twins. Childs Nerv Syst. 2004;20(8–9):635–9.
37. Kingston CA, McHugh K, Kumaradevan J, Kiely EM, Spitz L. Imaging in the preoperative assessment of conjoined twins. Radiographics. 2001;21(5):1187–208.
38. Logroño R, Garcia-Lithgow C, Harris C, Kent M, Meisner L. Heteropagus conjoined twins due to fusion of two embryos: report and review. Am J Med Genet. 1997;73(3):239–43.
39. Chen Y, Chen W, Wang Y, Wei Y, Huang J. Integrated multiomics reveal the molecular characteristics of

conjoined twin fetuses. Reprod Biomed Online. 2023;47(1):26–34.
40. Segal NL. The 2016 Satellite Meeting of the International Society of Twin Studies: An Overview/Tribute to Irving I. Gottesman/Research: MZ Twinning After Single Embryo Transfer; Twin Study of Mononucleosis; Cerebral Injury After Twin-To-Twin Transfusion Syndrome Surgery/Human Interest: Sixteen Twin Pairs Born in a Single Hospital; Death of an Identical Twin Playwright; Twin Themes in Advertising; Conjoined Twins Separated in Saudi Arabia; Murder of One Twin By Her Co-Twin Disproved. Twin Res Hum Genet. 2016;19(5):588–93.
41. Bhettay E, Nelson MM, Beighton P. Epidemic of conjoined twins in Southern Africa? Lancet. 1975;2(7938):741–3. https://doi.org/10.1016/s0140-6736(75)90725-4.
42. Milham S Jr. Symmetrical conjoined twins: an analysis of the birth records of twenty-two sets. J Pediatr. 1966;69(4):643–7. https://doi.org/10.1016/s0022-3476(66)80054-9.
43. Malvasi A, Tinelli A, Buia A, De Luca GF. Possible long-term teratogenic effect of isotretinoin in pregnancy. Eur Rev Med Pharmacol Sci. 2009;13(5):393–6.
44. Boreti S, Prasad N, Patell GS. Cephalothoracoomphalopagus: a rare type of conjoined twin. J Clin Neonatol. 2014;3(1):47–8. https://doi.org/10.4103/2249-4847.128737.
45. Spiers ZB, Biddle AJ, Gabor MJ, Lee E, Gabor LJ. Monocephalic thoracopagus tetrabrachius in twin lambs. Can Vet J. 2010;51(9):1037–9.
46. Aquino DB, Timmons C, Burns D, Lowichik A. Craniopagus parasiticus: a case illustrating its relationship to craniopagus conjoined twinning. Pediatr Pathol Lab Med. 1997;17(6):939–44.
47. Heuer GG, Madsen PJ, Flanders TM, Kennedy BC, Storm PB, Taylor JA. Separation of craniopagus twins by a multidisciplinary team. N Engl J Med. 2019;380(4):358–64. https://doi.org/10.1056/NEJMoa1805132.
48. Lasjaunias P, Kwok R, Goh P, Yeong KY, Lim W, Chng SM. A developmental theory of the superior sagittal sinus(es) in craniopagus twins. Childs Nerv Syst. 2004;20(8–9):526–37.
49. Mutchinick OM, Luna-Muñoz L, Amar E, Bakker MK, Clementi M, Cocchi G, da Graça DM, Feldkamp ML, Landau D, Leoncini E, Li Z, Lowry B, Marengo LK, Martínez-Frías ML, Mastroiacovo P, Métneki J, Morgan M, Pierini A, Rissman A, Ritvanen A, Scarano G, Siffel C, Szabova E, Arteaga-Vázquez J. Conjoined twins: a worldwide collaborative epidemiological study of the International Clearinghouse for Birth Defects Surveillance and Research. Am J Med Genet C Semin Med Genet. 2011;157C(4):274–87.
50. Spencer R. Conjoined twins: developmental malformations and clinical implications. Johns Hopkins University Press; 2003.
51. Sathekge MM, Venkannagari RR, Clauss RP. Scintigraphic evaluation of craniopagus twins. Br J Radiol. 1998;71(850):1096–9.
52. Konovalov AN, Vaĭchis CM. Uspeshnoe razdelenie kraniopagov [The successful separation of a craniopagus]. Zh Vopr Neirokhir Im N N Burdenko. 1991;2:3–10.
53. Rutka JT, Souweidane M, ter Brugge K, Armstrong D, Zuker R, Clarke H, Creighton R, McLeod E, Khoury A, Hoffman HJ. Separation of craniopagus twins in the era of modern neuroimaging, interventional neuroradiology, and frameless stereotaxy. Childs Nerv Syst. 2004;20(8–9):587–92.
54. Harvey DJ, Totonchi A, Gosain AK. Separation of craniopagus twins over the past 20 years: a systematic review of the variables that Lead to successful separation. Plast Reconstr Surg. 2016;138(1):190–200.
55. Staffenberg DA, Goodrich JT. Separation of craniopagus conjoined twins: an evolution in thought. Clin Plast Surg. 2005;32(1):25–34. viii
56. Huang WQ, Fang JY, Xiao LC, Jiang XP, Xia JH, Feng X, Jiang N. Anesthetic management for separation of craniopagus twins. Acta Anaesthesiol Scand. 2004;48(7):919–21.
57. Jansen O, Mehrabi VA, Sartor K. Neuroradiological findings in adult cranially conjoined twins. Case report. J Neurosurg. 1998;89(4):635–9.
58. Tannuri AC, Batatinha JA, Velhote MC, Tannuri U. Conjoined twins: twenty years' experience at a reference center in Brazil. Clinics (Sao Paulo). 2013;68(3):371–7.
59. Shafarenko MS, Zuker RM. Conjoined twin separation: review of 30-year case experience and lessons learned. Plast Reconstr Surg. 2022;150(1):133–44.
60. Giwangkancana G, Kusmayadi DD, Kadi F, Utariani A, Haryawan Z. The multidisciplinary perioperative management of conjoined twin separation surgery during the pandemic. J Multidiscip Healthc. 2022;15:2669–78.
61. Goodrich JT, Staffenberg DA. Craniopagus twins: clinical and surgical management. Childs Nerv Syst. 2004;20(8–9):618–24.
62. Mehollin-Ray AR. Prenatal and postnatal radiologic evaluation of conjoined twins. Semin Perinatol. 2018;42(6):369–80.
63. Dasan TA, N G B, Anvekar SM. A rare case of prenatally detected craniopagus twin. J Clin Diagn Res. 2015;9(4):TJ01–2.
64. Sharma UK, Dangol A, Chawla CD, Shrestha D. Antenatal detection of conjoined twin. JNMA J Nepal Med Assoc. 2007;46(167):133–5.
65. Sanhal CY, Ozekinci M, Mendilcioglu I, Sakinci M, Simsek M. Prenatal diagnosis of total type 1 vertical craniopagus with 3-dimensional sonography. J Ultrasound Med. 2014;33(1):179–81.
66. Rossi AC, Prefumo F. Additional value of fetal magnetic resonance imaging in the prenatal diagnosis of central nervous system anomalies: a systematic review of the literature. Ultrasound Obstet Gynecol. 2014;44(4):388–93.

67. Saleem SN. Fetal MRI: an approach to practice: a review. J Adv Res. 2014;5(5):507–23.
68. Cuillier F, Dillon KC, Grochal F, Scemama JM, Gervais T, Cerekja A, Piazze J. Conjoined twins: what ultrasound may add to management. J Prenat Med. 2012 Jan;6(1):4–6.
69. Bindlish A, Sawal A. A detailed description and discussion on conjoined twins. Cureus. 2022;14(9):e29526.
70. Sabur S, Nayyar R, Joung S. Counseling in fetal medicine: conjoined twins. Eur J Obstet Gynecol Reprod Biol. 2016; vol. 206. p. e98.
71. Lee M, Gosain AK, Becker D. The bioethics of separating conjoined twins in plastic surgery. Plast Reconstr Surg. 2011;128(4):328e–34e.
72. Grosek Š. A case of successful treatment and separation of conjoined twins in Croatia! Croat Med J. 2019;60(4):299–300.
73. Carreker C, De Jong H, Javor V, Fox L, Jacome J, Johns C, Springmeyer K, Davies J. Family support and media considerations with conjoined twins. Semin Perinatol. 2018;42(6):393–401.
74. Greco PS, Pitts D, Weadock WJ, Ladino-Torres M, Laventhal NT, Mychaliska G, Treadwell MC, Carver A. Conjoined twins: an obstetrician's guide to prenatal care and delivery management. J Perinatol. 2021;41(10):2424–31.
75. Campbell S. Separation of craniopagus twins: the Brisbane experience. Childs Nerv Syst. 2004;20(8–9):601–6.
76. Fontes RB, Smith AP, Muñoz LF, Byrne RW, Traynelis VC. Relevance of early head CT scans following neurosurgical procedures: an analysis of 892 intracranial procedures at Rush University Medical Center. J Neurosurg. 2014;121(2):307–12.
77. Thomas JM. Anaesthesia for conjoined twins. Childs Nerv Syst. 2004;20(8–9):538–46.
78. Winston KR, Rockoff MA, Mulliken JB, Strand RD, Murray JE. Surgical division of craniopagi. Neurosurgery. 1987;21(6):782–91.
79. Campbell S, Theile R, Stuart G, Cheng E, Sinnott S, Pritchard G, Isles A. Separation of craniopagus joined at the occiput. Case report. J Neurosurg. 2002;97(4):983–7.
80. Hirokazu T, Takayuki I, Yoshinori H, Kazunari K, Akio A, Keiji K. Separation surgery of pygopagus asymmetrical conjoined twins sharing U-shaped spinal cord: case report and literature review. Childs Nerv Syst. 2013;29(4):699–706.
81. Fieggen AG, Dunn RN, Pitcher RD, Millar AJ, Rode H, Peter JC. Ischiopagus and pygopagus conjoined twins: neurosurgical considerations. Childs Nerv Syst. 2004;20(8–9):640–51.
82. McHugh K, Kiely EM, Spitz L. Imaging of conjoined twins. Pediatr Radiol. 2006;36(9):899–910. quiz 1002-3
83. Leelanukrom R, Somboonviboon W, Bunburaphong P, Kiatkungwanklai P. Anaesthetic experiences in three sets of conjoined twins in King Chulalongkorn Memorial Hospital. Paediatr Anaesth. 2004;14(2):176–83.
84. Vagyannavar R, Bhattacharyya A, Misra G, Hashim M, Asmita. Craniopagus twins for magnetic resonance imaging. Saudi J Anaesth. 2017;11(4):509–10.
85. Yadav M, Chikkala R, Kulkarni D, Gopinath R. Anesthetic management of craniopagus conjoined twins in a remote location. Saudi J Anaesth. 2017;11(4):516–7.
86. Pai KM, Naidu RC, Raja A, Rai YS, Kumar N, Kini A, Joseph S, Hegde V, Ballal HS, Rao R, Sharma SV, Valakatte VK. Surgical nuances in the separation of craniopagus twins - our experience and a follow up of 15 years. Neurol India. 2018;66(2):426–33.
87. Mahmoud MA, Elshawady SB, Korkar GH, Hussein SM, Elserry TH, Mahmoud MWS. Separation of conjoined spinal cords in symmetrical pygopagus twins using intraoperative neuromonitoring: pearls and pitfalls. Childs Nerv Syst. 2023;39(7):1949–55.
88. Richard Winn H. Youmans and Winn neurological surgery – INK. Elsevier Health Sciences, ed 7. 2016; 1–4944.
89. Brizot Mde L, Liao AW, Lopes LM, Silva MM, Krebs V, Schultz R, Zugaib M. Gêmeos unidos: diagnóstico pré-natal, parto e desfecho após o nascimento [Conjoined twins: prenatal diagnosis, delivery and postnatal outcome]. Rev Bras Ginecol Obstet. 2011;33(5):211–8. Portuguese.
90. Afzal AR, Montero FJ. Conjoined Twins. 2023 Aug 8. In: StatPearls [Internet]. Treasure Island (FL): StatPearls Publishing; 2023 Jan–.
91. Lipsky K. Conjoined twins: psychosocial aspects. AORN J. 1982;35(1):58–61.
92. Sahu PK, Singh G, Gupta DK, Mahapatra AK, Kale SS. Pre- and postoperative rehabilitation of craniopagus conjoined twins: a case report. Phys Occup Ther Pediatr. 2021;41(6):637–54.
93. Murray PM. The history of informed consent. Iowa Orthop J. 1990;10:104.
94. Del Carmen MG, Joffe S. Informed consent for medical treatment and research: a review. Oncologist. 2005;10(8):636–41.
95. Murray B. Informed consent: what must a physician disclose to a patient? Virtual Mentor. 2012;14(7):563–6.
96. Beauchamp TL, Childress JF. Principles of biomedical ethics. New York: Oxford University Press; 2013. p. 121.
97. Pallocci M, Treglia M, Passalacqua P, Tittarelli R, Zanovello C, De Luca L, Caparrelli V, De Luna V, Cisterna AM, Quintavalle G, Marsella LT. Informed consent: legal obligation or cornerstone of the care relationship? Int J Environ Res Public Health. 2023;20(3):2118.
98. Deutsch, Spickhoff A. Medizinrecht: Arztrecht, Arzneimittelrecht, Medizinprodukterecht und Transfusionsrecht, 6th Auflage, Springer. 2008. p. 163–91.
99. Kundegraber S. Die ärztlicheAufklärungspflichtimLichte der neuestenJudikatur:

Aufklärungspflicht, Selbstbestimmungsrecht, PatientenwohleinSpannungsfeld? /eingereicht. von: Sonja Kundegraber (Magistra der Rechtswissenschaften, Linz. 2015;s. 39, 44–48.
100. Meisel A, Roth LH, Lidz CW. Toward a model of the legal doctrine of informed consent. Am J Psychiatry. 1977;134(3):285–9.
101. Berg JW, Applebaum PS, Lidz CW, et al. Informed consent: legal theory and clinical practice. Oxford: Oxford University Press; 2001. p. 1–340.
102. Kumar NK. Informed consent: past and present. Perspect Clin Res. 2013 Jan;4(1):21–5.
103. Alderson P, Sutcliffe K, Curtis K. Children's competence to consent to medical treatment. Hast Cent Rep. 2006;36(6):25–34.
104. Beauchamp TL, Childress JF. Principles of biomedical ethics. New York: Oxford University Press; 2001. p. 81–4.
105. Amer AB. Informed consent in adult psychiatry. Oman Med J. 2013;28(4):228–31.
106. Hall DE, Prochazka AV, Fink AS. Informed consent for clinical treatment. CMAJ. 2012;184(5):533–40.
107. Hakeri Hakan. TıpHukuku, Vol. 2 Seçkin Publishing. 2022. p. 446–7.
108. Samanta J, Samanta A. Medical law. Bloomsbury Publishing. 2015; p. 132–3.
109. Ulsenheimer K. Arztstrafrecht in der Praxis (Vol. 7). CF Müller GmbH, I §1. 2008;109-111a & 111c.
110. United Nations Convention on the Rights of the Child. 1989; art. 12.
111. Çakırca Sİ. Bebeklik Dönemi Aşı Uygulamalarının Velayet Hakkı Kapsamında Değerlendirilmesi. İstanbul HukukMecmuası. 2022;80(4):1105–38.
112. UN Committee on the Rights of the Child (CRC), General comment no. 5. General measures of implementation of the Convention on the Rights of the Child. 27 November 2003; CRC/GC/2003/5.
113. UN Committee on the Rights of the Child (CRC), General comment No. 14. On the right of the child to have his or her best interests taken as a primary consideration (art. 3, para. 1), 29 May 2013; CRC /C/GC/14.
114. Ingeborg Schwenzer, Basler KommentarZivilgesetzbuch I Art. 1-456 ZGB (3. Auflage, Helbing&Lichtenhahn. 2006; Art. 301-307 N. 4.
115. PeterTuor,BernhardSchnyder,JörgSchmit,Alexandra Jungo. Das SchweizersicheZivilgesetzbuch (Schulthess). 2015;43 N 50.
116. Kilkelly U. The right to respect for private and family life. A Guide to the Implementation of Article. 2003; 8, 200310-11.
117. Akrivopoulou CM. The right to family life in the framework of ECHR and EU case law. Int J Hum Rights Constit Stud. 2015;3(1):101–9.
118. Burchill R. Rights of the family and children. In: Defining civil and political rights. Routledge; 2016. p. 219–45.
119. Dyer C. Siamese twins to be separated against parents' will. BMJ. 2000;321(7260):529.
120. Waisel DB. Moral permissibility as a guide for decision making about conjoined twins. Anesth Analg. 2005;101(1):41–3.
121. Maher VF, Ford J. The heartbreak of parents patriae. JONAS Healthc Law Ethics Regul. 2002;4(1):18–22.
122. Annas GJ. Conjoined twins – the limits of law at the limits of life. N Engl J Med. 2001;344(14):1104–8.
123. Atkinson L. Ethics and conjoined twins. Childs Nerv Syst. 2004;20(8–9):504–7.
124. Lugosi CI. Playing God: Mary must die so Jodie may live longer. Issues Law Med. 2001;17(2):123–65.
125. Özsunay Ergun. Participation in the decision by the person who is in a situation that affects or limits his/her capacity to express will, Conference organised by the steering committee on bioethics (CDBI) of the Council of Europe Symposium on decision making process regarding medical treatment in end of life situations, 30 November – 1 December 2010. Strasbourg, France.
126. Meier P. The Swiss 2013 guardianship law reform-a presentation and a first assessment in the light of the convention on the rights of persons with disabilities. Elder L Rev. 2016;10:1.
127. Martin HE. Chang and Eng Bunker, "The original Siamese twins": living, dying, and continuing under the spectator's gaze. J Am Cult (Malden). 2011;34(4):372–90.
128. Métneki J, Varjassy P. Conjoined twins. In: Twin research for everyone. Academic Press; 2022. p. 85–112.
129. Mills E. Consciousness and topology. J Philos Res. 2020;45:189.
130. Craig JM. A twin tale to keep you up at night; 2017.
131. Wilkinson S. Separating conjoined twins: the case of Ladan and LalehBijani. In: Ethics, law and society. Routledge; 2019. p. 257–60.
132. Nejat F, Habibi Z, Goudarzi M, Azad MS, Moradi E, Heidari V, Kouchakzadeh L, et al. Emergencyseparation of craniopagustwins: case report. J Neurosurg Pediatr. 2017;20(4):307–13.
133. Hull C. Apparatus for production of three dimensional objects by stereolithography. US Patent. 1986; 4,575,330, 11.
134. Christensen AM, Humphries SM, Goh KY, Swift D. Advanced "tactile" medical imaging for separation surgeries of conjoined twins. Childs Nerv Syst. 2004;20(8–9):547–53.

Part III

Benign Disorders of the Scalp and Calvarium

Editor's Summary

In this "Part III: Benign Disorders of the Scalp and Calvarium," there are a variety of benign disorders discussed that affect the scalp alone or the scalp and calvarium. Benign lesions and neoplasms that involve the scalp and calvarium are addressed in Chap. 10 of this section. Lesions that are associated with and without atrophy of the scalp are discussed in the second chapter of this section, Chap. 11. Unfortunate complications that are associated with the scalp, namely, hypertrophic scarring and pressure sores, are highlighted in detail in Chap. 12. And this section concludes with the extremely important Chap. 13 that is often overlooked by surgeons which covers the metabolic disorders involving the scalp and calvarium. These disorders include rickets, hyperparathyroidism, acromegaly, Paget's disease, osteopenia, and osteoporosis to name a few.

Benign Lesions and Neoplasms of the Scalp and Calvarium

10

Joseph Kedra, Dan Draytsel, and Walter A. Hall

10.1 Introduction

In this chapter, we will explore a broad spectrum of pathologies that affect the scalp and underlying cranium. Understanding these lesions is crucial for accurate diagnosis, appropriate management, and ensuring optimal patient outcomes. While an exhaustive review of all benign lesions affecting the scalp and calvarium is beyond the scope of this chapter, we will consider the most clinically relevant lesions for the neurosurgeon and analyze the clinical presentation, diagnostic imaging, histopathology, and treatment strategies associated with these lesions. Some of the lesions discussed in this chapter can affect both the scalp and the calvarium simultaneously (e.g., epidermoid/dermoid cyst) while other pathologies discussed are only seen in either the scalp or the calvarium and do not cross domains. Additionally, vascular lesions such as hemangioma and arteriovenous malformations are discussed extensively elsewhere in this book and are therefore not included in this chapter.

J. Kedra · W. A. Hall (✉)
Department of Neurosurgery, State University of New York (SUNY) Upstate Medical University, Syracuse, NY, USA
e-mail: hallw@upstate.edu

D. Draytsel
Norton College of Medicine, State University of New York (SUNY) Upstate Medical University, Syracuse, NY, USA

10.1.1 Epidermoid and Dermoid Cysts

Dermoid and epidermoid cysts are benign masses arising from entrapment of the surface ectoderm. Histologically, epidermoid and dermoid cysts are distinguished by their contents with epidermoid cysts containing only stratified squamous epithelium while dermoid cysts contain more complex tissues such as hair, sebaceous and sweat glands, in addition to squamous epithelium. The glands within the dermoid cysts are functional which can result in the deposition on intraluminal keratin [1]. These lesions are likely present at birth but may not become apparent until the first two decades of life [2].

Epidermoid and dermoid cysts form along embryologic fusion lines. Very briefly, during embryogenesis, closure of the neural tube occurs during weeks 3–4 of gestation followed by complex folding along the midline [3]. During weeks 4–8 of gestation, there is ventral folding of the pharyngeal arches and the facial processes. Abnormal folding can occur along any of these fusion lines resulting in the formation of an epidermoid or dermoid cyst where the most common sites of which are periorbital (zygomaticofrontal suture), nasal (frontonasal suture and rhinion), intraoral (floor of mouth), scalp (anterior fontanelle and cranial sutures), and postauricular [4], with some studies suggesting that the fronto-temporal region is the most common [5].

M. Turgut et al. (eds.), *Lesions of the Scalp and Cranial Vault*,
https://doi.org/10.1007/978-3-031-88244-9_10

As mentioned, these cysts are benign as well as slow growing processes; therefore a watchful waiting approach to treatment may be taken. However, surgical management must be a consideration as epidermoid/dermoid cysts are not generally static and therefore tend to enlarge. With growth the cysts can erode into the calvarium and after enough time, they may further erode through the calvarium resulting in epidural extension. Additionally, as with any type of cyst, there is the possibility of infection resulting in abscess formation [6]. Diagnostic imaging is not routinely performed without high clinical suspicion for bony erosion or intracranial extension. However, given that these lesions occur mainly in the pediatric population, imaging modalities that do not utilize radiation such as magnetic resonance imaging (MRI) or ultrasonography would be best. With MRI, epidermoid/dermoid cysts classically show increased T1 signal intensity with variable T2 signal intensities owing to their fat content [7] (Fig. 10.1c–e). Using ultrasound, epidermoid/dermoid cysts have an oval appearance, with a hyperechoic surrounding wall and a hypoechoic internal structure [8].

While epidermoid and dermoid cysts may simply be cutaneous tumors with the potential to erode into the calvarium, intradiploic dermoid cysts do rarely occur. These lesions represent 0.04–0.7% of all cranial tumors and most frequently occur at the bregma (intersection of the coronal and sagittal sutures); however lateral fronto-temporal occurrence has been described [9]. Midline lesions such as these have a higher incidence of intracranial extension and should therefore warrant further diagnostic testing with computed tomography (CT) imaging. CT imaging will show a well-circumscribed exophytic bony lesion which while characteristic is not pathognomonic for a dermoid cyst (Fig. 10.1a–b). Regardless, given the risk for intracranial extension, infection, and sinus tract formation, the gold standard treatment for an intradiploic location is an en-bloc resection after which histopathologic analysis is able to provide a definitive diagnosis [10]. However, surgical intervention is not without risk as intra-operative rupture can lead to the development of a post-operative granulomatous infection [7]. Additionally, there has been a report of a post-operative CSF leak in a patient with previously unrecognized intracranial extension of the cyst prior to surgical resection [11].

10.1.2 Pilar (Trichilemmal) Cysts

Pilar or Trichilemmal cysts (TC) are relatively common scalp lesions originating from the trichilemmal or the exposed outer hair root sheath [12]. While it is a benign lesion, it is of clinical importance due to ability for transformation into a proliferating trichilemmal tumor (PTT), which can undergo malignant transformation into a malignant proliferating trichilemmal tumor (MPTT). Histologically, TCs and benign PTTs are marked by trichilemmal keratinization (the abrupt transition of a nucleated epithelial cell to an anucleate, keratinized cell without the formation of a granular layer) [13].

Clinically, TCs and PTTs are found predominantly in women over 60 years of age. These lesions generally present as smooth, rounded areas of scalp swelling with overlying hair loss. Patients presenting with multiple lesions have been described; however these lesions are generally solitary [14]. Additionally, TCs and PTTs are found in areas other than the scalp including but not limited to the face, neck, trunk, groin, and extremities; however lesions in these areas are not very common [13]. TCs and PTTs commonly range in size from 1 to 10 cm but can grow much larger [15]. Included in the differential diagnosis for TCs and PTTs are multiple malignant processes including squamous cell carcinoma (SCC), basal cell carcinoma (BCC), and angiosarcoma; therefore further diagnostic imaging is usually warranted.

Magnetic resonance imaging (MRI) is usually the diagnostic imaging of choice for TCs and PTTs. TCs and PTTs both show homogenous T1 hypo-intense signal while they can be differentiated on T2 weighted imaging with TCs showing homogenous T2 hyper-intense signal and PTTs showing heterogeneous T2 hyper-intense signal. Additionally, PTTs show heterogenous contrast enhancement due to the cystic and solid nature of the mass [16] (Fig. 10.2).

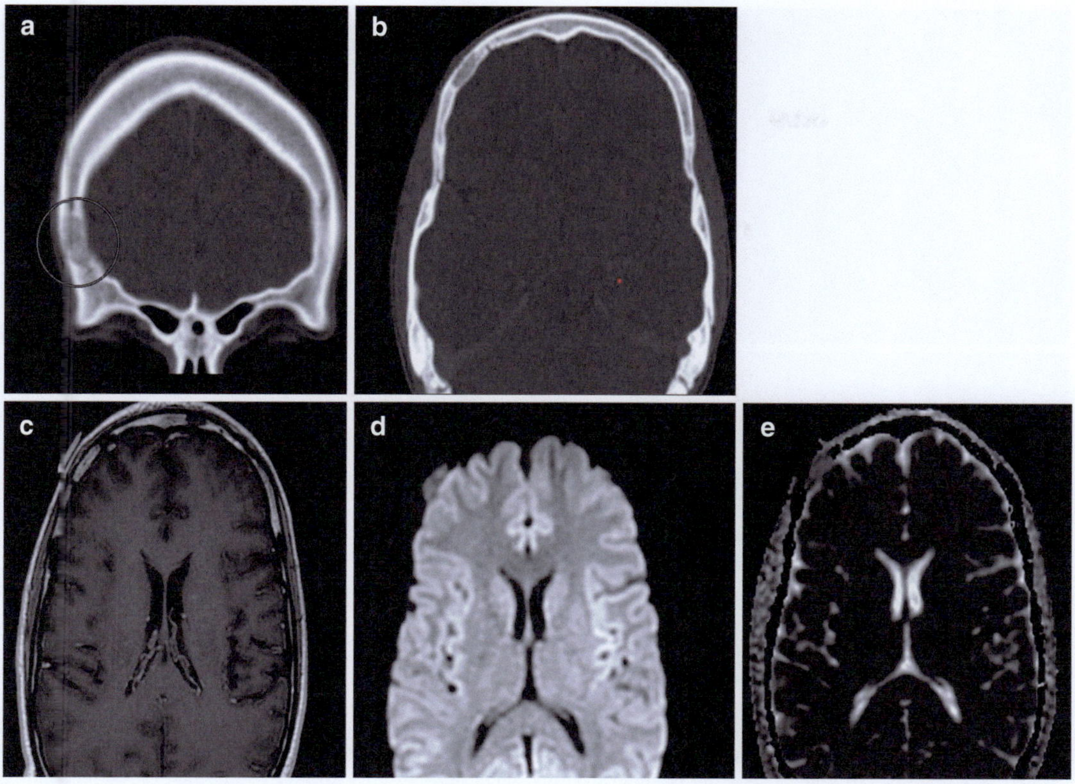

Fig. 10.1 CT and MRI imaging of a right frontal bone dermoid cyst. (**a–b**) Coronal and axial CT images of right frontal dermoid cyst showing some bony destruction of the right frontal bone without violation of the outer or inner tables of the bone. (**c**) Axial MRI T1 post contrast sequence of the right frontal dermoid cyst showing lack of contrast enhancement and iso-intensity to normal bone surrounding the cyst. (**d–e**) Axial MRI diffusion weighted imaging (DWI) and apparent diffusion co-efficient (ADC) showing slight DWI hyper intensity and increased ADC signal

As mentioned above, TCs are truly benign lesions while PTTs harbor the potential for malignant transformation. However, correlation between histologic appearance of the lesions and their clinical behavior has been difficult as some lesions that appear benign histologically (without areas of atypia) can act aggressive clinically and vice versa. One group has proposed a classification system for PTT which provides correlation between histologic appearance and clinical behavior. In this system, Group 1 PTTs are benign lesions that had no recurrence, displayed well-circumscribed margins, modest nuclear atypia, and no pathologic mitoses, necrosis, or vascular or neural invasion. Group 2 PPTs, low-grade malignant lesions that may recur, exhibit in addition irregular and locally invasive margins and involvement of the deep dermis and subcutis. Group 3 PPTs, high-grade malignant tumors with a tendency toward recurrence and lymph node metastasis, manifest invasive patterns of growth with prominent nuclear pleomorphism, atypical mitoses, necrosis, and possible vascular or neural invasion [14]. This grouping system can ideally guide management following surgical excision. Truly benign group 1 PTTs require only simple local excision. Group 2 PTTs should be treated with a wide local excision with approximately a 1 cm margins [17]. Group 3 lesions should be treated with wide local excision followed by adjuvant chemotherapy with cisplatin, Adriamycin, and Vindesine [18]. Following treatment, group 3 lesions show a 3.7% recurrence rate with time to recurrence ranging from 6 months to 10 years [19].

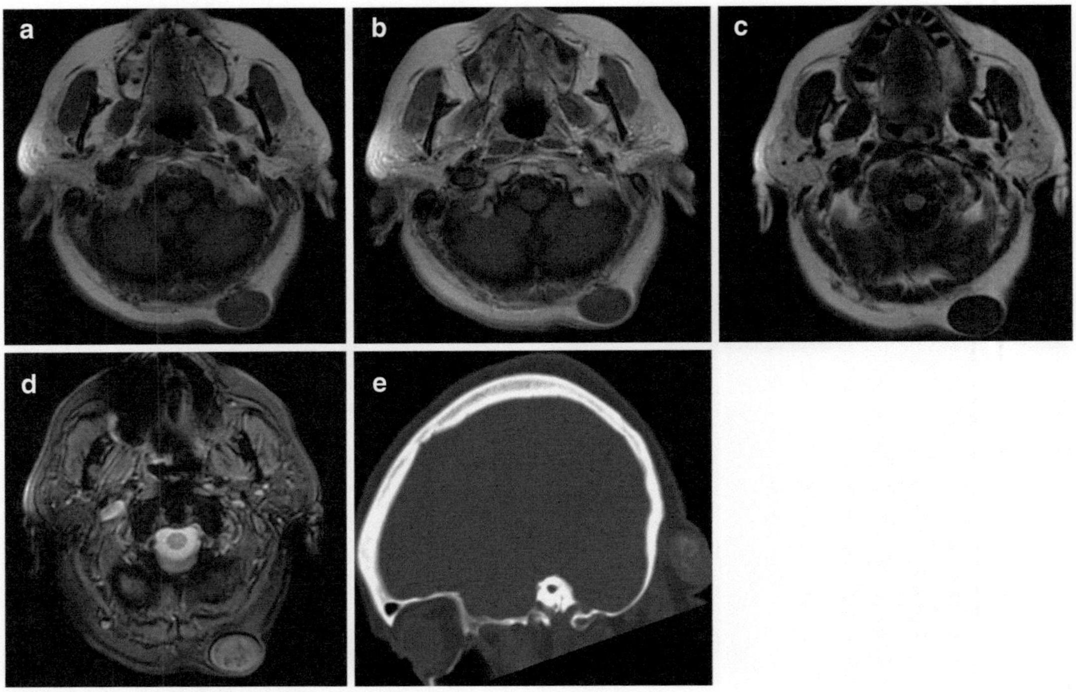

Fig. 10.2 CT and MRI imaging of a left occipital pilar cyst. (**a–b**) Axial MRI T1-weighted non-contrast enhanced (**a**) and post contrast (**b**) images showing iso-intensity to brain parenchyma and lack of contrast enhancement within the left occipital cyst. (**c**) Axial MRI FLAIR sequence showing homogenous hypo-intensity within the cyst. (**d**) Axial MRI GRE sequences showing heterogenous susceptibility artifact within the cyst corresponding to the calcification seen within the cyst on the sagittal CT image in panel (**e**)

10.1.3 Lipoma

Lipomas are an abnormal collection of mature fat cells either subcutaneously or intramuscularly and are one of the most commonly seen soft tissue tumors. Lipomas generally occur spontaneously but may also be post traumatic and occur at the site of previous trauma. Lipomas can be seen anywhere on the body but occur proximally more often than distally including in the scalp. Lipomas rarely occur in children with the peak incidence from age 40–60 years and demonstrating a slight male predominance [20]. Clinically lipomas typically present as a painless soft tissue mass. Given the often-asymptomatic nature of lipomas, their true incidence is likely underestimated.

Radiographically, US or MRI are the diagnostic imaging modalities of choice in the diagnosis of lipoma. Using US, lipomas appear as a homogenous hyperechoic mass. On MRI, lipomas show a homogenous isointense signal compared to fat on all sequences with the presence of occasional thin, fibrous septae [21]. Additionally, lipomas are deemed to be determinate lesions and can be diagnosed solely based on radiographic features on MRI [22].

Lipomas can be managed conservatively with observation; however if the mass is found to be increasing in size or poses a cosmetic issue, simple marginal resection is the treatment of choice. Following resection, local recurrence rates tend to be <5% [21, 23].

In addition to the subcutaneous variant, lipomas rarely occur as intraosseous tumors with intraosseous lipomas accounting for approximately 0.1% of all bone tumors [24]. Intraosseous lipomas are most often found in the calcaneus and metaphysis of long bones and much more rarely in the calvarium with calvarial intraosseous lipoma accounting for approximately 4% of all intraosseous lipomas [25]. The age distribution for intraosseous lipomas differs significantly from the subcutaneous variant with an age range of 4–85 years reported in the literature and no difference in their occurrence between males and females [26].

Intraosseous lipomas originate from hyperplasia of the bone marrow fat cells in trabecular bone leading to expansion of the medullary cavity of the bone. The unopposed growth of the bone marrow cells leads to necrosis, calcification, and ossification within the growing tumor. Additionally, these osteolytic changes can cause loss of trabecular bone and formation of new reactive bone [27, 28]. It was initially postulated that intraosseous lipomas were secondary lesions that originated either as part of the healing process following trauma or as part of a calcific reaction following bone infarction. These theories are generally regarded as incorrect currently as most patients do not have a history of trauma, furthermore bone calcification usually originates from the periphery and spreads inward while the calcification seen in intraosseous lipomas originating in the central adipocytes. Intraosseous lipomas are now regarded as primary and not secondary tumors and are not necessarily associated with any other processes [29, 30].

According to the classification system first proposed by Milgram in 1988 [24], intraosseous lipomas can be organized into three stages which can all be differentiated on CT. In stage 1 adipocyte hyperplasia occurs resulting in a low-density mass with cortical or medullary expansion being seen on CT imaging. Stage 2 is marked by the necrosis of the hyperplastic adipocytes and subsequent calcification. During stage 3, there is progression of the fat necrosis seen in stage 2 in addition to cyst and reactive bone formation resulting in primary trabecular bone absorption, central and peripheral calcification, and cystic areas that are seen on CT [31, 32]. Given that these lesions are primarily a soft tissue lesion, MRI is also of significant diagnostic utility. As expected, intraosseous lipomas will show high T1 and T2 signal intensity on MRI that is like that seen of subcutaneous fat on MRI [33] (Fig. 10.3).

There is no consensus as to the best treatment strategy for an intraosseous lipoma. As they are benign lesions, a conservative, watchful waiting approach with routine follow-up imaging is appropriate for many patients, specifically those that are asymptomatic and that do not have increased risk factor for fracture. For symptomatic patients, or those predisposed to fracture, surgical resection and bony reconstruction are recommended [34, 35]. Additionally, when the calvarium is involved, cosmesis must be considered when deciding on conservative versus surgical treatment. Recurrence of an intraosseous lipoma is extremely rare following surgical treatment for those reported in the literature, especially those occurring in the calvarium [36].

10.1.4 Intraosseous Meningioma

Meningioma is a relatively common benign cranial tumor arising from the dura mater. The majority of meningiomas are intradural and exist within the subdural space; however approximately 1–2% of meningiomas arise in the extradural space including the skin, nasopharynx, and skull [37, 38]. When meningiomas are present within he calvarium, they are called primary intraosseous meningiomas, which comprise approximately two-thirds of all extradural meningiomas [38]. By definition, meningiomas arise from meningo-epithelial cells; therefore the origin of extradural meningiomas is not clear. The leading theory is that primary intraosseous meningiomas rise from arachnoid cap cells on blood vessels which traverse the skull [39].

Clinically, primary intraosseous meningiomas present as firm, painless, slow growing scalp masses which may have a relationship to cranial sutures [40]. Calvarial intraosseous meningiomas are generally asymptomatic and are found incidentally, whereas skull base intraosseous meningiomas may present with neurologic symptoms due to their close proximity to the cranial nerves [41]. Unlike intradural meningiomas, intraosseous meningiomas show no sex predominance and occur equally in males and females [42]. Like intradural meningiomas, intraosseous meningiomas generally present later in life; however they have been found to have a second peak of incidence in the second decade of life [38].

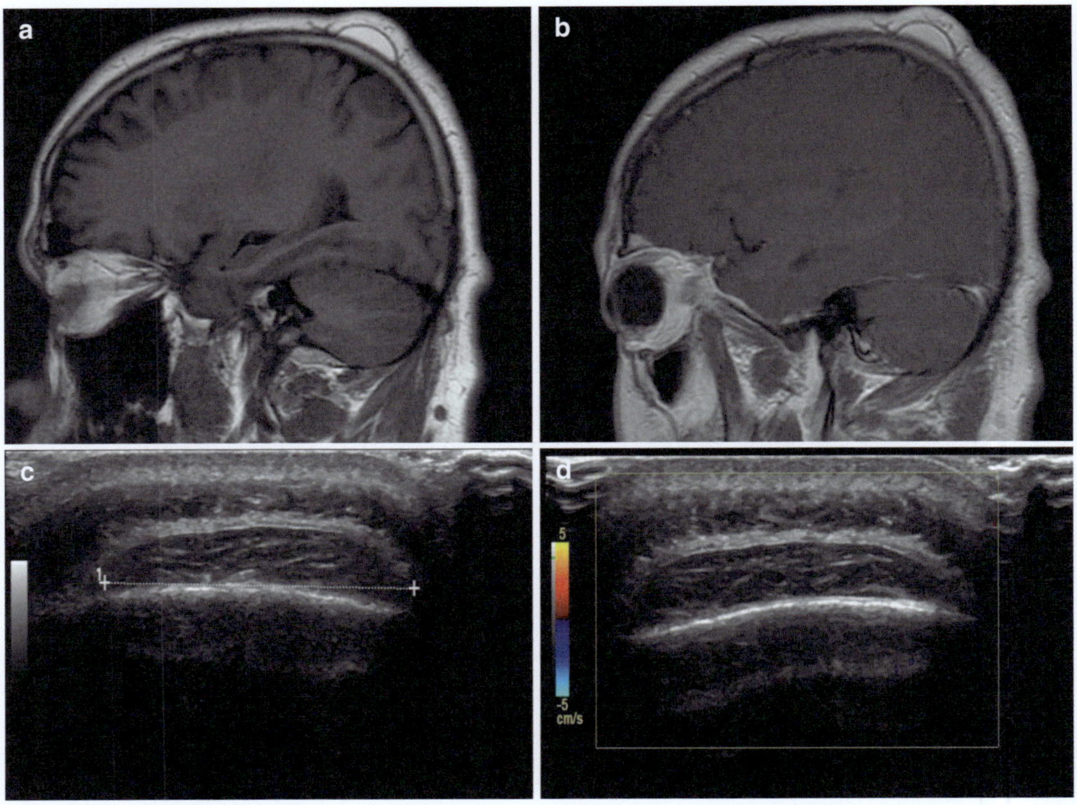

Fig. 10.3 MRI and ultrasound images of a parasagittal scalp lipoma. (**a–b**) Sagittal T1-weighted pre-contrast (**a**) and post contrast (**b**) showing a well demarcated lesion that is homogenously iso-intense to the subcutaneous fatty tissues without any post-contrast enhancement. (**c**) Ultrasound showing a well demarcated subcutaneous lesion iso-echoic to the surrounding subcutaneous tissue. (**d**) Doppler ultrasound showing no abnormal vasculature or blood flow to indicate malignancy

Like many other calvarial lesions, intraosseous meningiomas may be first identified on simple skull X-rays where the majority will demonstrate hyperostosis, thinning of the cortical bone, abnormal vascular markings, and irregular calcification [43]. CT imaging commonly shows a hyperdense, expansile lesion causing destruction of the cortical layers of the skull. These radiographic findings make intraosseous meningioma appear very similar to fibrous dysplasia (discussed elsewhere in this chapter) [44]. However, intraosseous meningiomas may appear as osteolytic lesions, instead showing a hypodense mass causing cortical destruction [45]. These masses are greatly similar to their intradural counterparts on MRI showing a T1 hypointense signal, T2 hyperintense signal, and avid homogenous contrast enhancement [40]. Histologically, intraosseous meningiomas appear similar to the intradural variant with their pathology often showing psammoma bodies and eosinophilic tumor cells with indistinct borders and nuclear pseudoinclusions grouped in a whorl pattern [44].

The gold standard, curative treatment for meningiomas is wide local excision of the mass when feasible. This result is more likely with calvarial intraosseous meningiomas than skull base meningiomas. Maximal resection is achieved with the use of neuronavigation and careful preoperative planning. The potential defect is mapped using a 3D CT to pre-fabricate a cranioplasty implant which can be placed during the index surgery limiting the number of return trips to the operating room for the patient [46]. Conversely, not all intraosseous meningiomas can be fully resected, either because of their proximity to or encroachment upon vital neural structures or invasion into parts of the skull that are either inaccessible or would be too morbid to resect In these cases, patients are followed with serial imaging to monitor for tumor growth. Of note, a much greater percentage of intraosseous meningiomas have some evidence of malignant transformation compared to intradural meningiomas (11% vs. 2%) [47, 48]. Therefore, patients that are unable to have a gross total resection must be carefully considered for adjuvant therapy with external beam radiation therapy or gamma knife radiosurgery, chemotherapy, hormonal therapy, or some combination thereof [41].

10.1.5 Osteoblastoma

Osteoblastoma is a benign growth of osteoblast cells, those which form bone, which usually occurs at the metaphysis of long bones and in vertebral bodies. Osteoblastoma of the calvarium makes up approximately 15–20% of all osteoblastoma cases [49]. Osteoblastoma generally occurs in younger people with approximately 80% of cases occurring in those younger than 35 years of age with no significant difference in incidence between males and females [50]. Clinically patient's generally present with complaints of an erythematous soft tissue swelling causing a dull, aching, and localized pain. Given these symptoms are non-specific in nature, further diagnostic testing is required to make a definitive diagnosis. CT is usually the initial diagnostic study of choice. Radiographically, osteoblastoma appears as a well circumscribed, cystic appearing lesion causing cortical erosion with a thin layer of newly formed bone surrounding the lesion. Depending on the size and age of the lesions, they may appear radiolucent, radioopaque, or have a more heterogenous appearance [51] (Fig. 10.4). Histologically, osteoblastoma demonstrates a trabecular network of osteoid, an unmineralized precursor to bone matrix, primarily made up of osteoblasts [52]. Additionally, multi-nucleated giants cells without atypia and numerous thin walled vascular channels are usually present [50].

Osteoblastoma is closely related to another benign bony lesion, osteoid osteoma. These lesions are essentially identical histologically and radiographically. They also produce the same clinical symptomatology and similar demographics profiles. Osteoblastoma and osteoid osteoma are therefore only differentiated based on size. Lesions <1.5 cm in size are classified as osteoid osteoma while lesions >2.0 cm are classified as osteoblastoma [53, 54]. However, osteoblastoma can show more local bony destruction when compared to osteoid osteoma, likely due to its larger size.

Like most benign lesions, the first option for management is observation; however within the differential diagnosis for lesions presenting similarly to osteoblastoma is osteosarcoma. Osteosarcoma is a malignant neoplasm affecting the bone which shows more aggressive bony destruction locally and has the potential for metastasis [55]. Therefore, definitive diagnosis is needed for appropriate treatment. Simple local resection of the lesion is the treatment of choice and provides tissue for a definitive diagnosis. With subtotal resection, the recurrence rate has been reported to be as high as 20% [56]; however most reports show negligible recurrence rates [57, 58]. Given the low recurrence rate and slow growing, benign nature of osteoblastoma, there is no role for post-operative radiation therapy, even with a subtotal resection.

10.1.6 Fibro-osseous Lesions

Fibro-osseous lesions are a group of lesions characterized by the replacement of normal bone with fibrous tissue, collagen, giant cells, and new blood vessels. Benign variants of fibro-osseous lesions include fibrous dysplasia and ossifying fibroma. Ossifying fibroma is typically found at the skull base and not within the calvarium and is therefore not discussed below.

Fibrous dysplasia is the result of the replacement of normal bone with fibrous connective tissue with varying degrees of mineralization. This entity accounts for 2.5–10% of all bone tumors [59]. Seventy percent of cases of fibrous

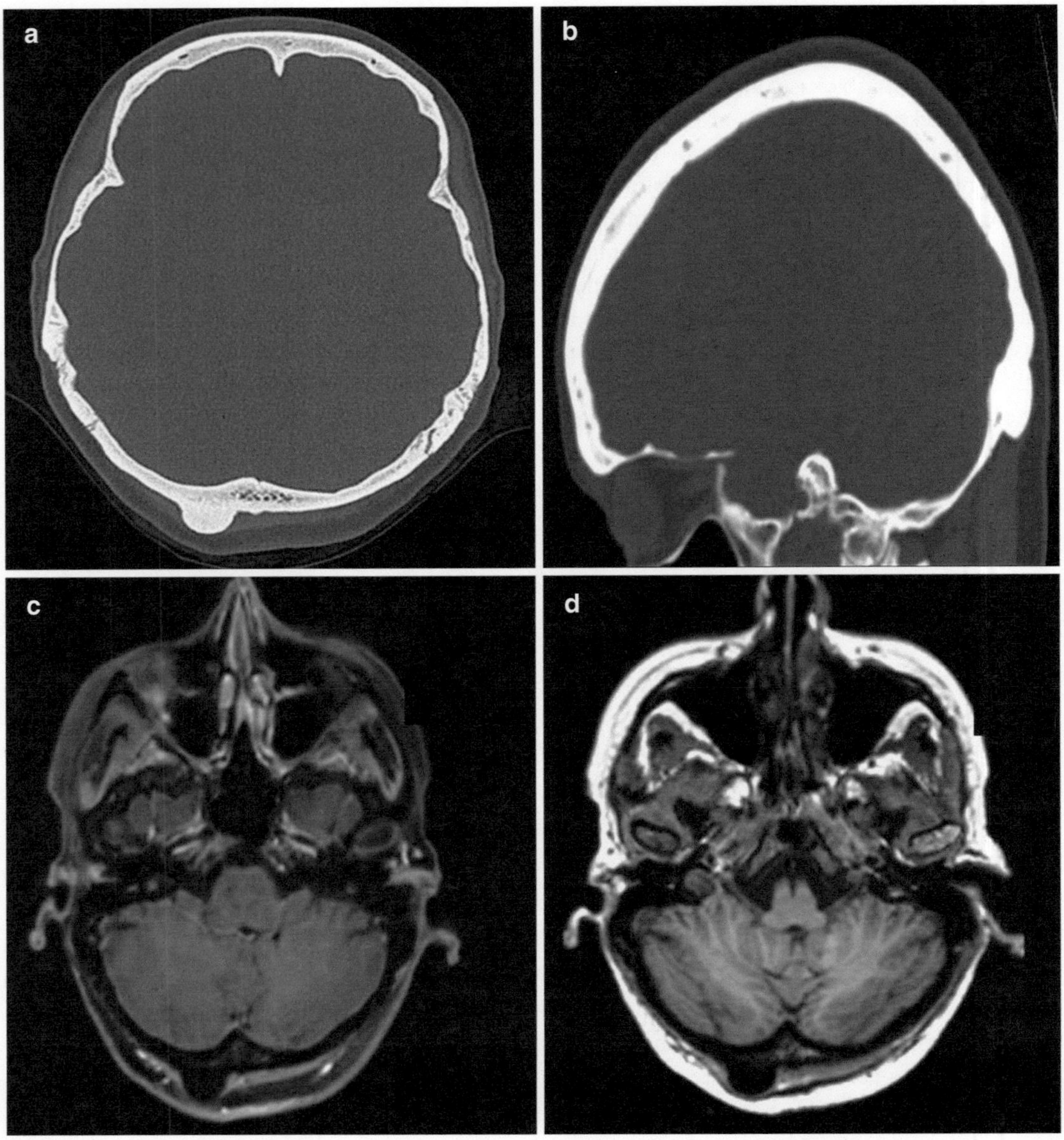

Fig. 10.4 CT and MRI images of a right occipital osteoid osteoma. (**a–b**) Axial and sagittal CT images showing an osteoid osteoma originating from the outer cortex of the right occipital bone. The lesion is homogenously radio-opaque and almost indiscernible from the normal adjacent bone. (**c–d**) Axial T1-weighted non-contrast (**c**) and post contrast (**d**) MRI images showing hypo-intensity within the lesion without any post-contrast enhancement

dysplasia are monostotic while 30% are polyostotic [60]. Fibrous dysplasia lesions are generally intradiploic, expansile lesions that affecting the outer table of the skull while sparing the inner table. While typically sporadic, fibrous dysplasia is also part of the constellation of symptoms seen in McCune-Albright syndrome along with precocious puberty, café au lait spots, and various endocrinopathies [61]. On CT, fibrous dysplasia appears as a mixed sclerotic and lytic lesion with a ground glass appearance. On MRI, fibrous dysplasia demonstrates low T1 and T2 signal intensity due to a high collagen content. Contrast uptake is generally heterogenous due to the variable fibro-osseous content [62] (Fig. 10.5).

Treatment of fibrous dysplasia involves a combined surgical and medical approach. Depending on the extent of the lesion (monostotic vs. polyostotic) and the anatomical location, fibrous dysplasia can be treated with radical, gross total resection followed by cranial reconstruction or limited resection and skeletal shaping and contouring [63]. When these lesions are in cosmetically challenging areas, they can require the combined efforts of both neurosurgeons and plastic surgeon to ensure a positive cosmetic outcome. Medical adjuncts have also been used in the treatment of fibrous dysplasia including steroids, tamoxifen, and bisphosphonates. These medications have varying levels of effectiveness with only bisphosphonates showing any benefit [64–66]. Therefore, the mainstay of treatment for fibrous dysplasia remains surgical resection of affected bone. Additionally, fibrous dysplasia has the potential for malignant transformation making timely treatment of the utmost importance. Approximately 0.5% of patients with fibrous dysplasia will show malignant transformation to osteosarcoma, chondrosarcoma, or fibrosarcoma. The risk for transformation is elevated to 4% for those with McCune-Albright syndrome [67].

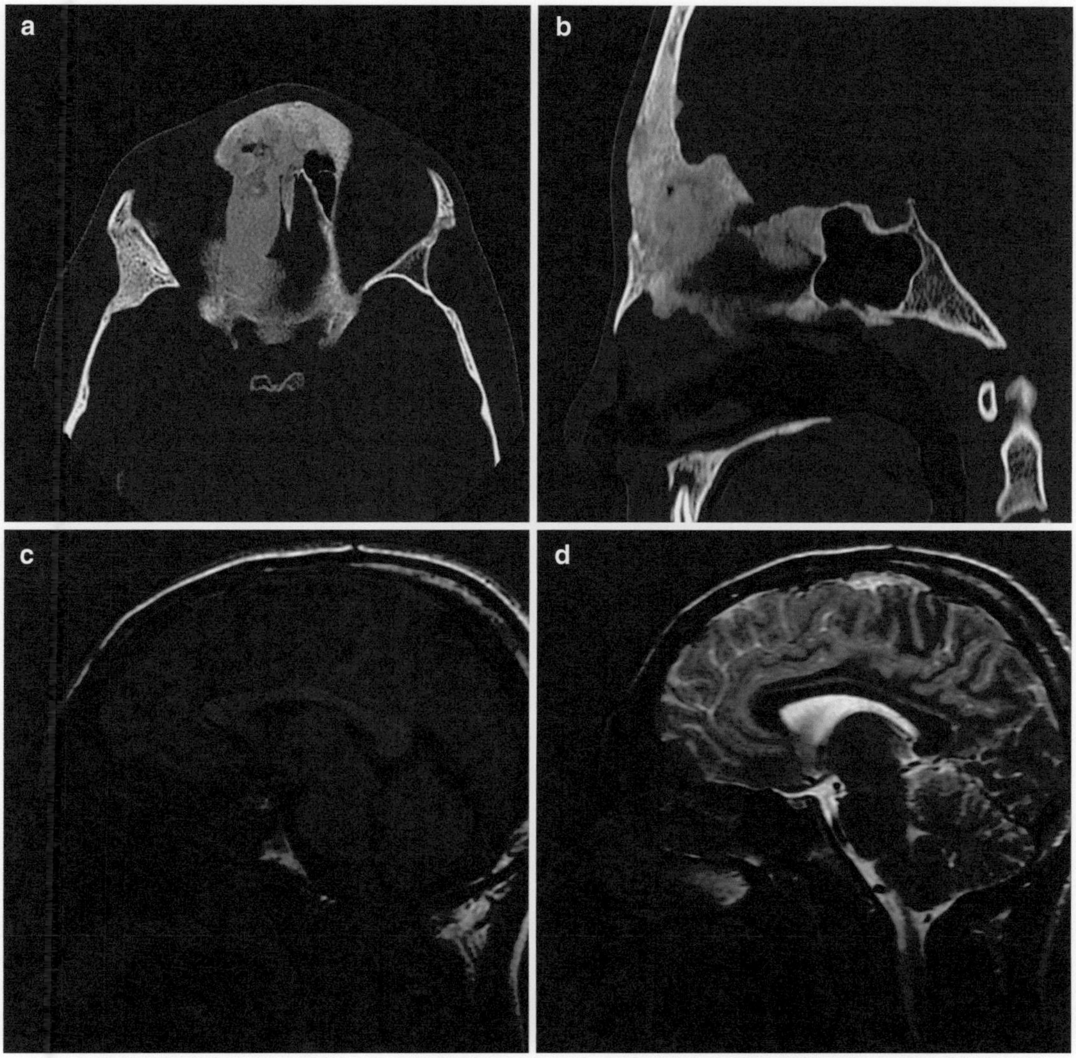

Fig. 10.5 CT and MRI images of right frontal bone and ethmoid bone fibrous dysplasia. (**a–b**) Axial (**a**) and sagittal (**b**) CT images of right frontal and ethmoid fibrous dysplasia showing mainly sclerotic bone compared to the adjacent normal frontal bone with a few lytic areas. (**c–d**) Sagittal T1 (**c**) and T2 (**d**) weighted MRI sequences showing both T1 and T2 signal hypo-intensity within the right frontal and ethmoid fibrous dysplasia

10.2 Conclusion

While the lesions described in this chapter are most commonly benign, they are not without clinical consequences that include pain, swelling, mass effect causing neurologic symptoms, cosmetic effects, and the risk of malignant transformation. Although surgical resection is the gold standard treatment for most of the lesions discussed, an accurate diagnosis and treatment of these lesions requires a multidisciplinary team approach, incorporating clinical, radiological, and histopathological findings to ensure optimal patient outcomes.

References

1. Reissis D, Pfaff MJ, Patel A, Steinbacher DM. Craniofacial dermoid cysts: histological analysis and inter-site comparison. Yale J Biol Med. 2014;87(3):349–57.
2. Pryor SG, Lewis JE, Weaver AL, Orvidas LJ. Pediatric dermoid cysts of the head and neck. Otolaryngol – Head Neck Surg. 2005;132(6):938–42.
3. Ahuja R, Azar NF. Orbital dermoids in children. Semin Ophthalmol. 2006;21(3):207–11.
4. Golden BA, Jaskolka MS, Ruiz RL. Craniofacial and orbital dermoids in children. Oral Maxillofac Surg Clin North Am. 2012;24(3):417–25.
5. Sorenson EP, Powel JE, Rozzelle CJ, Tubbs RS, Loukas M. Scalp dermoids: a review of their anatomy, diagnosis, and treatment. Child's Nervous Syst. 2013;29(3):375–80.
6. Agrawal A. Infected dermoid cyst presenting as scalp abscess. Infect Dis Clin Pract. 2008;16(5):311–2.
7. Wood J, Couture D, David LR. Midline dermoid cyst resulting in frontal bone erosion. J Craniofac Surg. 2012;23(1):131–4.
8. Riebel T, David S, Thomale UW. Calvarial dermoids and epidermoids in infants and children: sonographic spectrum and follow-up. Childs Nerv Syst. 2008;24:1327–32.
9. Rinna C, Reale G, Calafati V, Calvani F, Ungari C. Dermoid cyst: unusual localization. J Craniofac Surg. 2012;23(5):e392–4.
10. Vega RA, Hidlay DT, Tye GW, Fuller CE, Rhodes JL. Intradiploic dermoid cyst of the lateral frontotemporal skull: case report and review of the literature. Pediatr Neurosurg. 2013;49(4):232–5.
11. Bodkin PA, Bhangoo R, Walsh AR, Sgouros S. Beware of the midline scalp lump. J R Soc Med. 2004;97(5):239–41.
12. Jones EW. Proliferating epidermoid cysts. Arch Dermatol. 1966;94(1):11–9.
13. Satyaprakash AK, Sheehan DJ, Sangüeza OP. Proliferating trichilemmal tumors: a review of the literature. Dermatologic Surg. 2007;33(9):1102–8.
14. Ye J, Nappi O, Swanson PE, Patterson JW, Wick MR. Proliferating Pilar tumors: a clinicopathologic study of 76 cases with a proposal for definition of benign and malignant variants. Am J Clin Pathol. 2004;122(4):566–74.
15. Sau P, Graham JH, Helwig EB. Proliferating epithelial cysts. Clinicopathological analysis of 96 cases. J Cutan Pathol. 1995;22(5):394–406.
16. Kitajima K, Imanaka K, Hashimoto K, Hayashi M, Kuwata Y, Sugimura K. Magnetic resonance imaging findings of proliferating trichilemmal tumor. Neuroradiology. 2005;47(6):406–10.
17. Shet T, Rege J, Naik L. Cytodiagnosis of simple and proliferating trichilemmal cysts. Acta Cytol. 2001;45(4):582–8.
18. Hayashi I, Harada T, Muraoka M, Ishii M. Malignant proliferating trichilemmal tumour and CAV (cisplatin, adriamycin, vindesine) treatment. Br J Dermatol. 2004;150(1):156–7.
19. Takenaka H, Kishimoto S, Shibagaki R, Nagata M, Noda Y, Yasuno H. Recurrent malignant proliferating trichilemmal tumour: local management with ethanol injection. Br J Dermatol. 1998;139(4):726–9.
20. Johnson CN, Ha AS, Chen E, Davidson D. Lipomatous soft-tissue tumors. J Am Acad Orthop Surg. 2018;26(22):779–88.
21. Murphey MD, Carroll JF, Flemming DJ, Pope TL, Gannon FH, Kransdorf MJ. From the archives of the AFIP: benign musculoskeletal lipomatous lesions. Radiographics. 2004;24(5):1433–66.
22. Papp DF, Khanna AJ, McCarthy EF, Carrino JA, Farber AJ, Frassica FJ. Magnetic resonance imaging of soft-tissue tumors: determinate and indeterminate lesions. J Bone Joint Surg Am. 2007;89(Suppl 3):103–15.
23. Bjerregaard P, Hagen K, Daugaard S, Kofoed H. Intramuscular lipoma of the lower limb. Long-term follow-up after local resection. J Bone Joint Surg. 1989;71(5):812–5.
24. Milgram JW. Intraosseous lipomas. A clinicopathologic study of 66 cases. Clin Orthop Relat Res. 1988;231:277–302.
25. Milgram JW. Intraosseous lipomas: radiologic and pathologic manifestations. Radiology. 1988;167(1):155–60.
26. Campbell RS, Grainger AJ, Mangham DC, Beggs I, Teh J, Davies AM. Intraosseous lipoma: report of 35 new cases and a review of the literature. Skeletal Radiol. 2003;32(4):209–22.
27. Hirata M, Kusuzaki K, Hirasawa Y. Eleven cases of intraosseous lipoma of the calcaneus. Anticancer Res. 2001;21(6a):4099–103.
28. Goto T, Kojima T, Iijima T, Yokokura S, Motoi T, Kawano H, et al. Intraosseous lipoma: a clinical study of 12 patients. J Orthop Sci. 2002;7(2):274–80.
29. Bruni L. The "cockade" image: a diagnostic sign of calcaneum intraosseous lipoma. Rays. 1986;11(1):51–4.

30. Muthuphei MN. Intra-osseous lipoma of the calcaneus. South African medical journal =. Suid-Afrikaanse tydskrif vir geneeskunde. 1996;86(12):1554–5.
31. Radl R, Leithner A, Machacek F, Cetin E, Koehler W, Koppany B, et al. Intraosseous lipoma: retrospective analysis of 29 patients. Int Orthop. 2004;28(6):374–8.
32. Arslan G, Karaali K, Cubuk M, Senol U, Lüleci E. Intraosseous lipoma of the frontal bone. A case report. Acta Radiol (Stockholm, Sweden : 1987). 2000;41(4):320–1.
33. Petcevik Y, Arslan IB, Arslan Y. CT and MRI findings of the incidental intraosseous lipomatous lesions of the sphenoid bone. Head Neck. 2016;38(2):E41–4.
34. Sanjuan A, Dean A, Garcia B, Alamillos F, Roldan E, Blanco A. Condylar intramedullary intraosseous lipoma: contribution of a new case and review of the literature. J Clin Exp Dent. 2017;9(3):e498–502.
35. Wolfswinkel EM, Imahiyerobo TA, McComb JG, Sanchez-Lara PA, Urata MM. Proteus syndrome with a cranial intraosseous lipoma. J Craniofac Surg. 2017;28(8):e771–e3.
36. Han Z, Liu Y, Hao X, Li C, Tian Y. Large intraosseous lipoma of the skull: a case report and review of the literature. World Neurosurg. 2018;120:525–9.
37. Muzumdar DP, Vengsarkar US, Bhatjiwale MG, Goel A. Diffuse calvarial meningioma: a case report. J Postgrad Med. 2001;47(2):116–8.
38. Lang FF, Macdonald OK, Fuller GN, DeMonte F. Primary extradural meningiomas: a report on nine cases and review of the literature from the era of computerized tomography scanning. J Neurosurg. 2000;93(6):940–50.
39. Inagaki K, Otsuka F, Matsui T, Ogura T, Makino H. Effect of etidronate on intraosseous meningioma. Endocr J. 2004;51(3):389–90.
40. Arana E, Diaz C, Latorre FF, Menor F, Revert A, Beltrán A, et al. Primary intraosseous meningiomas. Acta Radiol (Stockholm, Sweden : 1987). 1996;37(6):937–42.
41. El Mahou S, Popa L, Constantin A, Jamard B, Cantagrel A, Mazieres B, et al. Multiple intraosseous meningiomas. Clin Rheumatol. 2006;25(4):553–4.
42. Tokgoz N, Oner YA, Kaymaz M, Ucar M, Yilmaz G, Tali TE. Primary intraosseous meningioma: CT and MRI appearance. AJNR Am J Neuroradiol. 2005;26(8):2053–6.
43. Changhong L, Naiyin C, Yuehuan G, Lianzhong Z. Primary intraosseous meningiomas of the skull. Clin Radiol. 1997;52(7):546–9.
44. Daffner RH, Yakulis R, Maroon JC. Intraosseous meningioma. Skeletal Radiol. 1998;27(2):108–11.
45. Rosahl SK, Mirzayan MJ, Samii M. Osteolytic intra-osseous meningiomas: illustrated review. Acta Neurochir. 2004;146(11):1245–9.
46. Westendorff C, Kaminsky J, Ernemann U, Reinert S, Hoffmann J. Image-guided sphenoid wing meningioma resection and simultaneous computer-assisted cranio-orbital reconstruction: technical case report. Neurosurgery. 2007;60(2 Suppl 1):ONSE173-4. discussion ONSE4
47. Younis G, Sawaya R. Intracranial osteolytic malignant meningiomas appearing as extracranial soft-tissue masses. Neurosurgery. 1992;30(6):932–5.
48. Partington MD, Scheithauer BW, Piepgras DG. Carcinoembryonic antigen production associated with an osteolytic meningioma. Case report. J Neurosurg. 1995;82(3):489–92.
49. Doshi SV, Frantz TD, Korol HW. Benign osteoblastoma of the temporal bone: case report and literature review. Am J Otolaryngol. 2001;22(3):211–4.
50. Lichtenstein L. Benign osteoblastoma; a category of osteoid-and bone-forming tumors other than classical osteoid osteoma, which may be mistaken for giant-cell tumor or osteogenic sarcoma. Cancer. 1956;9(5):1044–52.
51. Gellad FE, Hafiz MA, Blanchard CL. Osteoblastoma of the temporal bone: CT findings. J Comput Assist Tomogr. 1985;9(3):577–9.
52. Singer JM, Deutsch GP. The successful use of radiotherapy for osteoblastoma. Clin Oncol (Royal College of Radiologists (Great Britain)). 1993;5(2):124–5.
53. Dugert E, Lagleyre S, Brouchet A, Deguine O, Cognard C, Bonneville F. Osteoid osteoma invading the posterior labyrinth of the petrous bone. AJNR Am J Neuroradiol. 2010;31(9):1764–6.
54. Cervoni L, Innocenzi G, Raguso M, Salvati M, Caruso R. Osteoblastoma of the calvaria: report of two cases diagnosed with MRI and clinical review. Neurosurg Rev. 1997;20(1):51–4.
55. Lucas DR, Unni KK, McLeod RA, O'Connor MI, Sim FH. Osteoblastoma: clinicopathologic study of 306 cases. Hum Pathol. 1994;25(2):117–34.
56. Clutter DJ, Leopold DA, Gould LV. Benign osteoblastoma. Report of a case and review of the literature. Archiv Otolaryngol (Chicago, Ill : 1960). 1984;110(5):334–6.
57. Matsumoto K, Kakita K, Fukuma S. Large, benign osteoblastoma of the temporal bone – case report. Neurol Med Chir. 1989;29(5):444–8.
58. Hidaka H, Yamauchi D, Fujishima F, Watanabe M, Kato Y, Nomura K, et al. Osteoid osteoma of the temporal bone manifesting as first bite syndrome and a meta-analysis combined with osteoblastoma. Eur Archiv Oto-Rhino-Laryngol. 2017;274(2):607–16.
59. Gabbay JS, Yuan JT, Andrews BT, Kawamoto HK, Bradley JP. Fibrous dysplasia of the zygomaticomaxillary region: outcomes of surgical intervention. Plast Reconstr Surg. 2013;131(6):1329–38.
60. DiCaprio MR, Enneking WF. Fibrous dysplasia. Pathophysiology, evaluation, and treatment. J Bone Joint Surg Am. 2005;87(8):1848–64.
61. Dumitrescu CE, Collins MT. McCune-Albright syndrome. Orphanet J Rare Dis. 2008;3:12.
62. Kee TP, Liauw L, Sathiyamoorthy S, Lee HY, Tan GSL, Yu WY. Large solitary lytic skull vault lesions in adults: radiological review with pathological correlation. Clin Imaging. 2020;59(2):129–43.

63. Edgerton MT, Persing JA, Jane JA. The surgical treatment of fibrous dysplasia. With emphasis on recent contributions from cranio-maxillo-facial surgery. Ann Surg. 1985;202(4):459–79.
64. Weisman JS, Hepler RS, Vinters HV. Reversible visual loss caused by fibrous dysplasia. Am J Ophthalmol. 1990;110(3):244–9.
65. Chapurlat RD, Delmas PD, Liens D, Meunier PJ. Long-term effects of intravenous pamidronate in fibrous dysplasia of bone. J Bone Mineral Res. 1997;12(10):1746–52.
66. Mansoori LS, Catel CP, Rothman MS. Bisphosphonate treatment in polyostotic fibrous dysplasia of the cranium: case report and literature review. Endocrine Pract. 2010;16(5):851–4.
67. Ruggieri P, Sim FH, Bond JR, Unni KK. Malignancies in fibrous dysplasia. Cancer. 1994;73(5):1411–24.

Lesions with and Without Atrophy of the Scalp

11

George H. Bourdages and Walter A. Hall

11.1 Introduction

There are numerous pathologies of the human head presenting with tissue loss of varying degrees impacting the scalp or calvarium. Parry-Romberg syndrome, bilateral parietal osteodystrophy, Gorham disease, hyperostosis frontalis interna, chronic anemia, and renal osteodystrophy all result in atrophy of tissue layers pertaining to the skull or scalp. Initial presentation and symptomatology are variable; however notable cosmetic or neurologic sequalae can be seen in each disorder. A combination of a comprehensive clinical assessment combined with cranial imaging is necessary to assess the extent of disease involvement and the potential risks associated with each pathological process.

11.2 Parry-Romberg Syndrome

Parry-Romberg Syndrome is also known as progressive hemifacial atrophy [1]. It presents in the first two decades of life with slowly progressive loss of tissue involving the skin, subcutaneous areas, muscle, and osseous structures [1, 2]. The disease is more common in females, but can also occur in males [2]. The disease burden seems to correlate with the age of onset, such that younger patients often develop more severe deformities [2]. With the onset of the condition in the soft tissues, cosmetic changes are often the first presenting sign. In addition, ophthalmological and neurologic deficits have been reported that include enophthalmos, retinal changes, optic nerve and oculomotor dysfunction, headaches, and seizures [3, 4]. Neurologic complications are thought to arise due to both direct involvement and indirect factors secondary to local inflammation, erosion, and compression. With the etiology of the disease unclear and under debate, autoimmune, traumatic, neuro-vascular, infectious, or genetic causes are being considered. Arif et al. describe treatment options in their review, and with an auto-immune etiology as the favored cause, methotrexate and prednisone constitute the initial medical management. The surgical treatments that are discussed are centered around the correction of severe deformities.

11.3 Bilateral Parietal Osteodystrophy

Bilateral parietal osteodystrophy is a pathological thinning of the parietal bone relative to the rest of the calvarium. There are reports of bilateral parietal thinning of the skull dating back to the medieval period and even to the bronze age

G. H. Bourdages · W. A. Hall (✉)
Department of Neurosurgery, State University of New York (SUNY) Upstate Medical University, Syracuse, NY, USA
e-mail: hallw@upstate.edu

M. Turgut et al. (eds.), *Lesions of the Scalp and Cranial Vault*,
https://doi.org/10.1007/978-3-031-88244-9_11

[5, 6]. Classically, the disease is described as an oval shaped symmetric thinning of the parietal bones [7, 8]. The etiology of the disorder is unknown although it is thought to be due to resorption of the diploic bone in the involved area. There is some debate regarding the loss of the outer table of the skull and the decreased formation of bone rather than true bone resorption; however the inner table remains undisturbed [7, 9]. An early theory proposes that continuous external pressure can interrupt the vascular supply to the region resulting in the condition; however this seems unlikely because of the symmetric nature of the disease and the sparing of the scalp [10]. The disease presents most commonly in a painless fashion after the seventh decade in life with a prevalence estimated at about 0.5% with a preponderance for affecting females [11]. Often the disease is unrecognized since it is painless and generally asymptomatic. With the increased rate of cranial imaging performed in the modern era, the condition tends to be diagnosed incidentally. Traumatic injury is the most common symptomatic presentation and can be clinically devastating due to the reduced protection provided to the brain parenchyma. The literature describes multiple instances of fatal injuries and severe hemorrhages secondary to ground level falls and relatively minor trauma with a presumed impact to the parietal region [8, 12, 13]. Treatment is often conservative, and surgical options are reserved for patients that present with acute symptoms often secondary to a traumatic hemorrhage where the management is determined using traumatic brain injury guidelines.

11.4 Gorham Disease

Vanishing bone disease or Gorham disease is a pathological resorption of bone with angiomatosis and lymphatic proliferation. This rare disorder frequently affects the skull and upper extremities but can present in other bones that include the spine, lower extremities, and pelvis. Vascular and lymphatic proliferation can extend into soft tissues, including the scalp. In contrast to the prior disorders, Gorham disease is associated with painful osteolysis. The osseus resorption can progress to virtually complete loss of bone in the affected region [14]. Early descriptions of the disease date back to the 1800s [15]. The etiology is unknown and reports exist in nearly all age groups. Skull base osteolysis is a rare complication which carries a high risk of cranio-cervical instability, infection, and leakage of cerebrospinal fluid [16]. Maroufi et al reviewed the English literature for skull base osteolysis and found that meningitis and cerebrospinal leak occurred in 12 of 26 cases. Treatment options are variable and depend on the disease location and the presenting symptoms. Medical management includes bisphosphonates, and recently several case reports have demonstrated efficacy and safety using sirolimus [17–19]. Radiation therapy for the treatment of painful and large lesions can limit disease progression [20]. Surgery is considered for resecting and correcting functional deficits, providing stability, or repairing skull base cerebrospinal fluid leakage.

11.5 Hyperostosis Frontalis Interna

Hyperostosis frontalis interna is a condition where the inner table of the frontal bone thickens with an irregular contour. The scalp is generally spared. Unlike the other conditions described, this disorder is often a discrete entity that is not associated with systemic diseases or additional involved locations. The overgrowth is benign and commonly an incidental radiographic finding.

Although the etiology of the disease is unknown, it is more common in females and the elderly and is thought to be related to prolonged estrogen exposure [21, 22]. From a historical perspective, this condition is more apparent in the modern era and has only rarely been described in antiquity [23]. Symptoms are very rare, but cerebral atrophy, cognitive changes, headaches, seizures, and neuropsychiatric changes can be seen with excessive hyperostosis [24]. Surgical treatment is usually not necessary because of the incidental presentation and asymptomatic nature of the disease. However, medical management for any related issues is appropriate.

11.6 Chronic Anemia and Renal Osteodystrophy

Medical conditions such as chronic anemia and renal osteodystrophy can cause changes in various layers of the skull. Chronic anemia results in hyperplasia of the bone marrow, including that in the skull, resulting in a reduction of the thickness of the outer table of the skull and a widened region of cancellous bone. The proliferating bone marrow erodes the outer table and causes a classical "hair-on-end" appearance due to small bony spicules [21]. Congenital and acquired chronic anemias can also cause these imaging changes. In contrast, chronic renal disease influences the balance between bone production and resorption via increased levels of parathyroid hormone from hypocalcemia and hyperphosphatemia seen in chronic kidney disease. These changes cause the bony layers of the skull to coalesce with an apparent loss of the boundaries between the inner and outer tables creating a single "salt and pepper" appearance of the calvarium [21]. The changes in the calvarium from both conditions are generally symmetric and widespread and are uncommonly a focal or isolated process. Although the outer table is impacted by these pathologies, the scalp does not demonstrate significant atrophy.

11.7 Case Presentation

An 86-year-old female presented with a progressively worsening headache over a week. She was intubated in the emergency department for unresponsiveness and hypotension after a potential seizure and cranial computed tomography was obtained. The study revealed hyperostosis frontalis interna, a left frontal meningioma, and a right convexity acute on chronic subdural hematoma as seen in Fig. 11.1. She underwent a subdural evacuation port system placement with a decrease in the size of the subdural hematoma (Fig. 11.2). As is often the case, frontal hyperostosis was an incidental finding on imaging. Although it did not contribute to her presentation, it was important to recognize her pathology for treatment planning of the subdural hematoma. Placement of the subdural evacuation port system was intended to drain a region of chronic appearing hematoma and to avoid the frontal areas of the skull where excessive drilling may be required, and where traditional tactile feedback that is encountered between the inner and outer tables while drilling may be lost. The recognition of the hyperostotic bone and the surgical planning used to drain the subdural hematoma helped reduce the risk of iatrogenic injury to the patient while maximizing the potential for treatment success. Like most patients, she required no treatment for the hyperostosis frontalis interna and was asymptomatic from that pathology.

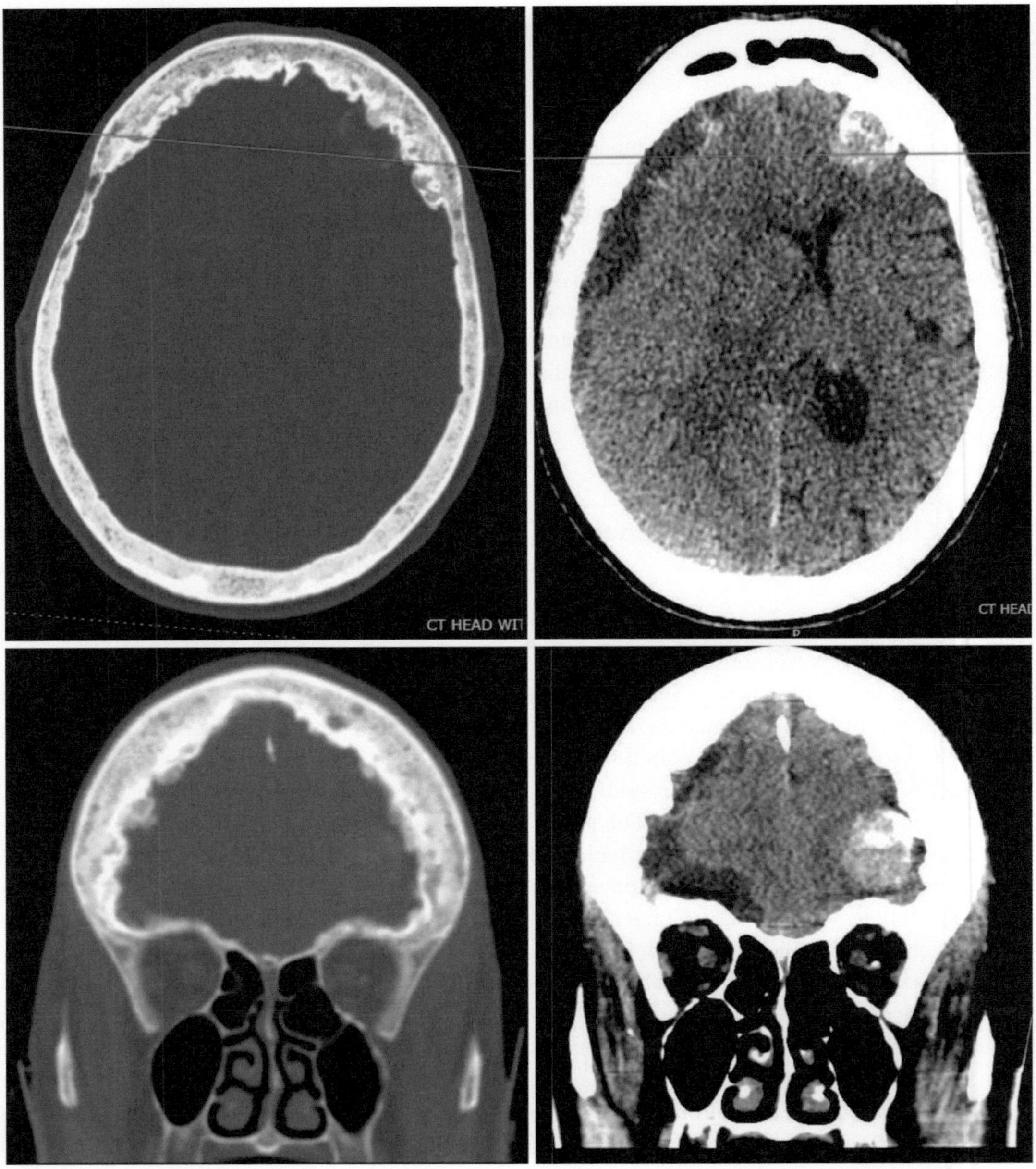

Fig. 11.1 Computed tomography of the head showing hyperostosis frontalis interna in a patient with a left frontal meningioma and right convexity acute on chronic subdural hematoma. The images on the left show the axial and coronal bone windows, while the right-side images reveal the axial and coronal soft tissue windows

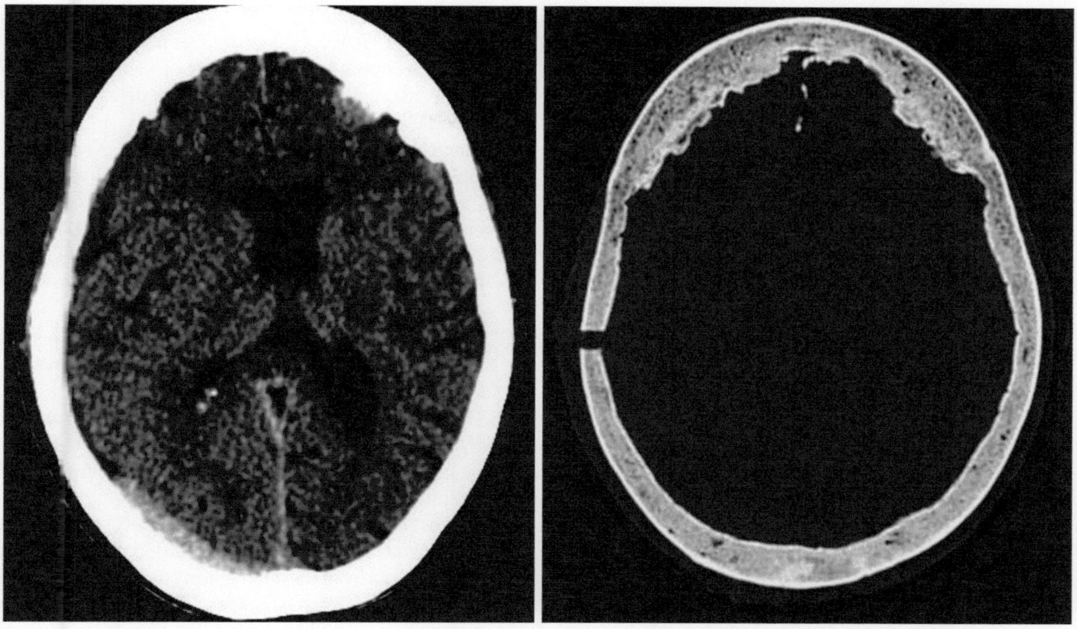

Fig. 11.2 Imaging from the same patient after burr hole placement for subdural evacuation port system drainage of the chronic subdural hematoma. Care was taken to avoid the frontal region of hyperostosis where excessive drilling may have been necessary and traditional tactile feedback between the layers of the skull would be impaired by the hyperostosis. The left-side computed tomography image shows the soft tissue window with a decrease in the size of the subdural hematoma and the right-side computed tomography image shows the bone window with hyperostosis frontalis interna and the burr hole placed for the procedure

11.8 Conclusion

Although the exact etiologies for Parry-Romberg syndrome, bilateral parietal thinning, Gorham disease, and hyperostosis frontalis interna are not known, various known principles help guide medical treatment options. Surgical treatment is considered in the presence of a severe symptomatic presentation. Ultimately, care of these complex disorders requires a multi-disciplinary approach with close attention to clinical and radiographic details.

References

1. El-Kehdy J, Abbas O, Rubeiz N. A review of Parry-Romberg syndrome. J Am Acad Dermatol. 2012;67(4):769–84.
2. Arif T, Fatima R, Sami M. Parry-Romberg syndrome: a mini review. Acta Dermatovenerol Alp Pannonica Adriat. 2020;29(4):193–9.
3. Bucher F, Fricke J, Neugebauer A, Cursiefen C, Heindl LM. Ophthalmological manifestations of Parry-Romberg syndrome. Surv Ophthalmol. 2016;61(6):693–701.
4. English SW, Ho ML, Tollefson MM, Wong-Kisiel LC. Focal epilepsy in a teenager with facial atrophy and hair loss. Semin Pediatr Neurol. 2018;26:68–73.
5. Tonina E, Larentis O, Tesi C, Fusco R, Campagnolo M, Licata M. A severe case of biparietal thinning in a medieval skull from a Northern Italy necropolis. J Craniofac Surg. 2022;33(1):70–5.
6. Dutta PC. Bilateral parietal thinning in bronze age skull. Br Med J. 1969;1(5635):55.
7. Cvetković D, Bracanović D, Djonić D, Živković V, Djurić M, Nikolić S. Biparietal osteodystrophy: macroscopic appearance, computed tomography imaging and microarchitectural analysis. Leg Med Tokyo Jpn. 2022;55:102025.
8. Mann RW, Kobayashi M, Schiller AL. Biparietal thinning: accidental death by a fall from standing height. J Forensic Sci. 2017;62(5):1406–9.
9. Yiu Luk S, Fai Shum JS, Wai Chan JK, San Khoo JL. Bilateral thinning of the parietal bones: a case report and review of radiological features. Pan Afr Med J. 2010;4:7.
10. Durward A. A note on symmetrical thinning of the parietal bones. J Anat. 1929;63(Pt 3):356–62.
11. Bruyn GW. Biparietal osteodystrophy. Clin Neurol Neurosurg. 1978;80(3):125–48.

12. Sioutas G, Karakasi MV, Kapetanakis S, Pavlidis P. Death due to fracture of thin calvarial bones after a fall: a forensic approach. Chin J Traumatol Zhonghua Chuang Shang Za Zhi. 2017;20(3):180–2.
13. Yılmaz MB, Egemen E, Ozbakır B, Tekiner A. Epidural hematoma after minor trauma on patient with biparietal osteodystrophy. J Korean Neurosurg Soc. 2013;53(1):57–8.
14. Nikolaou VS, Chytas D, Korres D, Efstathopoulos N. Vanishing bone disease (Gorham-Stout syndrome): a review of a rare entity. World J Orthop. 2014;5(5):694–8.
15. Ruggieri P, Montalti M, Angelini A, Alberghini M, Mercuri M. Gorham-Stout disease: the experience of the Rizzoli Institute and review of the literature. Skeletal Radiol. 2011;40(11):1391–7.
16. Maroufi SF, Habibi Z, Dabbagh Ohadi MA, Mohammadi E, Nejat F. Gorham-Stout disease of skull base leading to cranial settling and rhinorrhea: a case-based review. Childs Nerv Syst ChNS Off J Int Soc Pediatr Neurosurg. 2022;38(4):695–703.
17. Liu Y, Zhong DR, Zhou PR, Lv F, Ma DD, Xia WB, et al. Gorham-Stout disease: radiological, histological, and clinical features of 12 cases and review of literature. Clin Rheumatol. 2016;35(3):813–23.
18. Ricci KW, Hammill AM, Mobberley-Schuman P, Nelson SC, Blatt J, Bender JLG, et al. Efficacy of systemic sirolimus in the treatment of generalized lymphatic anomaly and Gorham-Stout disease. Pediatr Blood Cancer. 2019;66(5):e27614.
19. Liang Y, Tian R, Wang J, Shan Y, Gao H, Xie C, et al. Gorham-Stout disease successfully treated with sirolimus (rapamycin): a case report and review of the literature. BMC Musculoskelet Disord. 2020;21(1):577.
20. Agyeman K, Pretell-Mazzini J, Subhawong T, Kerr DA, Jose J. Gorham disease. Am J Orthop Belle Mead NJ. 2017;46(6):E458–62.
21. Gomez CK, Schiffman SR, Bhatt AA. Radiological review of skull lesions. Insights Imaging. 2018;9(5):857–82.
22. Hershkovitz I, Greenwald C, Rothschild BM, Latimer B, Dutour O, Jellema LM, et al. Hyperostosis frontalis interna: an anthropological perspective. Am J Phys Anthropol. 1999;109(3):303–25.
23. Raikos A, Paraskevas GK, Yusuf F, Kordali P, Meditskou S, Al-Haj A, et al. Etiopathogenesis of hyperostosis frontalis interna: a mystery still. Ann Anat Anat Anz Off Organ Anat Ges. 2011;193(5):453–8.
24. Khizar A, Shahzad W, Yadav PK. Hyperostosis frontalis interna presenting as a forehead scar in a young male. Clin Case Rep. 2023;11(4):e7256.

12 Hypertrophic Scarring and Pressure Sores of the Scalp

Zheng Yang and Qiying Wang

12.1 Hypertrophic Scars on the Scalp

Hypertrophic scars is a pathological phenomenon caused by excessive tissue repair and disordered extracellular matrix deposition after trauma, inflammation, surgery, or burns. It is a fibrous dysproliferative disease of the dermal reticular layer that manifests as chronic inflammation of the dermal reticular layer, excessive revascularization, and collagen fiber hyperplasia [1, 2].

12.1.1 Pathogenesis

In postnatal tissues, wound healing involves three phases—the inflammation phase, proliferation phase, and remodeling phase—which require very fine regulation. Whether these three stages are orderly and finely adjusted will directly lead to wound healing without scarring or excessive fibrosis. The current general understanding is that the persistence of acute inflammation is an important reason for the formation of hypertrophic scars. The pathological manifestation of hypertrophic scars is that these lesions are due to a disorder in the production or degradation of collagen-based extracellular matrix, or both, resulting in a large amount of collagen-based extracellular matrix deposition. In addition, the expression of fibronectin and hyaluronic acid in the extracellular matrix of hypertrophic scars is upregulated, the expression of core proteoglycans is downregulated, and elastin is absent. Changes in the composition of the extracellular matrix directly determine the flexibility and thickness of hypertrophic scars [1, 3–6].

12.1.2 Risk Factors

Many risk factors affect scar outcome by affecting chronic inflammatory processes within the dermis. These factors can be summarized into four categories, namely, genetic factors, systemic factors, local factors, and lifestyle factors. (1) Genetic factors: There are obvious racial differences in the incidence of hypertrophic scars. In addition, families with family members that are predisposed to developing hypertrophic scars/keloids are not uncommon. (2) Systemic factors: The level of a women's estrogen level is one of the known systemic risk factors, in addition to high blood pressure. (3) Local factors: In addition to repeated skin damage and infection, skin tension is also an important local risk factor. (4) Lifestyle: Some lifestyle factors also have a significant impact on the formation of hypertrophic

Z. Yang · Q. Wang (✉)
Department of Plastic Surgery, The First Affiliated Hospital of Zhengzhou University, Zhengzhou, Henan Province, China
e-mail: wangqiying@zzu.edu.cn

M. Turgut et al. (eds.), *Lesions of the Scalp and Cranial Vault*,
https://doi.org/10.1007/978-3-031-88244-9_12

scars and keloids, such as strenuous or heavy physical labor, a spicy diet, alcohol consumption, and excessive hot bath time [5].

12.1.3 Clinical Manifestations

Hypertrophic scars not only affect appearance but are also accompanied by varying degrees of itching, pain, and other abnormal sensations. Some hypertrophic scar tissue forms sinus tracts, abscess cavities, etc., causing repeated infections and affecting the patient's quality of life. The scalp has a large amount of hair, and the incidence of infection is greater in the scalp than in other parts of the body. Hypertrophic scars located on the scalp have high local tension and are accompanied by scarring alopecia, making them more difficult to treat than scars located in other parts of the body [7].

Surgeons often make a diagnosis of hypertrophic scars based solely on clinical manifestations, but for some benign tumors (such as pseudolymphoma, mixed cutaneous tumor, xanthogranuloma, leiomyoma, and dermatofibroma) and malignant tumors (such as protuberant cutaneous fibrosarcoma, squamous cell carcinoma and anochromic melanoma), the clinical manifestations are sometimes similar and difficult to differentiate, especially with dermatofibrosarcoma, squamous cell carcinoma and amelanotic melanoma.

Treatment strategies:

12.1.4 Early Preventive Measures

Prevention is the best treatment, and how to promote faster early wound healing is the primary measure for preventing scarring. Early wound closure through suturing, skin flap transfer, skin grafting, etc., can effectively prevent the occurrence of hypertrophic scars on the scalp. During the wound healing stage, the prevention of hypertrophic scars is more important than the treatment of hypertrophic scars [8–11].

Nonsurgical treatments: Conservative treatments for hypertrophic scars include topical silicone gel patches, topical corticosteroid patches, topical garlic extract gel, oral medications (such as propranolol and oxandrolone), intrascar injections of corticosteroids, intrascar injections of 5-fluorouracil, intrascar injections of botulinum toxin type A, intrascar injections of bleomycin, compression therapy, laser therapy and cryotherapy, etc. In addition to cryotherapy and topical corticosteroid patches, the therapeutic effects of the other methods mentioned above are supported by high-level (level I) evidence-based medical evidence [7, 9, 11–16].

12.1.5 Surgical Treatment

Surgical treatment is not the first treatment choice for hypertrophic scars. Surgical intervention is required for hypertrophic scars that are combined with sinus tracts or ulcers or for cosmetic purposes. Small areas of scalp scarring alopecia can be treated with hair follicle transplantation to achieve a good appearance [17]. For wounds formed after scalp hypertrophic scar resection, there are a variety of repair methods to choose from depending on the size of the wound, and these include soft tissue expansion, local flap transfer, adjacent axial flap, free flap transplantation, skin grafting, etc. The ideal repair method is to restore the wound coverage, reduce the displacement of anatomical landmarks, hide the incision, and preserve hair growth and the normal flow of the hair.

Among these treatments, soft tissue expansion technology can better balance wound coverage and aesthetics and is an ideal method for repairing hypertrophic scalp scars. This type of surgery needs to be performed in two stages. Expansion phase implantation is performed in the first phase. The implantation layer in the expansion phase is the subgaleal aponeurosis. The implantation location should be reasonably designed according to the size and location of the wound to avoid damaging the blood supply of the flap to be transferred. The capacity and shape of the flap used for the expansion phase needs to be reasonably selected in combination with the design of the flap used for the second phase. After implantation during the expansion period during the operation, deep sutures should be placed far from the incision, and the expansion bag should be closed in a "fence-like" manner to reduce the tension of the skin incision and avoid displacement during the expansion period after surgery and during the water injection period. After implantation in the expansion phase, water is regularly injected to expand the skin. The amount and frequency of each water injection are judged based on the volume during the expansion phase and the tension and blood supply of the expanded skin flap. In the second stage of surgery, the expansion phase is stopped, and the expansion flap is transferred and advanced to repair the remaining wounds after the removal of the hypertrophic scar from the scalp. The uneven appearance of the base after the expander is removed can be left alone, and the patient will gradually recover within 6 months after the operation. A scalp expansion flap is used to repair hypertrophic scalp scars. The color and texture of the expansion flap can meet the patient's requirements for appearance, use of this flap can effectively utilize the normal hairy area, and the use of this flap can help avoid postoperative scarring alopecia. An appropriate flap transfer direction can maximize the preservation of the hair flow direction.

12.2 Scalp Pressure Ulcers

The European Pressure Ulcer Advisory Panel (EPUAP) and the National Pressure Ulcer Advisory Panel (NPUAP) define pressure ulcers as "a pressure ulcer that develops on the skin or subcutaneous tissue that usually occurs at the bony prominences due to pressure, or combined with shearing and/or friction." In 2016, the NPUAP adjusted the name "pressure ulcers to pressure injuries." Pressure injuries refer to local injuries of the skin and deep soft tissues, usually at the site of bone protuberances, or they can be associated with medical devices, etc. These injuries may manifest as intact skin or open ulcers, which may be painful. Pressure injuries are caused by intense and/or prolonged pressure or pressure combined with shearing forces. The tolerance of soft tissue to pressure and shear forces may be affected by the microenvironment, nutrition, perfusion, complications, and the state of the soft tissue itself [2].

12.2.1 Risk Factors

Pressure injuries are primarily caused by intense and/or prolonged pressure or pressure forces combined with shear forces. The effect caused by an external force depends on both the size of the external force and the time it takes the tissue to react. In the past, many people believed that pressure injuries were more common in patients who were bedridden for a long time. However, in clinical practice, many patients often develop obvious pressure injuries in a short period of time, which may be caused by a higher intensity of local pressure or shear forces. Whether skin and soft tissue will be damaged under the action of pressure and shear forces also depends on the tissue's tolerance to external forces. Many factors affect the tolerance of soft tissue, including the microenvironment, such as temperature, relative humidity, pH, bacterial colonization, malnutrition, insufficient blood perfusion, complications such as diabetes and neurodystrophy, increased skin fragility, and soft tissue conditions such as increased skin fragility and local scar formation [18].

12.2.2 Pressure Ulcer Staging

The Daniel pressure ulcer staging system, the Shea pressure ulcer staging system, and the NPUAP pressure ulcer staging system were developed after the revision of the Shea staging system. The number of each stage is slightly different. In the NPUAP pressure ulcer staging system, ulcers can be divided into four stages according to the degree of injury and depth of involvement: unstageable pressure injury and deep tissue pressure injury [19–23].

Stage 1 pressure injury: The skin is intact, and erythema appears that does not turn white under finger pressure. Erythema caused by blanches with finger pressure or changes in sensation, temperature, or firmness may precede visible changes in the skin. Skin color changes do not include purple or maroon changes, which may indicate a deep tissue pressure injury.

Stage 2: Pressure injury: there is a partial cortical defect with exposure of the dermis. The wound base is active, pink or red, and moist and may appear as complete or damaged serous blisters. Fat and deep tissue are not exposed, and there is no granulation tissue, sloughing, or eschar.

Stage 3: Pressure injury: full-thickness skin loss. A stage 3 pressure injury refers to a full-thickness skin defect with exposed adipose tissue, usually granulation tissue or wound edge involution, and local sloughing and/or eschar may also be present. The depth of tissue damage varies depending on the anatomical site, with areas rich in fatty tissue likely to have deeper wounds. Submerged lacunae and sinus tracts may occur without exposure of the fascia, muscles, tendons, ligaments, cartilage, and/or bone. If an area of sloughing or an eschar obscures the extent of tissue loss, it is defined as a nonstageable pressure injury.

Stage 4 Pressure injury: There is full-thickness skin and tissue loss. A stage 4 pressure injury refers to an ulcer formed by a full-thickness skin and tissue defect, accompanied by visible or palpable fascia, muscle, tendon, ligament, cartilage or bone exposure, and there is local sloughing and/or eschar. It is usually accompanied by wound edge involution and hidden lacunae and/or sinus tracts. If an area of sloughing or an eschar obscures the extent of tissue loss, it is defined as a nonstageable pressure injury.

Unstageable pressure injury: There is full-thickness skin and tissue loss of an unknown extent. However, due to the local sloughing and/or eschar covering this type of lesion, it is difficult to determine the degree of the defect. If the sloughing and/or eschar are removed, it can be determined that it is a stage 3 or 4 pressure injury.

Deep tissue pressure injury: Deep tissue pressure injury indicates that the skin is intact or incomplete; the local area appears dark red, maroon, or purple and does not turn white under continuous finger pressure; or a black wound base or congested blisters can be seen after the epidermis is separated. Pain and temperature changes often precede changes in skin color. The changes in the color of darker skin may vary. This type of damage is caused by strong and/or sustained pressure and shear forces at the bone–muscle interface, which can progress rapidly and expose the actual extent of tissue damage or can be dissolved and absorbed without tissue loss. If necrotic tissue, subcutaneous tissue, granulation tissue, fascia, muscle, or other deep tissue is visible, it is defined as a full-thickness pressure injury to the skin (unstageable, stage 3, or 4). This injury cannot be used to describe vascular, traumatic, neurological, or dermatologically associated wounds [19].

12.2.3 Prevention and Treatment Measures

Malnutrition is closely related to the development, severity, and healing of pressure injuries. Comprehensive nutritional assessments of patients and the development of personalized nutritional care plans are increasingly valued by medical staff. For patients whose nutritional needs cannot be met by oral administration, appropriate enteral nutrition or parenteral nutrition support is selected based on the patient's wishes and feasibility [24, 25]. Scientific postural changes and early activities are equally important for the prevention of pressure injuries. During postural changes, the pressure on all bony prominences should be minimized, and the pressure should be distributed evenly to the maximum extent. In addition, preventing device-related pressure injuries requires regular monitoring of the tightness of medical devices [19, 26].

Nonsurgical treatment: Established pressure injuries should be scientifically evaluated and monitored and re-evaluated if necessary based on the healing status [27]. Through skin and wound cleaning, the injured area and surrounding skin should be kept clean; if an ulcerated wound forms, attention should be given to improving the dressing changes, removing necrotic tissue and biofilm, and providing good conditions for the growth of granulation. When changing dressings, appropriate wound dressings, such as hydrocolloid dressings, hydrogel dressings, calcium alginate dressings, and foam dressings, should be selected based on the stage of pressure injury and wound exudation, by following the principle of wet healing. In addition, nonsurgical treatments also include biological dressings, growth factors, biophysical treatments, etc. Concentrated platelet plasma has been gradually introduced for the treatment of pressure ulcers in recent years and has achieved certain results [19].

Surgical treatment: For pressure injuries involving deep wounds and severe damage, surgical treatment should be considered. Before surgery, it is necessary to comprehensively evaluate the possibility of a cure between the use of both conservative treatment and surgical intervention, as well as the patient's personal care goals, personal clinical status, personal motivation and ability to comply with the treatment plan, personal surgical risks, and other factors. Depending on the severity of the injury, surgery may be performed in stages if necessary. In the early stage, debridement and drainage are used to remove necrotic tissue, sinus tracts, biofilm, etc., and the wound can be rinsed thoroughly. When the wound conditions are suitable, second-stage damage repair is carried out. During this period, dressing changes need to be improved, or a closed negative pressure drainage device for the wound needs to be used. Defects in the skin and subcutaneous soft tissue should be directly pulled together and sutured without tension. For patients with no defects or dead spaces in the muscles and deep tissues, these tissues can be directly sutured together. For patients with severe skin and subcutaneous tissue defects, high tension lesions, deep tissue defects, and dead space formations, local skin flaps, axial skin flaps, free skin flaps, etc., can be used to repair scalp defects [28].

References

1. Knowles A, Glass DN. Keloids and hypertrophic scars. Dermatol Clin. 2023;41(3):509–17.
2. Kottner J, et al. Pressure ulcer/injury classification today: an international perspective. J Tissue Viability. 2020;29(3):197–203.
3. Jeschke MG, et al. Scars. Nat Rev Dis Prim. 2023;9(1):64.
4. Zhang T, et al. Current potential therapeutic strategies targeting the TGF-β/Smad signaling pathway to attenuate keloid and hypertrophic scar formation. Biomed Pharmacother. 2020;129:110287.
5. Lingzhi Z, Meirong L, Xiaobing F. Biological approaches for hypertrophic scars. Int Wound J. 2020;17(2):405–18.
6. Wang ZC, et al. The roles of inflammation in keloid and hypertrophic scars. Front Immunol. 2020;11:603187.
7. Worley B, et al. Treatment of traumatic hypertrophic scars and keloids: a systematic review of randomized control trials. Arch Dermatol Res. 2023;315(7):1887–96.
8. Choi C, et al. Management of hypertrophic scars in adults: a systematic review and meta-analysis. Australas J Dermatol. 2022;63(2):172–89.
9. Leszczynski R, et al. Laser therapy for treating hypertrophic and keloid scars. Cochrane Database Syst Rev. 2022;9(9):CD011642.
10. Barone N, et al. Current advances in hypertrophic scar and keloid management. Semin Plast Surg. 2021;35(3):145–52.
11. Ogawa R. The most current algorithms for the treatment and prevention of hypertrophic scars and keloids: a 2020 update of the algorithms published 10 years ago. Plast Reconstr Surg. 2022;149(1):79e–94e.
12. Nobari NN, et al. A systematic review of the comparison between needling (RF-needling, meso-needling, and micro-needling) and ablative fractional lasers (CO(2), erbium YAG) in the treatment of atrophic and hypertrophic scars. Lasers Med Sci. 2023;38(1):67.
13. Frech FS, et al. Hypertrophic scars and keloids: advances in treatment and review of established therapies. Am J Clin Dermatol. 2023;24(2):225–45.
14. Klifto KM, Asif M, Hultman CS. Laser management of hypertrophic burn scars: a comprehensive review. Burns. Trauma. 2020;8:tkz002.
15. Tosa M, Ogawa R. Photodynamic therapy for keloids and hypertrophic scars: a review. Scars Burn Heal. 2020;6:2059513120932059.
16. Juhasz M, Cohen JL. Microneedling for the treatment of scars: an update for clinicians. Clin Cosmet Investig Dermatol. 2020;13:997–1003.
17. Madura C, et al. The assessment of hair transplantation outcomes in Cicatricial alopecia. Int J Trichology. 2020;12(4):164–7.
18. Chung ML, et al. Risk factors for pressure injuries in adult patients: a narrative synthesis. Int J Environ Res Public Health. 2022;19(2)

19. Kottner J, et al. Prevention and treatment of pressure ulcers/injuries: the protocol for the second update of the international Clinical Practice Guideline 2019. J Tissue Viability. 2019;28(2):51–8.
20. Alderden JG, Shibily F, Cowan L. Best practice in pressure injury prevention among critical care patients. Crit Care Nurs Clin North Am. 2020;32(4):489–500.
21. Munoz N, et al. Malnutrition and pressure injury risk in vulnerable populations: application of the 2019 international Clinical Practice Guideline. Adv Skin Wound Care. 2022;35(3):156–65.
22. Pittman J, et al. Pressure injury prevention and management: a gap analysis using key stakeholder engagement. J Wound Ostomy Continence Nurs. 2022;49(5):416–27.
23. Haesler E, et al. Protocol for the development of the fourth edition of the prevention and treatment of pressure ulcers/injuries: clinical practice guideline using GRADE methods. Adv Skin Wound Care. 2024;37(3):136–46.
24. Munoz N, et al. The role of nutrition for pressure injury prevention and healing: the 2019 international Clinical Practice Guideline recommendations. Adv Skin Wound Care. 2020;33(3):123–36.
25. Munoz N, Posthauer ME. Nutrition strategies for pressure injury management: implementing the 2019 International Clinical Practice Guideline. Nutr Clin Pract. 2022;37(3):567–82.
26. Gefen A. The aetiology of medical device-related pressure ulcers and how to prevent them. Br J Nurs. 2021;30(15):S24–30.
27. Tschannen D, Anderson C. The pressure injury predictive model: a framework for hospital-acquired pressure injuries. J Clin Nurs. 2020;29(7–8):1398–421.
28. Bajaj J, et al. Rotational occipital scalp flap for occipital pressure ulcer. Neurol India. 2022;70(3):876–8.

Metabolic Disorders of the Scalp and Calvarium

13

Gökhan Sargın, Yaşar Barış Turgut, and Daphne J. Theodorou

13.1 Introduction

The calvarium comprising the superior part of the neurocranium is formed by portions of the frontal bone, the occipital bone, and the parietal bones [1]. Similar to a diverse array of disease processes affecting bones elsewhere in the body, various pathologic conditions may affect the calvaria including metabolic bone disease (i.e., rickets, Paget's disease), hematological disease processes (i.e., chronic anemia, thalassemia), and several endocrinological disorders (i.e., hyperparathyroidism, acromegaly). Indeed, variability of the disease states associated with different calvarial lesions may signify serious nosology mandating scrupulous differential diagnosis. Although asymptomatic calvarial lesions are often described as incidental findings on the imaging studies, patients may have symptoms of pain, neurological deficits, and mass.

Because disease of calvarial bones is uncommon and easily overlooked, systematic appraisal of the clinical and laboratory findings, coupled with analysis of the imaging findings can prove helpful in detecting abnormalities. The general purpose of imaging studies is to define the anatomic location of lesions primarily arising from the calvarial bones or infiltrating the skull secondary to other scalp or brain-based lesions, or systemic disease. Besides, familiarity with the imaging findings of metabolic disorders affecting the calvarial bones may be important so that they are not misdiagnosed as other types of pathologic conditions. Finally, an imaging diagnosis of calvarial involvement may prove helpful in the follow-up. Therefore in this chapter, a broad spectrum of metabolic disorders of the calvaria and scalp were reviewed to determine clinical and imaging patterns of involvement.

13.2 Rickets

In rickets, bone mineralization is impaired and unmineralized osteoids accumulate in the bone. The disease is often associated with decreased levels of vitamin D, phosphorus, calcium, or inhibition of mineralization in bone. Calcipenic rickets is most often associated with inadequate calcium intake due to deficiency of vitamin D, whereas phosphopenic rickets is due to abnormal absorption of phosphate from the intestines or abnormal excretion of phosphate from the kid-

G. Sargın (✉)
Department of Rheumatology, Aydın Adnan Menderes University Faculty of Medicine, Aydın, Türkiye
e-mail: gokhan_sargin@hotmail.com

Y. B. Turgut
Internal Medicine Clinic, Aydın State Hospital, Aydın, Türkiye

D. J. Theodorou
Department of Radiology, General Hospital of Ioannina, Ioannina, Greece

M. Turgut et al. (eds.), *Lesions of the Scalp and Cranial Vault*,
https://doi.org/10.1007/978-3-031-88244-9_13

neys. Rickets caused by vitamin D deficiency is seen rarely in developed countries [2, 3].

Patients may suffer from widespread bone pain, bone tenderness, fractures, hypotonia, tetany, muscle weakness, and muscle cramps. Kyphosis, wide wrists, rachitic rosary, appendicular skeleton deformities, valgus or varus deformity, and waddling gait may occur due to reduction in the vertebral body trabeculae, concave deformity of vertebrae, bone resorption at the distal end of the long bones, and abnormal configuration of the metaphyses. The secondary hyperparathyroidism can be detected in long-term and severe calcipenic rickets [2, 4]. Fontanels are fibrous and membrane-covered spaces that occur when the skull bones come together, of which there are six in the newborn. After birth, the size and closure time of the normal fontanels may vary. In the neonate calvaria, rickets is one of the most common causes of abnormal anterior fontanel size or delayed fontanel closure. In newborns with craniotabes, gentle exercise of thumb pressure on the occipital area causes the bone to collapse, reversibly bending out like a ping-pong ball. Although the "ping-pong ball" sign is considered normal in the first few months of life, persistence in later periods is considered a sign of rickets [2, 3].

Deformities are similar in both vitamin D-resistant rickets and classical rickets. Craniosynostosis, premature closure of the cranial sutures, may be seen in these patients. Although craniosynostosis can complicate nutrition-related rickets, the relationship between craniosynostosis and rickets is mostly associated with the familial forms of the disease. Craniosynostosis may be seen in X-linked hypophosphatemic rickets and vitamin D-resistant rickets due to 1-alpha hydroxylase deficiency. Early skull X-ray survey is recommended for children with these disease states of a genetic origin. Clinical findings of X-linked hypophosphatemia include bone deformation, bone pain, growth retardation, and rickets [2, 4, 5]. Sclerosis and thickening of the cranial vault, prominence in the forehead and decrease in height in the posterior of the skull, lambdoid suture synostosis, dolichocephaly, and Chiari I malformation have been reported in patients with X-linked hypophosphatemic rickets or autosomal dominant hypophosphatemic rickets (Figs. 13.1 and 13.2) [6].

The 25-hydroxyvitamin D 1-alpha-hydroxylase gene mutations cause vitamin D-resistant rickets. In these patients, the clinical findings of hypocalcemic rickets and craniosynostosis are observed in childhood, showing no improvement after treatment with vitamin D [2, 4, 5]. Deficiency in the anterior skull base length, the ramus height, and the skull base angle are considered morphological craniofacial derangements in hypophosphataemic vitamin D-resistant rickets [7]. Oncogenic osteomalacia is a paraneoplastic disease and is rare. It is characterized by normocalcemia, hypophosphatemia, phosphaturia, and osteomalacia. This condition is mostly caused by mesenchymal origin tumors that secrete fibroblast growth factor-23 [8, 9]. Oncogenic osteomalacia involving the occipital bone has been reported in the literature [9]. Physical examination, alkaline phosphatase, vitamin D, electrolytes like calcium, phosphate, and imaging studies can help diagnosis. Treatment is directed towards the underlying disease. In this context, hypophosphatemia, hypocalcemia, and vitamin D deficiencies need to be corrected, and the vitamin D and calcium levels need to be evaluated and monitored following treatment [2–4].

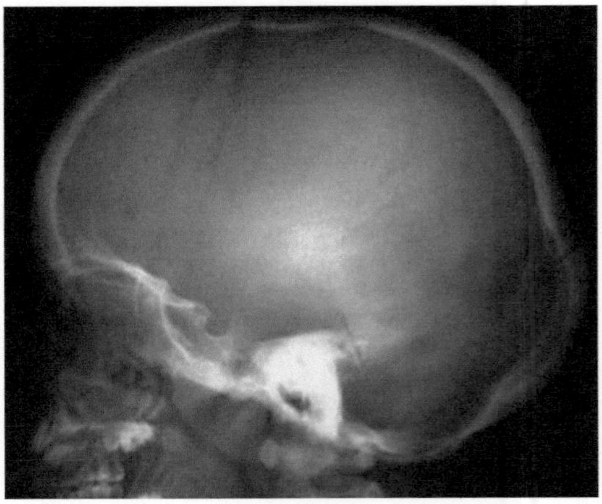

Fig. 13.1 Thickening and sclerosis of the skull, lateral cranial radiograph (Reproduced from Currarino G. Sagittal synostosis in X-linked hypophosphatemic rickets and related diseases. Pediatr Radiol 2007;37(8):805–12; with permission)

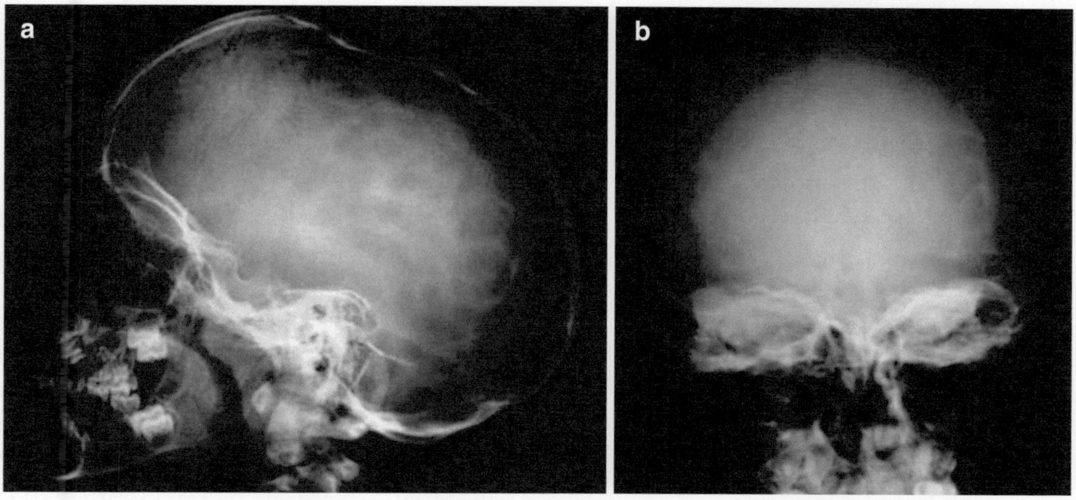

Fig. 13.2 (**a**) Prominence in the forehead and decrease in height in the posterior of the skull, lateral cranial radiograph. (**b**) Lambdoid suture synostosis, anteroposterior cranial radiograph (Reproduced from Currarino G. Sagittal synostosis in X-linked hypophosphatemic rickets and related diseases. Pediatr Radiol 2007;37(8):805–12; with permission)

13.3 Hyperparathyroidism

Calcium is an important cation that plays a critical role in intracellular and extracellular homeostasis. Vitamin D, parathyroid hormone (PTH), and calcitonin are significant in maintaining calcium balance. Hypercalcemia has clinical effects on the kidney, and the cardiovascular, neuromuscular, and gastrointestinal systems. Primary hyperparathyroidism may develop due to adenoma, hyperplasia, carcinoma of parathyroid gland, multiple endocrine neoplasias, or it may as well occur sporadically [10, 11]. Persistent and high levels of PTH may have a catabolic effect on cortical and trabecular bone. Intermittent administration of PTH may lead to an anabolic effect on bone [12].

In patients with osteitis fibrosa cystica, bone pain pathological fractures, and renal stones may develop as a result of hypercalcemia. Hypercalcemia can be a late manifestation of hyperparathyroidism in patients with parathyroid carcinoma. Radiological findings may include subperiosteal resorption of cortical bone, especially in the phalanges, various osteolytic lesions, loss of lamina dura in the teeth, osteoporosis, and a “salt and pepper” appearance in the skull. Bone densitometry may detect skeletal abnormalities before clinical findings occur [10, 13, 14].

Radiological findings are seen in less than 2% of the patients with hyperparathyroidism [14]. Prolonged and untreated hyperparathyroidism leads to excessive osteoclastic activity, bone resorption, and lytic lesions. The combination of trabecular bone resorption and granular tissue results in a “salt and pepper” appearance on the skull (Fig. 13.3) [15, 16]. Osteosclerosis and Brown tumors can be present on radiographs of the skull. Brown tumors are benign, non-neoplastic, lytic lesions seen in hyperparathyroidism. Deposits of hemosiderin and hemorrhage account for the characteristic brown color of lesions. Brown tumors involving the craniofacial are extremely rare, although they may occur in the extracranial skeletal system including clavicle, ribs, or femur [13, 17].

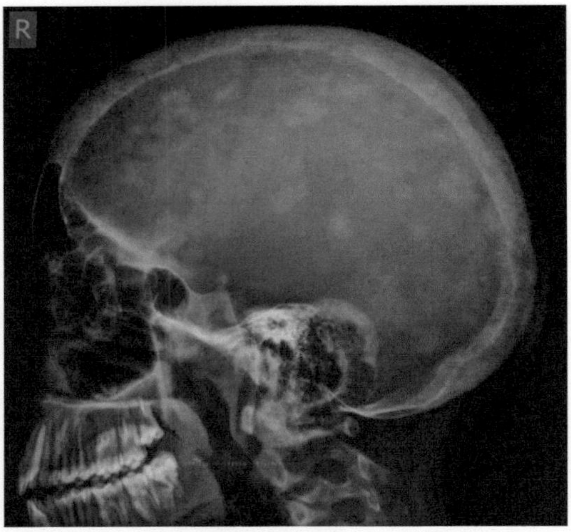

Fig. 13.3 Sclerotic areas and "salt and pepper" appearance in the skull, lateral cranial radiograph (Reproduced from Saini V, Gupta N, Mohan A, Gupta V, Kolluru K. Osteitis fibrosis cystica: classical case report of an uncommon presentation in a young female. Indian J Otolaryngol Head Neck Surg 2022;74:5319–23; with permission)

13.4 Renal Osteodystrophy

Chronic renal failure is defined as progressive deterioration of the kidney's electrolyte balance, and the metabolic and endocrine functions that results from decreased glomerular filtration. In chronic renal failure, there is decrease of urinary phosphate excretion, and in addition, the synthesis of active vitamin D decreases as does the calcium level. Low serum calcium levels in turn, increase PTH secretion, with ensuing secondary hyperparathyroidism. Profound metabolic changes in the bones of patients with chronic kidney disease are known as renal osteodystrophy [12, 18]. Indeed, renal osteodystrophy is a broad term denoting distinctive bone abnormalities in end-stage renal disease or chronic kidney disease. High bone turnover due to the elevated parathyroid hormone levels develops, with increasing numbers of osteoblasts and osteoclasts and improper mineralization. The radiographic findings of renal dystrophy are variable reflecting generalized bone density loss and cortical layers thinning. In advanced disease, there is loss of distinction between the inner and outer bony tables, with extensive trabecular resorption of the medullary bone and the development of granular tissue, creating a "salt and pepper" appearance of the skull (Fig. 13.4) [19]. Less commonly, Brown tumor, featuring purely osteolytic or multilobular cystic lesions may occur as previously stated in hyperparathyroidism [20, 21]. Adynamic bone disease is an additional condition caused by low osteoblastic activity in kidney disease. Bone pain, fracture, and osteomalacia may develop in these cases [21]. Some of the imaging features, however, may resemble those seen in hyperparathyroidism and rickets.

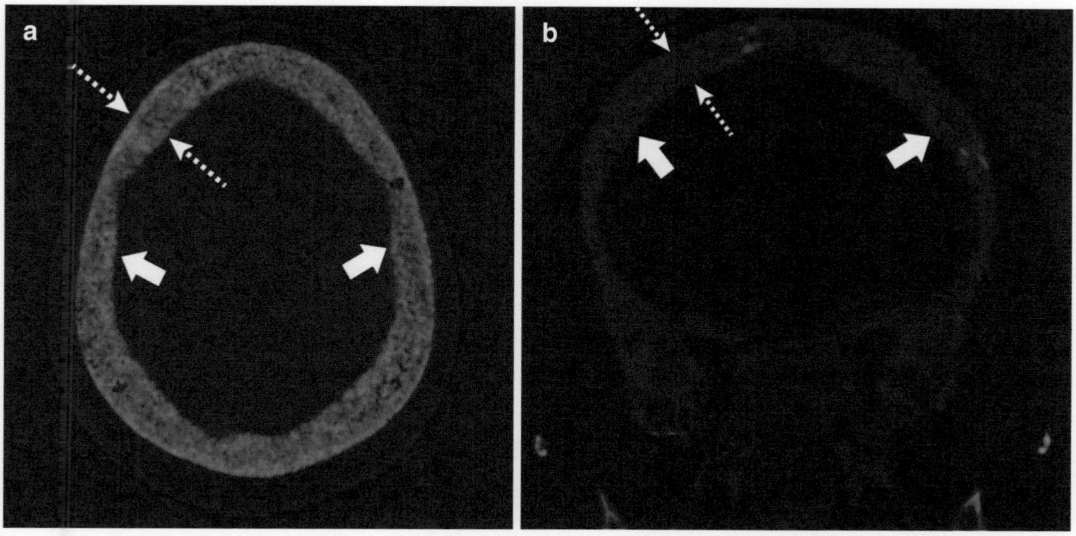

Fig. 13.4 Granular deossification and "salt and pepper" appearance (thick arrows), and distinction losses of the inner and outer tables (thin and dashed arrows), axial (**a**) and coronal (**b**) computed tomography (CT) (Reproduced from Gomez CK, Schiffman SR, Bhatt AA. Radiological review of skull lesions. Insights Imaging 2018;9:857–82; with permission)

13.5 Acromegaly

Acromegaly is associated with the abnormal, excessive growth hormone secretion duo to adenoma in the pituitary gland. Acromegaly can cause increased morbidity and mortality due to the detrimental metabolic effects imposed by hormonal hypersecretion, and the direct mass effect exercised on the pituitary gland by the growing adenoma. Acromegalic patients usually present with a rough face, acral enlargement, headache, fatigue, excessive sweating, and gonadal dysfunction. Coarsening of the facial features, frontal bossing, widening of the nose, thickening of the lips, macroglossia, and prominence of supraorbital protrusions are typical. Hydrocephalus, visual field defects, ophthalmoplegia, and various cranial nerve palsies may occur due to the local mass effect of macroadenomas. On CT images, there is calvarial thickening typically involving the inner table, and the sella turcica is enlarged [10, 20, 22]. Hyperostosis in the frontal region with enlarged paranasal sinuses, hypertrophic external occipital protrusion, and mandibular enlargement are among the typical findings seen on cranial radiographs, in patients with acromegaly (Fig. 13.5) [23].

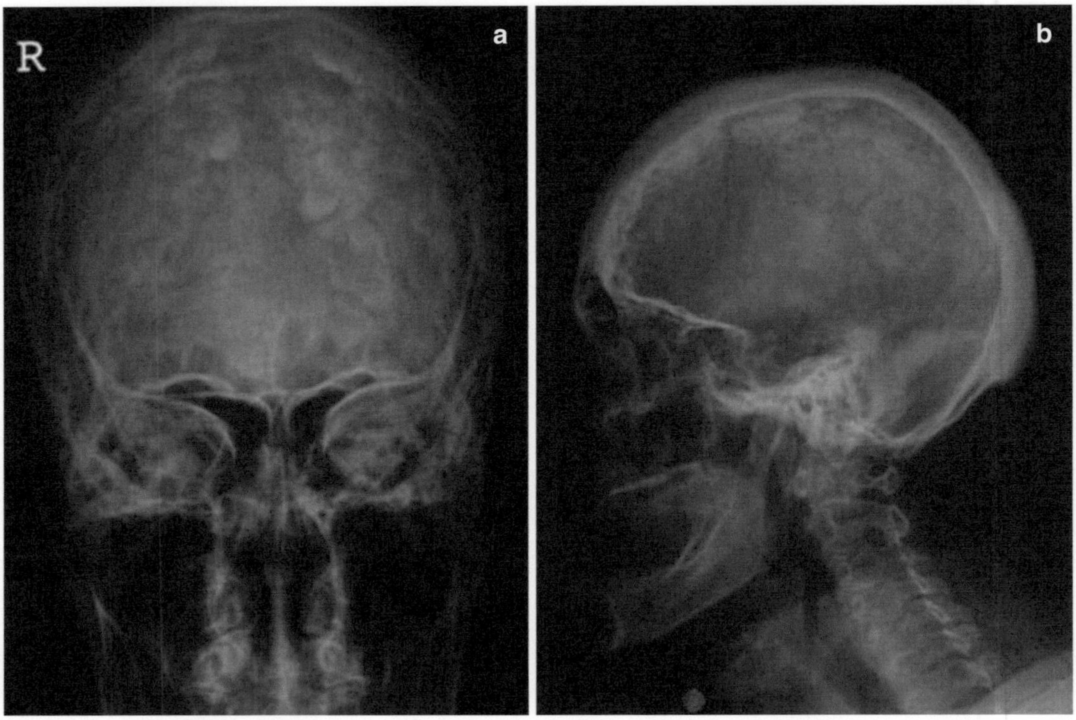

Fig. 13.5 Thickening of the skull, hyperostosis in the frontal region, enlarged sella turcica, hypertrophic external occipital protrusion, and mandibular enlargement, (**a**) anteroposterior (**b**) lateral cranial radiograph (Reproduced from Guglielmi G. Acromegaly. In: Baert AL (eds) Encyclopedia of Diagnostic Imaging. Springer, Berlin, Heidelberg, 2008; with permission)

13.6 Amyloidosis

Amyloidosis is a rare disease associated with the accumulation of abnormal amyloid fibrils and amorphous deposits, in protein structure. Amyloid fibrils can accumulate in the kidney, heart, skin, musculoskeletal system, gastrointestinal system, and the nervous system, causing clinical symptoms of serious disease. Systemic amyloidosis is associated with plasma cell dyscrasias and secondary amyloidosis is associated with inflammatory disorders and chronic infections. Interestingly, in localized amyloidosis, the dysfunction is limited to one organ only due to the abnormal buildup of amyloid at the production site [24, 25].

Among several plasma cell dyscrasias, multiple myeloma is the most serious disease. Amyloids detected in the bone structures are generally associated with plasma cell dyscrasias and multiple myeloma. Some people with multiple myeloma may develop primary or amyloid light chain amyloidosis, a protein structure [26]. Osteopenia, osteoporotic fractures, and osteolytic lesions are signs of bone involvement associated with considerable morbidity. Multiple, well-circumscribed lytic lesions can be seen on the skull radiographs of patients with multiple myeloma. These lesions appear in characteristic punched-out-raindrops (Fig. 13.6) [20, 27, 28].

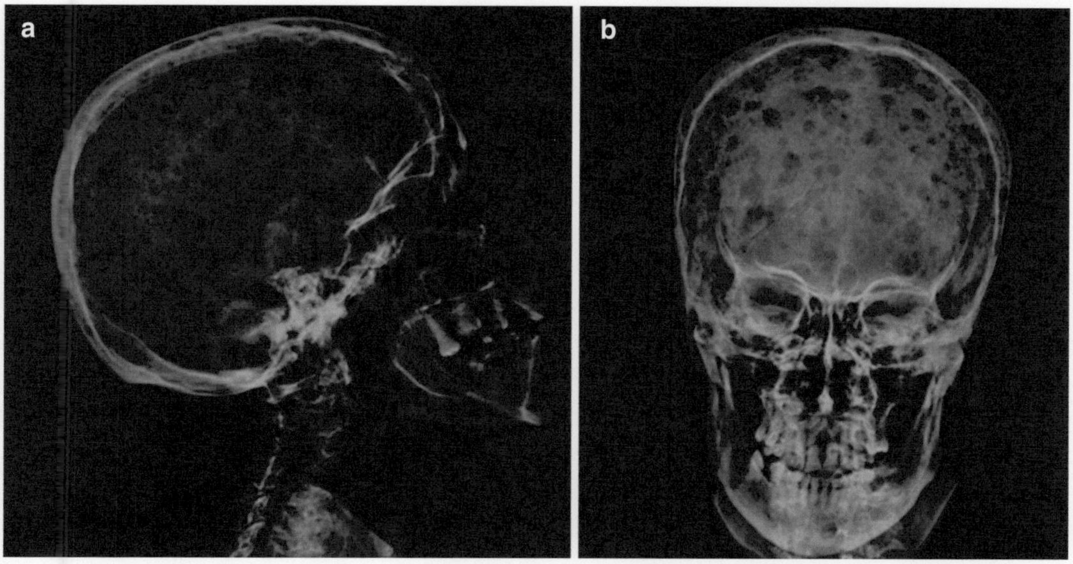

Fig. 13.6 Multiple, well-circumscribed lytic lesions, "punched-out-raindrops" appearance, (**a**) lateral and (**b**) anteroposterior cranial radiograph (Reproduced from Di Giuliano F, Picchi E, Muto M, Calcagni A, Ferrazzoli V, Da Ros V, Minosse S, Chiaravalloti A, Garaci F, Floris R, Muto M. Radiological imaging in multiple myeloma: review of the state-of-the-art. Neuroradiology 2020;62(8):905–23; with permission)

Primary solitary amyloidoses, also known as amyloidomas, are tumors containing amyloid that is deposited in the pituitary gland, cerebral hemisphere, and the temporal bones. Localized amyloid tumors, amyloidoma of the skull base, mass amyloid lesions involving the central nervous system, and diffuse infiltrating soft tissue amyloidosis in the pterygopalatine fossa are reportedly rare entities [29–32]. Amyloidomas may need to be considered in patients on long-term dialysis, individuals with plasma cell dyscrasias, and various inflammatory disease states. Several other pathologic conditions including the chondrosarcomas, benign or malignant mesenchymal neoplasms, metastatic tumors, plasmacytoma, and brown tumors of the calvarium may need to be considered in the broad differential diagnosis [33]. Amyloidoma can be seen on computed tomography of the skull as a giant heterogeneous mass with calcification (Fig. 13.7) [34]. Bone amyloidosis is very rare and may be mistaken as chondrosarcoma on plain radiographs or CT images. Lytic, destructive mass lesions with calcifications can be appreciated on radiographs or CT scans [29, 31, 32].

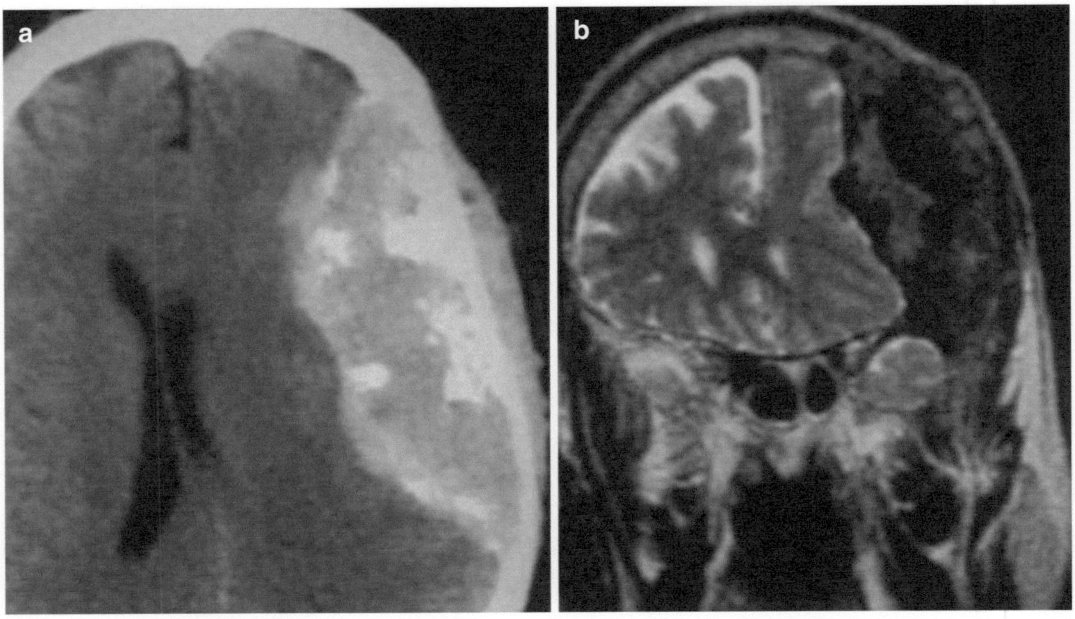

Fig. 13.7 Giant heterogeneous mass with calcifications, amyloidoma, CT (Reproduced from Pons Escoda A, Naval Baudin P, Mora P, Cos M, Hernandez Gañan J, Narváez JA, Aguilera C, Majós C. Imaging of skull vault tumors in adults. Insights Imaging 2020;11(1):23; with permission)

13.7 Paget's Disease

Paget's disease is the second most common metabolic bone disease after osteoporosis in the elderly population [35]. Patients may be present with bone deformity, pain, fracture, and nonspecific rheumatic complaints. Nocturnal, dull and aching pain is typical. The most important pathological hallmarks of Paget disease are increased focal osseous resorption followed by the apposition of disorderly new bone, reflecting an overall abnormal bone turnover. Paget's disease progresses in three phases: the osteolytic phase with increased osteoclastic activity, the mixed phase with both osteoclastic and predominant osteoblastic activity, and the blastic phase with declining osteoblastic activity [36, 37].

In Paget disease, cranial involvement is often asymptomatic and lesions are most commonly located in the occipital and frontal bones. In the cranial vault, round areas of osteolysis known as "osteoporosis circumscripta" can cross the suture lines (Fig. 13.8) [38]. Trabecular coarsening, cortical thickening, osseous widening, and "cotton-wool" bone appearance are characteristic features. In the skull, cortical thickening may cause platybasia and mechanical compression of the brainstem. With progression of sclerosis,

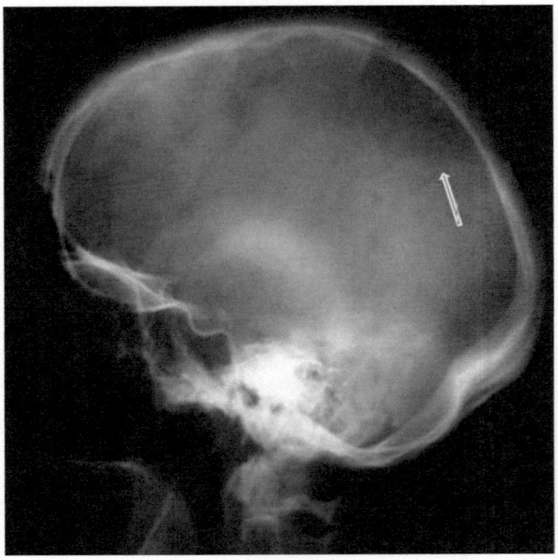

Fig. 13.8 Well-circumscribed region of reduced density (white arrow), lytic phase, osteoporosis circumscripta, lateral cranial radiograph (Reproduced from Winn N, Lalam R, Cassar-Pullicino V. Imaging of Paget's disease of bone. Wien Med Wochenschr 2017;167(1–2):9–17; with permission)

inner calvarial thickening table may occur, designated as a "tam-o'-shanter" skull. Rarely, sarcomatous transformation of the pagetic lesions may develop in the cranium [20, 38, 39].

The bone expansion in the skull can cause compression of the cranial nerves, with loss of hearing and an increase in hat size. Indeed, cranial nerve entrapment due to narrowing of the nerve foramina may cause serious neurological complications including various cranial nerve palsies, paraplegia, and quadriplegia. Deafness secondary to involvement of the 6th cranial nerve is common. Obstructive hydrocephalus, brain stem compression, and vertebrobasilar insufficiency may be observed less frequently [36, 37].

13.8 Phenytoin-Induced Hyperostosis

Phenytoin is a widely used anti-epileptic drug indicated for clinical administration both in pediatric and adult patients. Long-term phenytoin treatment, however, is associated with gross facial features, denoting overgrowth of the facial structures, gingival hyperplasia, and thickening of the cranium. Cranial computed tomography (CT) shows significant thickening of the calvaria (Fig. 13.9). Investigators have suggested that etiology relates to stimulation of osteoblast differentiation and proliferation [40, 41]. Thus far, the effectiveness of antiepileptic drug prophylaxis for post-traumatic seizures in pediatric patients is not clear. When it comes to the selection of antiepileptic drugs, it appears that in clinical practice, various factors including the preference of physician and the patient should be taken into consideration [42–44]. As such, use of phenytoin should be carefully evaluated for expected benefits and possible, serious side effects. The prophylactic use of anti-epileptics, including phenytoin, in pediatric patients with late post-traumatic seizures has been queried [45].

The detrimental effects of phenytoin on bone are related to the development of biochemical rickets, which is compensated by secondary hyperparathyroidism. Most importantly, high levels of PTH have different effects on the skeleton (osteoporosis-inducing, catabolic) in contrast to the calvarium (hyperostosis-inducing, proliferative) [46]. It appears that paradoxical, dual effect of PTH associated with phenytoin relates to the activation of complex biological mechanisms regulating bone turnover [47, 48]. Close monitoring of bone turnover biomarkers would probably be useful for the identification of medical risks related to anti-epileptic drug therapy [46].

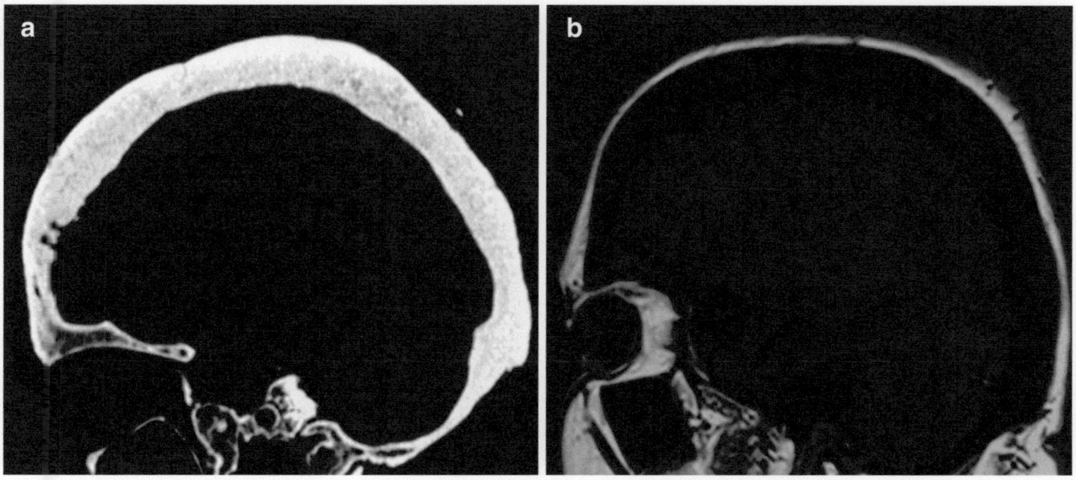

Fig. 13.9 (**a**) Sagittal reformatted CT image shows diffuse thickening of the calvarial bones (**b**) Corresponding T1-weighted magnetic resonance imaging (MRI) shows thickened calvaria (**b**)

13.9 Chronic Anemia

In patients with chronic anemia, hyperplasia of red marrow may cause various skull changes including outer table obliteration and diploic space widening. A coarse-grained or dotted pattern may be seen in the superior parietal region before diploic expansion. In the presence of hyperplastic bone marrow and destruction of the outer table, thin bony spicules may develop perpendicular to the outer table of the skull, assuming the typical "hair on tip" appearance. Such findings may be seen in other hematological diseases including sickle cell disease, thalassemia, and iron deficiency anemia [49–51]. The "goosebump appearance" has been associated with various anemic conditions, including sickle cell disease, spherocytosis, thalassemia major, and iron deficiency [52, 53].

Sickle cell anemia is recognized as a qualitative disorder of the synthesis of malfunctioning hemoglobin, manifest as hemolytic anemia, and bone infarction [54]. The conventional radiography may demonstrate enlargement of the medullary and the diploic space due to hyperplasia of the bone marrow. Magnetic resonance imaging (MRI) can prove useful to detect the early ischemia and osteonecrosis [55]. The trabecular structure, which is perpendicular to the inner plate of the skull, gives a characteristic "goosebump" appearance. In the presence of osteomyelitis, periosteal reaction, bone destruction, and areas of dead bone can be easily detected on CT images [55]. Radiologically, abscesses in the soft tissue and bone are observed as low-attenuation fluid collections with peripheral ring enhancement, with or without the formation of gas. Importantly, osteonecrosis and osteosclerosis that cannot be seen on radiographs can be detected on CT. [55].

MRI allows for early detection of profound bone marrow changes related to infarction, marrow hyperplasia, osteomyelitis, and osteonecrosis [55]. Over time, bone infarcts present as regions of serpiginous low signal intensity surrounding marrow of relatively unaltered signal intensity on T1-weighted images [55]. In the chronic phase, infarcted regions become hypointense on T1- and T2-weight images due to ensuing fibrosis and sclerosis in necrotic tissue.

13.10 Osteopenia

Osteopenia, defined as a mild form of osteoporosis, is characterized by decreased mineralization of bone tissue, owing to inadequate bone formation or excess resorption. Various congenital, toxic, metabolic, or idiopathic factors have been related to the complex pathophysiology of this process. Cortical and trabecular bone loss can lead to a radiologically heterogeneous appearance [56].

13.11 Thalassemia

Thalassemia, an autosomal recessive hematological disease, is characterized by a decrease in the rate of hemoglobin chain synthesis, thus leading to the production of abnormal hemoglobin molecules manifest as "microcytic anemia" [55, 57]. Characteristic imaging findings include expansion of the medullary component in the skull, with thinning of the cortical component due to proliferation of the marrow cavity, and loss of bone density because of predominant resorption of the cancellous bone. CT images of the calvaria may diplay characteristic "goosebumps" [55]. In patients with thalaemia major, the diploic area of the skull may be widely enlarged (Fig. 13.10). Although on the imaging studies thalassemia may present features that are similar to those observed in sickle cell disease, thalassemia relates to quantitative derangement of the globin synthesis, whereas sickle cell disease is a hematological disease associated with a qualitative disorder of the globin synthesis [55, 58].

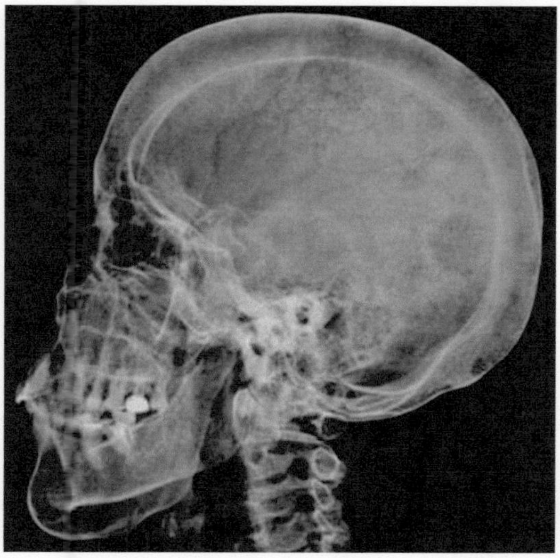

Fig. 13.10 Lateral radiograph of the skull shows diffuse widening of the diploic space

13.12 Osteopetrosis

Osteopetrosis is a rare inherited disorder related to malfunction of osteoclasts failing to resorb bone during the 9th week of pregnancy that causes calcified cartilage to accumulate in the medullary space [55, 59]. Etiologically, several genetic abnormalities associated with an imbalance in the bone resorption process may be responsible for osteopetrosis, although its exact mechanism is not clear. It has been suggested that in osteopetrosis, the number of osteoclasts may be normal or increased, but the acidification function is defective, or according to another hypothesis, mutation of the carbonic anhydrase gene may result in the formation of abnormally dense and fragile bone, and fractures [55, 60].

Different forms of osteopetrosis are classified according to mode of inheritance causing distinct molecular aberrations [55, 60]. The autosomal dominant type, termed Albers-Schönberg disease or osteopetrosis type 2, is the mildest form of human osteopotrosis. Patients can be asymptomatic, and the features of musculoskeletal involvement may be incidentally discovered on the imaging studies. Occasionally, bone fracture, arthritis, and osteomyelitis are seen in adolescent patients [55, 61]. The autosomal recessive type is the more severe form of osteopetrosis. Clinical findings including increased bone density, motor disabilities, and impaired hearing or vision due to compression of the cranial nerves are seen in patients starting at infancy [55]. Clinically, patients with osteopetrosis type 1 and 2 are usually immunocompromized and present with anemia, because of reduced production of blood cells and effacement of bone marrow. Further, it is possible to encounter osteopetrosis with an X-linked pattern of inheritance [55, 60]. Regardless of the exact molecular defects or location of the mutations, however, the radiological features in the skull suggesting osteopetrosis may include high inner table attenuation, widened diploe with low-attenuation, and an outer table of intermediate attenuation [55]. Periosteal reaction in the skull may be seen as fine, vertical trabeculations interspersed with radiolucent areas of bone marrow hyperplasia in the cranial vault, known as the "hair on tip" sign [55]. Diffuse increase in bone density, calvarial thickening, and poor sinus development are additional radiographic findings seen in osteopetrosis [62].

13.13 Conclusion

The calvarium and scalp can be affected by a number of systemic metabolic diseases. The spectrum of these conditions is broad and in each individual case the manifestations of disease may be different with regard to the location, size and extent, and type of calvarial involvement. Clinicians and radiologists alike may need to evaluate images of lesions in the cranium and correlate the radiologic appearances with the clinical, pathologic, and laboratory findings. Recognition of abnormalities can prevent misdiagnosis and may prove substantial in the planning of appropriate treatment.

References

1. Tubbs RS, Bosmia AN, Cohen-Gadol AA. The human calvaria: a review of embryology, anatomy, pathology, and molecular development. Childs Nerv Syst. 2012;28(1):23–31. https://doi.org/10.1007/s00381-011-1637-0.

2. Gentile C, Chiarelli F. Rickets in children: an update. Biomedicine. 2021;9(7):738.
3. Kiesler J, Ricer R. The abnormal fontanel. Am Fam Physician. 2003;67(12):2547–52.
4. Lips P, van Schoor NM, Bravenboer N. Vitamin D-related disorders. In: Rosen CJ, editor. Primer on the metabolic bone diseases and disorders of mineral metabolism. 8th ed. MA: Wiley-Blackwell Publishing; 2013. p. 613–23.
5. Di Rocco F, Rothenbuhler A, Cormier Daire V, Bacchetta J, Adamsbaum C, Baujat G, Rossi M, Lingart A. Craniosynostosis and metabolic bone disorder. A review. Neurochirurgie. 2019;65(5):258–63.
6. Currarino G. Sagittal synostosis in X-linked hypophosphatemic rickets and related diseases. Pediatr Radiol. 2007;37(8):805–12.
7. Al-Jundi SH, Dabous IM, Al-Jamal GA. Craniofacial morphology in patients with hypophosphataemic vitamin-D-resistant rickets: a cephalometric study. J Oral Rehabil. 2009;36(7):483–90.
8. Brociek-Piłczyńska A, Brodowska-Kania D, Szczygielski K, Lorent M, Zieliński G, Kowalewski P, Jurkiewicz D. A rare combination of tumor-induced osteomalacia caused by sinonasal glomangiopericytoma and coexisting parathyroid adenoma: case report and literature review. BMC Endocr Disord. 2022;22:31.
9. Mani MK, Panigrahi MK. Unusual calvarial tumour-oncogenic osteomalacia. Br J Neurosurg. 2017;31(4):495–6.
10. Carroll MF, Schade DS. A practical approach to hypercalcemia. Am Fam Physician. 2003;67(9):1959–66.
11. Goltzman D. Approach to hypercalcemia. In: Feingold KR, Anawalt B, Blackman MR, Boyce A, Chrousos G, Corpas E, de Herder WW, Dhatariya K, Dungan K, Hofland J, Kalra S, Kaltsas G, Kapoor N, Koch C, Kopp P, Korbonits M, Kovacs CS, Kuohung W, Laferrère B, Levy M, EA MG, McLachlan R, New M, Purnell J, Sahay R, Shah AS, Singer F, Sperling MA, Stratakis CA, Trence DL, Wilson DP, editors. Endotext [Internet]. South Dartmouth (MA): MDText.com, Inc; 2023. p. 2000.
12. Aguilar A, Gifre L, Ureña-Torres P, Carrillo-López N, Rodriguez-García M, Massó E, da Silva I, López-Báez V, Sánchez-Bayá M, Prior-Español Á, Urrutia M, Paul J, Bustos MC, Vila A, Garnica-León I, Navarro-González JF, Mateo L, Bover J. Pathophysiology of bone disease in chronic kidney disease: from basics to renal osteodystrophy and osteoporosis. Front Physiol. 2023;14:1177829.
13. Naji Rad S, Anastasopoulou C, Barnett MJ, Deluxe L. Osteitis Fibrosa Cystica. In: StatPearls [Internet]. Treasure Island (FL): StatPearls Publishing; 2023.
14. Pokhrel B, Leslie SW, Levine SN. Primary hyperparathyroidism. In: StatPearls [Internet]. Treasure Island (FL): StatPearls Publishing; 2022.
15. Lacativa PG, Franco FM, Pimentel JR, Patrício Filho PJ, Gonçalves MD, Farias ML. Prevalence of radiological findings among cases of severe secondary hyperparathyroidism. Sao Paulo Med J. 2009;127(2):71–7.
16. Saini V, Gupta N, Mohan A, Gupta V, Kolluru K. Osteitis fibrosis cystica: classical case report of an uncommon presentation in a young female. Indian J Otolaryngol Head Neck Surg. 2022;74:5319–23.
17. Psaila A, Conti L, Azzopardi AP, Coppini DV. A brown tumor secondary to hyperparathyroidism in the maxilla, skull, scapula, and femora. Proc (Baylor Univ Med Cent). 2020;34(1):163–5.
18. Lafage-Proust MH. Bone and chronic kidney disease. Semin Musculoskelet Radiol. 2023;27(4):463–70.
19. Gomez CK, Schiffman SR, Bhatt AA. Radiological review of skull lesions. Insights Imaging. 2018;9:857–82.
20. Khodarahmi I, Alizai H, Chalian M, Alaia EF, Burke CJ, Slasky SE, Wenokor C. Imaging spectrum of calvarial abnormalities. Radiographics. 2021;41(4):1144–63.
21. Tejwani NC, Schachter AK, Immerman I, Achan P. Renal osteodystrophy. J Am Acad Orthop Surg. 2006;14(5):303–11.
22. Wydra A, Stelmachowska-Banaś M, Czajka-Oraniec I. Skeletal complications in acromegaly. Reumatologia. 2023;61(4):248–55.
23. Guglielmi G. Acromegaly. In: Baert AL, editor. Encyclopedia of diagnostic imaging. Berlin, Heidelberg: Springer; 2008.
24. Girnius S. Overview of systemic and localized amyloidosis. Rev Health Care. 2013;4(4):231–47.
25. Picken MM. The pathology of amyloidosis in classification: a review. Acta Haematol. 2020;143(4):322–34.
26. Boccadoro M, Pileri A. Plasma cell dyscrasias: classification, clinical and laboratory characteristics, and differential diagnosis. Baillieres Clin Haematol. 1995;8(4):705–19.
27. Di Giuliano F, Picchi E, Muto M, Calcagni A, Ferrazzoli V, Da Ros V, Minosse S, Chiaravalloti A, Garaci F, Floris R, Muto M. Radiological imaging in multiple myeloma: review of the state-of-the-art. Neuroradiology. 2020;62(8):905–23.
28. Kristinsson SY, Minter AR, Korde N, Tan E, Landgren O. Bone disease in multiple myeloma and precursor disease: novel diagnostic approaches and implications on clinical management. Expert Rev Mol Diagn. 2011;11(6):593–603.
29. Ferreiro JA, Bhuta S, Nieberg RK, Verity MA. Amyloidoma of the skull base. Arch Pathol Lab Med. 1990;114(9):974–6.
30. Lee K, Mani N, Tan ZE, Slevin N. Successful use of radiotherapy for pterygopalatine fossa amyloidosis. Otolaryngol Head Neck Surg. 2016;155(2):353–5.
31. Simoens WA, van den Hauwe L, Van Hedent E, Warson F, Demaeseneer R, Williams D, De Schepper AM. Amyloidoma of the skull base. AJNR Am J Neuroradiol. 2000;21(8):1559–62.
32. Unal F, Hepgül K, Bayindir C, Bilge T, Imer M, Turantan I. Skull base amyloidoma. Case report. J Neurosurg. 1992;76(2):303–6.
33. Oruckaptan H, Karli Oğuz K, Işikay I, Ruacan S. Amyloidoma of the temporal bone and upper cervical spine; presentation of a rare clinical entity

with a brief literature review. Turk Neurosurg. 2009;19(2):159–62.
34. Pons Escoda A, Naval Baudin P, Mora P, Cos M, Hernandez Gañan J, Narváez JA, Aguilera C, Majós C. Imaging of skull vault tumors in adults. Insights Imaging. 2020;11(1):23.
35. Theodorou DJ, Theodorou SJ, Kakitsubata Y. Imaging of Paget disease of bone and its musculoskeletal complications: review. AJR Am J Roentgenol. 2011;196(6 Suppl):S64–75.
36. Bolland MJ, Cundy T. Paget's disease of bone: clinical review and update. J Clin Pathol. 2013;66(11):924–7.
37. Cook SJ, Wall C. Paget's disease of bone: a clinical update. Aust J Gen Pract. 2021;50(1-2):23–9.
38. Winn N, Lalam R, Cassar-Pullicino V. Imaging of Paget's disease of bone. Wien Med Wochenschr. 2017;167(1–2):9–17.
39. Lombardi AF, Aihara AY, Fernandes ADRC, Cardoso FN. Imaging of Paget's disease of bone. Radiol Clin North Am. 2022;60(4):561–73.
40. Ikedo D, Ohishi K, Yamauchi N, Kataoka M, Kido J, Nagata T. Stimulatory effects of phenytoin on osteoblastic differentiation of fetal rat calvaria cells in culture. Bone. 1999;25(6):653–60.
41. Marques P, Korbonits M. Pseudoacromegaly. Front Neuroendocrinol. 2019;52:113–43.
42. Bakr A, Belli A. A systematic review of levetiracetam versus phenytoin in the prevention of late post-traumatic seizures and survey of UK neurosurgical prescribing practice of antiepileptic medication in acute traumatic brain injury. Br J Neurosurg. 2018;32(3):237–44.
43. Hao X, Xu X, Li M, Xiao L, Wang Y, Li W, Wang C Sun T. Effectiveness of antiseizure medications therapy in preventing seizures in brain injury patients: a network meta-analysis. Front Pharmacol. 2022;13:1001363.
44. Xu JC, Shen J, Shao WZ, Tang LJ, Sun YZ, Zhai XF, Qi L, Li J, Zheng JY. The safety and efficacy of levetiracetam versus phenytoin for seizure prophylaxis after traumatic brain injury: a systematic review and meta-analysis. Brain Inj. 2016;30(9):1054–61.
45. Samara Q, Ifraitekh A, Jayyousi O, Sawan S, Hazaimeh E, Jbarah P. Use of antiepileptic drugs as prophylaxis against posttraumatic seizures in the pediatric population: a systematic review and meta-analysis. Neurosurg Rev. 2023;46(1):49.
46. Theng EH, Weinstein LS, Collins MT. Calvarial hyperostosis in primary hyperparathyroidism and other settings of increased cAMP signalling. Lancet. 2022;399(10328):956.
47. Koide M, Kinugawa S, Ninomiya T, Mizoguchi T, Yamashita T, Maeda K, Yasuda H, Kobayashi Y, Nakamura H, Takahashi N, Udagawa N. Diphenylhydantoin inhibits osteoclast differentiation and function through suppression of NFATc1 signaling. J Bone Miner Res. 2009;24:1469–80.
48. Martin TJ. PTH1R actions on bone using the cAMP/protein kinase A pathway. Front Endocrinol (Lausanne). 2022;12:833221.
49. Moseley JE. Skeletal changes in the anemias. Semin Roentgenol. 1974;9(3):169–84.
50. Sebes JI, Diggs LW. Radiographic changes of the skull in sickle cell anemia. AJR Am J Roentgenol. 1979;132:373–7.
51. Younghee Y, Woon-Jin M, Hyeong SA, Joon C, Myung HR. Imaging findings of various calvarial bone lesions with a focus on osteolytic lesions. J Korean Soc Radiol. 2016;74(1):43–54.
52. Ejindu VC, Hine AL, Mashayekhi M, Shorvon PJ, Misra RR. Musculoskeletal manifestations of sickle cell disease. RadioGraphics. 2007;27(4):1005–21.
53. Hollar MA. The hair-on-end sign. Radiology. 2001;221(2):347–8.
54. Kavanagh PL, Fasipe TA, Wun T. Sickle cell disease: a review. JAMA. 2022;328(1):57–68. https://doi.org/10.1001/jama.2022.10233.
55. Yao A, Taub JS, Gault AT, Naidich TP, Taub PJ. Systemic changes affecting the morphology of calvarial bone. J Craniofac Surg. 2019;30(1):e65–75.
56. Chang CY, Rosenthal DI, Mitchell DM, Handa A, Kattapuram SV, Huang AJ. Imaging findings of metabolic bone disease. Radiographics. 2016;36:1871–87.
57. Pines M, Sheth S. Clinical classification, screening, and diagnosis in beta-thalassemia and hemoglobin E/Beta-thalassemia. Hematol Oncol Clin North Am. 2023;37(2):313–25. https://doi.org/10.1016/j.hoc.2022.12.003.
58. Ferraresi M, Panzieri DL, Leoni S, Cappellini MD, Kattamis A, Motta I. Therapeutic perspective for children and young adults living with thalassemia and sickle cell disease. Eur J Pediatr. 2023;182(6):2509–19.
59. Stark Z, Savarirayan R. Osteopetrosis. Orphanet J Rare Dis. 2009;4:5. https://doi.org/10.1186/1750-1172-4-5.
60. Penna S, Villa A, Capo V. Autosomal recessive osteopetrosis: mechanisms and treatments. Dis Model Mech. 2021;14(5):dmm048940.
61. Wilson CS, Vellodi A. Autosomal recessive osteopetrosis: diagnosis, management and outcome. Arch Dis Child. 2000;83:449–52.
62. Yadav S, Chalise S, Chaudhary S, Shah GS, Gupta MK, Mishra OP. Osteopetrosis in two siblings: two case reports. BMC Res Notes. 2016;9:55.

Part IV

Traumatic, Vascular, and Infectious Lesions of the Scalp and Calvarium

Editor's Summary

In this "Part IV: Traumatic, Vascular and Infectious Lesions of the Scalp and Calvarium," there are six chapters that address traumatic, vascular, and infectious lesions of the scalp and calvarium. The wide variety of traumatic injury to the scalp and calvarium that is seen in both children and adults is covered in Chap. 14. Those iatrogenic lesions that affect the scalp and calvarium which can be surgical and nonsurgical are described in detail in Chap. 15. Interestingly, the scalp and the calvarium have their own separate types of vascular lesions and malformations that are very different in their nature. The vascular lesions and malformations involving the scalp are addressed in Chap. 16, whereas the intraosseous vascular lesions and malformations of the calvarium are covered in the subsequent Chap. 17. Classic infectious lesions involving the scalp and calvarium commonly caused by bacterial or fungal organisms represent the focus of Chap. 18. Inflammatory lesions associated with the immune system such as sarcoidosis, histiocytosis, and granuloma formation that affect the scalp and calvarium are discussed in the last chapter in this section, Chap. 19.

14 Traumatic Lesions of the Scalp and Calvarium

Brody Hooper, Cameron Shuman, and Timothy Beutler

14.1 Introduction

The scalp and calvarium are vital protective barriers that shield the intracranial structures from trauma and injury. Various kinds of traumatic injuries can occur and appropriate treatment will depend on the mechanism and severity of the injury. Minor injuries can be managed conservatively while more severe injuries may require surgical intervention. Understanding the anatomy and mechanism of injury is important for accurate diagnosis, prompt management, and optimal patient outcomes. This chapter will explore common injuries to the scalp and calvarium as well as special pediatric considerations and complications that can arise from treatment.

14.2 Scalp Injuries

14.2.1 Normal Anatomy of the Scalp

The scalp is comprised of five distinct layers. These include the skin, dense subcutaneous connective tissue, epicranial aponeurosis, loose areolar connective tissue, and periosteum (Fig. 14.1). Functionally, the scalp serves as a safeguard for the underlying skull, offering essential cushioning, insulation, and structural support. Abundant vascularity ensures a robust blood supply, facilitating the nourishment of its diverse layers. However, this rich vascularization also allows for significant bleeding in the event of injury. The layer of loose areolar connective tissue, often referred to as a "danger area," bears a particular risk of injury due to the presence of valveless emissary veins that connect superficial veins in the subaponeurotic space to intracranial venous sinuses.

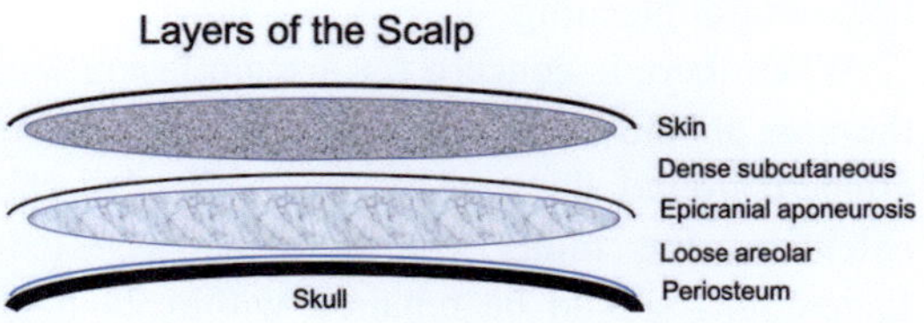

Fig. 14.1 Layers of the scalp from superficial to deep: skin, dense subcutaneous tissue, epicranial aponeurosis, loose areolar tissue and periosteum

14.2.2 Lacerations of the Scalp

Sharp injury to the scalp can result in lacerations. Scalp lacerations are among the most common kinds of injury to the scalp. They are frequently encountered in the emergency care setting and may require urgent treatment. When assessing injury to the scalp, it is important to consider the depth, size, shape, and mechanism of injury.

B. Hooper · C. Shuman · T. Beutler (✉)
Department of Neurosurgery, State University of New York (SUNY) Upstate Medical University, Syracuse, NY, USA
e-mail: beutlert@upstate.edu

M. Turgut et al. (eds.), *Lesions of the Scalp and Cranial Vault*,
https://doi.org/10.1007/978-3-031-88244-9_14

Severe injuries or injuries associated with high-velocity mechanisms may benefit from CT imaging of the head to rule out co-morbid intracranial injury. Because of the scalp's rich vascular supply, deep lacerations are at risk for significant hemorrhage and steps may need to be taken to urgently control blood loss. Small and superficial lacerations that do not completely penetrate through the skin layer may not require any invasive treatment and can be managed with local wound care. Direct pressure can be applied to the wound to obtain hemostasis and in some cases, local lidocaine with epinephrine can be used to help control bleeding.

When there is concern for a scalp laceration, the area should be thoroughly cleaned and hair clipped around the area of injury so that the extent of the injury can be fully assessed. Lacerations should be repaired within 24 h of injury to avoid risk of infection. The wound should be washed out with irrigation and any particulate matter within the wound should be removed. Deep and grossly contaminated wounds should be taken to the operating room for washout and closure (Fig. 14.2). Failure to remove particulate matter from the wound can result in infection and non-healing wounds with persistent drainage. Persistently draining wounds with exposed granulation tissue may need surgical excision of the granulation tissue and direct closure of the skin to allow for optimal wound healing (Fig. 14.3).

Scalp lacerations that penetrate through the skin layer or deeper will often require closure to obtain adequate hemostasis. However, the method of scalp closure may depend on the size and shape of the laceration. Staples can be an effective means to obtain hemostasis and closure of a laceration, particularly for linear lacerations that are actively bleeding. For complex lacerations that have a stellate-shaped injury to the scalp, simple interrupted monofilament sutures (typically 3-0 or 4-0 sutures) can be used to approximate the wound edges.

Large full-thickness scalp lacerations may benefit from multi-layered closure. Severe injuries may need to undergo definitive repair in the

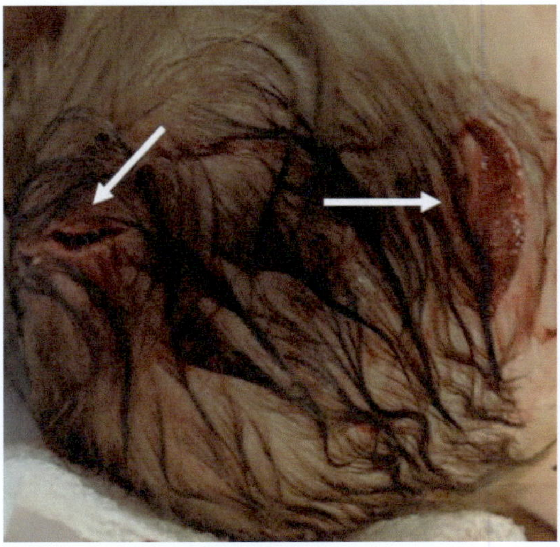

Fig. 14.2 Three-year-old boy who sustained multiple dog bite injuries to the head. Deep and contaminated lacerations required washout and closure in the operating room

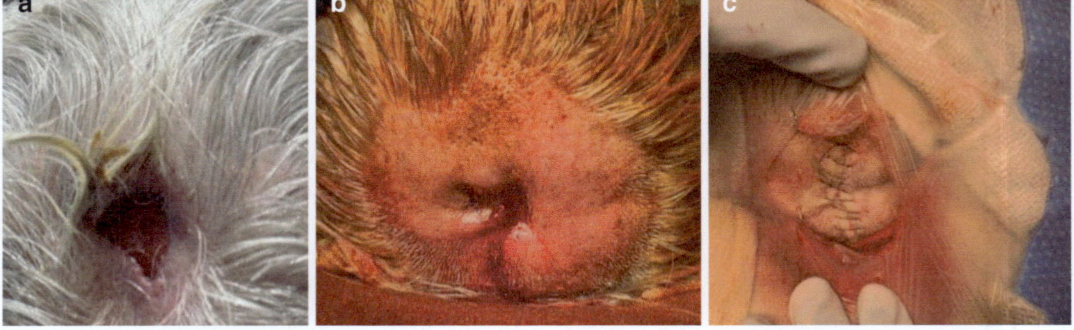

Fig. 14.3 Eighty-year-old woman with non-healing wound after mechanical fall. Failed conservative management with local wound care and oral antibiotics. Found to have a scalp granuloma (**a**, **b**) that required surgical excision (**c**)

operating room. In the most severe form of scalp injury, a degloving or an avulsion injury of the scalp can occur. These injuries would benefit from evaluation in the operating room and multilevel closure. Despite the scalp's rich vascular supply, a degloving or avulsion injury may not necessarily be able to be repaired directly if an extensive region of the scalp tissue is compromised. These wounds should be evaluated by specialists who have experience with scalp reconstruction and may need multiple operations including skin grafting for adequate healing.

14.2.3 Hematomas of the Scalp

Hematomas of the scalp can occur with or without scalp lacerations. They most commonly manifest as a result of blunt force trauma and are typically managed conservatively. Multiple layers of the scalp allow for hematomas to form in several different layers and it may be difficult to clinically distinguish between them. The most common kinds of scalp hematomas are caput succedaneum, subgaleal hemorrhage, and cephalohematomas (Fig. 14.4).

14.2.3.1 Caput Succedaneum

Caput succedaneum is a condition where edema and hemorrhage occur within the subcutaneous connective tissue layer of the scalp superficial to the epicranial aponeurosis. It is commonly seen in infants shortly after delivery and is associated with birth-related trauma to the scalp. This condition is considered benign and does not typically require any surgical treatment. Given the location of the injury, swelling can cross suture lines and midline. The swelling appears edematous and fluctuant consistent with a pitting edema. There may be some associated ecchymoses or petechiae around the injury. It is associated with extended labor, vertex delivery, and the use of forceps and vacuum-assisted delivery. Physical examination is typically diagnostic; nonetheless, it is important to distinguish it from other kinds of scalp hemorrhage. Caput succedaneum typically self-resolves within 48 h and rarely results in hyperbilirubinemia in newborns.

14.2.3.2 Subgaleal Hematoma

Subgaleal hematomas occur between the epicranial aponeurosis and the periosteum in the loose areolar connective tissue layer. These hemorrhages can cross suture lines similar to those found in caput succedaneum; however, they have the potential to become more diffuse. Subgaleal hematomas can become quite large as the space extends behind the orbit and into the back of the neck. They are associated with trauma and can occur throughout the lifespan. When they occur in adults, they are typically benign. In young children, hemorrhage into this space can be significant and result in hypotension and coagulopathy. Subgaleal hemorrhages in newborns have high mortality and morbidity. They are associated with seizures, skull fractures, and hyponatremia. Risk factors for newborns include vacuum and forceps-assisted

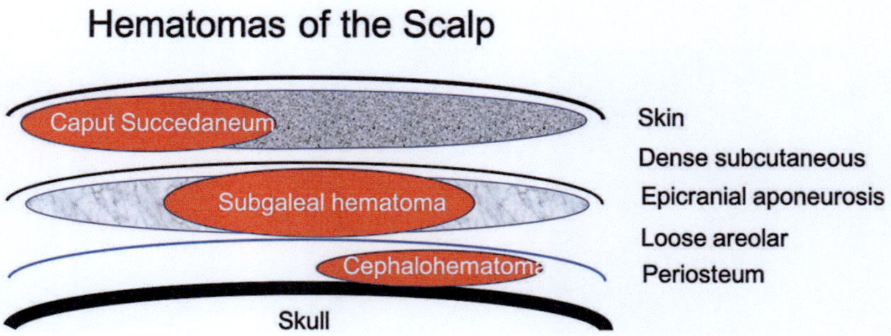

Fig. 14.4 Hematomas of the scalp depicted in relation to the anatomic layers of the scalp. Caput succedaneum occurs in the dense subcutaneous layer. Subgaleal hematomas are found in the loose areolar tissue layer. Cephalohematomas occur between the periosteum and the skull

delivery. Conservative management consists of a headwrap and interval monitoring of the head circumference. In the case of large hemorrhages, hemoglobin/hematocrit and sodium levels should also be monitored.

14.2.3.3 Cephalohematoma

A cephalohematoma is a collection of blood between the periosteum and the skull bone, typically resulting from birth trauma or assisted deliveries. This occurs due to the rupture of capillaries located below the periosteum. On clinical examination, the hematomas are firm and do not cross suture lines or midline. Typically, they have the potential to enlarge over the first 24 h but are rarely associated with intracranial hemorrhage. Newborns may have to be monitored for hyperbilirubinemia. Cephalohematomas can be present bilaterally making them more difficult to distinguish from caput succendaneum. They typically self-resolve within 2–6 weeks.

A rare complication of cephalohematoma is calcification where the blood clot transforms into a calcified mass over time. Calcified cephalohematomas are generally benign and asymptomatic; however, they can cause significant deformities that justify cosmetic concerns for children and parents. The development of a calcified cephalohematoma is exceedingly rare and the incidence rate is not well documented. One 25-year-long study at the University of Michigan found that ~40% of infants with calcified cephalohematomas required surgical correction [1]. They are often discovered incidentally on physical exams or imaging studies. On physical exam, they appear as a firm immobile painless mass. X-ray or CT imaging can be obtained to confirm the presence of calcification within the cephalohematoma and its extent. Treatment is primarily conservative with a focus on observation and reassurance. Parents should be reassured that the mass is benign and does not affect their child's health not development. Surgical intervention is rarely indicated and reserved for cases with severe cosmetic concerns or complications.

14.3 Burn Injuries of the Scalp

While not as common as other forms of traumatic injury, burn injuries to the scalp can also occur. Burn injuries may be due to thermal, electrical, or chemical exposures. When assessing a burn injury to the scalp, the extent of injury needs to be assessed. This often requires operative debridement until healthy tissue is encountered. In the case of full-thickness burn injuries that extend beyond the periosteum, the underlying bone may also require debridement. If the burn injury does not extend through the entire thickness of the skull, then the outer cortical table can be removed leaving the inner cortical table intact. Split-thickness skin grafting is often required for full-thickness burns injuries to completely heal. Treatment of burn injuries to the scalp and calvarium often will involve a multidisciplinary team and multiple operations. Figure 14.5 depicts a thermal burn injury that occurred secondary to

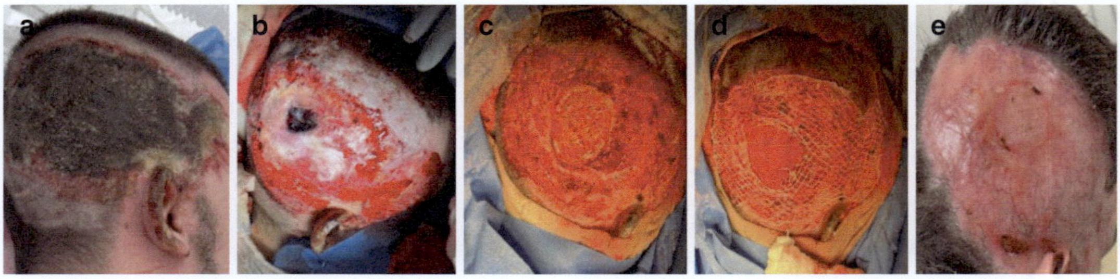

Fig. 14.5 Thirty-year-old man found down with extensive burn injury from frostbite (**a**). Underwent staged debridement of necrotic tissue. Injury extended into the bone (**b**) and required removal of outer table of the skull (**c**). Subsequent partial thickness skin grafting (**d**) and wound healing (**e**)

frostbite that extended into the outer table of the skull and required staged debridement and reconstruction.

14.4 Calvarial Injuries

14.4.1 Normal Anatomy of the Calvarium

The calvarium, also known as the skullcap or vault, forms a dome-shaped bone covering the brain. It is comprised of the frontal, parietal, temporal, occipital, and greater wing of the sphenoid bones and excludes the bone that forms the lower jaw and facial portions of the skull. Between the bones that form the calvarium are suture lines that allow for growth and flexibility during development. The primary function is to provide structural integrity and to safeguard the contents of the cranial cavity.

The bones of the calvarium are typically composed of three layers (Fig. 14.6). An outer cortical layer that lies directly beneath the periosteum, a middle cancellous layer, and an inner cortical layer that lies directly over the dura. The bone varies in thickness at various locations ranging from thin over the squamous temporal regions to thick in the frontal and parietal regions.

Traumatic injuries that affect the calvarium can vary in complexity in relation to the underlying anatomic and vascular structures. This results in a broad spectrum of clinical presentations that range from observable external signs, such as lacerations and hematomas, to more concealed internal injuries, including fractures and contusions. Therefore, a comprehensive evaluation of patients with head trauma becomes crucial, requiring a multidimensional approach that incorporates a detailed clinical history, a thorough physical examination, and judicious utilization of radiographic imaging modalities.

14.4.2 Skull Fractures

Skull fractures commonly occur after trauma when the force exerted on the skull compromises its structural integrity. Many of these injuries are high impact and high energy, but depending on patient-specific biomechanic properties, fractures can occur even after low-energy trauma, especially in young children and the elderly. Skull fractures primarily involve the parietal, temporal, occipital, and frontal bones, with the parietal bone being the most frequently affected. Notably, males aged 20–29 years are at the highest risk, with males being three times more susceptible than females [2]. Mechanisms of injury commonly include motor vehicle accidents (MVAs), physical assaults, falls, and sporting accidents.

During the initial assessment, a detailed history and physical examination are crucial to understanding the mechanism of injury. In addition to identifying fractures, clinicians must assess for lacerations, contusions, and hematomas, as these may serve as indicators of underlying injuries.

Patients with skull fractures may present with a variety of symptoms, including altered mental status, focal cranial nerve findings, draining of blood or cerebrospinal fluid (CSF), bruising, particularly around the eyes (periorbital ecchymosis; Raccoon sign) and ears (retroauricular ecchymosis; Battle's sign), changes in pupils (size, reactivity, regularity), confusion, headache, seizures, nausea and vomiting, visual disturbances, loss of consciousness, and head or neck pain. Prompt recognition of these signs is essential to provide

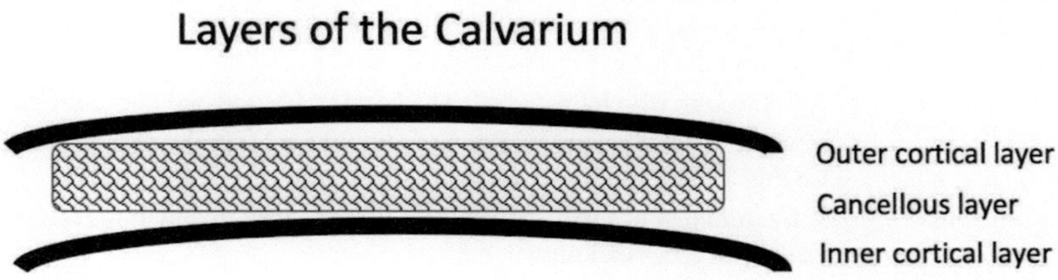

Fig. 14.6 Layers of the calvarium showing the relationship between the outer cortical, cancellous and inner cortical layers

timely intervention and optimize patient outcomes.

Diagnostic imaging is of paramount importance in the assessment of skull fractures. X-ray, MRI, and CT scans are frequently utilized, with CT imaging being particularly favored due to its widespread availability, cost-effectiveness, and ability to detect both bony injuries and soft tissue and intracranial lesions. Given the considerable force needed to cause a skull fracture, the availability of multidetector computed tomography (MDCT) with 3D reconstruction offers superior identification of clinically significant skull fractures, enhancing diagnostic accuracy, and aiding in comprehensive treatment planning.

Skull fractures are typically described based on a variety of parameters beyond the physical location including open vs closed, linear vs comminuted, and depressed vs non-depressed. An open fracture is a fracture that is associated with an overlying scalp laceration, while in closed injuries, the scalp remains intact. Linear fractures are fractures that extend in a single line, while comminuted fractures are complex and may involve multiple interconnected breaks in the bone. Fractures are considered depressed when the inner table is compressed inward towards the brain parenchymal and non-depressed with the normal alignment of the fractured bone maintained. Table 14.1 describes additional terms that are often used in classifying and describing skull fractures.

Managing skull fractures necessitates a multidisciplinary approach, with neurosurgeons playing a central role. Treatment strategies depend on the severity and complexity of the fracture, associated injuries, and the overall clinical status of the patient. Mild fractures without neurologic deficit and underlying brain injury can be managed conservatively and do not require any intervention. These fractures are typically described as closed, linear, and non-displaced fractures. Patients should be admitted for observation when there is a risk, suspicion, or unclear determination of brain injury. In more severe cases with intracranial involvement, elevated intracranial pressure, or neurological deficits, surgical intervention may be necessary. Neurosurgical procedures may include decompressive craniectomy, repair of dural lacerations, removal of intracranial hematomas, and fixation of complex fractures. Severe fractures can also extend from the calvarium into the facial structures and require a multidisciplinary approach with ENT and Facial Plastics teams for treatment and reconstruction (Fig. 14.7).

All open fractures should be washed out and irrigated free from debridement before the overlying scalp deficit is closed. Open depressed skull fractures with depression of the fragment greater than the thickness of the skull should go to the

Table 14.1 Classification of skull fractures

Fracture type	Description
Linear	A simple fracture line that runs in a straight or slightly curved pattern without significant displacement or involvement of nearby bones. Most common type. Typically do not require intervention.
Elevated	May be associated with significant intracranial injuries. Require neurosurgical consultation.
Depressed	A fracture that results in an inward displacement of bone fragments, causing a depression in the skull surface. Increased risk of infection and seizures reported.
Diastatic	A fracture that occurs along the cranial sutures, resulting in separation and widening of the suture lines. These fractures are most often seen in newborns and older infants.
Basilar	A fracture involving the base of the skull, typically extending through the ethmoid, sphenoid, or temporal bones. This is often considered the most serious type of skull fracture and almost always requires admission for observation status.
Comminuted	A fracture in which the bone is shattered or fragmented into multiple pieces.
Le Fort	Fractures of the facial skeleton that may extend into the cranial vault, classified into three types: Le Fort I, II, and III.
Growing	A fracture that occurs in infants and young children due to the incomplete fusion of cranial bones, leading to abnormal growth patterns.

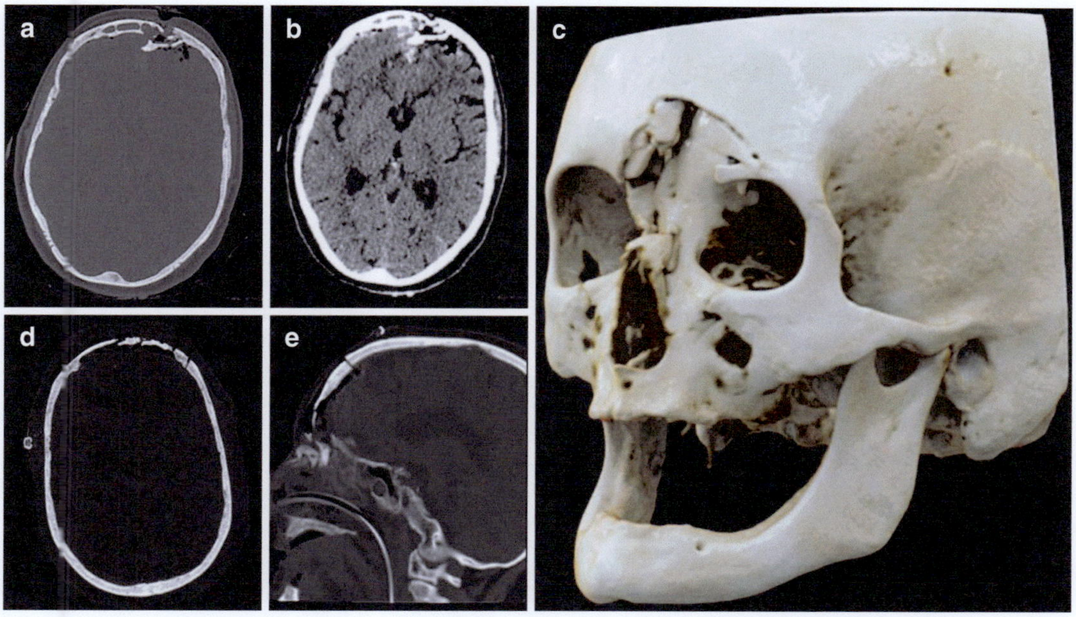

Fig. 14.7 Seventy-eight-year-old woman s/p 4 × 4 falling on her head. Comminuted frontal sinus fracture with associated dural laceration (**a–c**). Underwent bifrontal craniotomy for elevation of depressed skull fracture with cranialization of the frontal sinus and dural repair (**d**, **e**). Multidisciplinary approach needed during surgery as the patient also had extensive facial fractures

Operating Room for elevation to the depressed fracture fragment and repair of any underlying dural laceration to prevent infection. Early operative intervention is recommended along with antibiotics during the perioperative period. As long as there is no obvious sign of infection at the time of surgery, replacement of the primary bone fragment is recommended. Depressed skull fractures may be treated non-operatively if there is no clinical or radiographic evidence of dural laceration, no underlying intracranial hematoma, depression of the fragment < 1 cm, no frontal sinus involvement, no cosmetic deformity, and no wound infection or grossly contaminated wound. Figure 14.8 shows the initial and post-operative imaging for an open depressed skull fracture that underwent operative repair with replacement of the primary bone fragment at the time of the index surgery.

14.4.3 Penetrating Head Injuries

Penetrating traumas to the scalp and calvarium are rare but potentially life-threatening injuries caused by objects penetrating the skin and skull. They can occur after high-velocity projectiles, such as bullets, or non-missile penetrating injuries from accidents, falls, assaults, or other traumatic events. The severity of the injury depends on various factors, including the size, shape, and force of the penetrating object. They are often associated with open depressed, comminuted skull fractures. Management of penetrating brain injuries differs slightly from closed head injuries because of the elevated risk for infection and vascular injury. Figure 14.9 shows an example of a penetrating head injury caused by severe percussive trauma to the skull from a horse hoof injury to the head.

Penetrating brain injuries are rarer than closed-head injuries and often require careful management and vigilant monitoring in the Intensive Care Unit. Prognosis largely depends on the initial Glasgow Coma Scale and early detection of vascular and infectious complications [3]. Initial diagnosis can be derived from a variety of radiologic modalities including X-rays, CT, and MRI. Depending on the kind of injury, multiple modalities are often needed to determine the extent of injury. These imaging studies help identify the

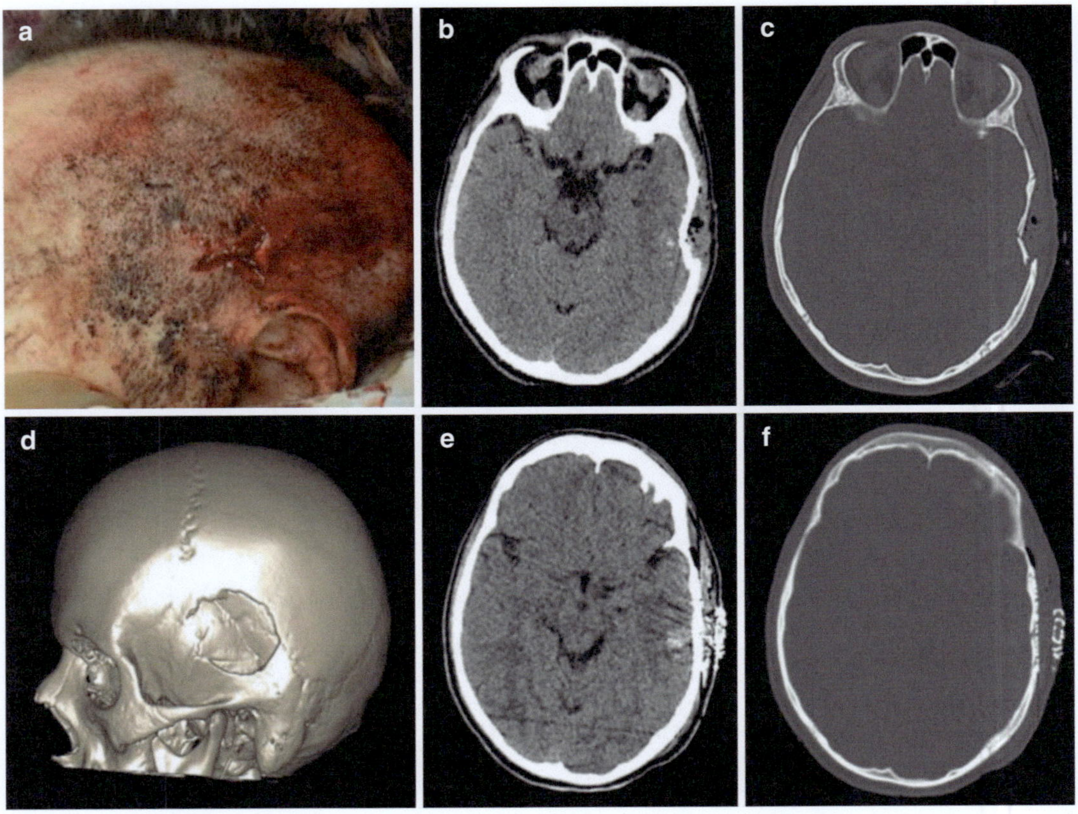

Fig. 14.8 Fifteen-year-old presented after a tree branch fell on his head (**a**). GCS 7 on arrival. CT with open depressed skull fracture (**b–d**). Underwent surgery for elevation, washout and direct repair (**e**, **f**). Primary bone replaced during surgery because there was concern for active infection

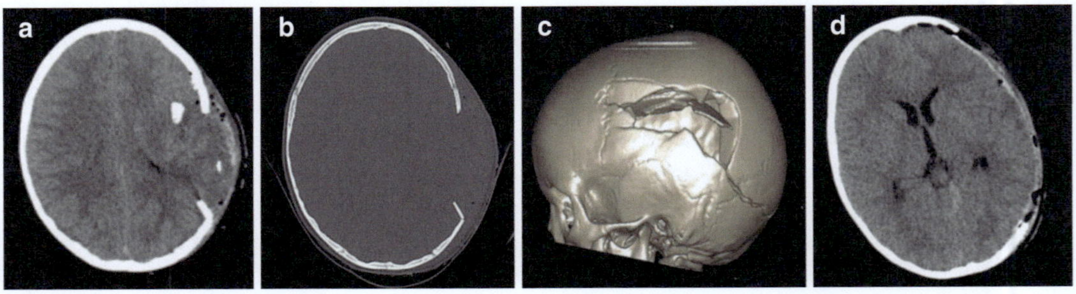

Fig. 14.9 Three-year-old with open depressed skull fracture after being kicked in the head by a horse (**a–c**). Underwent decompressive craniectomy with removal of bone fragments and washout (**d**)

penetration depth, location of foreign bodies, and potential intracranial injuries. CT is the preferred method to evaluate the initial soft tissue and bony injury but can be limited if there are retained metallic foreign bodies. Because vascular injuries can commonly occur, CT angiography or conventional digital subtraction angiography should be completed on all patients at the time of injury to screen for early vascular imaging. Repeat vascular imaging 7–10 days after initial injury should also be obtained to rule out the development of any delayed vascular complications.

Gunshot wounds (GSWs) represent a complex category of penetrating injuries involving the scalp and calvarium, resulting from the impact of projectiles discharged from firearms. These high-velocity projectiles cause extensive tissue damage and create intricate injury patterns, marked by variable entry and exit wounds, tissue fragmentation, and potential missile deformation (Fig. 14.10). Epidemiologically, GSWs to the head significantly contribute to traumatic brain injuries (TBIs), accounting for around 35% of TBI-related deaths with a staggering 90% fatality rate [4]. A collaborative approach involving neurosurgeons, public health organizations, law enforcement, and policymakers is essential for promoting firearm safety measures and raising awareness. Clinical presentations of GSWs vary based on factors such as bullet characteristics and trajectory, with complications including infection, cerebrospinal fluid leakage, and neurovascular deficits. Diagnostic imaging, especially CT and MRI, plays a critical role in assessing and planning treatment. Management depends on specific injuries, with neurosurgical intervention often required for penetrating brain injuries and intracranial hemorrhages. The risk of infection is high, necessitating prophylactic antibiotics. Long-term complications may include chronic pain, motor and/or sensory deficits, and cognitive impairments. Psychological trauma is also a concern, necessitating a holistic approach to care.

Nonmissile penetrating wounds can introduce foreign material and organisms, increasing the risk of infection. Thorough wound exploration and debridement are essential to remove any debris, foreign bodies, and necrotic tissue, thereby reducing the risk of complications. Depending on the nature of the injury and the presence of contamination, prophylactic antibiotics should be administered to prevent infection.

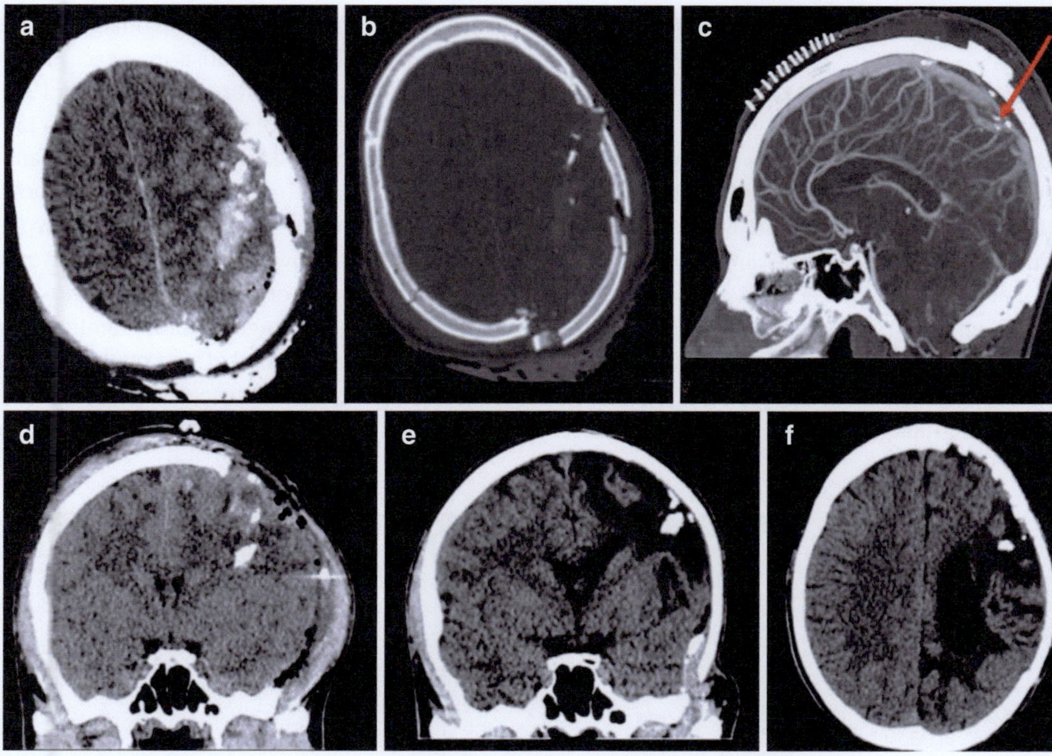

Fig. 14.10 Twenty-year-old man who sustained a gunshot wound to the head (**a**, **b**). Initial GCS on arrival to the ED was 7T but he quickly decompensated to a 3T with bradycardia. Vascular imaging concerning for non-occlusion thrombosis in sagittal sinus (**c**). Underwent emergent left sided decompressive craniectomy (**d**). Hospital course complicated by intracranial hypertension and sympathetic storming. Patient did well with mild residual aphasia and left sided weakness. He is able to ambulate independently. He subsequently underwent cranioplasty with PEEK implant (**e**, **f**)

The choice of antibiotics should be based on the suspected pathogens and local antimicrobial resistance patterns. The duration of antibiotic coverage is controversial and may vary based on the mechanism of injury.

Surgical exploration and washout are often needed in cases of penetrating injuries. Neurosurgical procedures may be performed to address any intracranial damage. Reconstructive surgery may be required for the scalp and calvarium. Depending on the co-morbidities and the extent of tissue damage, reconstruction options may either occur at the time of initial treatment or in a delayed fashion. During initial surgical management, it is crucial to debride accessible tissue and repair any associated dural or vascular injuries. Post-operative care should pay particular attention to monitoring for infection and delayed vascular complications.

14.5 Pediatric Considerations

14.5.1 Ping-Pong Fractures

Because the pediatric skull is still growing and not yet mature calvarium, there are some pediatric specific conditions that require additional discussion. Simple skull fractures are not uncommon amount children and the vast majority do not require any intervention. Some depressed skull fractures in young children can be managed conservatively. One of these fracture types is referred to as a ping-pong fracture (Fig. 14.11). In these cases, there is often not a distinct fracture line present, but the bone appears to be indented and pushed inwards. These fractures behave similarly to greenstick fractures in long bones and can sometimes resolve without surgical intervention.

14.5.2 Congenital Skull Depression

Congenital skull depressions, a rare developmental anomaly, emerge during fetal development or delivery and manifest as localized areas of flattened or sunken skull bones present at birth. While the exact cause of this condition remains elusive, it is thought to be linked to genetic factors, intrauterine positioning influenced by fetal limbs or maternal anatomy, and occasionally birth-related trauma. Complex deliveries, involving manual pressure from instruments such as forceps or digital pressure from the obstetrician's hands, may contribute to the development of these depressions. Its rarity and often asymptomatic nature make it challenging to establish the exact prevalence statistics, with a European study from 1986 reporting an incidence of 0.01% over 8 years [5]. Clinically, congenital skull depressions can manifest in two forms: deformed (depressed) without fracture or as fractures with depression. A physical examination following birth typically reveals these localized areas of cranial bone depression, and while generally benign, careful monitoring is essential to assess potential effects on the infant's growth and development, especially in cases of larger depressions that might pose a risk to the

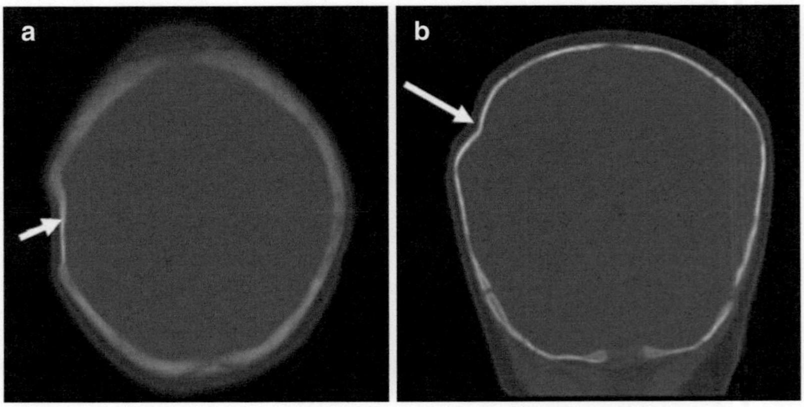

Fig. 14.11 Five-month-old presenting after a fall. Found to have a small depressed skull fracture. "Ping-pong" fracture. Greenstick type skull injury which can usually be managed conservatively. Most fractures will resolve without intervention

underlying cortex. Diagnostic evaluation involves plain film skull X-rays initially, with CT scans or MRI subsequently used for further assessment. The management approach is predominantly conservative, with regular pediatrician monitoring to ensure stability and absence of progression. Surgical intervention is exceedingly rare. Although congenital skull depressions are frequently asymptomatic and self-limiting, the cosmetic nature can be a source of significant concern for parents, prompting the need for physician recognition and monitoring.

14.5.3 Growing Fractures

Growing fractures, also referred to as pediatric skull fractures, are a unique subset of skull fractures affecting infants and young children, typically under the age of 3 years. These fractures have been described in medical literature for centuries, and identified by various names including expanding skull fractures, craniocerebral erosion, and leptomeningeal cysts. The distinctive characteristics of developing skulls render pediatric patients particularly susceptible to this phenomenon. The prevailing theory suggests that the pulsatile forces stemming from the expanding brain may contribute to the enlargement of skull fractures, typically linear at the time of injury, potentially leading to the extrusion of brain tissue or other neurological complications when accompanied by a lacerated dura mater. As such, early detection and appropriate management are paramount in these cases.

Growing fractures predominantly occur in children under the age of three and often stem from traumatic incidents such as falls, accidents, or abuse. Improperly closed dural lacerations following craniotomies can also result in growing skull fractures. While the incidence varies, it generally falls within the range of 0.05% to 1.6% [6]. Growing fractures most commonly affect the parietal bone, with less frequent occurrences observed in the frontal, parietal-occipital, and parietal-temporal regions, followed by the orbital roof and other less common locations, in descending order of occurrence rates [7].

Clinical considerations for growing fractures involve recognizing telltale signs after trauma, including swelling, bruising, tenderness, and visible depressions or bumps on the child's head. Many patients will exhibit a scalp mass, which can be a concerning feature for parents and caregivers. To evaluate the extent of the fracture and any associated brain injuries, a comprehensive medical assessment, including imaging studies like X-rays or CT scans, is essential. For milder fractures, a conservative approach entails careful observation and pain management. In contrast, more severe cases necessitate neurosurgical consultation and, in some instances, surgical intervention. The presence of CSF leaks poses an increased risk for serious infections. Early management in serious cases is pivotal for preventing potential neurological deficits. Surgical correction aims at preventing brain shift and progressive neurological deterioration through craniectomy and the repair of the dura and fracture.

14.5.4 Non-accidental Head Trauma/Child Abuse

Child abuse cases involving traumas to the scalp and calvarium are distressing and alarming occurrences. Child abuse is a serious public health issue, and physical abuse is one of its most concerning forms. Traumatic injuries to the scalp and calvarium in children due to intentional acts of violence, such as shaking, hitting, or blunt force trauma typically result in multiple, complexly characterized fractures involving more than one cranial bone whereas fractures due to accidents usually result in single, narrow or linear fractures often localized to the parietal bone [8, 9]. Identifying and managing these cases appropriately is essential to ensure the safety and well-being of the child.

Child abuse cases are often underreported, making it challenging to collect statistics. Nonetheless, research indicates that physical abuse is a significant cause of traumatic head injuries in children, with infants and toddlers being the most vulnerable age group. In the United

States, Child Protective Services (CPS) received reports of approximately 4.4 million child abuse cases in 2019, and physical abuse accounted for a substantial portion of these cases [10].

Healthcare professionals, including pediatricians, emergency room physicians, and nurses, must remain vigilant in recognizing signs of possible child abuse. Unexplained injuries, repeated injuries, changing caregiver histories, or delays in seeking medical care are red flags that may warrant further investigation. Children with suspected abusive head injuries must undergo a thorough medical evaluation, including a detailed history, physical examination, and neuroimaging studies (e.g., CT scans, MRI) to assess the extent of the scalp and calvarial trauma and to detect any associated intracranial injuries. Imaging studies may reveal findings such as skull fractures, subdural hematomas, epidural hematomas, or intracranial bleeding, which may be indicative of abusive head trauma. The medical management of child abuse cases involving traumas to the scalp and calvarium includes conservative management with detailed reporting in minor cases. In cases of severe head trauma with intracranial injuries, neurosurgical consultation is crucial to assess the need for surgical intervention and to ensure optimal management. If child abuse is suspected or confirmed, child protection measures are implemented to ensure the child's safety. This may involve temporary removal from the home, court orders for protection, or supervised visitation.

Child abuse cases can have significant emotional and psychological impacts on the affected child and their family. Providing appropriate psychological support and counseling is essential for their well-being and recovery. Healthcare professionals have a legal and ethical obligation to report suspected cases of child abuse to child protective services or law enforcement for further investigation.

14.6 Complications

14.6.1 Posttraumatic Osteolysis

Posttraumatic osteolysis of the scalp and calvarium is a rare pathological condition characterized by the localized dissolution and resorption of the bone following head trauma primarily in children. This condition is also known as "parietal cephalohematoma osteolysis" or "sinking skin flap syndrome." Typically, it arises after significant head injuries such as traumatic brain injuries, skull fractures, or hematomas. Although the exact pathophysiological mechanisms remain uncertain, it is believed to involve a combination of ischemic factors and inflammatory processes. The progressive loss of bone can lead to the inward displacement of the scalp, resulting in cosmetic deformity, neurological symptoms, and increased intracranial pressure.

Diagnosing posttraumatic osteolysis is challenging, as it typically becomes apparent weeks to months after the initial head injury. Patients may present with a sunken or depressed area on the scalp, often accompanied by pain, headaches, and neurological deficits. Initial evaluation involves plain X-rays of the skull, while more extensive imaging modalities such as CT scans or MRI may be essential for confirming the diagnosis and assessing the extent of bone loss. These imaging studies can also identify any concurrent intracranial abnormalities.

Mild cases of posttraumatic osteolysis may be managed conservatively through observation and symptomatic treatment. Pain relief measures and anti-inflammatory medications may be prescribed to alleviate discomfort. Surgical management is typically indicated in more severe cases characterized by significant bone loss, neurological symptoms, or cosmetic concerns. Several surgical options are available:

- **Bone Grafting**: In instances of focal bone loss, bone grafts can be employed to restore the contour of the calvarium. This may involve the use of autologous bone grafts or synthetic bone substitutes.
- **Cranioplasty**: In cases where a substantial area of bone loss is present, cranioplasty may be performed to reconstruct the calvarium using implants or custom-made prostheses.
- **Decompressive Craniectomy**: If increased intracranial pressure is due to the inward displacement of the scalp, a decompressive craniectomy may be considered to relieve pressure on the brain.

Posttraumatic osteolysis of the scalp and calvarium is an uncommon condition that requires a heightened level of suspicion, especially in patients with a history of significant head trauma. Early diagnosis, appropriate imaging, and meticulous neurological evaluation are pivotal in managing this condition effectively. While mild cases may be managed conservatively, surgical intervention may be imperative for severe cases marked by significant bone loss or neurological symptoms. The choice of surgical approach should be tailored to the extent of bone loss and associated symptoms.

14.6.2 Flap Osteonecrosis

Flap osteonecrosis of the scalp and calvarium is a relatively rare but significant complication that can develop following reconstructive surgeries, such as decompressive craniotomies, commonly employed to address defects resulting from various causes such as trauma, tumor resection, or other surgical interventions. Risk factors include bone incongruency, younger age (<18 years), and multiple fractures. Higher complication rates have also been noted specifically in cases of hemicraniectomy due to malignant MCA infarction [11]. This condition involves the demise of bone tissue due to impaired blood supply, potentially leading to bone deterioration and the risk of infection. Low-grade infections, such as those caused by Propionibacterium acnes, are also believed to play a role in flap necrosis after cranioplasty [12].

Clinical presentation of flap osteonecrosis typically involves persistent or worsening pain localized at the surgical site. Patients may also experience complications such as wound breakdown, drainage issues, and challenges with wound healing. To assess the extent of osteonecrosis and evaluate associated complications, imaging modalities like X-rays, CT scans, or MRI are invaluable tools. Laboratory studies can aid in determining the patient's overall health and systemic involvement, with wound cultures and biopsies performed to confirm the diagnosis or rule out infections or malignancies. Hyperbaric oxygen therapy may be considered as a treatment option to promote tissue oxygenation and repair.

Preventative measures play a crucial role in managing flap osteonecrosis, including regular wound cleaning and appropriate dressings to prevent infections and facilitate the healing process. Patients should be screened and educated about risk factors such as smoking, glycemic control, and proper diet to optimize wound healing. In cases where wound breakdown has occurred, debridement of necrotic tissue may become necessary.

For more severe cases of flap osteonecrosis, surgical intervention may be necessary. Options include flap revision or reconstruction, particularly in instances of partial flap necrosis, to enhance blood supply and salvage viable tissue. In cases where bone sequestration is present, surgical removal of non-viable bone may be required to prevent infection and expedite the healing process.

When caring for patients with cancer, one should consider osteoradionecrosis, which can occur after bone is exposed to radiation therapy. Close imaging surveillance using MRI can be sufficient to monitor the progression of this condition. While mild and uncomplicated cases are often asymptomatic, more severe instances can lead to pain, fractures, and infection.

14.7 Conclusion

Traumatic lesions of the scalp and calvarium present significant challenges for neurosurgeons and healthcare professionals. Understanding the complexities and unique characteristics of various traumatic injuries in these regions is essential for accurate diagnosis, effective management, and optimal patient outcomes.

The scalp and calvarium serve as vital protective barriers for the intracranial structures they encompass, making any assault on their integrity a major concern for patients and clinicians alike. Fractures, gunshot wounds, nonmissile penetrating traumas, and flap osteonecrosis are among the diverse traumatic lesions that can occur in these regions, each requiring specialized knowledge and expertise to manage effectively.

In the context of traumatic lesions affecting the scalp and calvarium in infants and young children, clinicians must be alert to the possibility of child abuse cases. These complex situations require specialized training in recognizing signs of abuse and implementing appropriate medical management, including child protection measures and psychological support.

Overall, managing traumatic lesions of the scalp and calvarium necessitates a comprehensive and systematic approach, combining clinical expertise, advanced imaging technologies, and a multidisciplinary team effort. Vigilance in recognizing red flags, early intervention, and a patient-centered approach are vital to ensure the best possible outcomes for patients affected by these challenging conditions.

By staying up-to-date with advancements in the field and embracing a holistic approach to care, neurosurgeons and healthcare professionals can continue making significant contributions to the successful treatment and recovery of patients with traumatic lesions of the scalp and calvarium, further advancing the field of neurosurgery and enhancing patient well-being.

References

1. Singhal G, Atri S, Suggala S, Jaluka D, Singhal S, Shrivastava A. Growing skull fractures; pathogenesis and surgical outcome. 2021;16:539–48.
2. Hobbs CJ. Skull fracture and the diagnosis of abuse. 1984;59:246–52.
3. Abdelhameid AK, Saro A. Non-missile penetrating brain injuries: cases registry in Sohag University Hospital. 2019;34:1–9.
4. Child Welfare Information Gateway. Child maltreatment 2019: summary of key findings. U.S. Department of Health and Human Services, Administration for Children and Families, Children's Bureau; 2021. https://www.childwelfare.gov/pubs/factsheets/canstats/
5. Ben-Ari Y, Merlob P, Hirsch M, Reisner SH. Congenital depression of the neonatal skull. 1986;22:249–55.
6. Taylor CA, Bell JM, Breiding MJ, Xu L. Traumatic brain injury–related emergency department visits, hospitalizations, and deaths — United States, 2007 and 2013. 2017;66:1–16.
7. Ottenhausen M, Kalasauskas D, Kramer A, Neuhoff J, Serrano L, Schwandt E, Ringel F. Bone flap necrosis due to low-grade infection with propionibacterium acnes. 2019;124:1–3.
8. Ewald C, Duenisch P, Walter J, Götz T, Witte OW, Kalff R, Günther A. Bone flap necrosis after decompressive hemicraniectomy for malignant middle cerebral artery infarction. 2014;20:91–7.
9. Ersahin Y, Gülmen V, Palali I, Mutluer S. Growing skull fractures (craniocerebral erosion). 2000;23:139–44.
10. Ulma RM, Sacks G, Rodoni B, Duncan AL, Buchman AT, Buchman BC, Vercler CJ, Kasten SJ, Muraszko K, Buchman SR. Management of calcified cephalohematoma of infancy: a single institution 25-year experience. 2020;8:38–9.
11. Gunshot Wound Head Trauma. https://www.aans.org/en/Patients/Neurosurgical-Conditions-and-Treatments/Gunshot-Wound-Head-Trauma#:~:text=U.S.%20Statistics&text=Gunshot%20wounds%20to%20the%20head%20are%20the%20cause%20of%20an,die%20in%20the%20emergency%20room.
12. Meservy CJ, Towbin R, McLaurin RL, Myers PA, Ball W. Radiographic characteristics of skull fractures resulting from child abuse. 1987;149:173–5.

Iatrogenic Lesions of the Scalp

15

Alexander E. Braley and Walter A. Hall

15.1 Introduction

Iatrogenic scalp lesions represent any lesions inadvertently created as a result of a direct or indirect action of the clinician or surgeon in an attempt to treat an underlying pathology or deformity. The source of these lesions can be from damage directly to the tissue during a procedure or due to the resultant effects from therapies intended to act distantly from the lesion. Iatrogenic scalp injuries can be caused by poorly planned skin incisions, defective or misused cranial fixation devices, radiation injury to the tissue, and chemotherapy impairing normal wound healing, to note some examples. The management for scalp lesions can range from simple observation and with supportive care all the way to placement of rotational free flaps or healing by secondary intention. The consideration of potential iatrogenic injuries should be performed by the clinician or surgeon to avoid these complications as they can lead to poor cosmesis or infection which can complicate the chosen treatment plan for local or systemic pathology. In addition, the emotional impact of the disfigurement can lead to the loss in confidence in the practitioner that results in damage to the relationship with the provider that may prevent the adherence to necessary therapies and a sense of general mistrust for future recommendations. Additionally, the risks of these complications must be anticipated and discussed with the patient to avoid potential medicolegal sequelae.

15.2 Scalp Overview

The scalp is a unique and complicated structure that provides protection for the cranium and the hair that it produces serves a tremendous role in human aesthetics. The scalp consists of five layers of tissue which each have a distinct architecture and function. These layers consist of the skin, subcutaneous tissue, galea aponeurosis, loose connective tissue, and the pericranium. The outermost layer is the skin, rich in hair follicles and sebaceous and sweat glands. Hair follicles in the skin that covers the rest of the body fail to grow to the same thickness, volume, or at the rate of the scalp. The skin of the scalp is the thickest compared to any other in the body, ranging from 3 to 8 mm [1]. The subcutaneous tissue provides padding for the scalp and along with the galea they are rich in their vascular supply which is necessary to support the numerically dense hair follicles found in the scalp. The galea aponeurosis is a layer of dense connective tissue that is an aponeurosis of the orbital and occipital fiber bundles of the occipitofrontalis muscle and the tem-

A. E. Braley · W. A. Hall (✉)
Department of Neurosurgery, State University of New York (SUNY) Upstate Medical University, Syracuse, NY, USA
e-mail: hallw@upstate.edu

M. Turgut et al. (eds.), *Lesions of the Scalp and Cranial Vault*,
https://doi.org/10.1007/978-3-031-88244-9_15

poroparietal fascia, laterally [1]. The galea is incredibly important during procedures involving the scalp as it is the primary source of tension during primary suture closure of the scalp. Failure to close the galea is significantly associated with wound dehiscence of scalp incisions. The loose connective tissue which is also called the innominate fascia allows the scalp to move independently from the overlying skull. The deepest layer is a thin sheet of tissue overlying the skull called the pericranium, which is similar to and contiguous with the outermost layer of dura found in the spine. The pericranium is important for protecting and nourishing the skull.

15.3 Etiology of Injury

Iatrogenic scalp injuries can be caused by a variety of factors, both intentionally and inadvertently. This event can occur sharply during the skin incision with a scalpel or may result accidentally during a malfunction of or slippage of the skull fixation clamp. Direct injury to the scalp can also occur due to tearing the tissue from over retraction, or by an inadvertent burn injury from electrocautery. Wounds may be full thickness or may be partial in thickness such as occurs with an abrasion. The implications for wound healing in either situation depend on the nature of the injury, the ability to reapproximate the skin, and whether or not the wound was contaminated during the injury. Head clamp injuries can lead to laceration, skull fracture, and even venous air embolisms [2, 3]. Lacerations secondary to head clamp migration are rare; however these injuries are occasionally hidden by hair coverage and are particularly susceptible to infection because most surgeons do not clean and prep those areas outside of the immediate surgical area.

Incision planning and execution are also critical to wound healing. Special attention should be given to the blood supply of an area of the scalp to be incised and other considerations should be made as to whether this incision is compatible with future surgeries that may need to be performed. For example, an external ventricular drain incision placement for a patient with an anterior communicating artery aneurysm should be made with the understanding that this incision may need to be converted into a bifrontal skin incision fit for a pterional craniotomy. Poor incision planning may lead to suboptimal incision angles or the inadvertent creation of ischemic areas, as in the undesirable situation of two parallel incisions perpendicular to the route of arterial supply with resultant ischemia in the tissue between incisions.

Skin breakdown can occur over a subcutaneously implanted device such as a deep brain stimulator (DBS) lead, cerebrospinal fluid shunt catheter or valve, or a pulse generator. These implants come with the added concern of having to decide whether to retain, remove, or replace the device [4–7]. Avoidance of skin breakdown is paramount for successful wound healing which can be accomplished using a lower profile device, assuring that the device is sufficiently buried under the subcutaneous tissue, avoiding thin skin areas, and countersinking devices when technically possible [4]. DBS leads have a low likelihood of wound erosion, with most studies reporting between a 1% and 5% rate of wound breakdown [4, 5]. However, if this complication is not identified promptly after implantation, the entire system may need to be removed and could also increase the risk of meningitis and brain abscess formation, and the wound breakdown site could require the placement of a flap for an adequate repair. Barrett et al described a surgical technique wherein patients with impending hardware exposure were electively taken to the operating room and a small patch of acellular dermal matrix was placed subcutaneously between the hardware and the scalp resulting in good healing results in 20 patients [4]. Another study in 2017 had good results retaining the DBS leads while utilizing a rotational flap for skin ulceration over DBS leads [6]. Exposed shunt hardware is more common in children, in part because children have thinner skin for implant coverage [7]. Infected CSF shunts can lead to wound breakdown and conversely, wound breakdown can lead to infected shunts [7]. Complications of shunt infection secondary to exposed hardware can lead to deeper brain infections such as ventriculitis and brain abscess development, which can be clinically devastating. In addition, although explanting a DBS lead can be costly and has its own risks, patients are not DBS dependent in the same way shunt patients are dependent on their CSF diversion; these patients must undergo days and sometimes weeks of CSF diversion via ventriculostomy in the ICU waiting for their infection to clear enough to reinsert a shunt [7].

An important consideration for any patient undergoing the surgical resection of a brain tumor or even in the patient with an unrelated history of cancer is the difficulty of healing a wound when the scalp is exposed to chronic chemotherapy and radiation therapy. Both of these treatment modalities are particularly detrimental to rapidly dividing cells such as those required for the process of wound healing. Careful consideration as to skin incision planning and surgical timing must be undertaken in these patients. Even when patients are no longer receiving chemotherapy, wound healing abilities may be weakened by chronic malnutrition or vitamin and protein deficiencies. Additional care should be taken in the monitoring and re-evaluation of patients at a higher risk for wound breakdown to more rapidly identify wound healing issues that can be accomplished with more frequent clinic visits for wound evaluation or by leveraging technology with HIPAA-compliant uploads of patient-provided photographs of their wound.

Radiotherapy uses ionizing radiation to target cancer cells, this treatment works by causing cascading ionization which damages the DNA causing strand breaks and cross linking that results in apoptosis [8]. Normal cells are similarly susceptible to injury from radiation therapy which creates the potential for iatrogenic injury to tissues. Skin is particularly susceptible to radiation injury, as the radiation must pass through the skin and connective tissue to arrive at the therapeutic target, and because the radiation will decrease collagen strength, decrease angiogenesis, and increase fibrosis [8, 9]. Radiation can affect scalp breakdown leading to desquamation, atrophy, ulceration, and wound healing issues [8, 10, 11]. Radiation will have both acute and long-term effects on wound healing [1, 9, 12]. Surgical repair of these complications can be very difficult to almost impossible depending on the extent of the injury. Because of this possibility, avoidance of radiation injury to tissues is paramount to reducing radiation-related wound complications. Radiation therapy for intracranial pathologies has become more targeted with less spillover affects to adjacent tissues; however radiotherapy for scalp lesions has a high risk for radiation-related wound issues [11]. Wound issues can vary from surface breakdown to full thickness necrosis of the scalp [11]. Postoperative radiation therapy should be performed at least 1 week after surgery as the most critical wound healing events occur within the first 5 to 7 days [12].

Chemotherapy is a broad term for chemical compounds administered that will kill or slow the progression of cancer cells. These agents act by a variety of mechanisms, some having little to no impact on wound healing, and others that can severely impact wound healing. An additional consideration with chemotherapy is the effect on leukocytes which are not only critical in preventing wound infections but play a significant role in wound remodeling [12]. Notably, although radiation therapy effects on wound healing can be permanent, chemotherapy affects can be transient provided the white blood cell count rebounds after stopping chemotherapy. To best avoid chemotherapy-induced wound healing issues, chemotherapy should be discontinued 2 weeks before surgery and held for at least 1 week after surgery [12]. With this consideration in mind, surgery can be timed between treatment cycles in certain circumstances.

15.4 Methods of Repair

Each type of scalp injury will necessitate a different method of achieving a satisfactory repair; however the goal should be an aesthetically acceptable repair that is most likely to achieve healing with as minimal a scar as possible with the lowest likelihood of infection. Hair shaving and prepping or reapplication of the prep may be necessary in cases of frank contamination. Surface abrasions or partial thickness scalp injuries may be amenable to topical dressings with antibiotic ointments and observation alone. Multiple layer injuries will require proper closure, with an emphasis on a strong galea aponeurotica closure and good skin approximation. If primary wound closure is not possible, healing by secondary intention is possible if no periosteum-deficient skull is exposed. Tissue expansion may be necessary in cases where primary approximation is not possible without undue tension across skin edges [1]. If this is not possible, a rotational or free flap may be indicated, and appropriate plastic or otolaryngology consultation should be sought [13]. When primary closure is possible, suture or staples are appropriate for skin closure depending on physician and patient preference. Hair transplantation may be necessary depending on the location and extent of the scalp injury and patient preference [1]. The utilization of local flaps may not be possible if the radiation therapy affected adjacent tissue sources [1, 10].

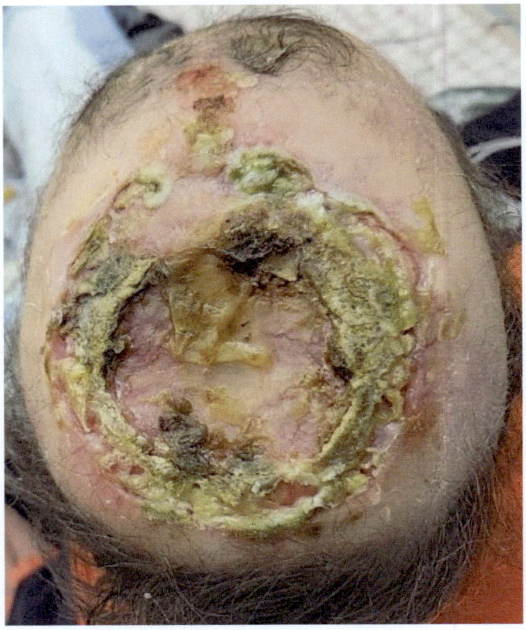

Fig. 15.1 Sixty-eight-year-old patient who suffered significant radiation necrosis after resection and radiation in Southeast Asia. Patient underwent free flap surgery which unfortunately failed after 3 months and suffered subsequent infection. After treating underlying infection, patient will require another complex flap at a later date

15.5 Conclusion

Iatrogenic scalp wounds are an unfortunate complication of therapies and interventions aimed at treating pathologies of the head and neck. These issues can range from poor wound healing secondary to systemic chemotherapy or fractionated radiation therapy or to accidental laceration during surgery or patient positioning. Great care must be taken to address these injuries to avoid wound infections, patient dissatisfaction, poor cosmesis, and medicolegal ramifications (Figs. 15.1, 15.2, and 15.3).

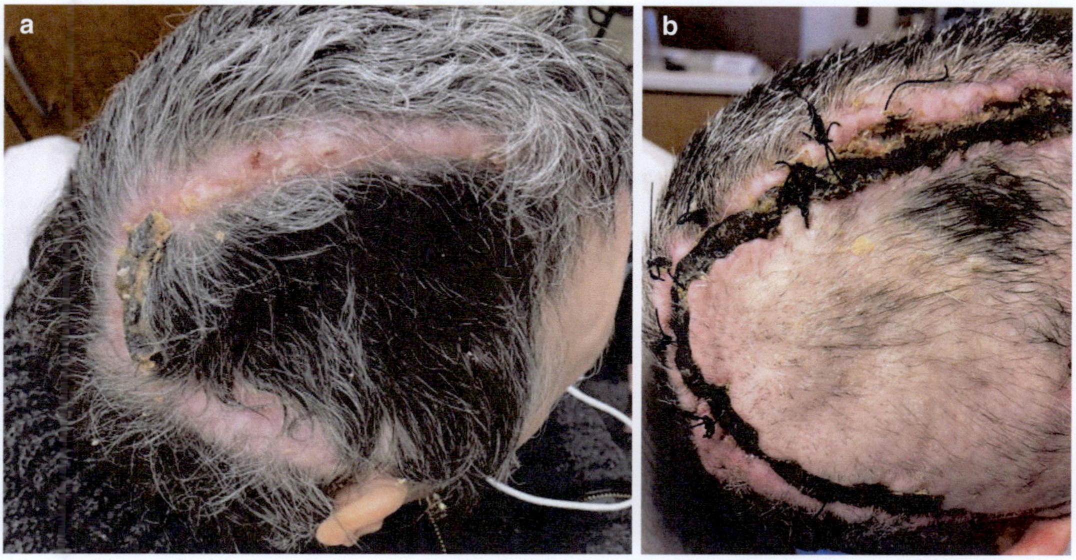

Fig. 15.2 (a) 52-year-old female patient that underwent a right decompressive craniectomy secondary to stroke with associated cocaine use that developed post operative dehiscence and wound infection requiring washout and closure. Wound was complicated further with eschar (b) which would require a complex scalp flap for definitive correction. This illustrates the importance of vascular supply to wound healing

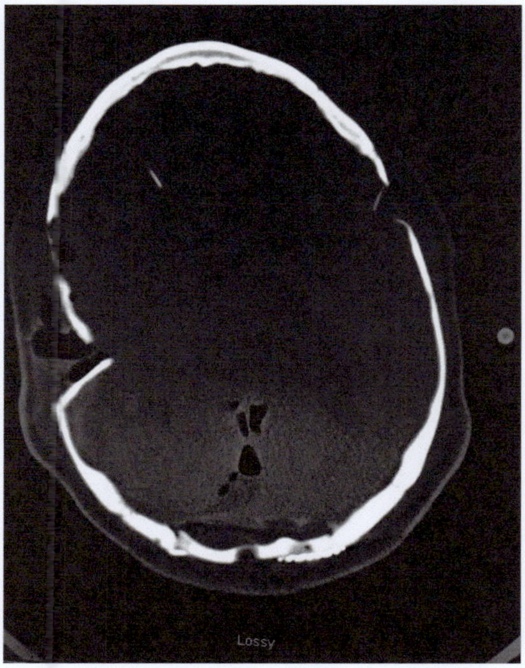

Fig. 15.3 Post operative CT scan demonstrating bilateral skull fractures secondary to head clamp fixation after posterior fossa craniectomy. Patient also had scalp lacerations (not pictured) that were repaired in the OR with elevation of the skull fractures

References

1. Leedy JE, Janis JE, Rohrich RJ. Reconstruction of acquired scalp defects: an algorithmic approach. Plast Reconstr Surg. 2005;116:1114. https://doi.org/10.1097/01.prs.0000179188.25019.6c.
2. Khandelwal A, Gupta S, Prabhakar H, Burman S. Venous air embolism following application of Mayfield head clamp: a word of caution. Indian J Anaesth. 2018;62:1002–3. https://doi.org/10.4103/ija.IJA_477_18.
3. Moutaoukil M, Bensghir M, Eddik S, Jaafari A, Ahtil R, Meziane M, Haimeur C. Embarrure suite à l'utilisation de la têtière de Mayfield chez l'adulte: À propos d'un cas et revue de la literature. Pan Afr Med J. 2016;24 https://doi.org/10.11604/pamj.2016.24.129.8367.
4. Barrett TF, Rasouli JJ, Taub P, Kopell BH. Technical note: preemptive surgical revision of impending deep brain stimulation hardware erosion. World Neurosurg. 2018;111:41–6. https://doi.org/10.1016/j.wneu.2017.12.045.
5. Blomstedt P, Hariz MI. Hardware-related complications of deep brain stimulation: a ten year experience. Acta Neurochir. 2005;147:1061–4. https://doi.org/10.1007/s00701-005-0576-5.
6. Staudt MD, Pourtaheri N, Lakin GE, Soltanian HT, Miller JP. Surgical management of deep brain stimulator scalp erosion without hardware removal.

Stereotact Funct Neurosurg. 2017;95:385–91. https://doi.org/10.1159/000484323.
7. Suryaningtyas W, Ranuh IGMAR, Parenrengi MA. Shunt exposure as a ventriculoperitoneal shunt complication: a case series. Int J Surg Case Rep. 2021;79:484–91.
8. Dormand E-L, Banwell PE, Goodacre TE Radiotherapy and wound healing
9. Tibbs MK. Wound healing following radiation therapy: a review. Radiother Oncol. 1997;42:99–106. https://doi.org/10.1016/S0167-8140(96)01880-4.
10. Karalashvili L, Mardaleishvili K, Uhryn M, Chakhunashvili D, Kakabadze Z. Current condition and challenges in treatment of non-healing wound after radiation therapy (review). Georgian Med News. 2018:23–8.
11. Kim YH, Aye MS, Fayos JV. Therapeutic radiology radiation necrosis of the scalp: a complication of cranial irradiation and methotrexate. Radiology. 1977;124(3):813–4.
12. Drake D, Oishi S. Wound healing considerations in chemotherapy and radiation therapy. Clin Plast Surg. 1995;22:31–7.
13. Espinosa MC, Hohman MH, Sunthosh S. Oral and maxillofacial surgery, facial laceration repair. Continuing Education Activity. 2023.

Vascular Lesions and Malformations of the Scalp

16

Haydn Hoffman, Hanish Polavarapu, and Grahame C. Gould

16.1 Introduction

Vascular lesions of the scalp are rare and may involve any combination of the arteries, capillaries, and veins. When diagnosing a scalp lesion, recognition of a vascular origin is important so that the appropriate work-up and treatment can be planned. Frequently endovascular techniques are employed to diagnose lesions through catheter angiography, reduce blood flow in preparation for surgery, or cure with embolization. Many lesions require definitive treatment through surgical excision, which may be performed by neurosurgeons or head and neck surgeons with training in complex scalp reconstruction. This chapter will review a variety of scalp vascular lesions with emphasis on arteriovenous malformations (AVMs) and sinus pericranii (SP).

16.2 Vascular Anatomy

The scalp is supplied by the superficial temporal (STA), occipital (OA), posterior auricular, supraorbital, and supratrochlear arteries. The STA is a terminal branch of the external carotid artery (ECA) that originates in the parotid gland, crosses over the zygomatic arch, and enters the layer between the temporalis muscle and galea. It divides into frontal and parietal branches. The OA is a proximal branch of the ECA that travels posteriorly and superiorly deep to the digastric muscle before penetrating the fascia between the sternocleidomastoid and trapezius muscles. The OA and vertebral artery have anastomoses through C1 and C2 segmental branches, and recognition of these is critical when performing embolization. The posterior auricular artery is a small ECA branch that travels toward the mastoid region and supplies the scalp behind the ear. It gives rise to a stylomastoid branch that supplies the facial nerve in the stylomastoid foramen. Nontarget embolization of this branch can cause facial nerve palsy. The supraorbital and supratrochlear arteries are branches of the ophthalmic artery that supply the anterior scalp. The superficial scalp veins follow the same course and are named after their arterial counterparts.

16.3 Arteriovenous Malformation

AVMs are high-flow abnormal connections between arteries and veins without intervening capillaries. When located on the scalp, they are known as “cirsoid aneurysms” and may present as a palpable pulsatile mass or with headache, tinnitus, and bleeding. They may be congenital or

H. Hoffman (✉) · H. Polavarapu · G. C. Gould
Department of Neurosurgery, State University of New York (SUNY) Upstate Medical University, Syracuse, NY, USA
e-mail: haydnhoffman@gmail.com

M. Turgut et al. (eds.), *Lesions of the Scalp and Cranial Vault*,
https://doi.org/10.1007/978-3-031-88244-9_16

there may be a history of trauma or surgery. They are prone to slow or rapid growth but do not usually regress [1]. The OA and STA are the most common arterial supplies. A variant of scalp AVMs located in the temporalis muscle exists. Temporalis scalp AVMs are typically supplied by the deep temporal artery, have a more diffuse appearance on DSA, and have striated muscular bundles mixed in with the nidus [2].

Diagnosis can be made with computed tomography angiography (CTA) or magnetic resonance angiography (MRA), but digital subtraction angiography (DSA) is required to confirm the diagnosis, characterize the arterial supply and drainage patterns, and to out intracranial involvement. Treatment typically involves surgical resection with preoperative endovascular embolization to reduce blood loss. However, resolution with embolization alone has been reported [3]. Percutaneous injection of liquid embolics is another option [4]. Outcomes are excellent with high rates of complete occlusion and low rates of morbidity and mortality.

16.4 Case 1: Scalp Arteriovenous Malformation

A 20-year-old female presented with recurrent episodes of bleeding from a slowly enlarging subcutaneous scalp mass in the midline parieto-occipital region. CTA demonstrated numerous engorged scalp vessels adjacent to the mass, suggestive of AVM (Fig. 16.1). DSA confirmed the presence of a large scalp AVM supplied by bilateral STA, OA, middle meningeal artery (MMA), and posterior meningeal artery (PMA) feeders. The patient underwent two staged embolizations with Onyx that targeted the left STA, OA, and MMA. Following the second embolization, the AVM was resected by a facial plastics and reconstructive surgical team. The excised region of

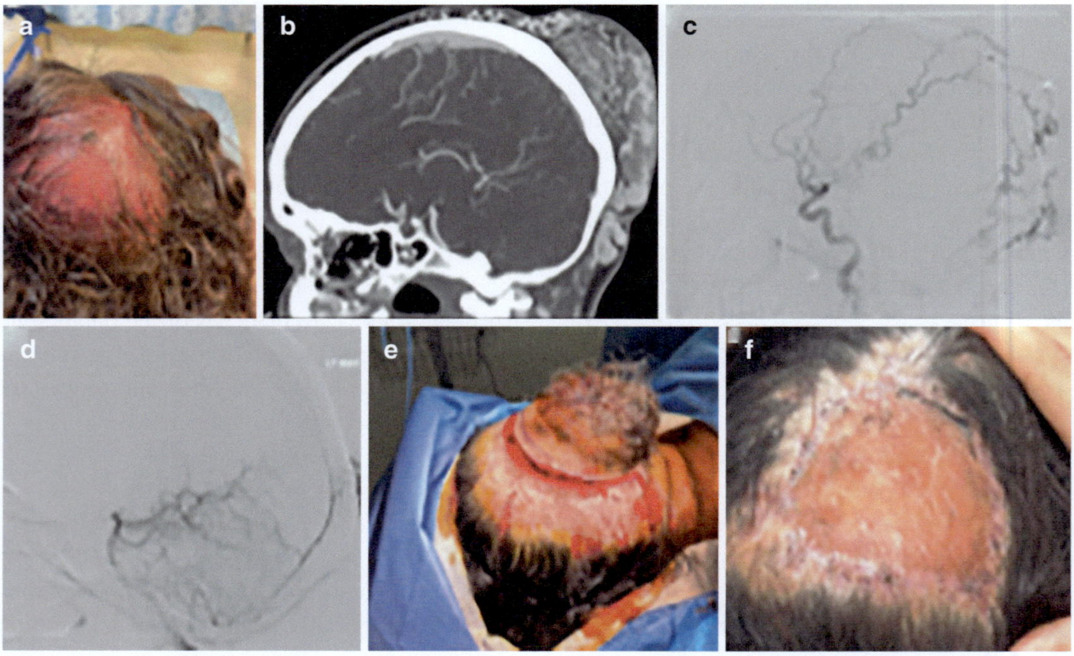

Fig. 16.1 (**a**) Erythema and swelling overlying the scalp AVM; (**b**) sagittal CTA demonstrating hypertrophied occipital and superficial temporal artery branches coalescing on the nidus; (**c**) left lateral common carotid angiogram demonstrating hypertrophied occipital and superficial temporal artery branches supplying the AVM; (**d**) left lateral vertebral angiogram showing supply to the AVM from a posterior meningeal artery; (**e**) Following a second embolization procedure the patient underwent excision of the AVM; (**f**) Expected healing of the split thickness skin graft 1 month after placement

scalp was repaired with a split thickness skin graft harvested from the thigh. The patient remained neurologically intact after the embolizations and the graft had healed well at 1 year follow-up.

This case demonstrates the progressively symptomatic nature of scalp AVMs. The patient's lesion was first diagnosed 5 years before treatment. It remained stable and asymptomatic before enlarging and continuing to bleed. Growth of scalp AVMs during puberty is believed to be related to hormones that increase vascular endothelial growth factor. The case also shows how scalp AVMs may be supplied by intracranial dural vessels such as the MMA and PMA. Finally, this case demonstrates the multidisciplinary nature of treatment among neurosurgery, interventional neuroradiology, and otolaryngology that is often required for scalp AVMs.

16.5 Scalp Arterial Aneurysms

Aneurysms or pseudoaneurysms may arise from any scalp artery, but STA is most common due to its superficial location. The STA may be most susceptible to injury as it crosses the superficial temporal line because it no longer has the cushion of the temporalis muscle and is only separated from the skull by periosteum [5]. Scalp aneurysms typically present as a pulsatile mass that may or may not be painful. Most cases are pseudoaneurysms that are post-traumatic or iatrogenic; however, several spontaneous true aneurysms related to vascular risk factors such as hypertension and hyperlipidemia have been reported [6]. Diagnosis can be made with CTA or MRA. These studies may reveal an intracranial aneurysm, which often accompany true aneurysms of the scalp [7]. The natural history is benign despite a propensity for growth, and treatment is usually only needed for cosmetic reasons. Aneurysm rupture with subgaleal hematoma is extremely rare; in a literature review of 32 cases, no patients presented with aneurysm rupture [6]. The treatment of choice is usually surgical excision, given this can easily be performed under local anesthesia by ligating the STA proximal and distal to the lesion. However, endovascular embolization with coils, ultrasound-guided thrombin injection, and manual compression has also been described [5]. Embolization may be favored when the frontal STA branch is involved due to its proximity to the frontal branch of the facial nerve. Liquid embolics such as Onyx are typically not used due to the possibility of causing a tattooing effect on the skin.

16.6 Sinus Pericranii

SP is a rare venous anomaly involving a connection between the intracranial and extracranial venous systems that results in a venous varix on the external table of the skull. They are usually discovered during childhood or young adulthood. The typical presentation is a midline, soft, nonpulsatile, compressible, subcutaneous mass that enlarges with activity and supine position. They are frequently associated with intracranial developmental venous anomalies. SP is often asymptomatic and usually does not increase in size, so treatment is often for cosmetic reasons. Diagnosis can be made with ultrasound or magnetic resonance imaging (MRI), but DSA is required when treatment is being considered. DSA differentiates dominant- and accessory-type SPs. Dominant type is characterized by cerebral venous drainage predominantly through the SP, while accessory type is when minimal or no cerebral venous outflow occurs through the extradiploic vessels [8]. In a case series of 15 patients, dominant type was observed in approximately half (46%) [8]. Dominant type should not be treated due to the risk of causing a venous infarction. Treatment involves embolization through transvenous endovascular techniques or with direct puncture [9]. This can be followed by surgical excision, but lesions may regress following embolization alone [9]. Observation is reasonable for stable, asymptomatic lesions, and spontaneous resolution has been reported.

16.7 Case 2: Sinus Pericranii

An otherwise healthy 8-month-old boy presented with a soft scalp mass in the midline suboccipital region that was more noticeable on crying. MRI demonstrated a 3.5 cm enhancing vascular mass with connection to the right transverse sinus through emissary veins (Fig. 16.2). DSA confirmed an accessory SP. The lesion was asymptomatic, so no treatment was pursued. At 8 years old, the patient presented again after minor head trauma, at which point the lesion was larger and painful. MRI showed that the lesion had expanded to 5.5 cm.

The patient underwent transfemoral venography for attempted endovascular embolization of the SP. The small transosseous channels to the SP could not be accessed with a microcatheter, so embolization with direct puncture was performed. An ultrasound-guided direct puncture of the lesion was achieved with an 18g lumbar puncture needle. Onyx-34 was injected from three needle positions under fluoroscopy to confirm no embolysate penetrated intracranially. Following embolization, repeat venography showed significantly reduced filling of the SP. A tight headwrap was placed for 24 h. At 3-week follow-up, the mass was almost completely gone on physical examination, and 1 year follow-up MRI demonstrated near complete resolution of the SP.

This case is unique because the SP was located in the occipital region, whereas the frontal and parietal regions are most common. It also demonstrates the complementary nature of direct puncture and transvenous access. Finally, venography performed adjacent to the transosseous connection initially did not demonstrate the lesion. However, when the lesion was manually compressed and released just prior to injection of contrast, this enabled visualization of the lesion as it refilled.

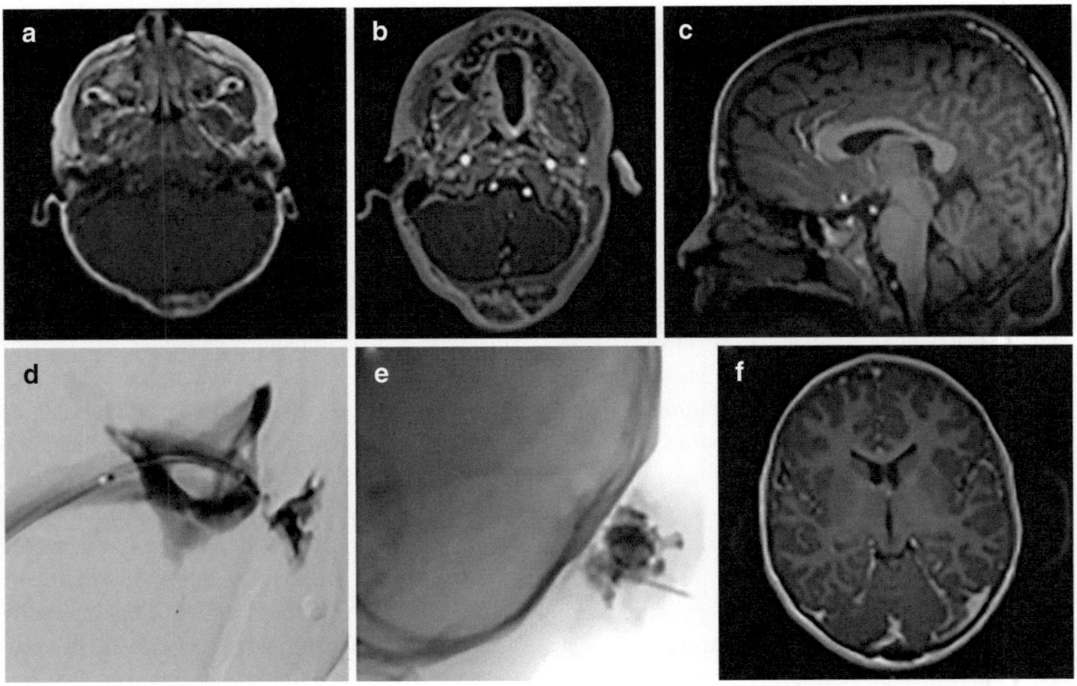

Fig. 16.2 (**a**) Axial T1 MRI with contrast at age 8 months shows a 3.5 cm enhancing subcutaneous vascular mass with connection to the right transverse sinus through emissary veins, consistent with sinus pericranii; repeat axial (**b**) and sagittal (**c**) T1 MRI with contrast shows enlargement of the lesion to 5.5 cm; (**d**) lateral venogram performed from the right transverse sinus demonstrates filling of the sinus pericranii through transosseous veins; (**e**) embolization of the sinus pericranii through direct puncture with Onyx. A distal access catheter is present in the transverse sinus for control venograms throughout embolization. (**f**) Axial T1 MRI with contrast shows near-complete resolution of the lesion 1 year after embolization

16.8 Hemangioma

Scalp hemangiomas are benign vascular tumors that are more commonly seen in infancy and childhood. They usually present as small, soft, compressible masses that may grow rapidly during the first year of life but often regress spontaneously by 5–7 years of age. Although most lesions are only of cosmetic concern, larger lesions may cause bleeding, ulceration, ocular compression, consumptive coagulopathy, or high output cardiac failure due to arteriovenous shunting [10, 11]. The diagnosis can be made clinically but MRI is recommended. For midline lesions, MRI helps evaluate for a connection to the superior sagittal sinus and for other central nervous system abnormalities. DSA can clarify the venous drainage pattern when MRI is inconclusive.

Treatment options include medication, endovascular embolization, and surgical excision. Medical treatment includes steroids or propranolol, which have been administered topically, systemically, and intralesionally [12]. Endovascular embolization with Onyx, coils, and polyvinyl alcohol particles has been described, and lesion regression following embolization without need for surgery has been reported [11]. Endovascular embolization may be a desirable stand-alone option in infants who have developed high output cardiac failure, which has been performed as early as 2 days of age [13]. When pursuing surgery, this should be delayed until an older age when greater blood loss can be tolerated.

16.9 Conclusion

A variety of vascular conditions can occur in the scalp, and the natural history of these is typically benign. Although the STA and OA are the most common contributing arteries, detailed understanding of all the vasculature involved is necessary before pursuing treatment. In the case of SP, knowledge of the venous involvement is also critical. MRA and CTA provide valuable anatomical information, but DSA provides a deeper understanding of the flow through the lesion in a time-resolved manner. When reviewing these studies, it is important to remember that many patients with congenital scalp vascular lesions often have coexisting intracranial vascular abnormalities. In many cases, treatment may involve a combination of endovascular and open surgical techniques, highlighting the multidisciplinary nature of these lesions. Outcomes are generally favorable with high rates of cure and low rates of morbidity or recurrence. The literature is mostly comprised of small case series. Publication of multi-institutional cohorts and meta-analyses may aid in surgeons' understanding of the natural history and optimal treatment of these rare lesions.

References

1. Li D, Heiferman DM, Rothstein BD, Syed HR, Shaibani A, Tomita T. Scalp arteriovenous malformation (Cirsoid Aneurysm) in adolescence: report of 2 cases and review of the literature. World Neurosurg. 2018;116:e1042–6. https://doi.org/10.1016/j.wneu.2018.05.161.
2. de San R, Pedro J, Cuartero Perez B, Ferri Niguez B, Vicente VS, V. Arteriovenous malformations of the temporalis muscle: a comprehensive review. Oper Neurosurg (Hagerstown). 2018;14(4):325–40. https://doi.org/10.1093/ons/opx149.
3. Talafha M, Al Sharie S, Abu-Hamdiyah OJ, Araydah M, Al-Husinat L, Varrassi G. A rare case of scalp arteriovenous malformation in an adolescent patient. Cureus. 2023;15(4):e37952. https://doi.org/10.7759/cureus.37952.
4. Shi Y, Liu P, Liu Y, Quan K, Li P, Li Z, et al. Case report: endovascular treatment of two scalp arteriovenous malformation cases via direct percutaneous catheterization: a case series. Front Neurol. 2022;13:945961. https://doi.org/10.3389/fneur.2022.945961.
5. Stapleton CJ, Fusco MR, Thomas AJ, Levy EI, Ogilvy CS. Traumatic pseudoaneurysms of the superficial temporal artery: case series, anatomy, and multidisciplinary treatment considerations. J Clin Neurosci. 2014;21(9):1529–32. https://doi.org/10.1016/j.jocn.2014.02.004.
6. Kawai H, Hamasaki T, Imamura J, Tomonori N, Odashiro T, Yamahata H, et al. Three cases of spontaneous superficial temporal artery aneurysm with literature review. Neurol Med Chir (Tokyo). 2014;54(10):854–60. https://doi.org/10.2176/nmc.cr2013-0033.
7. Karsy M, Raheja A, Guan J, Osborn AG, Couldwell WT. Scalp arteriovenous malformation with concomitant, flow-dependent malformation and aneurysm. World Neurosurg. 2016;90(708):e5–9. https://doi.org/10.1016/j.wneu.2016.03.047.

8. Gandolfo C, Krings T, Alvarez H, Ozanne A, Schaaf M, Baccin CE, et al. Sinus pericranii: diagnostic and therapeutic considerations in 15 patients. Neuroradiology. 2007;49(6):505–14. https://doi.org/10.1007/s00234-007-0211-7.
9. Hoffman H, Koutsouras GW, Oh J, Suryadevara N, Gould GC. Percutaneous embolization of sinus pericranii. J Neurointerv Surg. 2023;15(8):828. https://doi.org/10.1136/jnis-2022-019117.
10. Khan IS, Kiehna EN, Satti KF, Ehtesham M, Ghiassi M, Singer RJ. Surgical management of large scalp infantile hemangiomas. Surg Neurol Int. 2014;5:41. https://doi.org/10.4103/2152-7806.129560.
11. Wolfe SQ, Farhat H, Elhammady MS, Moftakhar R, Aziz-Sultan MA. Transarterial embolization of a scalp hemangioma presenting with Kasabach-Merritt syndrome. J Neurosurg Pediatr. 2009;4(5):453–7. https://doi.org/10.3171/2009.6.PEDS08363.
12. Cho YK, Ryu DW, Chung HY, O TM, Blei F, Waner M. Surgical management of scalp infantile hemangiomas. J Craniofac Surg. 2015;26(4):1169–72. https://doi.org/10.1097/SCS.0000000000001561.
13. Shah SS, Snelling BM, Sur S, Ramnath AR, Bandstra ES, Yavagal DR. Scalp congenital hemangioma with associated high-output cardiac failure in a premature infant: case report and review of literature. Interv Neuroradiol. 2017;23(1):102–6. https://doi.org/10.1177/1591019916669089.

Intraosseous Vascular Lesions and Malformations of the Calvarium

17

Arya Nabavi, Katja Kniese, and Bogdan-Marius Corbu

17.1 Introduction

Vascular intraosseous lesions are rare. Of 133 calvarial lesions reported over the course of 13 years from a single institution, about 8% pertain to this chapter (9 hemangiomas and 1 aneurysmatic bone cyst) [1]. Heckl et al. [2] retrieved reports of 103 cavernomas of the skull in a review covering 25 years. In regard to other entities of this chapter, the state of the literature becomes even more sketchy with further cases augmented by the accumulation of previous case reports. Their basic common feature is the rather wide setting of the boundary condition for the search, to accumulate enough patients. Another feature is the indistinct and wide variety of labels. Therefore, it is necessary to scrutinize not just the cumulative publication but their respective sources. Not infrequently this results in a correction of the numbers reported, particularly, since most of the vascular entities encountered in the literature are reported for the skull base which has a different phylogenetic and ontogenetic root than the vault [3].

Still, despite the lack of data, some features can be extracted. However, it has to be emphasized that there are no "typical" features, which would allow a definite diagnosis of the skull lesions. This is accentuated in the radiological literature on the differential diagnosis of skull vault lesions. Radiological reviews of specific imaging features mostly consist of precise descriptions of assumed typical appearances, while the "exceptions to the rule" appear almost more numerous [4–8]. It remains certain that the most frequent benign calvarial lesion is the osteoma, followed by the hemangioma. These two entities also harbor the most distinguishing imaging features. But even hemangiomas, which are considered to have a typical computed tomography (CT) appearance show a significant variability [2, 4–6, 9–11] and may even show different appearances (see case in Fig. 17.3) and particularly in the pediatric population [12, 13].

Of course, general rules apply as derived from general skeletal pathology. The rapidity of the growth determines the features. Slow-growing or benign lesions display rather defined borders, occasionally with a sclerotic frame. Fast-growing lesions, mostly malignant, show uneven poorly defined borders, a wide transition area, and reaction of the adjacent soft tissue [4–8].

Even with these hallmarks of diagnosis, only histopathology provides certainty [7, 14–16]. In summary the sparsity of data precludes a definite statistically valid characterization of the "normal case" by imaging. It is more important to be aware that there is a huge bandwidth of lesions, particularly of the juvenile age.

A. Nabavi (✉) · K. Kniese · B.-M. Corbu
Department of Neurosurgery, Nordstadt Hospital KRH, Hannover, Germany
e-mail: arya.nabavi@krh.de

M. Turgut et al. (eds.), *Lesions of the Scalp and Cranial Vault*,
https://doi.org/10.1007/978-3-031-88244-9_17

In addition, there is disagreement in regard to the classification of vascular lesions. Neurosurgical and histopathological descriptions dominate the literature on intracranial lesions. However, in including all vascular anomalies, vascular, cranio-maxillofacial, and plastic surgeons as well as radiologists adhere increasingly on the International Society for Study of Vascular Anomalies (ISSVA) definition [17, 18]. The ISSVA differentiates into malformations and tumors. Particularly in regard to hemangiomas, this adds another term to the already numerous names of this lesion [2, 19–22]. Since this chapter does not intend to add to the inconsistencies, the synonyms will be cited. However, the systematic approach suggested by the ISSVA has merits and is increasingly alluded to in the literature. Particularly with genetic characterization [18], potential common entities and division of previously pooled cases, just as we are experiencing in the WHO classification of CNS tumors, may yield further insight.

This chapter concentrates on intraosseous low-flow and high-flow malformations and tumor-like lesions with vascular components. Vascular tumors of intermediate dignity (i.e., epitheloid hemangioma and pseudomyogenic hemangioendothelioma) and malignant variants (i.e., epitheloid hemangioendothelioma and angiosarcoma) [18, 23] are usually beyond the intraosseous confines when diagnosed [5, 6, 8] and their imaging indicative of malignant growth [16].

17.2 Specific Lesions

17.2.1 Hemangiomas

The lesions generally referred to in the neurosurgical literature as hemangiomas are also referred to as cavernomas, cavernous hemangioma, intraosseous cavernomas, and more recently in the radiological literature based on the ISSVA classification intraosseous venous malformation [5, 8, 22]. For the present chapter, the term of hemangioma is retained for practicability, and since, histopathology and clinical practice retain this term. But, even with the simplicity of one term, histologically capillary and cavernous forms are distinguished [14].

Hemangiomas of the skull are the second most frequent benign lesion after osteoma. The so-called "globular" type, protruding from the bone, is situated in the skull base, while the "sessile" type is situated between the inner and outer table and is more frequent in the skull vault [7, 24].

With up to 10% of skull vault lesions [16], hemangiomas are the most frequent intraosseous vascular lesion. Over all they account for about 0.7% of all bone tumors with a predilection for the spinal column [14].

In a literature overview of 25 Years Heckl et al. [2] identified 103 histologically proven cases. Interestingly a more recent review [11] with a longer time span found only 93 cases between 1845 and 2015. This may in part be due to the abovementioned indistinct terminology of the lesion at hand. Nevertheless, in contrast to the significantly rarer lesions discussed below, it is possible to ascribe serviceable clinical and imaging characteristics. Contrary to the lesions of the younger population (e.g., aneurysmal bone cyst (ABC), lymphangioma, angioma), hemangioma occurrence increases with age and peaks between the 4th and 6th decade of life [2, 7, 11, 16, 20, 25]. The studies concur that a majority of the lesions is located within the frontal bones (approx. 40%), while temporal and parietal evenly combine to approx. 30% [2, 11] . This corresponds well to the localizations found in subsequently reported cases. Also, the range of clinical symptoms from incidental findings to expanding protrusions tender to palpation is comparable. The location determines clinical symptoms and growth pattern. At the skull base, the so-called "globular" expansile lesion expanding beyond the bone can cause multiple nerve dysfunctions. At the vault the interosseous "sessile" form (Fig. 17.1), expanding within the confines of the outer and inner table, may cause a local bulge with tenderness. Headache seems to be one of the leading symptoms; however, it remains unclear whether these headaches are generated by these lesions. When the lesion expanded beyond the inner table (see case), it is conceivable that dural irritation may be caused by the lesion (Fig. 17.2c).

Hemangiomas are primarily solitary lesions; however, in 15% of the cases, multiple skull lesions were encountered [5, 19]. Also, they may also occur sequentially during follow-up after surgical removal of the first lesion [26].

Bone pathologists differentiate between two entities, when multifocal disease is encountered. Multiple primary hemangiomas present with a collection of lesions, individually behaving like solitary lesions. Cystic angiomatosis, with multifocal lytic skeletal tumors, may also have visceral involvement [25].

17.2.2 Imaging

While every clinician immediately identifies the distinct imaging features with expansile well-circumscribed sunburst radiating internal bone trabeculae appearance with intact but thinned internal and external tables on CT as hemangioma, there is a substantial variability [11]

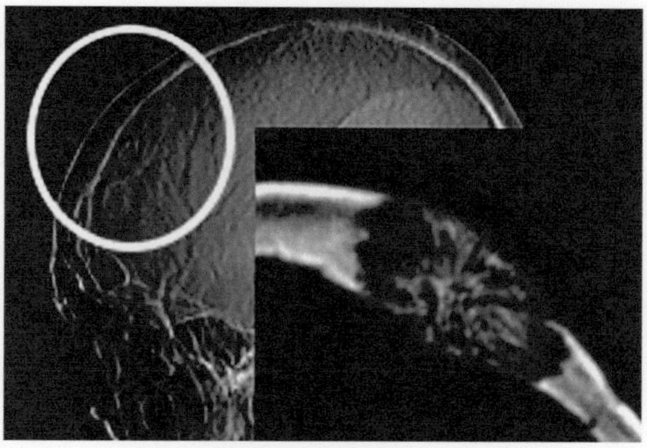

Fig. 17.1 Imaging work-up. Intraosseous venous malformation/hemangioma background: CT scout. Inlay: typical appearance of radiating trabecula in axial scan of area within white circle

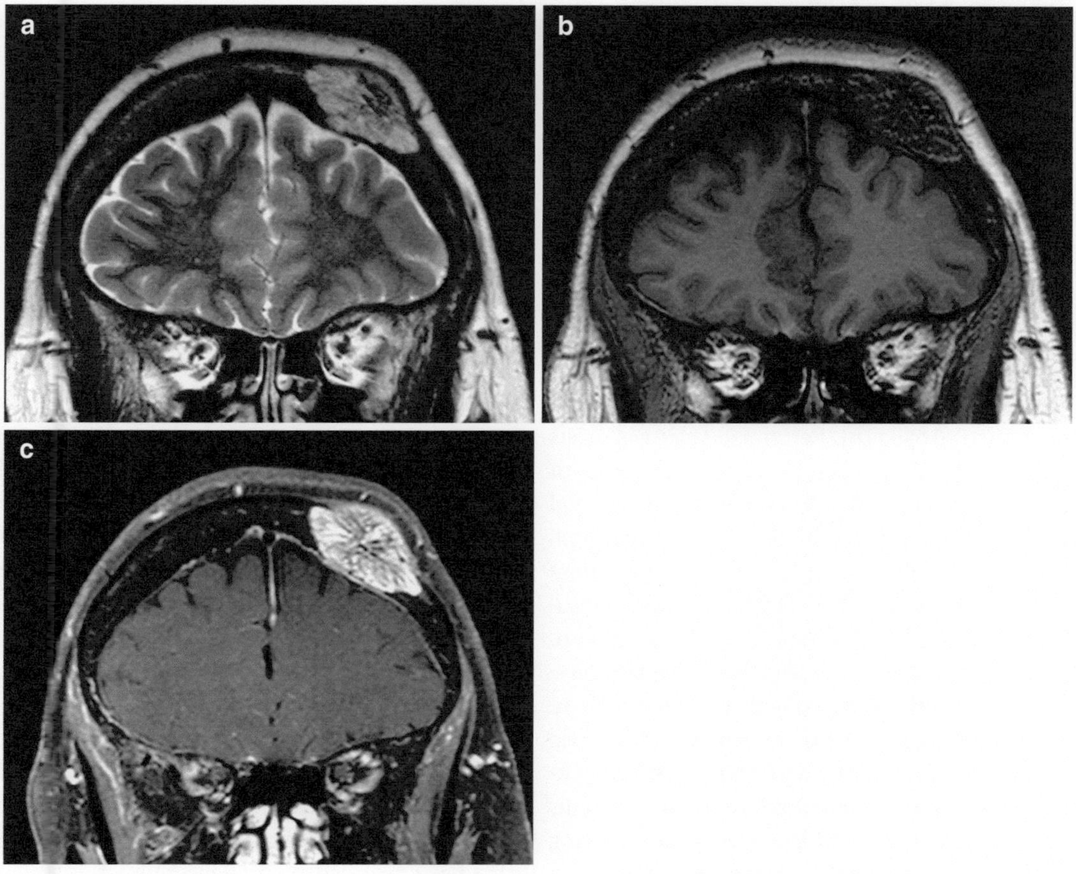

Fig. 17.2 (**a**) T2WI of same frontal intraosseous venous malformation/hemangioma, (**b**) T1WI, (**c**) T1WI+c

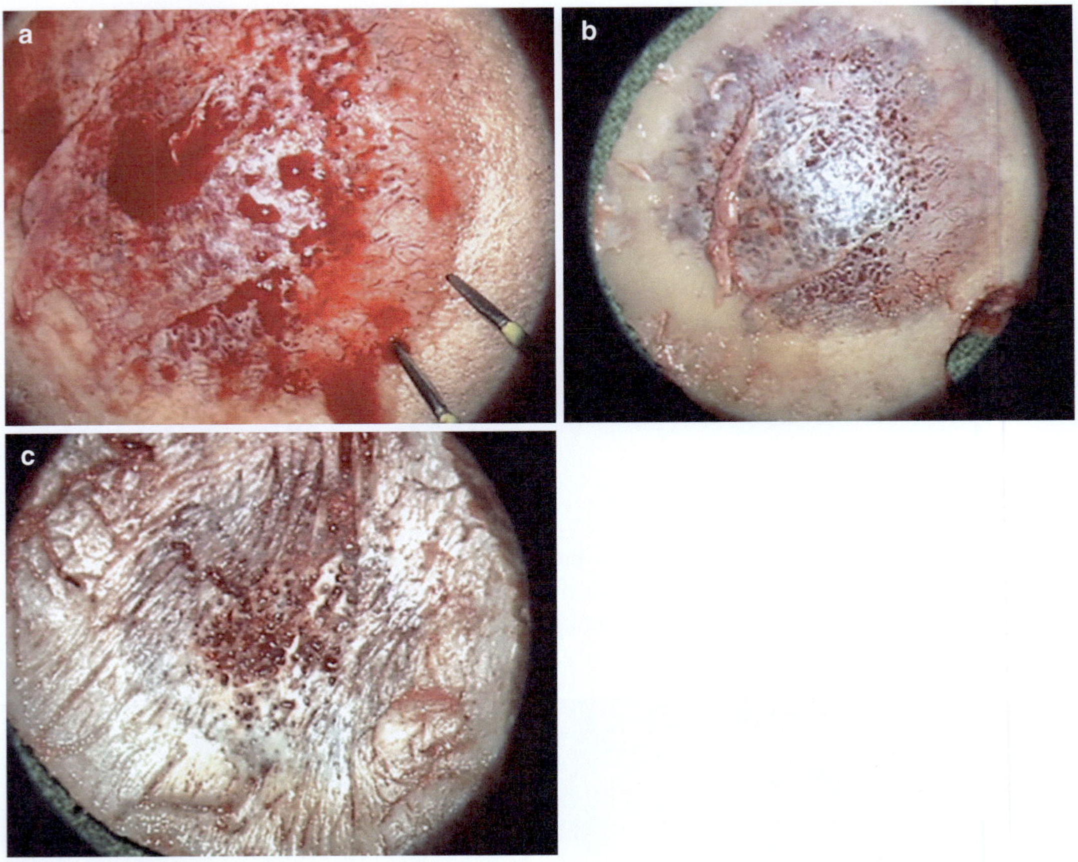

Fig. 17.3 Intraoperative images (**a**) Before craniotomy. Note attached Galea, (**b**) After craniotomy: visible decolorizing due to devascularization, (**c**) Inner table with mulberry appearance. Dura was unaffected, but it seems feasible, that dural irritation may have led to the leading symptom: headache, which resolved after surgery

(Figs. 17.1, 17.2, 17.3, and 17.4). The so-called honeycomb- or web-like trabecular pattern occurs in half of the patients and sunburst striations in 10–15% [16]. Peripheral sclerosis exists only in one third [16]. A surrounding area of decalcification [7] as well as a dural tail sign and [10] spiculae [6], medullary space expansion, and cortical thinning [22] may mimic more aggressive lesions [27]. Generally, MRI signal intensity depending on venous stasis and accompanying thrombosis is isointense to hyperintense on T1 (thrombus being bright) and hyperintense on T2 and FLAIR with interspersed flow void signals [5, 22]. Employing further imaging technology such as scintigraphy and more various MR-sequences, e.g., diffusion-weighted imaging (DWI) or dynamic contrast-enhanced MRI [28], yield further information. Still the differential diagnoses for intradiploic skull masses remain numerous, spanning the range from benign to aggressive and metastatic lesions. While the combination of patient history, symptoms and physical examination in conjunction with the imaging provides a solid basis for ruling out various differential diagnosis, it cannot supersede histopathological verification (Fig. 17.4).

17.2.3 Genetics

As to the classification, it remains interesting to discuss whether the reported hemangioma cases in the pediatric population [12, 13], which have also been reported with spontaneous regression

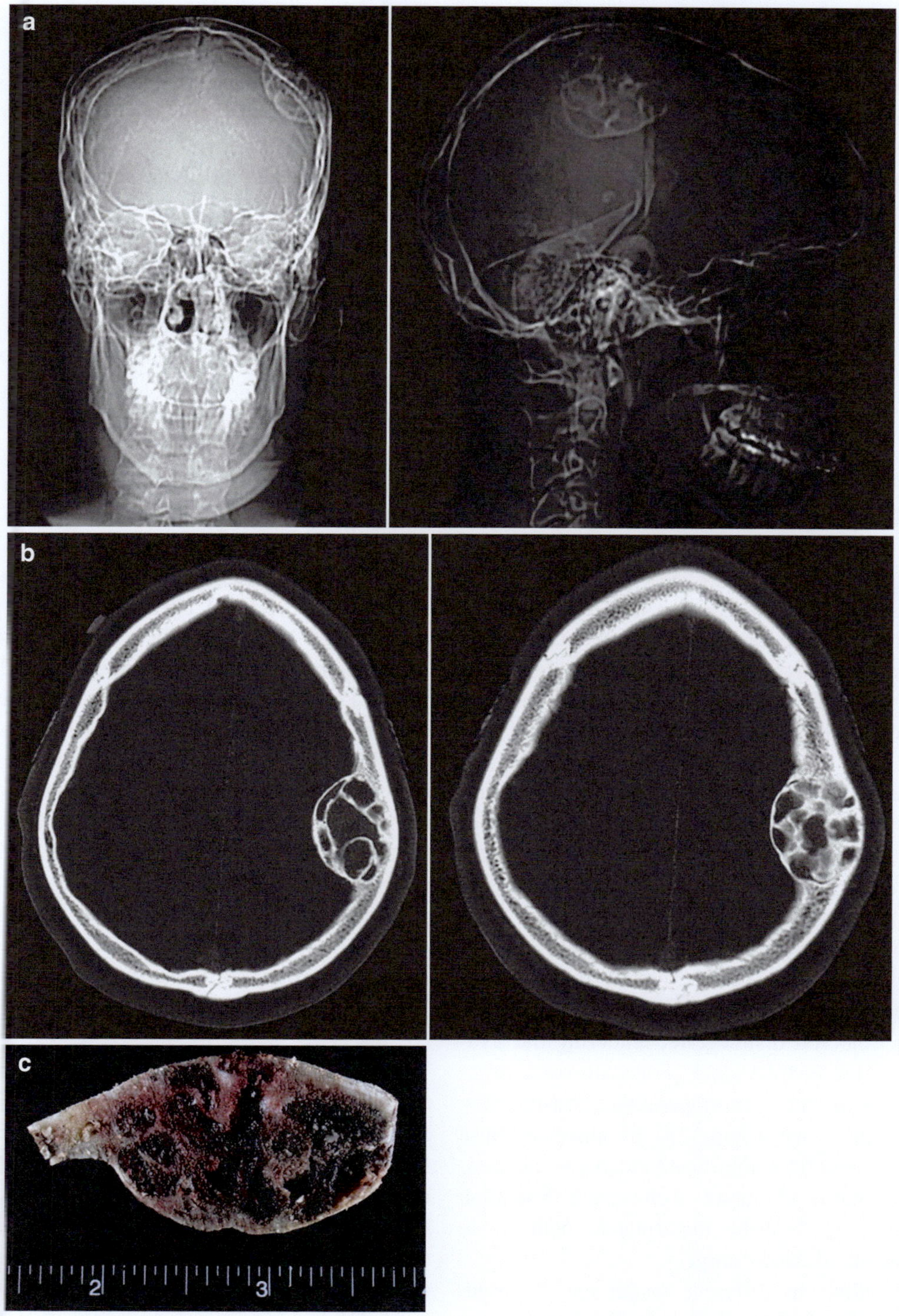

Fig. 17.4 (**a**) Atypical imaging findings in an intraosseous venous malformation/hemangioma: CT Scout which show a multilobulated osseous lesion. This could also be the appearance of an aneurysmal bone cyst (ABC). However, remarkable is the distinct cyst borders, which appear hyperdense. In an ABC these walls would be thinner and less prominent. (**b**) Axial slices of the hemangioma/intraosseous venous malformation. Interestingly, this proven hemangioma has features, which would also be fitting for an aneurysmal bone cyst, with the multiple cysts of different sizes. However, as a major differentiating point, the cyst walls are not as thin, as to be expected from an ABC, (**c**) Pathology specimen (courtesy of H. Ostertag, Hannover)

[22], are actually related to the entities in the adults or whether, as suggested by the current reported case and attempts at classification, we are indeed dealing with two separate entities: neoplastic and malformation. This might also apply to further differentiate Gorham-Stout disease which manifests with massive osteolysis and is presently considered a variant of hemangioma/lymphoma [25]. While presently there are no specific known genetic alterations [11], further analysis may yield a more comprehensive bases for the pathological and clinically reasonable characterization of these lesions [29, 30].

17.2.4 Surgery

Total surgical removal of the lesion is curative. Image-guided craniotomy assists in identifying the margins. To avoid small remnants in bony lesions, I always drill beyond the apparent margin. As with other bone tumors, the drilling "sound and feel" becomes different, once normal bone is reached. The drilling should be more radical in the marrow, while a thinned and narrow portion of the inner table can be retained, once beyond the border of the lesion. High-speed drilling with a diamond tip will destroy the cells thermally beyond the drilled area, keeping the calcifications. On polymethylmethacrylat (PMMA) reconstruction it should be borne in mind that these areas may decalcify with time and disintegrate, rendering the fixation of the PMMA slack. For vault reconstruction with the "intraoperative cast-molding technique," see Chap. 23. In children these lesions may have significant extension, necessitating more elaborate techniques. Nasrallah et al. [31] describe hyperplastic outer table replacement during surgery.

Bleeding in different magnitudes is mentioned. With large lesions, or in the vicinity of the sinuses, prior endovascular treatment may be contemplated. However, with the vascular supply mostly from the external cranial arteries, tributaries should be controllable on approach.

17.3 Lymphangioma

While this disease mostly occurs in soft tissue, the calvarium can be afflicted. This is remarkable, since anatomical studies have failed to demonstrate lymphatic vessels in normal bone [32]. Considered to be congenital they are generally encountered in newborn or young children [7]. Lymphangiomas are attributed to defects in the connection between lymphatic and venous system [14]. Histologically benign, they can expand into symptomatic space-occupying lesions. When within bones, they develop into a cystic expansile defect with intradiploic vascular channels composed of lymph vessels with dilated cystic spaces filled with clear fluid [7, 15, 16]. Expansion may cause a visible and palpable swelling which may become symptomatic by compressing adjacent structures. While imaging is described as mostly radiolucent [25, 33, 34], Berkman et al. [35] present a CT of their case with central hyperdense and radiating spiculae with surrounding radiolucency. This emphasizes the large variability in imaging encountered in vascular lesions of the skull [4, 5, 8]. The histological diagnosis may be challenging, as it is founded on very attenuated and barely discernable endothelial cells [14] which can be difficult to detect, resulting in the misreading as "normal bone" [25].

17.4 Aneurysmal Bone Cysts (ABCs)

These lesions commonly occur in the extremities and the spine (3–6% of tumors of the bone [16]). Skull involvement is rare at 3–6% of all skull lesions [7, 16], including the skull base with the most frequent location being the orbital bones. Gan et al. [36] have provided a thorough overview on the literature focused on skull lesions which encompasses the case reports from 1965 to 2004. Of 43 lesions, including their own cases, 31 are skull vault lesions, (frontal 6, temporal 8, parietal 4, and occipital 13). In a recent study on a 13-year single institution, one skull vault lesion is reported [1]. ABCs are most frequent in the younger population, the majority detected in patients younger than 20 years [23, 25]. In the extremities, thinning of the bone and the wasting of the internal structure cause fragility, leading to fractures as the primary manifestation. In the skull the expansile lesion may compress surrounding tissues causing symptoms. The leading symptom is swelling which is tender to palpation [36–39].

They are characterized by bloated bony margins and multiple large cystic portions without apparent internal bony structure. There may be fibrous septa, but mostly these cysts are filled with blood and various breakdown products of blood [14, 25]. Accordingly, CT shows extended, bloated, thin walled, bony cysts of different sizes, resulting in a "soap bubble" appearance [15]. MRI detects the diversity of blood in various stages of decomposition with non-cystic, solid regions suggestive of associated neoplasia [6, 40].

While these lesions are generally considered tumor-like lesions, recent cytogenetic investigations suggest a neoplastic origin [25, 41–43]. Sophisticated genetic analysis [44] will help to determine whether this is applicable to all locations.

The present working hypotheses attribute the formation of ABC either to reactive processes initiated by trauma associated with local hemodynamic disturbances [15] or secondary to primary neoplasms of the bone (e.g., giant cell tumor, chondroblastoma, fibrous dysplasia) [14, 25, 45, 46]. The later association mandates ample collection of specimen when removing such a lesion particularly in light of the cytogenetic findings [42].

Treatment of choice for ABC is complete surgical excision. Apparently in the extremities incomplete resection appears to be more frequent than for the cranial vault. Gan et al. detected 1 out of 32 cases in their literature review [36]. In the cranial vault, complete excision of the lesion, even when adherent to the dura, should be achievable, even if dural reconstruction in addition to the cranioplasty is necessary. The defect should be closed with either a split calvarial graft in small or with mesh, PMMA, or bone transplant. Computer aided design (CAD) cranial vault reconstruction in older patients may be done in a follow-up surgery. A variety of other treatment modalities have been attempted with mediocre results, albeit still applicable if surgery is not possible. However, mostly these therapies were used for ABCs of the extremities. With increasing capabilities for genetic classification, the potential for targeted immune- and chemotherapies [47] increases. Cases of spontaneous regression have also been reported [48]. Despite such rare events and particularly in light of potential neoplastic origin or co-occurrence, resection remains the treatment of choice.

17.5 High-Flow Intraosseous Malformations

17.5.1 Arteriovenous Malformation (AVM)

Arteriovenous malformations are generally presumed to be a congenital intertwining of primordial shunting vessels that did not evolve into capillary bed, thus draining arterial blood directly into venous channels [14, 25, 49]. Commonly such a nidus is located in soft tissue. However, intraosseous arterio-venous malformations (AVM's) exist and are mostly found in skeletal bones [14, 25]. Those in the skull have a predilection for the skull base. Only one case with truly intraosseous AVM of the vault was reported [50]. Symptoms in this case were a bump which, after a stable phase, increased in size over a short period of time. The non-tender bluish mass presented with a bruit. While the nidus appeared within the vault, engorged veins projected into the skin. Angiography detected only influx from external carotid branches. Venous drainage was only toward the skin. The CT showed enlarged intraosseous spaces and a thickened calvarium. Multiple embolizations and finally surgical removal with reconstruction of the vault with mesh and PMMA were performed.

Resection with prior embolization should be considered in symptomatic lesions. However, in addition general treatment options of skeletal intraosseous AVMs [51] can be discussed.

17.5.2 Intraosseous Dural Arteriovenous Fistula (DAVF)

Dural arteriovenous fistula (DAVF) is considered an acquired disease, based on post-thrombotic changes and fistulous shunting from arteries into veins. They encompass approximately 10–15% [49, 52] of all intracranial arteriovenous malformation. As AVMs of the brain occurs with an incidence of 1.34/100.000 [49], this would place DAVF at about 0.1/100.000.

Considering only DAVFs with the fistula within bone, Howard et al. [53] found 24 cases; however, most of these are within the skull base. Only two cases were located within the skull vault [53]. Others have to be discarded since the afflicted vasculature is only protruding into bone due to the enlargement. Truly intraosseous fistulae in the diploic system [54], as identified by the image documentation [55–59], present with a myriad of symptoms. They are generally determined by the involvement of the cortical venous system, with headache, confusion, pulsatile tinnitus, and hemorrhage. These lesions were treated endovascularly with transosseous [58, 59] or transarterial [56, 57] cannulation and embolization and one operation [55]. Standard Imaging with MRI and angiography will be diagnostic. As with most fistulae, detection depends on attentive scrutiny of the images and careful history taking.

17.6 Summary

The skull vault is afflicted by a myriad of diseases. However, numbers are small. Particularly within the scope of this chapter are intraosseous vascular lesions and malformations which altogether may include no more than 16–20% of calvarial lesions (hemangioma with 9–10, ABC with 3–6% as the most frequent with the others amounting at best to 1%). Therefore, general rules are difficult to deduce. Imaging allows a reasonable hypothesis but does not entirely rule out different diagnosis. The mainstay of treatment is surgical resection, which intents gross total removal, which is curative. In high-flow vascular malformations, endovascular treatment is an integral part, often also used standalone. Molecular profiling and sequencing may yield a basis for a more thorough understanding of the pathogenesis of intraosseous vascular lesions and malformations.

Acknowledgment With deep gratitude the authors thank C. Nimsky (Marburg), R. Wirtz and B. Schmitz (Ulm), J. Hensler (Kiel), G. Barest, A. Mian and A. Norbash (UCSD), and H. Ostertag (Hannover).

References

1. Nasi-Kordhishti I, Hempel JM, Ebner FH, Tatagiba M. Calvarial lesions: overview of imaging features and neurosurgical management. Neurosurg Rev. 2021;44(6):3459–69.
2. Heckl S, Aschoff A, Kunze S. Cavernomas of the skull: review of the literature 1975–2000. Neurosurg Rev. 2002;25(1–2):56–62. discussion 6–7
3. Morriss-Kay GM. Derivation of the mammalian skull vault. J Anat. 2001;199(Pt 1–2):143–51.
4. Colas L, Caron S, Cotten A. Skull vault lesions: a review. AJR Am J Roentgenol. 2015;205(4):840–7.
5. Gomez CK, Schiffman SR, Bhatt AA. Radiological review of skull lesions. Insights Imaging. 2018;9(5):857–82.
6. Pons Escoda A, Naval Baudin P, Mora P, Cos M, Hernandez Ganan J, Narvaez JA, et al. Imaging of skull vault tumors in adults. Insights Imaging. 2020;11(1):23.
7. St. Clair EG, IE MC. Skull tumors. In: Winn HR, editor. Youman´s & Winn neurological surgery, vol. 2. 7th ed. Elsevier; 2016. p. 5227–70.
8. Khodarahmi I, Alizai H, Chalian M, Alaia EF, Burke CJ, Slasky SE, Wenokor C. Imaging spectrum of calvarial abnormalities. Radiographics. 2021;41(4):1144–63.
9. Cervoni L, Artico M, Delfini R. Intraosseous cavernous hemangioma of the skull. Neurosurg Rev. 1995;18(1):61–4.
10. Politi M, Romeike BF, Papanagiotou P, Nabhan A, Struffert T, Feiden W, Reith W. Intraosseous hemangioma of the skull with dural tail sign: radiologic features with pathologic correlation. AJNR Am J Neuroradiol. 2005;26(8):2049–52.

11. Yang Y, Guan J, Ma W, Li Y, Xing B, Ren Z, et al. Primary intraosseous cavernous hemangioma in the skull. Medicine (Baltimore). 2016;95(11):e3069.
12. Martinez-Lage JF, Torroba MA, Cuartero Perez B, Almagro MJ, Lopez Lopez-Guerrero A, de la Rosa P. Cavernous hemangiomas of the cranial vault in infants: a case-based update. Childs Nerv Syst. 2010;26(7):861–5.
13. Prasad GL, Pai K. Pediatric cranial intraosseous hemangiomas: a review. Neurosurg Rev. 2018;41(1):109–17.
14. Atkins KA, Mills SE. Diseases of the bones and joints. In: Barnes L, editor. Surgical pathology of the head and neck. 2: informa; 2009. p. 951–94.
15. Doran SE, Gebarski SS, Hoff JT. Tumors of the skull. In: Youmans JR, editor. Neurological surgery. 4: W. B. Saunders; 1996. p. 2998–3023.
16. Hamilton HB, Voorhies RM. Tumors of the skull. In: Wilkins RHR, editor. Neurosurgery. II. 2nd ed. McGraw-Hill; 1996. p. 1503–28.
17. Hassanein AH, Mulliken JB, Fishman SJ, Greene AK. Evaluation of terminology for vascular anomalies in current literature. Plast Reconstr Surg. 2011;127(1):347–51.
18. Kunimoto K, Yamamoto Y, Jinnin M. ISSVA classification of vascular anomalies and molecular biology. Int J Mol Sci. 2022;23(4)
19. Bastug D, Ortiz O, Schochet SS. Hemangiomas in the calvaria: imaging findings. AJR Am J Roentgenol. 1995;164(3):683–7.
20. Bizzozero L, Solaining Talamonti C, Villa F, Brusamolino R, Collice M. Cavernous hemangioma of the skull. Case report and review of the literature. J Neurosurg Sci. 1997;41(4):419–21.
21. Liberale C, Rozell-Shannon L, Moneghini L, Nocini R, Tombris S, Colletti G. Stop calling me cavernous hemangioma! A literature review on misdiagnosed bony vascular anomalies. J Investig Surg. 2022;35(1):141–50.
22. Strauss SB, Steinklein JM, Phillips CD, Shatzkes DR. Intraosseous venous malformations of the head and neck. AJNR Am J Neuroradiol. 2022;43(8):1090–8.
23. van DGP IJ, Bovee J. Vascular tumors of bone: the evolvement of a classification based on molecular developments. Surg Pathol Clin. 2017;10(3):621–35.
24. Schneider RC, Gabrielsen TO, Hicks SP. Calvarial hemangioma. The value of selective external carotid angiography in surgical excision of the lesion. Neurology. 1973;23(4):352–6.
25. Nielson GP, Rosenberg AE. Diagnostic pathology: bone. 3rd ed. Elsevier; 2021.
26. Buhl R, Barth H, Dorner L, Nabavi A, Rohr A, Mehdorn HM. De novo development of intraosseous cavernous hemangioma. J Clin Neurosci. 2007;14(3):289–92.
27. Liu H, Chang X, Shang H, Li F, Zhou H, Xue X. Diffuse cavernous hemangioma of the skull misdiagnosed as skull metastasis in breast cancer patient: one case report and literature review. BMC Cancer. 2019;19(1):172.
28. Kurokawa R, Kurokawa M, Holmes A, Baba A, Bapuraj J, Capizzano A, et al. Skull metastases and osseous venous malformations: the role of diffusion-weighted and dynamic contrast-enhanced MRI. J Neuroimaging. 2022;32(6):1170–6.
29. Arbajian E, Magnusson L, Brosjo O, Wejde J, Folpe AL, Nord KH, Mertens F. A benign vascular tumor with a new fusion gene: EWSR1-NFATC1 in hemangioma of the bone. Am J Surg Pathol. 2013;37(4):613–6.
30. Kar S, Baisantry A, Nabavi A, Bertalanffy H. Role of Delta-Notch signaling in cerebral cavernous malformations. Neurosurg Rev. 2016;39(4):581–9.
31. Nasrallah IM, Hayek R, Duhaime AC, Stotland MA, Mamourian AC. Cavernous hemangioma of the skull: surgical treatment without craniectomy. J Neurosurg Pediatr. 2009;4(6):575–9.
32. Edwards JR, Williams K, Kindblom LG, Meis-Kindblom JM, Hogendoorn PC, Hughes D, et al. Lymphatics and bone. Hum Pathol. 2008;39(1):49–55.
33. Di Emidio P, Chibbaro S, Mirone G, Balercia P. Double skull lymphangioma. Case report and review of the literature. Orbit. 2009;28(5):293–6.
34. Kopperman M, Antoine JE. Primary lymphangioma of the calvarium. Am J Roentgenol Radium Therapy, Nucl Med. 1974;121(1):118–20.
35. Berkmann MZ, Bek S, Özcan D. Lymphangioma of the skull: a case report. Turk Neurosurg. 2001;11:56–9.
36. Gan YC, Hockley AD. Aneurysmal bone cysts of the cranium in children. Report of three cases and brief review of the literature. J Neurosurg. 2007;106(5 Suppl):401–6.
37. Ameli NO, Abbassioun K, Azod A, Saleh H. Aneurysmal bone cyst of the skull. Can J Neurol Sci. 1984;11(4):466–71.
38. Daszkiewicz P, Roszkowski M, Grajkowska W. Aneurysmal bone cyst of skull and vertebrae in children. Analysis of own material and review of the literature. Folia Neuropathol. 2004;42(1):25–30.
39. Ikeda H, Niizuma H, Yoshimoto T. Aneurysmal bone cyst of the skull. Surg Neurol. 1986;25(2):145–8.
40. Lin SP, Fang YC, Chu DC, Chang YC, Hsu CI. Characteristics of cranial aneurysmal bone cyst on computed tomography and magnetic resonance imaging. J Formos Med Assoc. 2007;106(3):255–9.
41. Obermeier KT, Schmockel E, Otto S, Haidari S. Frequency of translocation of USP-6 in the aneurysmal bone cyst of the jaw. J Oral Pathol Med. 2023;52(2):145–9.
42. Oliveira AM, Chou MM, Perez-Atayde AR, Rosenberg AE. Aneurysmal bone cyst: a neoplasm driven by upregulation of the USP6 oncogene. J Clin Oncol. 2006;24(1):e1. author reply e2
43. Panagopoulos I, Gorunova L, Andersen K, Lobmaier I, Lund-Iversen M, Micci F, Heim S. Fusion of the lumican (LUM) gene with the ubiquitin specific peptidase 6 (USP6) gene in an aneurysmal bone cyst carrying a

t(12;17)(q21;p13) chromosome translocation. Cancer Genomics Proteomics. 2020;17(5):555–61.
44. Sekoranja D, Bostjancic E, Salapura V, Mavcic B, Pizem J. Primary aneurysmal bone cyst with a novel SPARC-USP6 translocation identified by next-generation sequencing. Cancer Genet. 2018;228–229:12–6.
45. Kaloostian SW, Vartanian TK, Ordookhanian C, Vartanian T, Kaloostian PE. Concomittant fibrous dysplasia with aneurysmal bone cyst formation within the skull, humerus and rib. J Surg Case Rep. 2018;2018(7):rjy180.
46. Rappaport ZH. Aneurysmal bone cyst associated with fibrous dysplasia of the skull. Neurochirurgia (Stuttg). 1989;32(6):192–4.
47. Kurucu N, Akyuz C, Ergen FB, Yalcin B, Kosemehmetoglu K, Ayvaz M, et al. Denosumab treatment in aneurysmal bone cyst: Evaluation of nine cases. Pediatr Blood Cancer. 2018;65(4)
48. Borni M, Kolsi F, Cherif I, Boudawara MZ. Spontaneous rapid regression of a juvenile primary aneurysmal bone cyst of the skull: a case report and literature review. Radiol Case Rep. 2022;17(5):1634–9.
49. Choi JH, Mohr JP. Brain arteriovenous malformations in adults. Lancet Neurol. 2005;4(5):299–308.
50. Al-Smadi A, Shokuhfar T, Johnston A, Alden TD, Bowman R, Shaibani A. The rare case of a large complex intraosseous cranial arteriovenous malformation with successful multidisciplinary management. J Neurosurg Pediatr. 2017;20(6):591–7.
51. Kim R, Do YS, Park KB, Kim DI, Heo SH, Park HS, et al. Therapeutic outcomes of embolotherapy of extremity bone intraosseous arteriovenous malformation with ethanol, coils, and n-butyl cyanoacrylate. J Vasc Surg. 2021;73(6):2090–7 e5.
52. Newton TH, Cronqvist S. Involvement of dural arteries in intracranial arteriovenous malformations. Radiology. 1969;93(5):1071–8.
53. Howard BM, Manupipatpong S, Dion JE, Tamargo RJ, Gailloud P, Hui FK. Classification and management considerations for intraosseous dural arteriovenous fistulae. Neurosurgery. 2023;93(2):387–98.
54. Garcia-Gonzalez U, Cavalcanti DD, Agrawal A, Gonzalez LF, Wallace RC, Spetzler RF, Preul MC. The diploic venous system: surgical anatomy and neurosurgical implications. Neurosurg Focus. 2009;27(5):E2.
55. Hori E, Kuwayama N, Harada J, Kubo M, Yamamoto H, Endo S. Connection between a dural artery and a dural vein in a dural arteriovenous fistula of the cranial vault. Neurol Med Chir (Tokyo). 2007;47(1):26–8.
56. Ishaque AH, Keough MB, Alrohimi A, Rempel JL, Dobrowolski P, Chow MM. Intraosseous dural arteriovenous fistula causing contralateral intracerebral hemorrhage. Can J Neurol Sci. 2021;48(6):886–8.
57. Shim JH, Yoon SM, Shim JJ, Kim RS. A case of intraosseous dural arteriovenous fistulas involving diploic vein treated with transarterial onyx embolization. J Korean Neurosurg Soc. 2011;50(3):260–3.
58. Tokuyama K, Kiyosue H, Hori Y, Nagatomi H. Diploic arteriovenous fistulas with marked cortical venous reflux. Interv Neuroradiol. 2020;26(3):254–9.
59. White AC, Folzenlogen ZA, Harland TA, Case DE, Roark CD, Kumpe DA, Seinfeld J. Intraosseous cannulation of a calvarial diploic vein for embolization of a symptomatic dural arteriovenous fistula: a technical case report. Oper Neurosurg (Hagerstown). 2020;18(4):E132–E7.

Infectious Lesions of the Scalp and Calvarium

18

Ali Akhaddar

18.1 Introduction

Scalp and cranial vaults may be infected by various microorganisms including bacteria, fungi, and parasites. Classically, the majority of scalp and skull vault infections encountered in neurosurgical practices include scalp abscesses and cranial osteomyelitis. These disorders have a worldwide distribution and affect both sexes at any age and race [1–4]. Pure dermatologic, hair, and cutaneous infectious diseases will not be discussed in this section.

Scalp infections may involve any of its five anatomic layers. The majority of infections of the scalp are superficial, minor, and limited, such as erysipelas, non-necrotizing cellulitis, impetigo, furuncles, folliculitis, and scalp abscesses, but they can extend deeply and induce more serious complications such as necrotizing fasciitis and cranial osteomyelitis [2, 5–13].

Cranial osteomyelitis is defined as an inflammatory condition of both skull bones (osteitis) and their corresponding bone marrow (myelitis). Unlike the skull base, cranial osteomyelitis is often described in the calvaria [1].

The hair-bearing nature of the scalp may often hide scalp and/or calvarial lesions longer than those arising in other sites in the human body.

Because of the significant proximity of the scalp and cranial vault with intracranial structures, the seriousness of these infectious diseases is related to their intracranial extensions and potentially life-threatening complications. Management of cranial bone infections continues to pose a significant challenge to contemporary neurosurgeons worldwide [1, 4].

A summary of the main forms of scalp abscesses and cranial vault osteomyelitis is provided in this chapter.

18.2 Infectious Lesions of the Scalp

18.2.1 Epidemiology and Etiology

Scalp abscesses are unusual purulent collections mostly involving the subgaleal space between the aponeurosis (epicranium or galea) and the

A. Akhaddar (✉)
Department of Neurosurgery, Avicenne Military Hospital of Marrakech, Mohammed V University in Rabat, Rabat, Morocco
e-mail: akhaddar@hotmail.fr

M. Turgut et al. (eds.), *Lesions of the Scalp and Cranial Vault*,
https://doi.org/10.1007/978-3-031-88244-9_18

pericranium (external periosteum). Classically, scalp abscesses have been reported to occur following:

(a) Direct extension from contiguous site of infection (e.g., otorhinologic infection, oro-odontogenic infection, scalp lesion)
(b) Post-traumatic or postsurgical direct inoculation (e.g., contaminated wound, surgical site infection)
(c) Hematogenous dissemination from a remote source of infection (e.g., septicemia)

In developing countries, paranasal sinusitis, dermatologic lesions, and cranial osteomyelitis remain the most common source of scalp abscesses [5, 7]. On the other hand, postsurgical (e.g., craniotomy, scalp monitors, cosmetic surgery) and post-traumatic conditions have become the predominant sources in developed countries. Forms secondary to hematogenous dissemination are rare.

18.2.2 Clinical Features

The initial evaluation of patients with scalp infections should include a detailed past medical history and clinical exam. History would include questions about recent underlying diseases, medications, infections, injuries, and history of malignancies or surgeries [5–10, 12, 14]. Clinicians should pay special attention to the scalp by examining it thoroughly, as the infectious lesions may be hidden by hair (Fig. 18.1).

Local signs include tender and fluctuating swelling, erythema, and local heat. Pus formation, purulent tract, and discharge with or without foul odor are highly suggestive (Figs. 18.2, 18.3, and 18.4). General and regional signs such as fever, chills, fatigue, irritability, headache, and lymphadenopathy may be seen.

Concomitant deep underlying infection may induce more serious clinical signs and symptoms such as meningitis, high intracranial hypertension, and focal neurologic deficits [1, 2].

18.2.3 Diagnosis

Computed tomography (CT) scan, magnetic resonance imaging (MRI), and laboratory investigations remain the best methods of subgaleal abscess evaluation.

On imaging, the appearance is that of a subgaleal (extracranial) collection with post-contrast

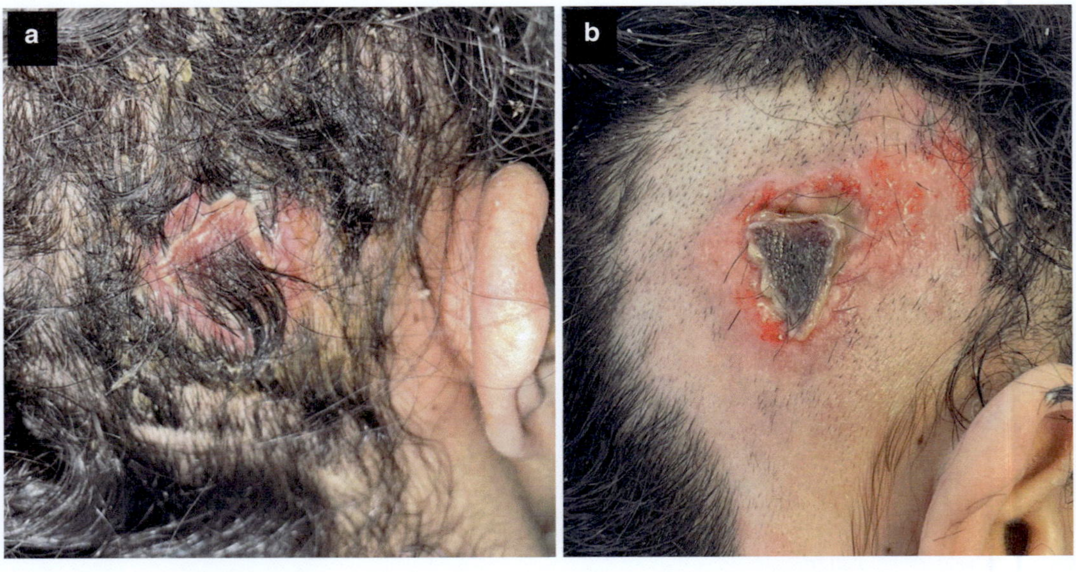

Fig. 18.1 Clinical pictures of a post-traumatic neglected nonhealing wound before (**a**) and after shaving (**b**) (courtesy of Doctor Achraf Moussa, M.D). Note that the wound was hidden by hair

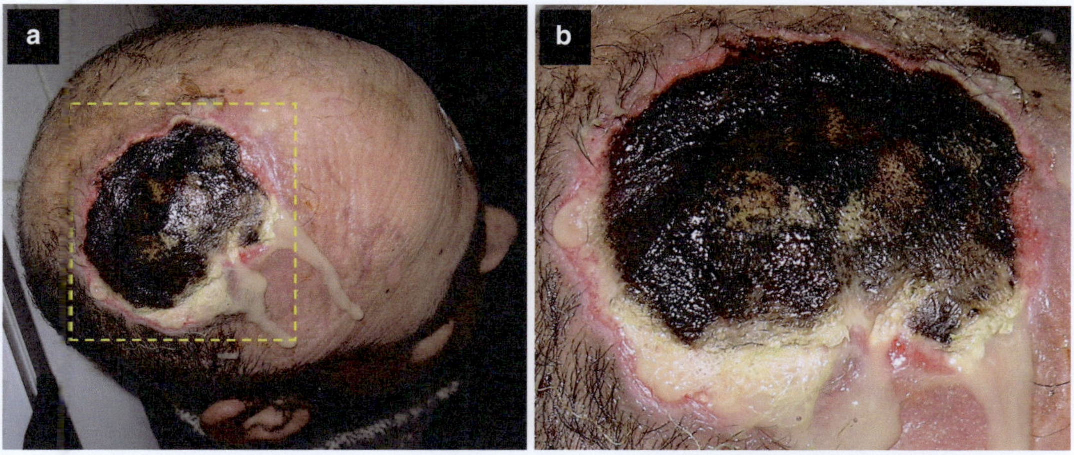

Fig. 18.2 Clinical pictures of post-traumatic infectious scalp necrosis on the parietal region (**a**, **b**)

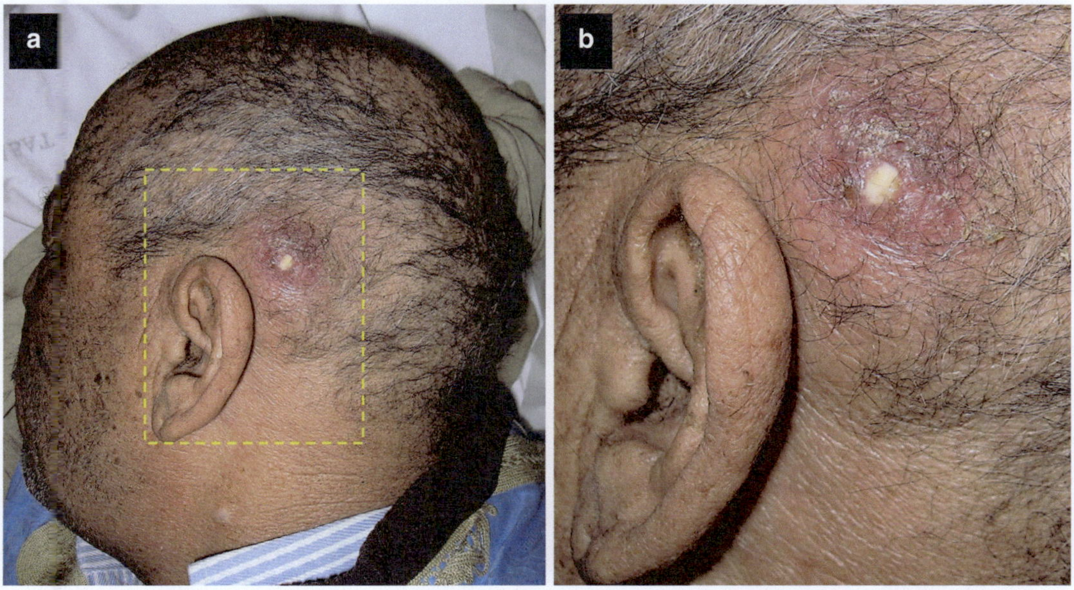

Fig. 18.3 Clinical pictures of a temporo-retroauricular subgaleal scalp abscess with purulent tract (**a**, **b**)

peripheral enhancement (Figs. 18.5 and 18.6). Ultrasound examination may help in excluding other scalp collections or neoplasms.

Peripheral white blood cell count and inflammatory biomarkers such as erythrocyte sedimentation rate and C-reactive protein level are not specific and highly variable in their expression [7, 11, 13]. Blood dosage of procalcitonin is more specific for sepsis and bacterial infection.

The samples obtained find gram-positive skin flora such as *Staphylococcus* species and *Streptococcus* species but *gram-negative bacilli* are not rare (e.g., *Escherichia coli*). The occurrence of polymicrobial and anaerobic infections may also occur. After identification of the pathogen agent(s), antimicrobial susceptibility testing is performed in vitro to predict the in vivo success/failure of antimicrobial therapy [1, 2, 14].

More rarely fungal (e.g., *Aspergillus* species, *Cryptococci*, *Coccidiomycetes*) and parasitic pathogens (e.g., hydatidosis) may be involved [3, 15].

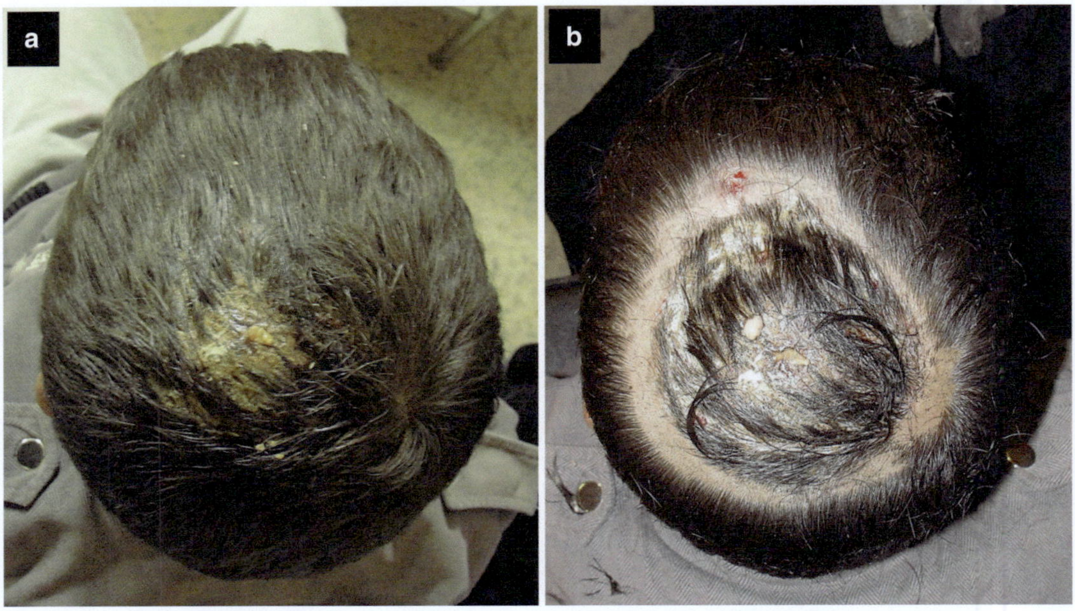

Fig. 18.4 Clinical pictures of a scalp abscess at the vertex secondary to a neglected tinea (dermatophytes) (**a**, **b**)

18.2.4 Treatment Options

Superficial and limited collection may be treated with antibiotics alone. While the subgaleal abscess should be drained [2].

Whenever possible, surgical treatment allows:

- Obtaining sample collections for microbiologic identification and cultures
- Removing purulent and necrotic tissues
- Cleaning the abscess cavity with antiseptic solutions
- Putting a drain
- Closing the wound if possible

Most traditional antimicrobial agents are administered parenterally for the first 2 weeks, followed by suitable oral therapy for at least 4 weeks. Definitive antimicrobial therapy was prescribed after the results of antibiotic susceptibility tests [1, 2, 16].

Specific bacterial and fungal pathogens must be treated with the appropriate anti-infectious agents.

Other sources of infections, underlying conditions, and predisposing causes should always be considered.

18.2.5 Outcomes

The majority of patients progress favorably. However, some cases require more serious clinical, biological, and imaging monitoring especially those with cranial and intracranial complications. Sequels are rare (chronic scalp fistula, discomfort, and facial keloid scar) and may need reconstructive procedures (*c.f. Chap. 25* about Principles of Surgery and Reconstructive Procedures for Lesions of the Scalp and Calvarium).

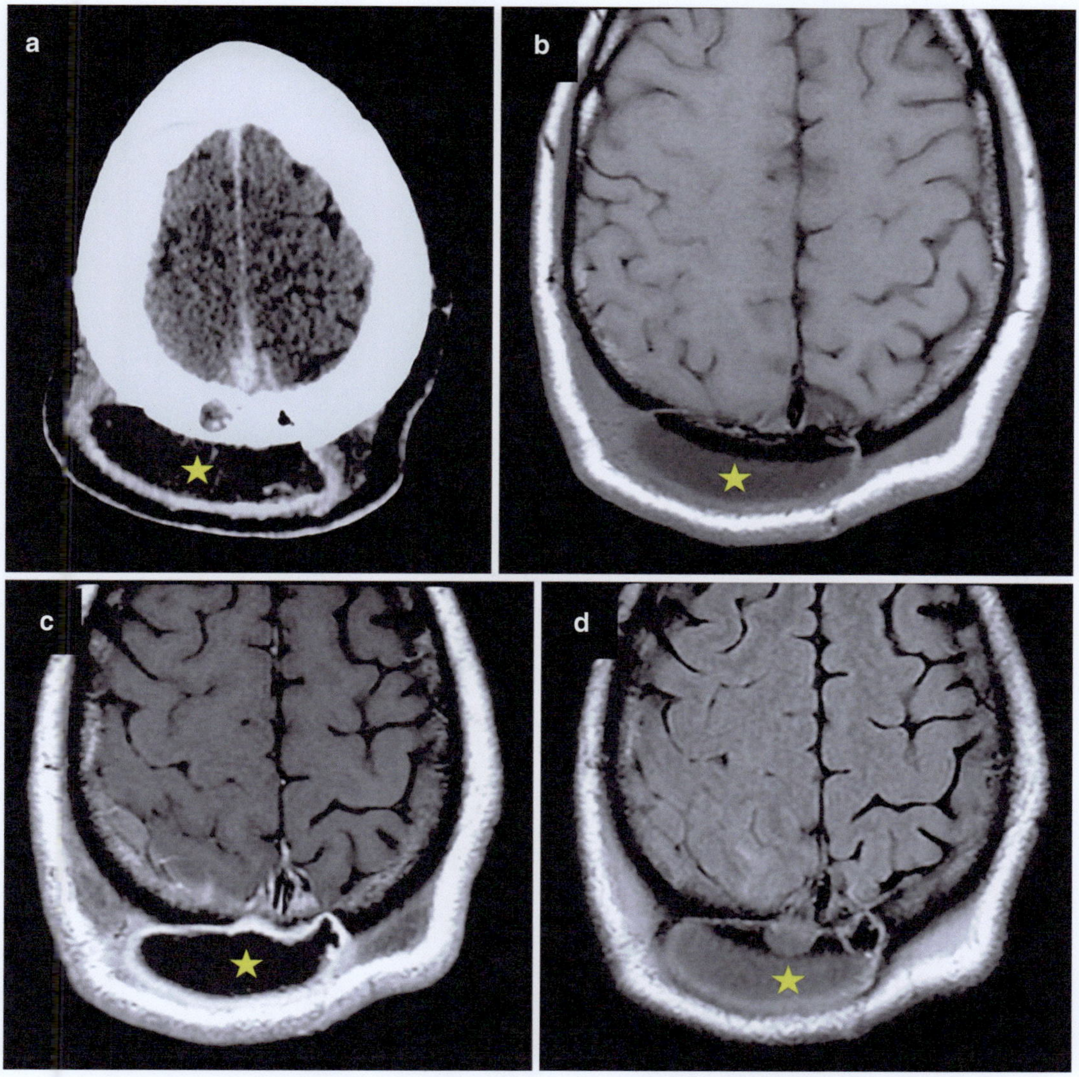

Fig. 18.5 Parietal subgaleal abscess (stars) as seen on axial CT-scan (**a**), T1-weighted MRI before (**b**) and after gadolinium injection (**c**) as well as on FLAIR sequence (**d**)

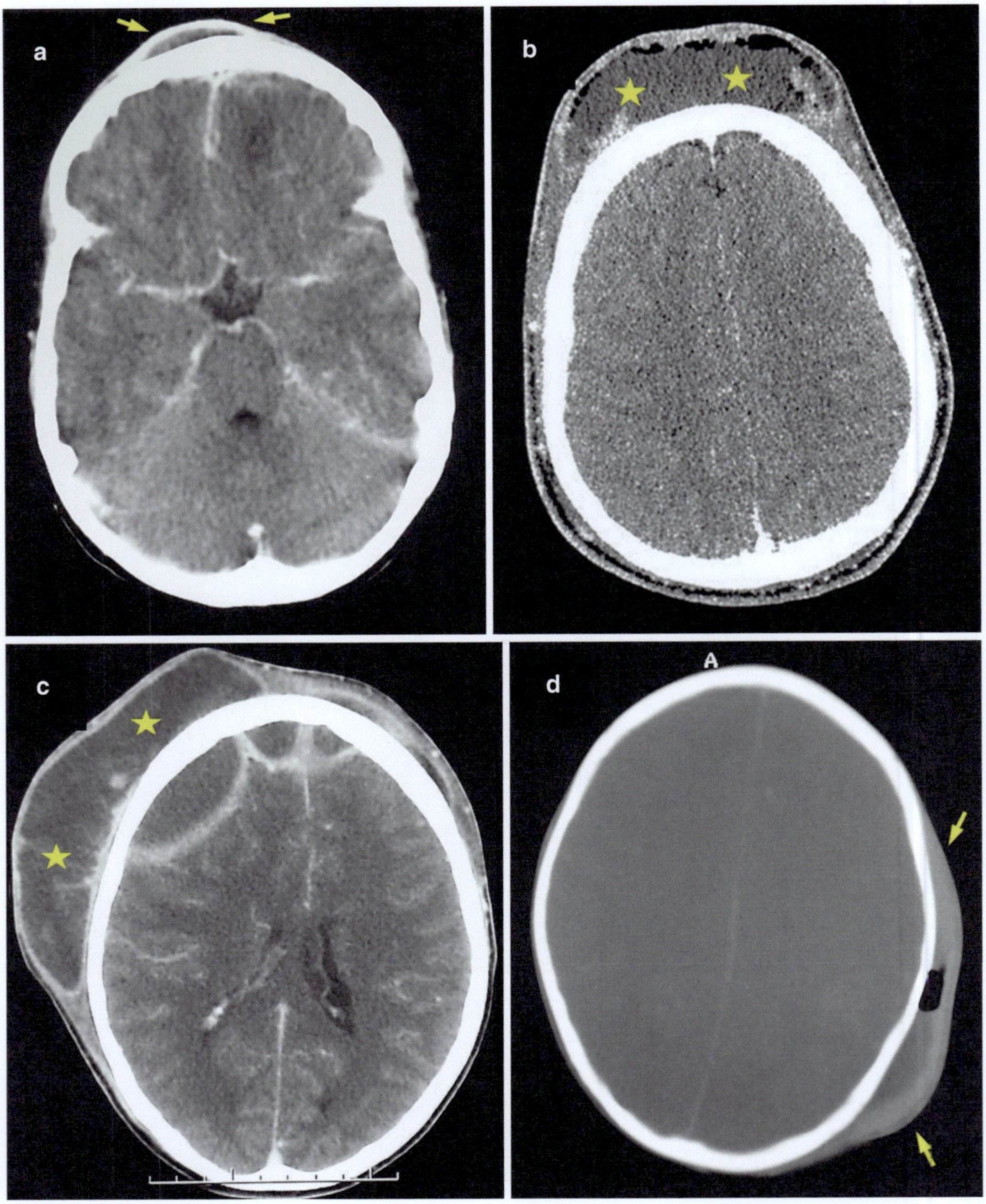

Fig. 18.6 Different forms and localizations of scalp abscesses as seen on axial CT-scan (**a**–**d**). Limited collection (arrows) (**a**, **d**) and large collections (stars) (**b**, **c**)

18.3 Infectious Lesions of the Cranial Vault

18.3.1 Epidemiology and Etiology

Most cranial osteomyelitis begins as an acute form, but it may change to a chronic infection. Like subgaleal scalp abscesses, cranial vault infection is often related to three main sources of infection: (**a**) direct extension from a contiguous site of infection, (**b**) post-traumatic or postsurgical direct inoculation, and more rarely (**c**) hematogenous dissemination [1, 4].

For many authors, cranial vault osteomyelitis is often "the transitional point between a primary extracranial infection and its secondary intracranial extension" [1].

The localization and progression of this infectious disease can be summarized (Fig. 18.7) as follows [1]:

- Type 0: initial cranial bone involvement
- Type I: limited to cranial bone
- Type II: extracranial extension
- Type III: intracranial extension
- Type IV: cranial, extracranial, and intracranial involvement

In developed nations, postsurgical craniotomy infections have become the predominant cause of cranial vault osteomyelitis. However, in developing countries, paranasal sinusitis and scalp infections remain the most common source of cranial bone infections.

The gravity of cranial vault osteomyelitis is related to its intracranial extensions and consequently the occurrence of meningitis, empyema, or brain abscess [1, 14, 17].

18.3.2 Clinical Features

Cranial vault osteomyelitis may have various clinical presentations. However, in the majority of cases, the clinical picture resembles that of a scalp abscess with local and general signs. Tenderness out of proportion of soft tissue lesions suggests cranial bone osteomyelitis rather than scalp abscess (Fig. 18.8). In acute forms, the duration of symptoms is less than 1 month, whereas in chronic infections, the duration of symptoms is several months. The cranial bone may sometimes be exposed with concomitant purulent and necrotic tissues.

Pott's puffy tumor is an uncommon form of cranial osteomyelitis, mostly a complication of frontal paranasal sinusitis especially in adolescent males presenting with a forehead subperiosteal abscess, frontal bone infection, and possible intracranial or orbital extensions (Fig. 18.9) [16, 18].

Seizures, signs of raised intracranial pressure, and focal neurologic deficits are related to intracranial extensions and deep complications [4].

18.3.3 Diagnosis

Cranial X-ray is usually the first diagnostic tool on which cranial bone infections are identified, but its use is decreasing due to the availability of more accurate imaging techniques, such as computed tomography (CT) and magnetic resonance imaging (MRI).

In the acute stage of presentations, CT scan exploration reveals areas of rarefaction and loss of diploic bone trabeculae, demineralization, erosion, or thinning of the cortical bone table. Association of extracranial soft tissue abscesses is not rare. In chronic forms, there is diploic bone sclerosis and cortical bone thickening mixed with areas of skull table destruction and radiolucency. Sequester formations are highly suggestive of chronic osteomyelitis. On CT scan, the skull bones are best assessed using a bone algorithm or at least bone windows (Figs. 18.9, 18.10, and 18.11).

MRI can show a lesion within the diploic space before it alters the bony architecture and can give greater detail about its internal content. However, enhancement patterns of bony and extracranial soft tissues are highly variable, especially in post-traumatic and postoperative forms. Nevertheless, MRI is useful in demonstrating intracranial lesions such as epidural abscesses, subdural empyemas, and brain abscesses (Fig. 18.12).

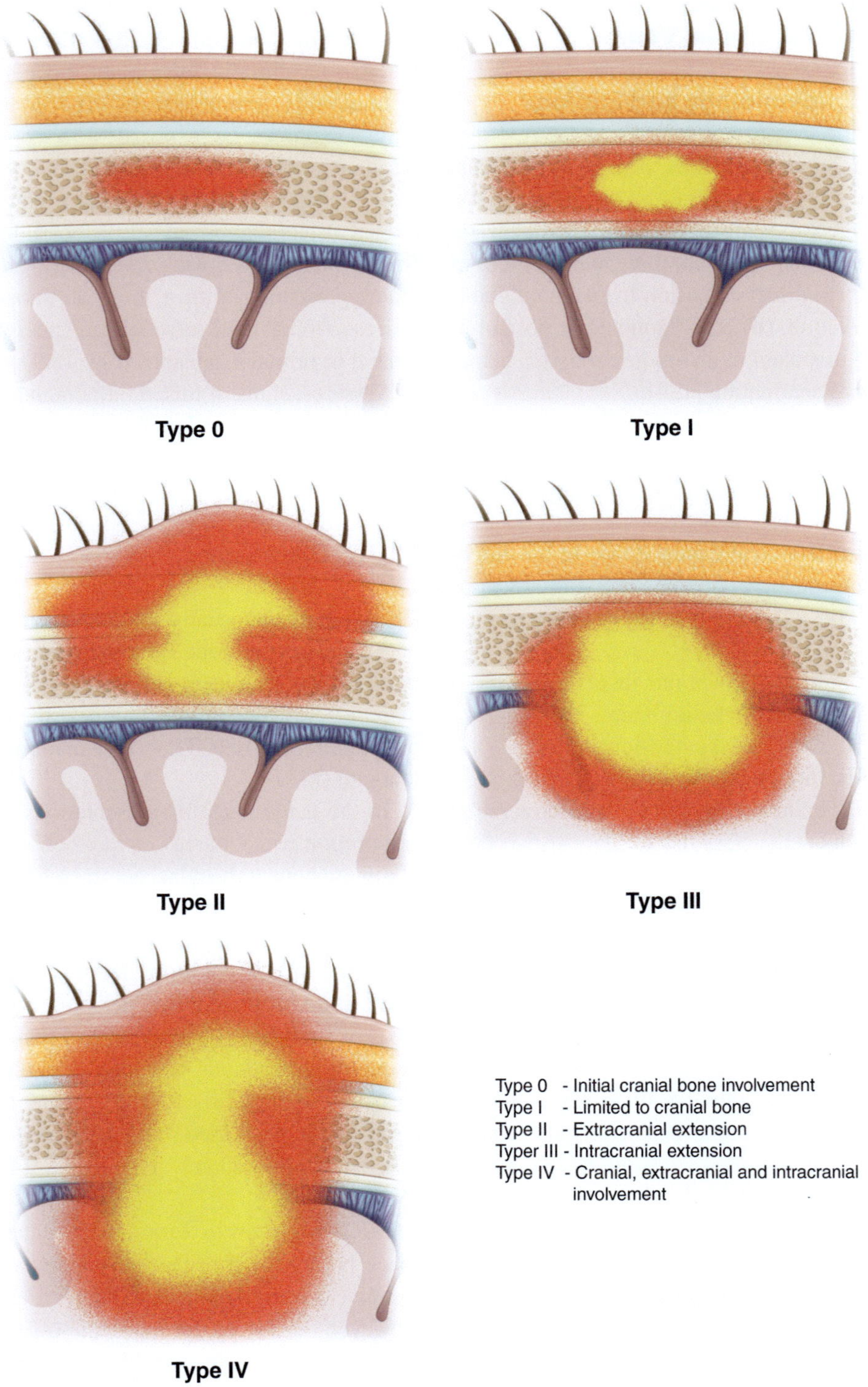

Fig. 18.7 Classification of cranial osteomyelitis: a staging system for skull osteomyelitis based on the location of cranial infection and its extension (Type 0: initial cranial bone involvement. Type I: limited to cranial bone. Type II: extracranial extension. Type III: intracranial extension. Type IV: cranial, extracranial, and intracranial involvement)

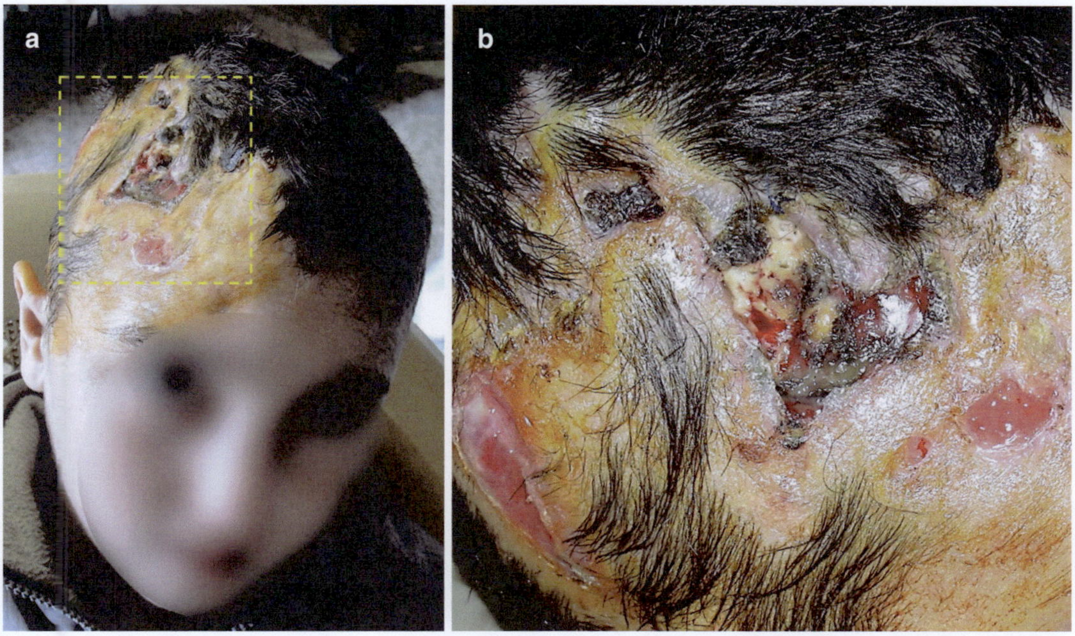

Fig. 18.8 Frontoparietal cranial osteomyelitis (**a**, **b**) due to a severe craniocerebral injury

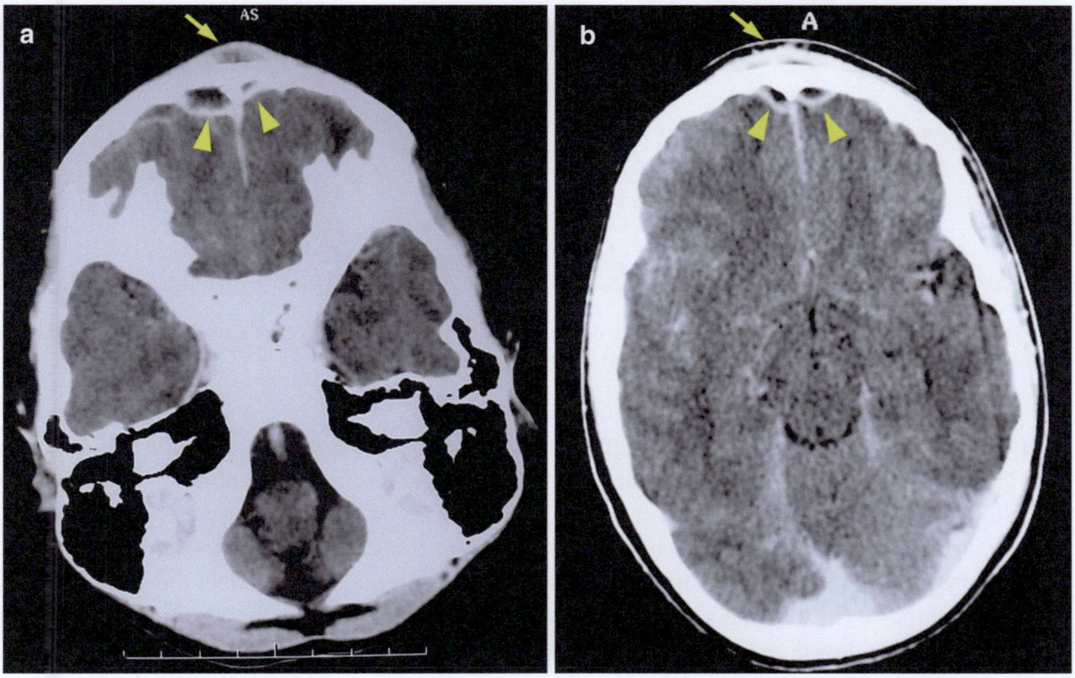

Fig. 18.9 Pott's puffy tumor in two patients (**a**, **b**). Note the frontal subperiosteal abscess (arrows) and the concomitant parameningeal empyemas (arrowheads)

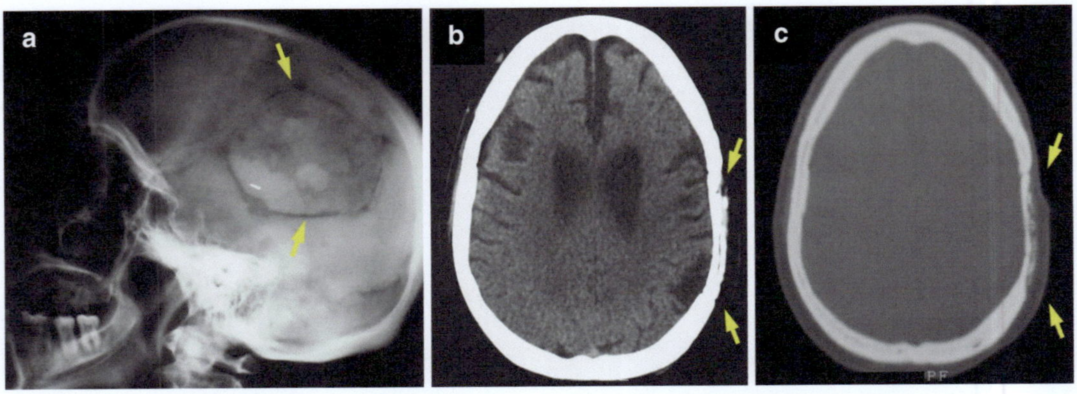

Fig. 18.10 Postoperative chronic parietal cranial osteomyelitis (arrows) as seen on lateral plain radiography (**a**) and axial CT-scan on parenchymal (**b**) and bone (**c**) windows

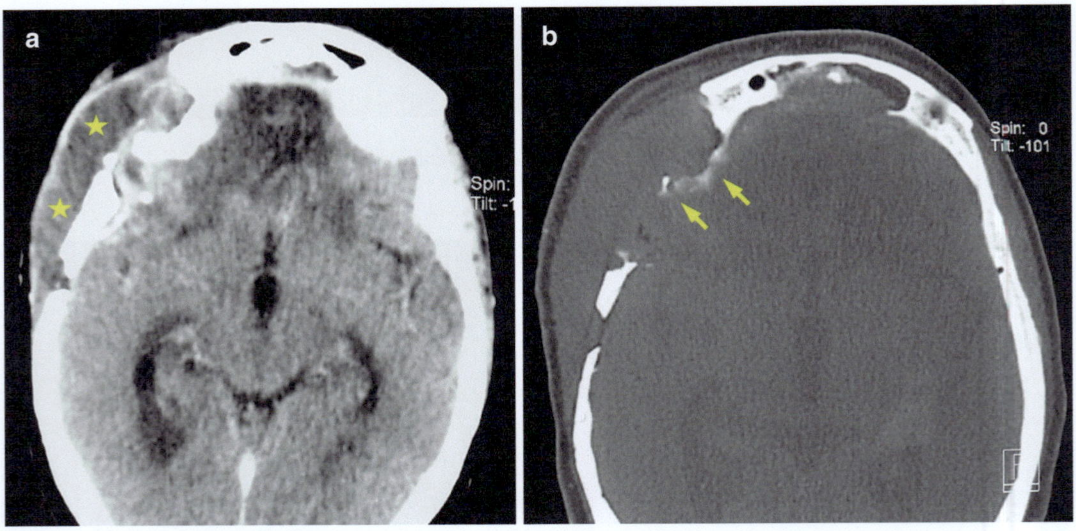

Fig. 18.11 Postoperative frontotemporal cranial osteomyelitis (arrows) with concomitant subgaleal scalp abscess (stars) as seen on axial CT-scan on parenchymal (**a**) and bone (**b**) windows

Bone scans (e.g., SPECT or FDG-PET) are very sensitive for detecting bone infection, especially in the acute stage of the disease.

Like in cases with scalp infections, classic biologic parameters (peripheral white blood cell count, erythrocyte sedimentation rate, and C-reactive protein level) are not specific and highly variable in their expression. However, the blood dosage of procalcitonin is more specific for sepsis and bacterial infection.

Aerobic and anaerobic bacteria are the main microorganisms involved especially *Streptococcus* species, *Staphylococcus* species, *Bacteroid* species, and *Fusobacterium* species. These pathogen agents reflect the various bacteria encountered in paranasal air sinus infection and endogenous skin flora [4].

The occurrence of polymicrobial infections is not rare. However, fungal and parasitic pathogens are rarely involved [15, 19].

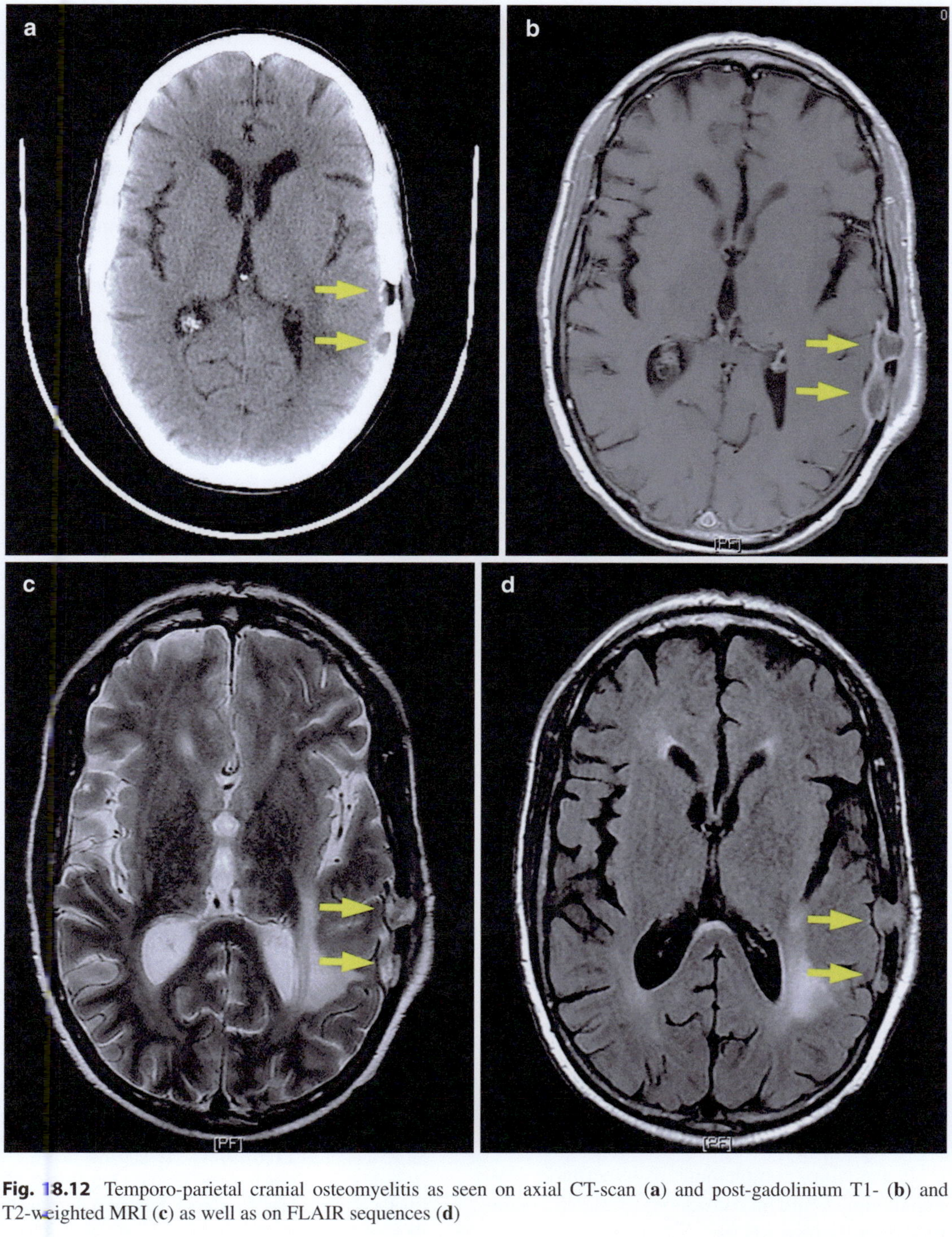

Fig. 18.12 Temporo-parietal cranial osteomyelitis as seen on axial CT-scan (**a**) and post-gadolinium T1- (**b**) and T2-weighted MRI (**c**) as well as on FLAIR sequences (**d**)

Anatomopathologic studies may be helpful for differentiating acute forms from chronic ones [1].

18.3.4 Treatment Options

Antibiotic therapy should include broad-spectrum antibiotic medications against aerobic and anaerobic bacteria with adequate penetration into the cranial bones. Treatment should be optimized according to the results of antibiotic susceptibility tests. Considering the cranial vault bony structures, antibiotics should be given for at least 2–3 months [1, 4, 14, 20].

Specific pathogens such as tuberculosis, mycosis, and hydatidosis must be treated with appropriate anti-infectious drugs [15, 19].

Overall, clinicians and biologists must work together closely to choose the most appropriate anti-infectious treatment for the patient.

Cases with limited and mild osseous infection can be managed with a prolonged course of antibiotics alone. However, more extensive and serious forms (especially those with intracranial involvement and/or cranial vault defect due to bony destruction) require surgical debridement to eliminate areas of necrosis and sequester followed by a cranioplasty in a second surgical intervention (following complete resolution of the infection) [21, 22]. Some authors use an extradural closed drainage system. Management of concomitant intracranial suppurations should be taken into account as well as the primary source of infection [17].

Patients with Pott's puffy tumors may need a multidisciplinary approach to treat the primary source of infection and its cranial and intracranial complications [16, 18].

If available, complementary hyperbaric oxygen therapy could be considered for the treatment of refractory forms [1].

Please refer to *Chap. 25* about Principles of Surgery and Reconstructive Procedures for Lesions of the Scalp and Calvarium.

18.3.5 Outcomes

Close clinical, biological, and neuroimaging monitoring (every 4–8 weeks until the infections have been completely resolved) is important to ensure adequate response to treatment. The outcome is related to the severity of the infection, poor medical condition, serious comorbidities, and the delay in diagnosis.

Sequels are rare but can be disabling such as seizures, permanent neurologic deficit, chronic fistula, and facial keloid scar [1].

18.4 Conclusion

As infections of the scalp and calvaria are unusual diseases, their recognition is often delayed with sometimes subsequent local and regional complications.

Quick positive diagnosis and initiation of appropriate therapies is the key to decreasing the potential neurological and esthetic complications associated with these diseases. The majority of scalp abscesses and cranial osteomyelitis remain preventable. Correct prevention and treatment of risk factors and causes that may lead to these infectious diseases are the best ways to close the door to pathogens invasion.

References

1. Akhaddar A, editor. Cranial osteomyelitis. Diagnosis and treatment. 1st ed. Cham, Switzerland: Springer International Publishing; 2016. https://doi.org/10.1007/978-3-319-30268-3.
2. Akhaddar A. Scalp abscesses. In: Atlas of infections in neurosurgery and spinal surgery. 1st ed. Cham, Switzerland: Springer International Publishing; 2017. https://doi.org/10.1007/978-3-319-60086-4_3.
3. Akhaddar A. Cranial vault lesions. In: Turgut M, Challa S, Akhaddar A, editors. Fungal infections of the central nervous system. 1st ed. Cham, Switzerland: Springer International Publishing; 2019. https://doi.org/10.1007/978-3-030-06088-6_16.
4. Mortazavi MM, Khan MA, Quadri SA, Suriya SS, Fahimdanesh KM, Fard SA, Hassanzadeh T, Taqi

MA, Grossman H, Tubbs RS. Cranial osteomyelitis: a comprehensive review of modern therapies. World Neurosurg. 2018;111:142–53. https://doi.org/10.1016/j.wneu.2017.12.066.
5. Amponsah EK, Sodnom-Ish B, Nguyen TTH, Kim SM. Odontogenic necrotizing fasciitis of face and scalp. J Craniofac Surg. 2021;32(6):e547–8. https://doi.org/10.1097/SCS.0000000000007528.
6. Barry J, Fridley J, Sayama C, Lam S. Infected subgaleal hematoma following blunt head trauma in a child: case report and review of the literature. Pediatr Neurosurg. 2015;50(4):223–8. https://doi.org/10.1159/000433442.
7. Jones H, Trinidade A, Jaberoo MC, Lyons M. Periorbital cellulitis, subgaleal abscess and superior sagittal sinus thrombosis: a rare combination of complications arising from unilateral frontal sinusitis. J Laryngol Otol. 2012;126(12):1281–3. https://doi.org/10.1017/S0022215112002228.
8. Lee MH, Votto SS, Read-Fuller AM, Reddy LV. Necrotizing fasciitis of the scalp stemming from odontogenic infection. Proc (Baylor Univ Med Cent). 2019;33(1):110–2. https://doi.org/10.1080/08998280.2019.1675419.
9. Liu H, Li Z, Yang L, Yang X, Zhang Y, Chen J. A 9-day-old neonate with giant scalp abscess: A case report. Medicine (Baltimore). 2019;98(48):e17830. https://doi.org/10.1097/MD.0000000000017830.
10. Masson R, Jeong CY, Ma E, Crew AB, Fragoso NM, Shi VY, et al. Treatments for dissecting cellulitis of the scalp: a systematic review and treatment algorithm. Dermatol Ther (Heidelb). 2023; https://doi.org/10.1007/s13555-023-01018-7.
11. Nabri M, Alharbi M, Al-Sayyid A, Alabdrabalrasol K, Hassan K, Al-Jehani H. Sub-galeal abscess: a rare sequel of an infected scalp sebaceous cyst. Int J Surg Case Rep. 2020;76:30–2. https://doi.org/10.1016/j.ijscr.2020.09.063.
12. Salloum S, Sit W, Walton MM, Kamian K. Infected subgaleal hematoma in a 4-month-old girl. Am J Emerg Med. 2021;39:250.e5–6. https://doi.org/10.1016/j.ajem.2020.05.090.
13. Thadchanamoorthy V, Dayasiri K. Subgaleal abscess following Staphylococcal cellulitis in a 10-month-old child: a diagnostic challenge for the clinician. Cureus. 2021;13(1):e12591. https://doi.org/10.7759/cureus.12591.
14. Akhaddar A, Hall W, Boucetta M. Subgaleal and brain abscesses due to Salmonella enteritidis following craniotomy for giant cell glioblastoma multiforme: a case report and literature review. Surg Neurol Int. 2019;10:37. https://doi.org/10.25259/SNI-31-2019.
15. Demir MK, Yapıcıer O, Hasanov T, Yılmaz B, Kılıç T. Hydatid disease: MR imaging of calvarium and superior sagittal sinus involvement. Neuroradiol J. 2018;31(3):320–3. https://doi.org/10.1177/1971400918764130.
16. AlSarhan H, Jwery AK, Mohammed AA. Pott's puffy tumour of the frontal and Parietal bones with subgaleal abscess as a complication of acute sinusitis – a case report. J Pak Med Assoc. 2021;71(Suppl 8(12)):S170–3.
17. Prasad GL. Cranial melioidosis presenting as osteomyelitis and/or extra-axial abscess: literature review. World Neurosurg. 2020;134:67–75. https://doi.org/10.1016/j.wneu.2019.10.058.
18. Rohde RL, North LM, Murray M, Khalili S, Poetker DM. Pott's puffy tumor: a comprehensive review of the literature. Am J Otolaryngol. 2022;43(5):103529. https://doi.org/10.1016/j.amjoto.2022.103529.
19. Dawar P, Gupta DK, Sharma BS, Jyakumar A, Gamanagatti S. Extensive calvarial tuberculosis presenting as exophytic ulcerated growth on scalp in an infant: an interesting case report with review of literature. Childs Nerv Syst. 2013;29(7):1215–8. https://doi.org/10.1007/s00381-013-2097-5.
20. Staudt MD, Etarsky D, Ranger A. Infected cephalohematomas and underlying osteomyelitis: a case-based review. Childs Nerv Syst. 2016;32(8):1363–9. https://doi.org/10.1007/s00381-016-3084-4.
21. Cerveau T, Rossmann T, Clusmann H, Veldeman M. Infection-related failure of autologous *versus* allogenic cranioplasty after decompressive hemicraniectomy – a systematic review and meta-analysis. Brain Spine. 2023;3:101760. https://doi.org/10.1016/j.bas.2023.101760.
22. Sadhwani N, Garg K, Kumar A, Agrawal D, Singh M, Chandra PS, et al. Comparison of infection rates following immediate and delayed cranioplasty for postcraniotomy surgical site infections: results of a meta-analysis. World Neurosurg. 2023;173:167–175.e2. https://doi.org/10.1016/j.wneu.2023.01.084.

19 Inflammatory Lesions of the Scalp and Calvarium

Sophia Silas, Rajiv Mangla, Christine E. Fuller, and Satish Krishnamurthy

19.1 Introduction

Inflammatory lesions are injuries to the cells, tissues, and organs which results from the body's own immune system and its defenses. Lesions of this type are common in autoimmune diseases, where the body's immune system attacks itself in a hyperreactive manner. These lesions can also occur through bacterial, viral, and fungal infections and through idiopathic mechanisms that are not fully understood.

Lesions to the scalp and calvarium are obvious threats, as the scalp is the outermost barrier covering the muscles and calvarium below, while the calvarium protects the dura and the brain within. Therefore, any lesions to either structure could threaten the safety of the underlying anatomy. Both structures hold an additional aesthetic importance. Some lesions may require aggressive curettage as management for patient health. This can impact the visual structure of the head and face and thereby impact self-image and patient satisfaction with their treatment.

In this chapter, we briefly discuss some examples of common inflammatory lesions that affect the scalp and calvarium. The conditions we discuss are sarcoidosis, Langerhans cell histiocytosis, granulomas (both in general and briefly discussing mucormycosis and giant cell arteritis), psoriasis, and tinea capitis.

S. Silas (✉)
College of Medicine, State University of New York (SUNY) Upstate Medical University, Syracuse, NY, USA
e-mail: silass@upstate.edu

R. Mangla
Department of Radiology, State University of New York (SUNY) Upstate Medical University, Syracuse, NY, USA

C. E. Fuller
Department of Pathology, State University of New York (SUNY) Upstate Medical University, Syracuse, NY, USA

S. Krishnamurthy
Department of Neurosurgery, State University of New York (SUNY) Upstate Medical University, Syracuse, NY, USA

19.2 Sarcoidosis

19.2.1 Etiology

Sarcoidosis is a multisystem inflammatory disease. It is characterized by its hallmark pathology of noncaseating epithelioid cell granulomas that can develop in virtually all organ systems and tissues. These granulomas form alongside many multinucleated giant cells, which are surrounded by lymphocytes such as activated T helper 1 cells [1, 2].

The exact etiology of this disease is unknown. Current theories suggest that these granulomatous formations are an exaggerated immune response to an antigenic exposure, such as killed

M. Turgut et al. (eds.), *Lesions of the Scalp and Cranial Vault*,
https://doi.org/10.1007/978-3-031-88244-9_19

or partially degraded pathogens [3]. This exaggerated response could be made more likely through genetic factors. One example includes a human leukocyte antigen (HLA) gene allele called *DQB1*0602*, which has been shown to confer both increased susceptibility to sarcoidosis and predilection in radiographic progression of the disease [4]. Several studies [4, 5] have found an increased risk of sarcoidosis through family history, where having at least one first-degree relative with sarcoidosis increases an individual's risk of developing it by 3–3.7-fold.

19.2.2 Prevalence

Sarcoidosis affects both sexes, though most studies report women being affected more than men [4, 6, 7]. Incidence for sarcoidosis varies geographically, but it is roughly 16.5 per 100,000 men and 19 per 100,000 women [6]. The average age of those afflicted ranges from 25 to 40 for both sexes, with an increased risk in women over the age of 50 [3, 6, 8].

Black patients – especially females – are consistently reported to be most affected by sarcoidosis [4, 7, 8]. Black patients are more commonly diagnosed than white patients, with the relative rate of sarcoidosis in black patients compared to white patients being 4:1 [4]. The annual incidence of sarcoidosis ranges between 11 and 24 cases per 100,000 individuals per year in Scandinavian countries and at 18 and 71 cases per 100,000 individuals per year for African Americans [2]. Furthermore, black patients face more financial barriers, greater delays in seeking care, more new organ development, more hospitalizations, and worse outcomes when dealing with sarcoidosis [4]. All of this contributes to black patients (females in particular) having a greater mortality due to sarcoidosis than any other racial/ethnic group [2]. Explanations for these disparities center on the implicit racial bias built into the medical system, with physicians potentially discounting the symptoms of black patients and black patients potentially delaying care out of medical mistrust or discrimination [4].

19.2.3 Clinical Presentation

10–15% of patients present with sarcoidosis of the head and neck, affecting the skin, scalp, and/or bone [7]. Osseous involvement is less common than skin, with multiple studies [3, 8, 9] reporting widely varying rates of incidence ranging from 0.5 to 30%. The majority of osseous sarcoidosis presents asymptomatically, so it is typically discovered accidentally rather than because of the lesion(s) causing any major symptoms [3, 9]. Osseous lesions can occur in the skull, long bones, and axial skeleton. These lesions can be osteolytic, cystic, and/or punched out [8].

Skull involvement of sarcoidosis is very rare, but several cases of calvarial sarcoidosis have been reported. Lesions of the skull are typically osteolytic, usually multiple in number, and have well-demarcated margins [10]. These lesions are typically devoid of reactive or sclerotic alterations, and it is important to note that these lesions rarely cause permeative destruction of the bone [11]. Though osseous lesions are generally asymptomatic, calvarial sarcoidosis could manifest with headaches and tenderness over the vertex of the skull [9, 10]. The range of differential diagnoses for these types of lesions is extensive, encompassing multiple myeloma, metastatic bone disease, lymphoma, infections, and osseous hemangiomas [11].

Skin lesions from sarcoidosis can be categorized into "specific" and "nonspecific." Those that are "nonspecific" lack granulomas on biopsy. Lesions that are "specific" have noncaseating granulomas present in skin biopsies. "Specific" lesions are linked with worse results and pose more of a challenge when it comes to treatment. When the scalp is affected by sarcoidosis, it is considered an uncommon "specific" lesion. Most manifestations are papules and plaques. The papules are widely diffused, of a red-brown to purplish color, and are typically less than 1 cm in diameter. They are considered a sign of good prognosis of sarcoidosis, and these lesions often self-resolve without scarring. However, papules could also eventually progress into plaques, which have an ovular or circular shape with defined edges. Plaques are of similar coloration to the papules, firm to the touch, and occasionally scaly in texture. Patients with plaques are more likely to have a chronic disease course, and the lesions are more likely to cure with persistent scarring [6].

19.2.4 Management

Both partial and complete remission of sarcoid lesions can spontaneously occur in some cases [10]. Remission can occur within 2 years in 50% of patients. However, the chance of complete remission decreases if the disease course lasts more than 5 years [2]. For those who do not achieve a spontaneous remission, treatment focuses on mitigating or preventing further damage. Choice in therapy depends on disease presentation and severity.

For cutaneous involvement alone, monthly intralesional triamcinolone injections are effective. Regularly applied topical treatments such as corticosteroids or a hydrocolloid occlusive dressing can also be used [6].

The first-line therapy for severe sarcoidosis is the use of systemic corticosteroids, which may reduce formation of granulomas or soft tissue edema. This treatment course is indicated for bone involvement since osseous manifestations occur in advanced and chronic forms of the disease. However, there are no firm guidelines for dosage or timeline of treatment [3].

In the cases of refractory or chronic and active sarcoidosis, corticosteroids should be used in conjunction with at least one steroid-sparing agent. If these options fail, alternative immunosuppressants or TNF-α antagonists can be considered [2]. Ongoing research focuses on the use of TNF-α antagonists because TNF-α seems to play a key role in the pathogenesis of sarcoidosis. However, one study [7] noted that a patient treated with adalimumab, a TNF-α antagonist, for psoriatic arthritis then developed sarcoidosis of the hypopharynx. The patient's sarcoidosis was resolved upon discontinuation of the drug. Other studies [2] have noted similar cases, where TNF-α antagonists may have induced sarcoid-like diseases.

In cases where granuloma formation threatens vital structures, surgical intervention can become necessary [7]. This can occur in end-stage disease when major organs, such as the heart or lungs, are failing due to loss of function and the patient requires a transplant [2].

19.3 Langerhans Cell Histiocytosis

19.3.1 Etiology

Langerhans cell histiocytosis (LCH), formerly known as histiocytosis X, is a rare disease with great variation in clinical presentation. It has been classified into three major syndromes: eosinophilic granuloma, Hand-Schüller-Christian's disease, and Letterer-Siwe disease. It can also present as a fourth rarer syndrome, known as Hashimoto-Pritzker syndrome [12, 13].

LCH and all of its subcategorical syndromes are characterized by the clonal proliferation of Langerhans cells (Fig. 19.1a). These cells are a key component of the immune system because they express a variety of surface markers that assist in the immune response [14, 15]. The markers, such as CD1a (Fig. 19.1b), S100, and CD207 (langerin), can be used to confirm a diagnosis of LCH alongside clinical presentation and history [16]. Birbeck granules, visible on electron microscopy, were historically the gold standard for diagnosing LCH and are still used for identification [17].

In LCH, these cells undergo unregulated, clonal proliferation. They subsequently accumulate in various tissues, such as the bones, skin, and lungs [14, 18]. The exact cause of this uncontrolled proliferation is unknown. Older theories posit an infectious cause, where the accumulation of Langerhans cells is an overexaggerated immune response to some unknown antigen [15]. However, no offending organism has been isolated [14]. One study [16] did suggest the possibility of Epstein-Barr viral infection (EBV) being a potential causative agent in some cases of LCH. They noted several case studies of simultaneous EBV infection and LCH manifestation, in

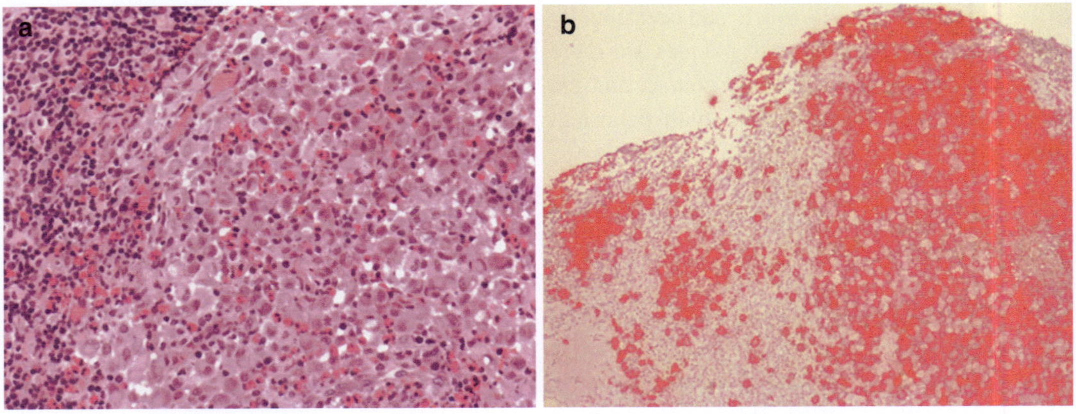

Fig. 19.1 (**a**) Photomicrograph of typical Langerhans cell histiocytosis lesion composed of a mixture of small mature lymphocytes, eosinophils, and Langerhans cells with abundant pink cytoplasm and irregular-shaped nuclei. (**b**) Langerhans cells are strongly positive with immunostain targeting CD1a (red stain)

which the patients went into remission of their LCH upon treatment of their EBV infections through antiviral therapy.

More recently, several oncogenic mutations, such as *BRAF V600E* and *MAP2K1*, have been identified in a majority of cases of LCH [19–22]. The presence of the *BRAF* mutation was seen in 57% of LCH cases [21, 22]. This discovery supports the more recent stance that LCH should be reframed a myeloid neoplasm rather than a disease of only autoimmune origins – a stance which the Histiocyte Society also supports [22]. In 2021, the National Comprehensive Cancer Network published clinical guidelines classifying LCH as a histiocytic neoplasm. Thus, LCH could be considered a type of cancer with inflammatory qualities and symptoms [23].

19.3.2 Prevalence

LCH has an annual incidence of around two to five cases per 1 million children [20, 22, 24], though one study [25] states higher range at five to ten cases per million children. LCH most often affects children under the age of 15, and it is slightly more prevalent in males than females [14, 22]. LCH among adults has an incidence of one to two cases per 1 million [20, 24, 25], though this lower incidence may be due to underdiagnosis [22].

Registry studies of LCH report that in comparison to non-Hispanic populations, there is increased incidence in Hispanic populations [19, 25]. One possible explanation for this is that the germline *SMAD6* variant, which is associated with increased risk of LCH, is present in higher rates in Hispanic populations than in non-Hispanic populations [25].

19.3.3 Clinical Presentation

The sites most commonly affected by LCH include the bone, lung, skin, liver, and central nervous system [14]. Of bone involvement, the skull is one of the most frequent sites of lesions, as well as the mandible, spine, and pelvis [18].

Current classifications of LCH depend on location, number of lesions, and risk of organ involvement. Therefore, LCH can be classified as single system or multisystem, unifocal or multifocal within a single system, and risk of organ involvement [24]. In clinical presentation, there are three classic syndromes of LCH and an additional less common presentation. The classic syndromes are eosinophilic granuloma (unifocal), Hand-Schüller-Christian disease (multisystemic), and Letterer-Siwe disease (disseminated) [20]. Hashimoto-Pritzker syndrome (unifocal or multifocal, congenital) is an additional and rare presentation [17]. Due to the clinical variation in the syndromes of LCH, each will be discussed independently in respect to more specified prevalence, presentation, and symptoms.

19.3.3.1 Eosinophilic Granuloma

Eosinophilic granuloma is a benign manifestation of LCH. It is the most common subtype, representing 60–80% of LCH cases [13]. It is limited to the bones or lungs, and it is commonly found in children younger than 15 years of age. Osseous lesions are usually asymptomatic, but they could present with pain, swelling, or deformity [15].

The calvarium is frequently affected [14], and lesions most commonly occur in the parietal or frontal regions (Fig. 19.2) [10]. These lesions typically have sharp borders, giving it a characteristic "punched-out" appearance with beveled edges due to unequal involvement of the inner and outer tables of the skull [10, 14, 15]. Some lesions may present with a "button sequestrum," in which the center of the osteolytic lesion has a residual piece of intact bone in the center. Lesions may have permeative and aggressive bone destruction and mimic malignant tumors of the skull [10]. Patients with skull involvement can experience headache, limitation of motion, localizing pain and swelling, hearing loss, and more [20].

19.3.3.2 Hand-Schüller-Christian Disease

Hand-Schüller-Christian disease is a chronic form of LCH with variable prognosis. It is commonly associated with skull lesions, diabetes insipidus, and exophthalmos. About 15–20% of cases of LCH are classified as Hand-Schüller-Christian disease [14]. It typically occurs in children under 10 years of age, though it can present in adults. Males are affected more commonly than females [15].

This subtype is characterized by multiple bone lesions that mostly occur in the skull or vertebral bodies. Calvarial lesions present in over 60% of patients affected by Hand-Schüller-Christian

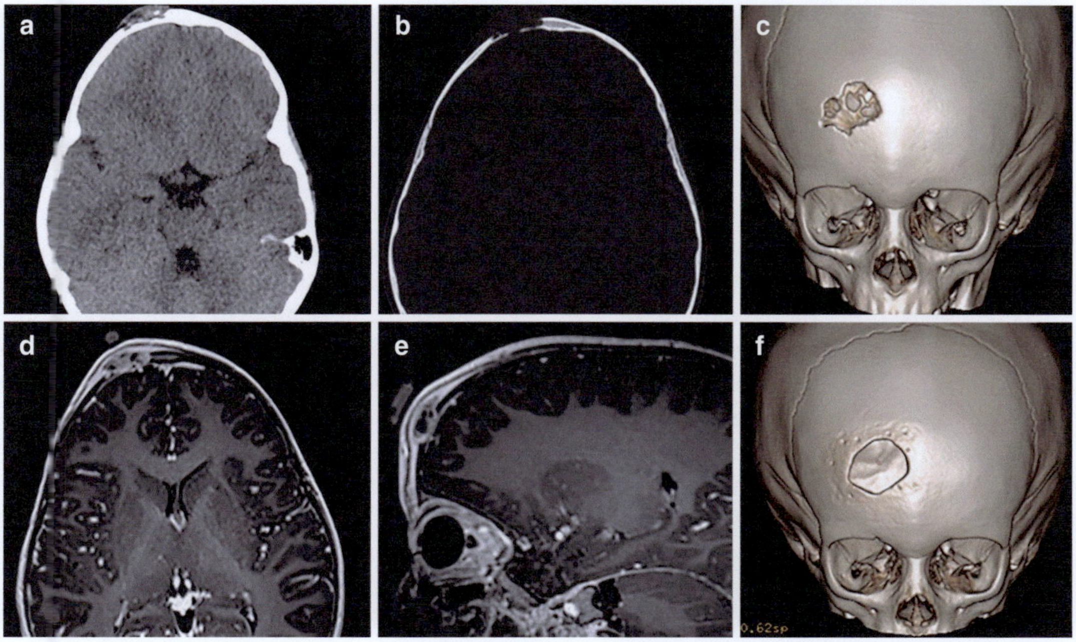

Fig. 19.2 32-month-old female who presented with a bump in right forehead with local pain. Axial CT soft tissue (**a**), axial CT bone window (**b**), and 3D volume rendering images (**c**) show a lytic lesion in the right frontal bone. Post-contrast T1 axial and sagittal images (**d** and **e**) show enhancement and involvement of underlying dura. Patient underwent elective resection and reconstruction with cranioplasty and duroplasty (**f**). Patient has recovered well and remained disease-free

disease. These lesions are frequently multiple in number and can cause injury to the underlying neural tissue. The skin can also be affected, as a scaly seborrheic rash can present at hair lines, hands, and feet [15].

19.3.3.3 Letterer-Siwe Disease

Letterer-Siwe disease is the most aggressive form of LCH and the least common of the classic syndromes, representing less than 10% of cases of LCH [14]. Patients affected are typically less than 2 years of age, and males are affected more commonly than females [15]. It presents with multi-organ involvement. Organs involved include bone marrow, lymph nodes, skin, liver, spleen, and gastrointestinal tract [14]. Most patients present with multiple destructive lesions in the skull. These lesions can be accompanied with brain damage, and the skin can develop a widespread, papular, and crusting hemorrhagic rash [15].

19.3.3.4 Hashimoto-Pritzker Syndrome

Hashimoto-Pritzker syndrome, also called congenital self-healing reticulohistiocytosis (CSHR), is a rare, benign, and congenital manifestation of LCH [17]. It manifests as self-resolving skin lesions during the newborn period in an otherwise healthy infant [17, 26, 27]. Underreporting of this disease may occur and contribute to its rarity, because spontaneous resolution often occurs before a dermatologist can assess the lesions [27].

Skin lesions from Hashimoto-Pritzker syndrome can be congenital or appear within days or weeks of birth. The skin lesions present as multiple red-brown papules, nodules, or vesicles that can occur anywhere on the body [17]. Though they are typically multiple, singular lesions comprise approximately 30% of cases of Hashimoto-Pritzker syndrome [26]. The lesions spontaneously resolve within several months of presentation, though self-healing may be accelerated by biopsy [26]. After healing, they may leave behind post-inflammatory hyperpigmentation [17].

19.3.4 Management

In some cases LCH can resolve spontaneously [14]. For cases which do not spontaneously resolve, the type of management depends on the site and extent of disease involvement. More conservative treatment can be used for less severe disease manifestations, and asymptomatic patients may be kept under observation until the disease worsens [12].

Unifocal bone lesions that are easily accessible can be treated with steroid injection and/or curettage. When using curettage, LCH does not require a complete excision with clean margins. Aggressive surgical excision can be associated with prolonged healing and deformity [25], especially with larger lesions [13]. Limited curettage of the skull usually results in resolved lesions without the need of prostheses [28]. Therefore, it is recommended to avoid surgical excision in lesions >5 cm in children [13].

For multifocal bone manifestations or lesions involving CNS sites, systemic chemotherapy is typically required. Due to the aggressive nature of these manifestations, risk of disease recurrence and risk of invasion into neurological tissue is increased [13]. Though there are no official or standard treatments, initial therapy for pediatric patients typically uses vinblastine/prednisone [24]. Though this combination can be tolerated in pediatric populations and is typically a first-line therapy, it may have higher toxicity in adult patients and therefore may not be an option [25, 28]. More recent studies [13] have reported less toxicity and lower recurrence in patients treated with cytarabine or cladribine, along with high overall response rates [28].

Adult patients face challenges in management, as there is currently no standard of care for multisystem disease management for adult patients with LCH. Because of this, ongoing research is looking into the use of targeted therapies specifically for adult patients. Early adult trials of MAPK pathway-directed targeted therapy with gene inhibition of BRAFV600E or MEK have found near complete high response rates among patients regardless of site of disease [25, 28]. However, these targeted therapies do not appear to be curative, as patients almost universally relapse with cessation of therapy [25].

There are no current guidelines regarding surgical treatment for multifocal bone lesions or lesions involving CNS sites. Surgical excision has been used for accessible lesions that invaded the dura or compressed brain matter, while systemic chemotherapy was used as an alternative if excision was not possible [13].

19.4 Granulomas

19.4.1 Etiology

Granulomas are aggregations of immune cells that sequester specific, persistent stimuli with the goal of "walling off" the stimuli. Initially, an inflammatory trigger sets off the body's immune system. This inflammatory trigger can be either infectious or noninfectious. Infectious granulomas can be caused by bacteria and fungi, while noninfectious granulomas can be the product of autoimmune diseases (such as sarcoidosis, as previously discussed), neoplasia, and foreign bodies, such as sutures or biomedical implants [29].

An individual macrophage will attempt to phagocytize the offending stimulus, but it will fail to do so. Upon its failure, different immune cells such as additional macrophages, epithelioid cells, and multinucleated giant cells, aggregate into marked, focal lesions surrounding the stimulus – a granuloma [30]. By creating granulomas, the immune cells can "wall off" the offending stimuli from the rest of the body and potentially mitigate further damage [31].

Granuloma macrophages can undergo further morphological changes as the disease/stimulus progresses, which may have effects on histological presentation. They can undergo epithelioid transformation, in which adjacent immune cells link together through interdigitating membranes, or they can become foam cells by accumulating oxidized lipids [29, 32]. The granulomas can also form multinucleated giant cells by fusing their membranes [29, 30, 32].

Moreover, granulomas can undergo morphological changes that affect clinical presentation. They can undergo necrosis, in which tissue death occurs within the granuloma [30]. Necrosis does not develop in all granulomas, even when they become large – such as those caused by sarcoidosis or Crohn's disease. Other granuloma-causing diseases, such as tuberculosis or other infectious agents, do undergo necrosis. The exact reason for this difference in necrosis and its manifestation is not currently understood [29, 32].

Granulomas can also undergo fibrosis, which occurs when an excessive amount of connective tissue is constructed [32]. This overgrowth of connective tissue can lead to permanent widespread loss of tissue function [30]. Both the loss of tissue function and the enduring damage of fibrosis is evident in both sarcoidosis and tuberculosis, where fibrosis in the lungs can reduce respiratory function [29, 32].

We will briefly discuss two examples of granulomatous diseases – one infectious and one noninfectious (not counting sarcoidosis, a noninfectious granulomatous disease which we have discussed above). These examples are mucormycosis, also called zygomycosis, and giant cell arteritis. For readers interested in some additional granulomatous conditions that can affect the scalp and/or calvarium, see reference Table 19.1.

19.4.1.1 Mucormycosis

Mucormycosis – also called zygomycosis – is a rare and infectious granulomatous disease. It is one of the most rapidly progressive and lethal forms of fungal infections in humans, with a mortality rate of around 25–62% in its rhino-orbital-cerebral form and 25% in its cutaneous form. Patients who have uncontrolled diabetes mellitus or are immunosuppressed are at much higher risk of infection [43].

Primary cutaneous mucormycosis, one of several clinical subtypes of mucormycosis infections, has a rapid and acute course. Infection can occur through direct inoculation through areas of trauma. When deep invasion of tissue occurs, the infection can spread to underlying muscles, tendons, and bone [43].

Table 19.1 Brief overview of additional granulomatous conditions of the scalp and/or calvarium with references provided for interested readers

Disease	Etiology	Clinical presentation	Management	References
Chronic granulomatous disease	Primary immunodeficiency due to a mutation of NADPH oxidase that results in recurrent bacterial and fungal infections and excessive inflammatory reactions	Infections can affect the skin, airways, lymph nodes, liver, brain, and bones. Chronic inflammatory cell reactions of lymphocytes and histiocytes can result in granuloma formation anywhere in the body	Early and aggressive use of parenteral antibiotics or antifungal therapy should be started if infection is suspected, even before culture results are available. Surgical drainage and/or excision of abscesses are usually necessary	[33–35]
Granuloma annulare	Unknown but thought to have an immunologic mechanism with precipitating factors such as physical trauma, insect bites, drugs, and sunburn	Isolated papules and plaques of the scalp. Subcutaneous variant is typically non- or slightly mobile nodules. Biopsy may show necrobiosis surrounded by palisading histiocytes, with mucin deposition and degraded collagen	Lesions can regress over time if left alone, yet they can also reoccur. Topical and intralesional corticosteroids are first-line therapies, though phototherapy is an additional option	[33, 36–38]
Inflammatory pseudotumor (also named in literature as plasma cell granuloma, inflammatory myofibroblastic tumor, histiocytoma, xanthoma, etc.)	Unknown. Trauma, foreign bodies, and infections, such as *actinomyces* and EBV, have been suggested as potential factors	Potentially tender enlarging mass(es) that can extend into deeper structures anywhere in the body. Biopsy may show spindle cells, plasma cells, and lymphocytes	Some lesions can spontaneously regress. Treatment consists of corticosteroids, surgical resection, or a combination of both	[39–42]

Cutaneous infection of the scalp is rare but has been noted in the past. It typically manifests as a necrotic eschar tissue, surrounded by erythema and infiltration [44]. The lesions progressively become necrotic in a matter of days if untreated, and they often progress to necrotizing fasciitis [43]. Gangrene formation may occur in longer durations of infection [44].

The first choice of treatment is amphotericin-B, which is highly effective against cutaneous mucormycosis [43, 44]. Other drugs, such as posaconazole or isavuconazole, could be considered as step-down therapies or salvage therapies [43]. Surgical debridement of all necrotic tissue is necessary to treat the disease and is known to improve survival. Moreover, repeated debridements are required to keep a clean and viable surgical margin, which increases the effectiveness of antifungal therapy [43].

19.4.1.2 Giant Cell Arteritis

Giant cell arteritis (GCA) is a form of autoimmune systemic vasculitis that presents with granulomatous inflammation of large and medium-sized vessels. Its etiology is unknown, though age, genetics, and infections have been proposed causes [45, 46]. Reports of prevalence [45, 46] range from 30.4 to 50 per 100,000 people. It primarily affects middle-aged individuals with a peak incidence over the age of 70 years. Non-Hispanic Caucasians are affected most often, and there is a gender predilection with a female-to-male ratio of 2:1 in the Caucasian population [45].

GCA primarily affects the medium and large arteries. Histologically, they present with granulomas composed of epithelioid cells, lymphocytes, and multinucleated giant cells (Fig. 19.3) [45]. These inflammatory manifestations typically occur in branches of the external carotid arteries [46].

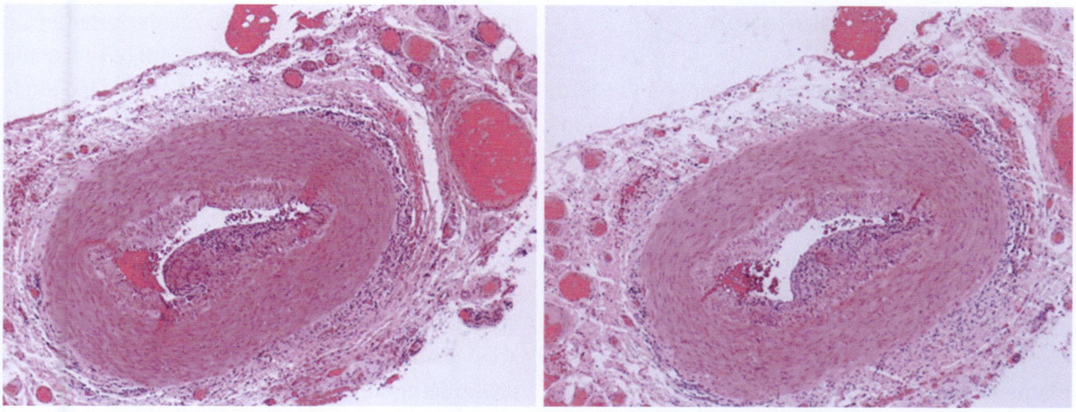

Fig. 19.3 Photomicrograph of cross section of temporal artery with multilayer inflammatory infiltrative including few multinucleated giant cells within intima. Note also associated fragmentation of the internal elastic lamina

Most clinical presentations of GCA are new-onset headache in the temporal region, tenderness upon palpation of the temporal artery, jaw claudication, scalp tenderness, and allodynia [45, 47]. Reports of patients affected by permanent loss of vision range from 10 to 30% [46, 47]. Necrosis of the scalp can occur in severe GCA, and it is considered a poor prognosis that is associated with high rates of mortality ranging from 20.2 to 38% [46].

The treatment of choice for GCA is corticosteroid therapy. However, abrupt exacerbation of GCA symptoms can be seen in 30–50% of cases even with ongoing corticosteroid therapy [45]. When there is a strong suspicion of GCA, it is recommended to start glucocorticoids immediately in order to prevent irreversible damage to vision. Biologic agents such as TNF blockers, rituximab, and ustekinumab are currently under investigation through several small clinical trials with varying results. So far, only tocilizumab has shown effectiveness at decreasing relapses and steroid use and has thus been FDA approved for use in GCA [47].

19.5 Psoriasis

19.5.1 Etiology

Psoriasis is a common inflammatory skin disease that typically affects the scalp. It is a polygenic disorder that can be triggered by a variety of factors, such as physical trauma (e.g., surgical incisions), streptococcal infections, some medications (e.g., anti-cytokine therapy), and smoking [48, 49].

There is a genetic predisposition to psoriasis. Many psoriasis susceptibility loci (*PSORS*) have been identified, such as one predominant risk gene called HLA-C*06:02. A meta-analysis found more than 1000 genes were differently expressed in lesioned psoriatic skin compared to unlesioned skin [48]. One example of altered gene expression includes an increased expression of Janus kinase (JAK) signal transducer and activated transcription (STAT) pathway in psoriatic lesions [50].

19.5.2 Prevalence

Worldwide, the prevalence of psoriasis is 2–3%, though it tends to be higher in Scandinavian populations and lower in some areas of Asia and Africa [48]. Though psoriasis can manifest at any age, patients commonly present with psoriasis prior to 35 years of age. Furthermore, the prevalence of psoriasis increases with age. There is no clear agreement on whether psoriasis has a gender predilection, as one meta-analysis found [51].

19.5.3 Clinical Presentation

Psoriatic lesions can occur anywhere on the skin, though almost 80% of patients experience lesions on the scalp [50]. The scalp is the first site of involvement in up to 25% of patients [52]. Of all patients with scalp psoriasis, 81% can experience scalp lesions for more than 5 years, and 48% can experience lesions affecting more than half of the entire scalp area [49]. Scalp psoriasis is characterized by demarcated chronic erythematous plaques covered by silver-white scales [48, 49]. The lesions can advance from the scalp and onto the face [49].

Psoriatic lesions can demonstrate intense scaling and persistent pruritus, which impairs quality of life for many patients [50]. Furthermore, lesions in visible areas such as the scalp can cause significant psychological stress to the patient [50] and adversely affects the quality of life [52]. Around 31% of patients with scalp psoriasis have indicated distress due to the condition [49], and the prevalence of depression, anxiety, and suicidality is increased in patients with psoriasis [48].

19.5.4 Management

When treating scalp psoriasis, topical corticosteroids are the first choice for treatment for short-term use. Other treatments, such as coal tar shampoos and salicylic acid, are also commonly used [49, 52]. Systemic treatments are only used in treatment-resistant cases [49]. These treatments can include biologic agents, which current research has been focusing on. One group of agents is TNF-α inhibitors, such as adalimumab. Adalimumab is the first fully human monoclonal antibody to inhibit TNF-α through binding to TNF-α and preventing interaction with its receptor. Adalimumab has been effective at treating scalp psoriasis, demonstrating a significant reduction in pruritus and improvement in symptoms [50].

Paradoxically, TNF-α inhibitors may actually induce new-onset or worse manifestations of psoriasis in some patients. This effect is independent of underlying disease and can resolve after termination of treatment. The mechanism of this manifestation is not fully understood [48]. One study [53] noted that, regardless of presence of history of psoriasis, some patients (mostly females) had developed psoriatic lesions when treating inflammatory bowel disease with TNF-α inhibitors such as adalimumab.

TNF-α inhibitors may potentially be associated with other complications, outside of psoriatic manifestation. TNF-α is an important pro-inflammatory cytokine that helps defend against infections and has anti-tumor activity [48]. Therefore, use of TNF-α inhibitors can increase risk of opportunistic infections of bacterial, viral, or fungal origins [54]. TNF-α inhibitors are associated with increased risk of activation of latent tuberculosis infection, and tuberculosis associated with TNF-α inhibitors is more likely to be life-threatening [48].

The development of brain abscesses in patients treated with adalimumab has been reported in case studies. One such case study [54] found that a patient with psoriatic arthritis being treated with adalimumab developed a brain abscess in the left frontal lobe of the brain. This abscess was discovered 2 days after the patient's third injection of adalimumab, in which the patient had an episode of sudden-onset general convulsions. The patient had no history of neurosurgeries or brain trauma, and it was suspected that the brain abscess had originated from an untreated dental infection. After undergoing a left frontal craniotomy and abscess drainage, along with systemic antibiotics, the patient developed drug rash with eosinophilia and systemic symptoms (DRESS), of which adalimumab has been reported as an inciting factor. After switching the patient's systemic antibiotics, they recovered and reported no neurological signs, though a follow-up MRI did reveal residual granulomatous tissue. A second case study [55] reported a similar manifestation, in which a patient treated with adalimumab for Crohn's disease developed a brain abscess in the left temporal lobe after starting the medication 17 days prior to admission.

These case studies are not a definitive confirmation that adalimumab is linked with brain abscesses. However, this increase in opportunistic infections should be kept in consideration for patients being treated with TNF-α inhibitors, particularly those presenting with altered mental status or neurological signs [55]. This holds especially true for patients being treated with TNF-α inhibitors after neurosurgery or penetrating head trauma, as both are predisposing factors for brain abscesses [54]. Moreover, additional investigations and research are necessary to fully understand the mechanisms of TNF-α inhibitors and any potential side effects they could elicit [48].

19.6 Tinea Capitis

19.6.1 Etiology

Tinea capitis, known commonly as ringworm, is a fungal infection most commonly caused by *Trichophyton tonsurans* and *Microsporum canis*. It is a dermatophyte, meaning that it is a fungus that requires keratin for growth. As such, it affects the scalp, eyelashes, and eyebrows [56]. The introduction of griseofulvin and public health interventions brought infection under control in Europe and North America in the mid-twentieth century, but cases have risen in these areas in the last 10–20 years [57, 58].

There are many predisposing factors to tinea capitis infection. Some factors include poor hygiene, crowded living conditions, immunodeficiency, household exposure, and lower socioeconomic status [59, 60]. These predisposing factors have resulted in tinea capitis being labeled as a "poor person's disease," thus creating long-lasting stigma about the disease [58].

19.6.2 Prevalence

Tinea capitis occurs worldwide. It most commonly affects children. Adults and infants can also be affected, though much less commonly. Reports of prevalence ranges from 6 months to 12 years of age [57], with peak incidence between 3–7 years of age [56, 59]. In the United States, the prevalence in prepubertal children ranges from 3 to 8% [56]. Reports vary over whether there is a gender predilection in the pediatric population [59]. In adults, tinea capitis is more common in females [56].

Tinea capitis is a disease that has frequently and historically become an epidemic. This can be noted in immigrant children who arrived on Ellis Island in the 1900s, children in France and Russia between the 1930s and 1950s, and children in Morocco in the 1950s [58]. Cases of tinea capitis have risen in the last 10–20 years [57]. However, the exact incidence of tinea capitis epidemics currently ongoing throughout the world cannot be accurately noted, as the disease is not commonly reported to public health agencies [58].

19.6.3 Clinical Presentation

Tinea capitis can be classified as noninflammatory or inflammatory. Noninflammatory is typically less severe and less painful. Inflammatory, also known as kerion, can be very painful and visually concerning [56].

Histologically, noninflammatory tinea capitis presents with spores and/or hyphae within or surrounding the hair shafts, fungi within stratum corneum, and a perifollicular mononuclear infiltrate in the dermis. Multinucleated giant cells can be present in the dermis if the hair follicles are disrupted. Kerion presents with a perifollicular inflammatory infiltrate with spongiosis [56]. In the early phases, kerion has infiltrates of neutrophils, lymphocytes, and plasma cells, while the later phases have fibrotic scars [56, 59].

Clinically, noninflammatory tinea capitis typically manifests as fine scaling, with single/multiple scaly plaques of circular alopecia, diffuse or patchy fine, white scaling of the scalp, or single/multiple plaques of well-demarcated areas of alopecia with broken-off hairs at the scalp surface [56]. Kerion initially presents as a painful, suppurative folliculitis that can cover all or most of the scalp, though it usually manifests in the occipital region [56, 59]. It then progresses to diffuse, patchy alopecia with scattered pustules or low-grade folliculitis, a painful indurated lesion, or a painful and suppurative boggy edematous plaque, with pustules, thick crusting, or nodules [56].

19.6.4 Management

The first-choice treatment for tinea capitis is oral antifungal agents, such as griseofulvin, terbinafine, itraconazole, and fluconazole [56, 57, 60]. Topical antifungal agents alone are not recommended, as they cannot penetrate deep enough to the root of the hair follicles [56]. They can, however, be used as adjuvant therapy to oral antifungals so as to potentially increase the cure rate, decrease shedding, and reduce risk of transmission [56]. Surgical drainage of kerion should not be performed [56, 59].

Oral antifungal agents, specifically griseofulvin, were only introduced in 1959. Prior to this, radiation therapy to remove hair followed by topical antimycotic ointments was the standard treatment for tinea capitis [58, 61, 62]. The Keinback-Adamson method was widely used, in which the scalp was divided into five regions with one or two regions irradiated each day [58, 62]. In the twentieth century, radiation therapy was used in several tinea capitis elimination campaigns worldwide. Israel, between 1946 and 1960, used ionizing radiation to treat around 17,000 children. Yugoslavia, in the 1950s, used radiation therapy to treat around 50,000 children, aged 5–15 years [58].

Though not known immediately at the time of these elimination campaigns, we now know that radiation is associated with late-occurring, deleterious health outcomes, such as inducing cancer years after treatment was first administered [58]. There is a latency period between use of radiation therapy and the appearance of neoplasms. Reports of the length of this period vary among sources, though most range between 4 and 47 years [58, 61]. These long-term effects of radiation can be seen now in elderly populations.

Many studies [61–64] have reported radiation-induced meningiomas, sarcomas, and glioblastomas in elderly patients who were treated for tinea capitis in their childhood. Some of these patients, at the time of presentation, ranged in age from 56 to 78 years [62, 64]. Radiation therapy for tinea capitis has a higher prevalence of calvarial tumors than other locations of the skull. This is due to the radiation being directed primarily to the scalp rather than the skull base [62].

These late-developing neoplasms can be seen especially in patients originating in countries where mass tinea capitis elimination campaigns occurred. For example, within the Israeli population, a retrospective cohort study found a 9.5-fold increase in meningioma incidence in patients treated with radiation therapy [62].

Though radiation therapy for tinea capitis has not been used in decades, physicians should still maintain vigilance for the late-term deleterious effects – cancer especially – caused by radiation when treating elderly patients who were treated for tinea capitis in their childhood [58]. This holds especially true for patients originating in countries where mass elimination campaigns occurred, such as Israel [63] or Serbia [58]. In 2023, patients from these areas presenting with neoplasm will most likely range from 70 to 90 years of age [58].

19.7 Conclusion

In this chapter, we have briefly discussed a variety of common inflammatory lesions of the scalp and calvarium. Sarcoidosis is characterized by epithelioid cell granulomas that can affect virtually any organ system, with people of African descent facing a greater burden than Caucasians. Lesions of the skull present as sclerotic/osteolytic, cystic, and/or punched out, while lesions of the scalp can be "specific" or "nonspecific." Some cases can spontaneously resolve, though corticosteroids are largely the medication of choice for those which persist. TNF-α antagonists are also a choice, though their paradoxical effects on sarcoidosis need more research.

Historically, LCH has been known as a hyperactive immune response, though recent studies propose reclassifying it as a neoplasm. It is a disease with a broad range of clinical subtypes, ranging from benign and affecting only neonates to severe multisystemic manifestations. Therefore, treatments vary, with some cases necessitating a "wait-and-see" approach and others requiring systemic chemotherapy or curettage.

Granulomas manifest in too many diseases to count, and they act as a last-ditch effort to wall off offending stimuli that macrophages cannot phagocytize. Granulomas are commonly differentiated between whether they are necrotizing or non-necrotizing and whether they have fibrosis. Mucormycosis is a highly lethal fungal infection that manifests with necrotizing granulomas, and giant cell arteritis is a type of autoimmune systemic vasculitis that primarily affects the large and medium vessels, such as those in the scalp.

Psoriasis is a common and well-known inflammatory lesion of the skin that commonly affects the scalp. Many different medications have been tested on psoriasis, with TNF-α inhibitors such as adalimumab being one. This medication has been associated with paradoxical affects, such as causing new manifestations of psoriasis in patients with no personal or family history of it. It has also been noted in several cases of brain abscesses, causing some concern over its usage.

Tinea capitis, commonly referred to as "ringworm," is an inflammatory lesion of the scalp. It is common in the pediatric population, though historical efforts at eradication have lessened its burden. Notably, past eradication attempts focused on use of radiation therapy, which is associated with late-term neoplasm development. The elderly population, especially those hailing from countries that went through epidemics and subsequent elimination campaigns, should be watched for these late-term manifestations.

This discussion is not all-encompassing but rather is meant to give a brief overview of some of the most common inflammatory lesions of the scalp and calvaria. For those interested in a deeper look into the conditions we have discussed as well as less common inflammatory lesions, you will find useful additional information in our references.

References

1. Sreeja C, Priyadarshini A, Premika, Nachiammai N. Sarcoidosis – a review article. J Oral Maxillofac Pathol. 2022;26(2):242–53.
2. Franzen DP, Brutsche M, Nilsson J, Böni C, Daccord C, Distler O, et al. Sarcoidosis – a multisystem disease. Swiss Med Wkly. 2022;152:w30049.
3. Kucharz EJ. Osseous manifestations of sarcoidosis. Reumatologia. 2020;58(2):93–100.
4. Hena KM. Sarcoidosis epidemiology: race matters. Front Immunol. 2020;11:537382.
5. Spagnolo P, Maier LA. Genetics in sarcoidosis. Curr Opin Pulm Med. 2021;27(5):423–9.
6. Koneti J, Cherukuri SP, Gadde S, Kalluru R, Chikatimalla R, Dasaradhan T. Sarcoidosis and its dermatological manifestations: a narrative review. Cureus. 14(8):e28053.
7. Badhey AK, Kadakia S, Carrau RL, Iacob C, Khorsandi A. Sarcoidosis of the head and neck. Head Neck Pathol. 2014;9(2):260–8.
8. Sève P, Pacheco Y, Durupt F, Jamilloux Y, Gerfaud-Valentin M, Isaac S, et al. Sarcoidosis: a clinical overview from symptoms to diagnosis. Cells. 2021;10(4):766.
9. Landsberger D, Rav'e D, Friedman G. The skull in chronic sarcoidosis. Postgrad Med J. 1988;64(757):875–7.
10. Gomez CK, Schiffman SR, Bhatt AA. Radiological review of skull lesions. Insights Imaging. 2018;9(5):857–82.
11. Thirunavukarasu V, Thirunavukarasu C, Willis T, Tsahtsarlis A. Osseous sarcoidosis with a solitary lytic skull lesion: a case report. J Neurol Surg Rep. 2019;80(2):e27–9.
12. Kumar YP, Agrawal J, Mohanlakshmi J, Kumar PS. Langerhans cell histiocytosis revisited: case report with review. Contemp Clin Dent. 2015;6(3):432–6.
13. Lam S, Reddy GD, Mayer R, Lin Y, Jea A. Eosinophilic granuloma/Langerhans cell histiocytosis: pediatric neurosurgery update. Surg Neurol Int. 2015;6(Suppl 17):S435–9.
14. Azouz EM, Saigal G, Rodriguez MM, Podda A. Langerhans' cell histiocytosis: pathology, imaging and treatment of skeletal involvement. Pediatr Radiol. 2005;35(2):103–15.
15. Hoover KB, Rosenthal DI, Mankin H. Langerhans cell histiocytosis. Skeletal Radiol. 2007;36(2):95–104.
16. Foster KW, Robinson SK, Tung-Hahn E, Gibbons G, Cruse CW, Mudaliar K, et al. Multifocal Langerhans cell histiocytosis: a unique presentation of eosinophilic granuloma with intracranial extension, massive lymphadenopathy, and Epstein-Barr viral infection in an adolescent female. Case Rep Dermatol. 2021;13(1):28–35.

17. Lee YH, Talekar MK, Chung CG, Bell MD, Zaenglein AL. Congenital self-healing reticulohistiocytosis. J Clin Aesthet Dermatol. 2014;7(2):49–53.
18. Zhong WQ, Jiang L, Ma QJ, Liu ZJ, Liu XG, Wei F, et al. Langerhans cell histiocytosis of the atlas in an adult. Eur Spine J. 2010;19(1):19–22.
19. Ribeiro KB, Degar B, Antoneli CBG, Rollins B, Rodriguez-Galindo C. Ethnicity, race, and socioeconomic status influence incidence of Langerhans cell histiocytosis. Pediatr Blood Cancer. 2015;62(6):982–7.
20. Reisi N, Raeissi P, Harati Khalilabad T, Moafi A. Unusual sites of bone involvement in Langerhans cell histiocytosis: a systematic review of the literature. Orphanet J Rare Dis. 2021;16:1.
21. Badalian-Very G, Vergilio JA, Degar BA, MacConaill LE, Brandner B, Calicchio ML, et al. Recurrent BRAF mutations in Langerhans cell histiocytosis. Blood. 2010;116(11):1919–23.
22. Allen CE, Merad M, McClain KL. Langerhans-cell histiocytosis. N Engl J Med. 2018;379(9):856–68.
23. Langerhans cell histiocytosis in children | Histiocytosis Association [Internet]. 2020 [cited 2023 Jun 1]. https://histio.org/histiocytic-disorders/langerhans-cell-histiocytosis-in-children/
24. Kobayashi M, Tojo A. Langerhans cell histiocytosis in adults: advances in pathophysiology and treatment. Cancer Sci. 2018;109(12):3707–13.
25. Gulati N, Allen CE. Langerhans cell histiocytosis: version 2021. Hematol Oncol. 2021;39 Suppl 1(Suppl 1):15–23.
26. de Lima LPN, Amorim CV, Marinho RM, Cintra ML, de Souza EM. Congenital solitary reticulohistiocytosis (Hashimoto - Pritzker). An Bras Dermatol. 2022;97(6):778–82.
27. Zanuncio VV, de Carvalho LR, Guedes ACM, Silva CMR, Gontijo B. Case for diagnosis. An Bras Dermatol. 2013;88(6):1001–3.
28. Goyal G, Tazi A, Go RS, Rech KL, Picarsic JL, Vassallo R, et al. International expert consensus recommendations for the diagnosis and treatment of Langerhans cell histiocytosis in adults. Blood. 2022;139(17):2601–21.
29. Williams O, Fatima S. Granuloma. In: StatPearls [Internet]. Treasure Island (FL): StatPearls Publishing; 2023. [cited 2023 Jul 2]. http://www.ncbi.nlm.nih.gov/books/NBK554586/.
30. Williams GT, Williams WJ. Granulomatous inflammation – a review. J Clin Pathol 1983 ;36(7):723–733.
31. The formation and function of granulomas | Annual Review of Immunology [Internet]. [cited 2023 Jun 1]. https://www.annualreviews.org/doi/10.1146/annurev-immunol-032712-100022?url_ver=Z39.88-2003&rfr_id=ori%3Arid%3Acrossref.org&rfr_dat=cr_pub++0pubmed
32. Pagán AJ, Ramakrishnan L. The formation and function of granulomas. Annu Rev Immunol. 2018;36(1):639–65.
33. Nwawka OK, Nadgir R, Fujita A, Sakai O. Granulomatous disease in the head and neck: developing a differential diagnosis. RadioGraphics. 2014;34(5):1240–56.
34. Kumar G. Lytic lesion of skull: a rare presentation of chronic granulomatous disease. BMJ Case Rep. 2020;13(9):e235423.
35. Roos D. Chronic granulomatous disease. Br Med Bull. 2016;118(1):50–63.
36. Ran Cai Z, Mamet F, Kokta V, Coulombe J. Subcutaneous nodules in children: don't forget deep granuloma annulare: a case report. SAGE Open Med Case Rep. 2020;8:2050313X20935713.
37. Sabuncuoğlu H, Oge K, Söylemezoğlu F, Sağlam A. Subcutaneous granuloma annulare of the scalp in childhood: a case report and review of the literature. Turk Neurosurg. 2007;17(1):19–22.
38. Joshi TP, Duvic M. Granuloma annulare: an updated review of epidemiology, pathogenesis, and treatment options. Am J Clin Dermatol. 2022;23(1):37–50.
39. Kansara S, Bell D, Johnson J, Zafereo M. Head and neck inflammatory pseudotumor: case series and review of the literature. Neuroradiol J. 2016;29(6):440–6.
40. Park SB, Lee JH, Weon YC. Imaging findings of head and neck inflammatory pseudotumor. AJR Am J Roentgenol. 2009;193(4):1180–6.
41. Patnana M, Sevrukov AB, Elsayes KM, Viswanathan C, Lubner M, Menias CO. Inflammatory pseudotumor: the great mimicker. AJR Am J Roentgenol. 2012;198(3):W217–27.
42. Fukunaga A, Yoshida K, Otani M, Ogawa Y, Horiguchi T, Ishihara M, et al. Plasma cell granuloma extending from the extracranial to the intracranial space associated with Epstein-Barr virus infection —case report. Neurol Med Chir. 1998;38(5):292–6.
43. Steinbrink JM, Miceli MH. Clinical review of mucormycosis. Infect Dis Clin N Am. 2021;35(2):435–52.
44. Harman M, Uçmak D, Dal T. A rare case of mucormycosis in the scalp. Acta Medica Port. 2013;26(6):754–7.
45. Thomas DC, Thomas P, Pillai DP, Joseph D, Lingaiah U, Mathai BC, et al. Giant cell arteritis: a case-based narrative review of the literature. Curr Pain Headache Rep. 2022;26(10):725–40.
46. Prieto-Peña D, Castañeda S, Atienza-Mateo B, Blanco R, González-Gay MÁ. A review of the dermatological complications of giant cell arteritis. Clin Cosmet Investig Dermatol. 2021;14:303–12.
47. Winkler A, True D. Giant cell arteritis: 2018 review. Mo Med. 2018;115(5):468–70.
48. Grän F, Kerstan A, Serfling E, Goebeler M, Muhammad K. Current developments in the immunology of psoriasis. Yale J Biol Med. 2020;93(1):97–110.
49. van de Kerkhof PC, Franssen ME. Psoriasis of the scalp. Diagnosis and management. Am J Clin Dermatol. 2001;2(3):159–65.
50. Papadimitriou I, Bakirtzi K, Katoulis A, Ioannides D. Scalp psoriasis and biologic agents: a review. Skin Appendage Disord. 2021;7(6):439–48.

51. Parisi R, Iskandar IYK, Kontopantelis E, Augustin M, Griffiths CEM, Ashcroft DM. National, regional, and worldwide epidemiology of psoriasis: systematic analysis and modelling study. BMJ. 2020;369:m1590.
52. Handa S. Newer trends in the management of psoriasis at difficult to treat locations: scalp, palmoplantar disease and nails. Indian J Dermatol Venereol Leprol. 2010;76(6):634–44.
53. Cullen G, Kroshinsky D, Cheifetz AS, Korzenik JR. Psoriasis associated with anti-tumour necrosis factor therapy in inflammatory bowel disease: a new series and a review of 120 cases from the literature. Aliment Pharmacol Ther. 2011;34(11–12):1318–27.
54. Lo YP, Desale S, Wu PY. Brain abscess in a patient with psoriatic arthritis treated with adalimumab. Medicine (Baltimore). 2020;99(10):e18954.
55. Atsawarungruangkit A, Dominguez F, Borda G, Mavrogiorgos N. Listeria monocytogenes brain abscess in Crohn's disease treated with adalimumab. Case Rep Gastroenterol. 2017;11(3):667–71.
56. Leung AKC, Hon KL, Leong KF, Barankin B, Lam JM. Tinea capitis: an updated review. Recent Patents Inflamm Allergy Drug Discov. 2020;14(1):58–68.
57. Hay RJ. Tinea capitis: current status. Mycopathologia. 2017;182(1):87–93.
58. Shvarts S, Sevo G, Tasic M, Shani M, Sadetzki S. The tinea capitis campaign in Serbia in the 1950s. Lancet Infect Dis. 2010;10(8):571–6.
59. John AM, Schwartz RA, Janniger CK. The kerion: an angry tinea capitis. Int J Dermatol. 2018;57(1):3–9.
60. Le TK, Cohen BA. Tinea capitis: advances and a needed paradigm shift. Curr Opin Pediatr. 2021;33(4):387–91.
61. Chowdhary A, Spence AM, Sales L, Rostomily RC, Rockhill JK, Silbergeld DL. Radiation associated tumors following therapeutic cranial radiation. Surg Neurol Int. 2012;3:48.
62. Umansky F, Shoshan Y, Rosenthal G, Fraifeld S, Spektor S. Radiation-induced meningioma. Neurosurg Focus. 2008;24(5):E7.
63. Robinson RG. A second brain tumour and irradiation. J Neurol Neurosurg Psychiatry. 1978;41(11):1005–12.
64. Piccirilli M, di Norcia V, Frati A, Salvati M. Glioblastoma in irradiated elderly patients: two case reports. Neurosurg Rev. 2005;28(3):226–8.

Part V

Malignant Neoplasms and Secondary Malignancies of the Scalp and Calvarium

Editor's Summary

In this "Part V: Malignant Neoplasms and Secondary Malignancies of the Scalp and Calvarium," there are four chapters that provide an extensive discussion of the neoplastic involvement of the scalp and calvarium. In back-to-back chapters, malignant neoplasms and secondary malignancies first involving the scalp and then the calvarium are covered in Chaps. 20 and 21, respectively. Those hematologic malignancies that involve the scalp and calvarium most often the diploic space are addressed in Chap. 22. An interesting group of patients that develop aggressive intracranial tumors such as meningiomas, lymphomas, and metastases that extend outward through the calvarium and into the scalp are described in Chap. 23.

20 Malignant Neoplasms and Secondary Malignancies of the Scalp

Zheng Yang, Dengpan Song, and Qiying Wang

20.1 Squamous Cell Carcinoma of the Scalp

Scalp squamous cell carcinoma (SCC) is a relatively common malignant tumor originating from squamous epithelial cells. It is highly destructive and can develop rapidly [1, 2]. It can not only locally erode and destroy surrounding normal tissue structures but also metastasize through lymphatic vessels. Squamous cell carcinoma is a common malignant skin tumor. It is more common in elderly individuals and is more common in men than in women [2]. In severe cases, scalp squamous cell carcinoma can invade the periosteum, the skull, and even the cranium, causing bone destruction, damage to the meninges, and even parenchymal brain damage. Therefore, early detection and treatment are important for the treatment of scalp squamous cell carcinoma [3].

Z. Yang · Q. Wang (✉)
Department of Plastic Surgery, The First Affiliated Hospital of Zhengzhou University, Zhengzhou, Henan Province, China
e-mail: wangqiying@zzu.edu.cn

D. Song
Department of Neurosurgery, The First Affiliated Hospital of Zhengzhou University, Zhengzhou, Henan Province, China

International Joint Laboratory of Nervous System Malformation, Zhengzhou, Henan Province, China

20.1.1 Risk Factors

Risk factors for the development of squamous cell carcinoma include long-term ultraviolet exposure; radioactive or thermal radiation damage; stimulation by chemical carcinogens; viral, fungal, or mycobacterial infections; and chronic or hereditary skin lesions. In addition, unhealthy lifestyles such as smoking and drinking, scars, and chronic ulcers are also risk factors for squamous cell carcinoma [4]. Pathogenesis: (1) The pathogenesis of squamous cells carcinomas include the involvement of cell cycle-related gene changes, such as TP53 mutations, NOTCH1 downregulation or loss, cyclin-dependent kinase inhibitor 2A (cyclin-dependent kinase inhibitor 2A, CDKN2A), RB1 deletion and somatic mutations, overexpression of the CCND1 and MYC gene, etc.; (2) Abnormal RAS, AKT, and receptor tyrosine kinase signaling pathways. changes in squamous cell differentiation pathways; (3) Abnormal epigenetic regulation; and (4) changes in the tumor microenvironment, etc. [5–7].

20.1.2 Clinical Manifestations

The clinical manifestations of squamous cell carcinoma vary among different stages of development. At the early onset of the disease, skin lesions may present as local erythema, papules, or nodules. The skin lesions gradually increase in

M. Turgut et al. (eds.), *Lesions of the Scalp and Cranial Vault*,
https://doi.org/10.1007/978-3-031-88244-9_20

size and may be accompanied by desquamation, ulcers, bleeding, etc. The lesions invade deep tissues, including the skull or even the intracranium. The invaded tissues stick together to form indurations with poor mobility, accompanied by pain and other sensory abnormalities. If infection and necrosis occur in the affected area, there will be a significant odor. If the lesion involves the brain, the patient will have neurological symptoms. If the disease metastasizes to lymph nodes, the patient will have enlarged lymph nodes in the lymph node drainage area (Fig. 20.1a and b).

20.1.3 Pathological Classification

The pathological classification includes the following: (1) squamous cell carcinoma in situ, in which the tumor does not grow through the basement membrane; (2) in invasive squamous cell carcinoma, the infiltrative growth of the tumor breaks through the basement membrane, and there are multiple histological subtypes: desmoplastic SCC, acantholytic SCC, spindle cell SCC, squamous adenocarcinoma, sarcomatoid differentiated SCC, etc.; and (3) special subtypes of squamous cell carcinoma: keratoacanthoma and verrucous carcinoma.

20.1.4 Tumor Grading and Staging

The Brigham and Women's Hospital (BWH) tumor T staging system is based on four clinical and pathological risk factors for grading and is simple and easy to use. The risk factors include the following: (1) tumor diameter ≥2 cm, (2) poorly differentiated histology, (3) perineural invasion, and (4) tumor invasion beyond the subcutaneous fat layer (excluding bone invasion). This system classifies tumors into stages T1 (0 risk factors), T2a (one risk factor), T2b (two to three risk factors), and T3 (four risk factors or bone invasion). The American Joint Committee

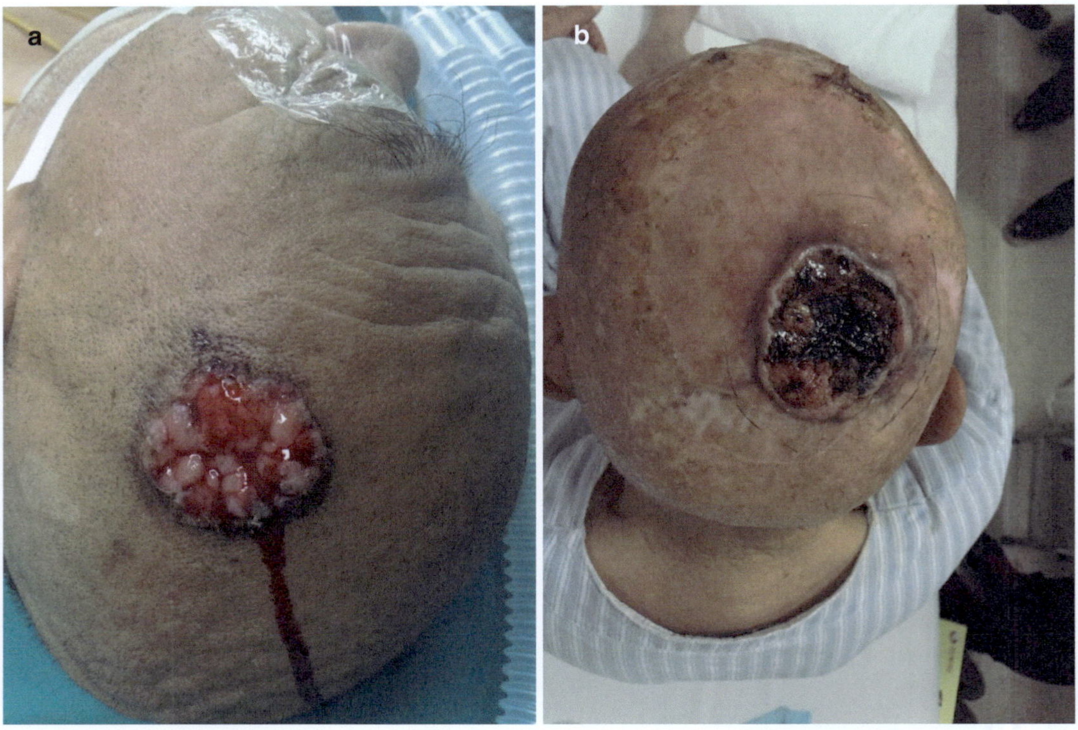

Fig. 20.1 (**a**) An elderly male patient with squamous cell carcinoma of the scalp; the mass had a cauliflower appearance and easily bled and ruptured. (**b**) An elderly female patient with scalp squamous cell carcinoma, a crater ulcer, and attachment of necrotic tissue

on Cancer (AJCC) TNM staging system (8th edition) is used to stage cutaneous squamous cell carcinoma (cSCC). This system includes the assessment of lymph node metastasis and distant metastasis and can play a supplementary role when the BWH system is used [2, 8–16].

20.1.5 Management of SCC

Surgical treatment is the most common method for treating scalp squamous cell carcinoma. In principle, the diseased tissue should be completely removed as much as possible [1]. Due to the special location of the scalp, it is necessary to consider both the scalp's function and appearance for complete removal of the tumor. The width of the resection range is generally 1–2.5 cm from the edge of the lesion. The resection margin needs to be clarified via pathological examination. If the postoperative pathology shows a positive resection margin, the possibility of a standard resection and a subsequent resection margin evaluation will be sought if the patient can tolerate it. The depth of resection depends on the degree of invasion of the disease. If the invasion is too deep, the subcutaneous tissue, muscle layer, periosteum, and bone tissue need to be removed together. With lesions that invade the skull, any dura mater that is eroded by the disease also needs to be removed.

Mohs surgery and slow Mohs surgery can preserve normal tissue to the greatest extent possible and meet the patient's functional and aesthetic needs [17]. Among these techniques, Mohs surgery relies on intraoperative frozen pathology examination and needs to be performed in hospitals with qualified conditions. After slow Mohs surgery is used to remove the diseased tissue, the pathological tissue is embedded as a whole to clarify the resection margin, and the wound is left open until the resection margin is clarified before the wound is closed.

The use of sentinel lymph node biopsy has mixed results in the prognostic judgment of cSCC, and most scholars still recommend sentinel lymph node biopsy for patients with cSCC stage T3 and above according to the American Joint Committee on Cancer (AJCC) staging system (8th edition) and for patients with stage T2b/T3 disease according to the Burrows–Wheeler–Whehn (BBH) staging system. Risk factors for positive sentinel lymph node biopsy include increased tumor diameter and thickness, vascular or lymphatic invasion, perineural invasion, and the coexistence of multiple high-risk factors. Therapeutic regional lymph node dissection is the preferred surgical treatment for patients with lymph node metastasis. The feasibility and extent of surgery should be evaluated by clinicians experienced in regional lymph node dissection.

Nonsurgical treatment: Patients with advanced or metastatic cSCC mainly receive chemotherapy, retinoic acid drugs, immunotherapy, targeted therapy, etc. [18–20]. Also, nonsurgical treatment is used for some patients with advanced cSCC or for other reasons and for those patients who cannot undergo curative treatment. Palliative care, including nonradical surgery, radiotherapy, electrodesiccation, chemical cauterization, and other therapies, aims to control the spread of tumors, relieve symptoms, and improve patients' quality of life. In addition, supportive care, psychological therapy, nutritional support, and skin lesion care can also significantly improve the quality of life of patients. For pain caused by cSCC, the World Health Organization's stepped therapy for pain should be followed, starting with nonsteroidal anti-inflammatory drugs and switching to opioids when the patient's pain control is not good.

20.2 Basal Cell Carcinoma of the Scalp

Basal cell carcinoma (BCC) is the most common malignant skin tumor [9]. It is more common in elderly individuals and has a higher incidence rate in men than in women. Basal cell carcinoma of the skin grows slowly and rarely metastasizes, but it can also grow locally invasively, destroy tissues and organs, cause organ dysfunction, and even endanger the patient's life [3].

20.2.1 Risk Factors

Ultraviolet exposure is the most important environmental risk factor. People with light-colored skin, and multiple sunburns and older people are prone to BCC [21, 22]. Other risk factors include a family history of skin cancer, immunosuppression (including HIV infection and organ transplantation), ionizing radiation, and chemical carcinogens (especially arsenic exposure). In addition, patients with certain genetic diseases, including xeroderma pigmentosum and cutaneous albinism, have an increased risk of developing BCC. Previous studies have suggested that abnormal activation of the Hh (Hedgehog) signaling pathway is closely related to the occurrence of BCC [23].

20.2.2 Clinical Manifestations and Classification

Clinically, it can be divided into five main types: nodular, superficial, morphea-like/infiltrative, pigmented, and fibroepithelioma [24]. Among these types, nodular BCC is the most common and occurs mostly on the face. It manifests as raised light red or smooth papules, plaques, and nodules that are of the patient's skin color, and they may be accompanied by telangiectasia and often have pearl-like raised edges. Central ulcers may appear when the number of skin lesions increases. There is also a cystic subtype within this type, which appears as blue–purple cystic nodules with cool liquid content. Superficial type BCCs usually occur on the trunk and appear as light red patches or rashes with clear borders and linear bulges. The clinical manifestations of morphea-like CC and infiltrative BCC are similar. These lesions are flat, slightly atrophic, or ill-defined plaques with a hard texture, they are colored light red or are skin color, and they may be associated with telangiectasia. The identification of the two requires the help of tissue pathology. Pigmented BCC usually contains obvious pigments and appears as black papules, patches, or nodules. Fibroepithelioma type B CC is relatively rare clinically, and the typical skin lesions are smooth, light-red nodules or plaques [9, 25] (Fig. 20.2).

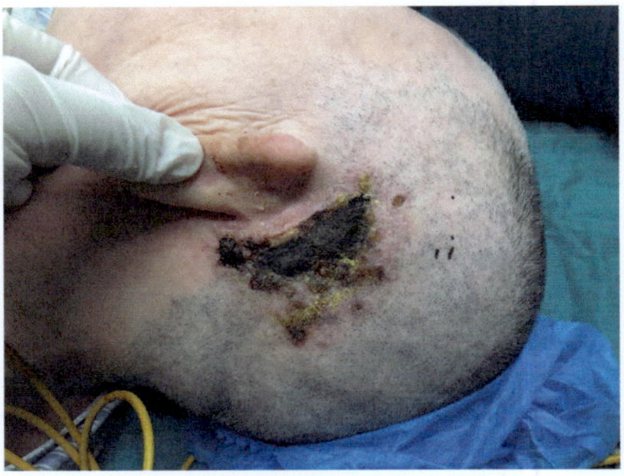

Fig. 20.2 An elderly patient with basal cell carcinoma of the scalp, necrotic tissue and a blood scab covered with erythema papulosis

In addition, two kinds of multiple BCCs are the main manifestations of this syndrome: Gorlin syndrome (nevoid basal cell carcinoma syndrome) and Bazex syndrome (Bazex–Dupré–Christol syndrome). Nevoid BCC syndrome (NBCCS), also known as Gorlin syndrome, is clinically rare, is related to PTCH1 or SUFU gene mutations, and is inherited in an autosomal dominant manner. Typical clinical manifestations include multiple BCCs, odontogenic keratocysts, bone dysplasia, palmar and plantar punctate depressions, and abnormal calcifications, which are easily accompanied by other benign or malignant tumors, such as brain tumors and myogenic tumors. Bazex syndrome is a clinically rare disease that has an X-linked dominant inheritance. The characteristic clinical manifestations are congenital sparse hair, follicular skin atrophy, milia, and multiple BCCs.

20.2.3 Tumor Grade and Staging

In view of the low malignancy of BCC and the rare occurrence of distant metastasis, TNM staging is not commonly used [3, 26]. The National Comprehensive Cancer Network (NCCN) guidelines provide a risk classification for recurrence. The risk of recurrence depends on the clinical and histopathological subtypes as well as tumor location, size, patient age, immune status, sex, and treatment methods used. These findings were combined with domestic and foreign diagnosis and treatment guidelines for high-risk and low-risk BCC patients. Patients can be divided into high risk and low risk of recurrence based on these factors, and the risk of recurrence can used to guide treatment plans. Patients who have any of the following high-risk factors are classified into the high-risk category: with any sized lesions on the head, neck, hands, feet, pretibial and anogenital lesions, or any lesions ≥2 cm that are on the trunk or extremities, ill-defined borders, recurrent tumors, immunosuppression, previous radiotherapy, an infiltrative growth pattern, and peripheral nerve involvement. Those who did not meet the criteria were considered to have a low risk of recurrence. According to the above classification, scalp BCC, regardless of size, is classified as a high-risk category [9, 13, 24, 27–30].

20.2.4 Management of BCC

Primary complete surgical resection with negative margins is the most effective method for treating BCC. Scalp BCC surgery can include standard surgical excision or Mohs/slow Mohs surgery, depending on the risk of recurrence. The standard surgical resection margins for scalp BCC can range from 5 to 15 mm, depending on the size, location, and histological subtype of the tumor and the surgeon's experience. The depth of resection should ensure a clean undercut margin. The scalp incision can be as deep as the fascia and galea, and if necessary, it can be as deep as the periosteum. Because the clinical characteristics of high-risk BCC are highly variable, there is no uniform standard for surgical margin selection. Surgical margins should be designed individually based on the specific conditions of the tumor and patient during treatment. During standard surgical resection, the surgical incision should be repaired after ensuring negative margins. The surgical incision can be directly closed for repair, or it can be repaired using adjacent or distant tissue flaps or skin grafts. Mohs surgery and slow Mohs surgery will not be described in detail [21].

Surgery is the main treatment for BCC. However, nonsurgical treatment can be selected when the patient will not tolerate surgery, the tumor is located at a difficult surgical site, the tumor cannot be completely removed by surgery, or the tumor relapses after surgery and reoperation are not suitable. Nonsurgical treatments include radiotherapy, photodynamic therapy, topical drug therapy, cryotherapy, laser therapy, and targeted therapy [31]. The FDA approved the hedgehog pathway inhibitors vismodegib, sonidegib, and patidegib for the treatment of advanced BCC. Hedgehog Inhibitor (HHI) can also be used as a preoperative neoadjuvant or postoperative adjuvant treatment for some BCCs that are difficult to treat.

20.3 Dermatofibrosarcoma Protuberans of the Scalp

Dermatofibrosarcoma protuberans (DFSP) is a relatively rare, low-grade malignant soft tissue dermal tumor that originates from fibrous tissue cells in the dermis and can invade subcutaneous tissue [32, 33]. These tumors have no clear capsule. Dermatofibrosarcoma protuberans mostly occurs in young and middle-aged people. It easily relapses after surgical resection and rarely metastasizes. The early clinical manifestations of DFSP are nonspecific and painless, and hard nodules protruding from the body surface are often the first symptoms. The tumor slowly grows into a nodule or a massive, red, or light red tumor, which resembles a scar or keloid and is difficult to distinguish with the naked eye. When the skin lesions are small, they are easily misdiagnosed as cysts or rashes; some patients have a clear history of trauma or surgery, which are the patients who are most likely to be misdiagnosed as having scars or keloids; in some patients, the lesions do not protrude from the skin and are easily misdiagnosed as pigmented nevi [32, 34, 35].

The most common site of occurrence is the trunk (50%), but it is less commonly found in the limbs (20–35%), the head and neck (10–15%), and the vulva and breast, which are even less common. However, in head and neck cancer patients, the recurrence rate (50–75%) is very high.

20.3.1 Clinical Manifestations and Classification

DFSP can be divided into many types based on histopathological characteristics, and they are mainly the classic type (accounting for approximately 90%) and the nonclassical type [36]. Classic DFSP shows typical radial or storiform manifestations, with cancer tissue growing around like crab legs and even infiltrating the fat layer to form a honeycomb-like structure. There are more than a dozen subtypes of atypical DFSP, and the common subtypes are pigmented, myxoid, and sarcomatous. Among these types, sarcomatous dermatofibrosarcoma protuberans is a subtype of atypical DFSP in which sarcomatoid changes occur in the tumor. Fibrosarcomatous DFSP (FS-DFSP) is obviously malignant both pathologically and clinically, and its recurrence and metastasis rates are significantly greater than those of classic DFSP. It has also been reported that DFSP can undergo type transformation after multiple recurrences, from classic DFSP to FS-DFSP (Fig. 20.3a–c).

20.3.2 Clinical Diagnosis

The diagnosis of DFSP currently relies mainly on pathological examination. Classic DFSP has a typical tissue morphology with radial or storiform structures visible microscopically [37]. Immunohistochemistry for CD34 is the most significant factor in diagnosing DFSP, with high sensitivity but low specificity. The combined detection of multiple immunohistochemical staining factors, such as vimentin, S-100, CD117, and SMA, can be used for the differential diagnosis of DFSP and other soft tissue tumors. In terms of genetic testing, important progress has been made in the detection of the DFSP COLIA1-PDGFB fusion gene, providing a more accurate method for the diagnosis of DFSP [36, 38].

20.3.3 Management of DFSP

Surgical treatment: The current main treatment method for DFSP is surgical resection, and the incision margin should be confirmed to be negative [38–42]. However, due to the infiltrative growth of DFSP, there is often a 2 cm wide extension of the tumor beyond the visible tumor boundary. The tumor margin is often difficult to define, and it has been reported that it may even be as wide as 10 cm [43–45]. The NCCN recommends a resection margin of 2–4 cm, and it is recommended that the resection depth is at the level of the periosteum of the skull to obtain a negative resection margin. Mohs surgery and slow Mohs surgery can ensure negative margins while preserving as much normal tissue as possible, which has a positive effect on reducing the difficulty of wound repair and preserving a good appearance [46]. If the resection range is too large, local flap reconstruction is needed. In these cases, pathological examinations should be performed to confirm negative

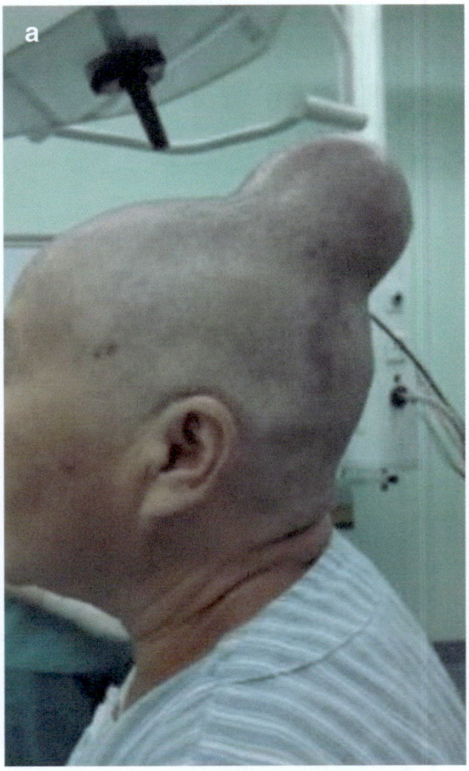

Fig. 20.3 (**a**) A 57-year-old female with dermatofibrosarcoma protuberans of the scalp, with a prominent body surface and exophytic growth. (**b**) Enhanced MR image showing lesions invading the cap aponeurosis, periosteum and skull. (**c**) CT indicating a mass in the left top of the scalp, skull discontinuity, and obvious bone defects

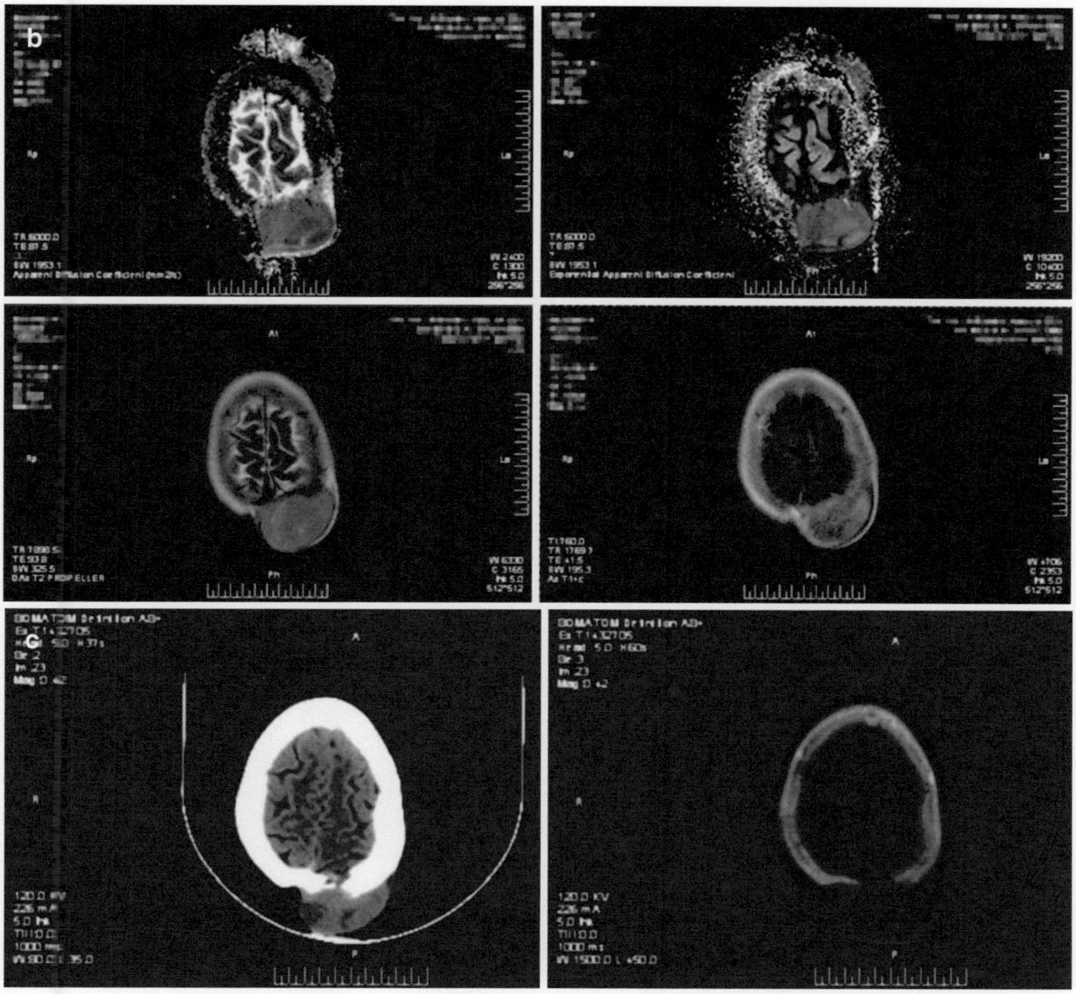

Fig. 20.3 (continued)

resection margins. For recurrent DFSP, the resection margin should be more than 5 cm away from the tumor to reduce recurrence as much as possible. Lymphatic metastasis of DFSP is extremely rare, so preventive regional lymph node dissection is not required during surgery. If preoperative color ultrasound shows regional lymph node enlargement, pathological examination of the lymph nodes can be performed, and if positive, lymph node dissection can be performed.

Nonsurgical treatment: DFSP is sensitive to radiotherapy. In clinical practice, a comprehensive surgical treatment model and postoperative radiotherapy are often used, especially for patients who cannot achieve negative margins due to local anatomical factors. Traditional chemotherapy is not effective for treating DFSP. In terms of targeted therapy, PDGF-β receptor blockers, such as imatinib, have been approved by the FDA for use in patients with unresectable DFSP [47, 48].

20.4 Malignant Melanoma of the Scalp

Cutaneous malignant melanoma (CMM) is a common and highly malignant tumor in clinical practice. It originates from melanocytes and can occur in the skin, mucosa, uvea, meninges, and other parts of the body. In recent years, the incidence of cutaneous malignant melanoma has been increasing [49]. CMM is usually transformed from skin melanoma nevi. CMM can metastasize through the blood and lymph in the early stage. It is highly invasive and highly metastatic and has a high fatality rate. Early detection, early diagnosis, and early treatment can improve patient prognosis and survival [50] (Fig. 20.4a and b).

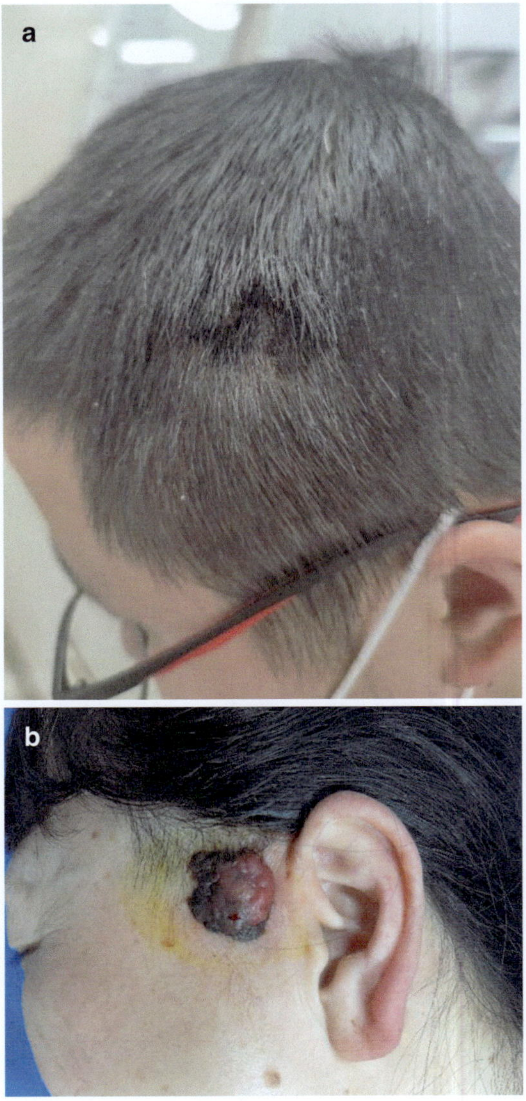

Fig. 20.4 (**a**) A 31-year-old male with malignant melanoma of the scalp, located in the temporal region, with a black surface covered with hair, which is insidious onset and not easily be found. (**b**) A middle-aged female with malignant melanoma of the scalp, located in the left temporal sideburns, local eminence, uneven color

20.4.1 Risk Factors

Factors such as excessive ultraviolet exposure, sex, age, and race are considered independent risk factors for cutaneous malignant melanoma. The number of melanocytic nevi on the skin, a family history of CMM, and genetic factors are also important factors leading to its occurrence [49, 51].

20.4.2 Early Detection

The early detection of CMM occurs mainly through the inspection of lesions by an attending doctor. The ABCDE rule for evaluating skin lesions is as follows: A is asymmetry (asymmetry), B is irregular edges (border), C is an uneven color (color), D is a diameter >6 mm (diameter), and E is lesion elevation or progression (elevation/evolving). Ugly duck syndrome. Dermoscopy can further improve the diagnostic accuracy. The gold standard for clinical diagnosis is skin pathology, and the biopsy needs to include lateral margins of 1–3 mm and the full thickness of the lesion.

20.4.3 Pathological Types

The four most common histological types of cutaneous melanoma are the acrofreckle type, malignant freckle type, superficial spread type, and nodular type. Rare histological types include desmoplastic melanoma, melanoma originating from blue, melanoma of a nevus, melanoma originating from giant congenital nevi, childhood melanoma, nevoid melanoma, etc. [52].

20.4.4 Tumor Grade and Stage

The NCCN staging system for melanoma is based on the American Joint Committee on Cancer (AJCC) TNM staging system [53], which classifies melanoma using three primary factors:

1. T (Tumor) Stage: Depth and characteristics of the primary tumor
   (a) Tis: Melanoma in situ (confined to the epidermis, no invasion of dermis)
   (b) T1: Tumor ≤1.0 mm thick
   - T1a: <0.8 mm, without ulceration
   - T1b: <0.8 mm, with ulceration
   - 0.8–1.0 mm, with or without ulceration

   (c) T2: Tumor >1.0–2.0 mm thick
   - T2a: Without ulceration
   - T2b: With ulceration

   (d) T3: Tumor >2.0–4.0 mm thick
   - T3a: Without ulceration
   - T3b: With ulceration

   (e) T4: Tumor >4.0 mm thick
   - T4a: Without ulceration
   - T4b: With ulceration

2. N (Node) Stage: Lymph node involvement
   (a) N0: No regional lymph node involvement
   (b) N1: One metastatic lymph node or in-transit, satellite, and/or microsatellite metastases with no tumor-involved nodes
   - N1a: One metastatic lymph node clinically occult (detected by sentinel lymph node biopsy (SLNB)), without in-transit, satellite, and/or microsatellite metastases
   - N1b: One metastatic lymph node clinically detected, without in-transit, satellite, and/or microsatellite metastases
   - N1c: No regional lymph node disease, with in-transit, satellite, and/or microsatellite metastases

   (c) N2: Two to three metastatic lymph nodes or in-transit, satellite, and/or microsatellite metastases with one tumor-involved node
   - N2a: Two to three metastatic lymph nodes clinically occult (detected by SLN biopsy), without in-transit, satellite, and/or microsatellite metastases
   - N2b: Two to three metastatic lymph nodes, at least one of which was clinically detected, without in-transit, satellite, and/or microsatellite metastases
   - N2c: One metastatic lymph node clinically occult or detected, with in-transit, satellite, and/or microsatellite metastases

   (d) N3: ≥4 metastatic lymph nodes, matted nodes, or in-transit, satellite, and/or microsatellite metastases with ≥2 tumor-involved nodes, or any number of matted nodes without or with in-transit, satellite, and/or microsatellite metastases
   - N3a: ≥4 metastatic lymph nodes clinically occult (detected by SLN biopsy), without in-transit, satellite, and/or microsatellite metastases
   - N3b: ≥4 metastatic lymph nodes, at least one of which was clinically detected, or presence of any number of matted nodes, without in-transit, satellite, and/or microsatellite metastases
   - N3c: ≥2 clinically occult or clinically detected and/or presence of any number of matted nodes, with in-transit, satellite, and/or microsatellite metastases

3. M (Metastasis) Stage: Distant metastasis
   (a) M0: No evidence of distant metastasis
   (b) M1a: Metastasis to distant skin, subcutaneous tissue, or distant lymph nodes
   (c) M1b: Metastasis to the lungs
   (d) M1c: Metastasis to non-central nervous system (CNS) visceral organs
   (e) M1d: Metastasis to the central nervous system (CNS)

Overall Stages (AJCC 8th Edition):

- Stage 0: Tis, N0, M0
- Stage IA: T1a, N0, M0
- Stage IB: T1b-T2a, N0, M0
- Stage IIA: T2b-T3a, N0, M0
- Stage IIB: T3b-T4a, N0, M0
- Stage IIC: T4b, N0, M0
- Stage III: Any T, N1-N3, M0
- Stage IV: Any T, any N, M1

The NCCN Guidelines align with these stages and provide treatment recommendations based on the stage, including surgery, sentinel lymph node biopsy, immunotherapy, targeted therapy, and radiation therapy. TNM staging before the first treatment is highly valuable for treating CMM and is the basis for standardized tumor treatment. Therefore, before radical surgical treatment is performed on patients with scalp CMMs, a pathological diagnosis should be obtained through biopsy, and CMMs should be staged based on pathological examination, imaging examination, etc., to determine subsequent surgical treatment strategies and comprehensive treatment strategies [54–56].

20.4.5 Management of CMM

Surgical treatment: Extensive resection of the lesion as soon as possible after diagnosis is currently the preferred treatment for early-stage CMM [57]. Complete tumor resection can significantly reduce local recurrence and melanoma-specific mortality. The safe margin for wide resection of the primary tumor is determined based on the depth of tumor invasion in the biopsy pathology report: (1) melanoma in situ, margin 0.5–1.0 cm; (2) tumor thickness ≤1.0 mm, margin 1 cm; (3) tumor thickness 1.1–2.0 mm, resection margin 1–2 cm; (4) tumor thickness 2.1–4.0 mm, resection margin 2 cm; and (4) tumor thickness >4.0 mm, resection margin 2 cm. The depth of resection refers to the width of the skin resection margin, which must include the full thickness of the skin and deep fascia or a considerable thickness of the subcutaneous tissue. The deep myofascia/periosteum can be retained as appropriate. However, for primary lesions with deep infiltration (Breslow thickness > 4 mm), severe ulceration, and other adverse factors, myofascial resection can be considered [58].

One-step resection of melanoma: The preoperative measurement of tumor thickness is through clinical judgment, dermoscopy, and high-frequency ultrasound. It is recommended that for tumors in situ and with a thickness <2 mm, the resection margin should be 1 cm. If the thickness is >2 mm, the resection margin should be 2 cm. A sentinel lymph node biopsy is recommended for tumors with a thickness >2 mm.

Lymph node biopsy and dissection: CMMs can metastasize through lymph nodes in the early stage. The lymphatic return in the head and neck is complex and usually involves multiple lymph node return areas. The risk of regional lymph node metastasis is closely related to the thickness of the primary lesion [59]. The MSLT-1 study revealed that patients with moderate depth of invasion (Breslow thickness of 1.2–3.5 mm) and no clinical signs of metastasis are suitable candidates for sentinel lymph node biopsy. Research on lymph node metastasis of cutaneous melanoma with shallow invasion depth (B reslow < 1 mm) shows that when the following risk factors are present, the positive rate of sentinel lymph node (SLN) increases to 5–18%: (1) a Breslow thickness > 0.75 mm, (2) combined with an ulcer, (3) lark grade IV, (4) nodular growth, (5) increased mitotic figures, and (6) disappearance is evident. Therefore, when patients with a shallow invasion depth have certain risk factors, SLNB should still be considered. For patients with a thick invasion depth (Breslow thickness > 4 mm), the MSLT-1 study suggested that SLNB did not significantly improve the long-term survival of patients with lymph node metastasis. If the SLNB result is positive, complete lymph node dissection (CLND) should be performed in the lymph node drainage area. Neck lymph node dissection: Drainage of the head and neck skin is complicated, and surgery needs to be performed by an experienced head and neck specialist. The dissection procedures for thyroid cancer can be a reference. The number of lymph nodes dissected should be ≥ 15.

Nonsurgical treatment: Nonsurgical treatment for CMM includes radiotherapy, chemotherapy, targeted therapy, and immunotherapy. With recent in-depth research, remarkable results have been achieved with targeted therapy and immunotherapy [60].

20.5 Scalp Scar Cancer

Scar cancer is a cancerous change in scar tissue. It is most common in old scars that are healed by deep burns without surgery, but it can also occur in chronic osteomyelitis fistulas, venous stasis ulcers, pressure ulcers, and other types of wounds that have a delay in healing or scars that have repeatedly ruptured [61, 62]. Among these complications, scarring caused by burns can result in ulcers, which can become cancerous. This type of ulcer was first reported by Marjolin in 1828; therefore, this type of ulcer is called a Marjolin ulcer The incidence of malignant transformation of skin scars ranges from 1 to 2%, they occur mostly in men, and the incubation period ranges from months to years. Those lesions with a latent period of less than 1 year are classified as acute scar cancers, which are clinically rare, accounting for approximately 4.6% of the total number of scar cancers; those lesions with a latent period of greater than or equal to 1 year are classified as chronic scar cancers, accounting for approximately 95.4% of the total number of scar cancers. The treatment of scar cancer emphasizes early detection and early surgery [63, 64].

20.5.1 Pathogenesis

Chronic irritation plays an important role in the development of scar cancer [65]. Nthumb summarized previous studies and speculated that the pathogenesis of scar cancer may include the following: (1) chronic irritation of scar ulcers that have delayed healing and are left unhealed; (2) necrotic tissue in wounds releases tissue toxins and endogenous growth-promoting factors as auxiliary carcinogens, which induce cell mutations; (3) poor blood circulation and a lack of lymphatic circulation in scar tissue make it difficult for normal function of immune surveillance functions, leading to the gradual growth of cancer cells, which is the so-called immune immunity effect produced by the scar barrier; (4) genetic factors. The human leukocyte antigen DR4 has been confirmed to be related to tumor development. Mutations in the p53 and Fas genes are conducive to the malignant transformation of scar tissue. Patients with immune deficiency are at high risk for developing scar cancer; and (5) environmental factors. Scar ulcers that do not heal are more likely to become cancerous under the influence of external factors such as ultraviolet rays, radiation, and chemicals [66].

20.5.2 Clinical Manifestations

Initially, patients initially experience local abnormal sensations, such as local itching, hyperalgesia, etc. of their scars; ulcers may appear after ulceration; and small papules may gradually enlarge and ulcerate. The lesions are eroded and ulcerated for a long time and do not heal for a long time, gradually leading to the formation of erosive ulcers or cauliflower-like lesions accompanied by pain and secretions. The wounds are prone to bleeding and also have a foul odor when they are infected. Scar cancer can be divided into the following types: (1) crater-like: The ulcer has an uneven base, a crater-shaped edge, and a hard texture and are mostly squamous cell carcinomas. (2) Cauliflower-like: the ulcer is papillary hyperplasia, with an uneven surface and everted edges. Like cauliflower: these are mostly squamous cell carcinomas. (3) Erosion-like: the base of the ulcer is uneven, and the border is not well defined, the lesions appears as if the patient has been bitten by an insect, and these lesions are mostly basal cell carcinomas.

20.5.3 Pathological Classification

Scar cancer was initially referred to as squamous cell carcinoma of burn scars. With the emergence of sporadic reports of cases of malignant transformation of other cells in burn scars and other nonburn surface scar malignant transformation cases, scar cancer now refers to all tumors originating from malignant tumors of body surface scars. All cellular components within scars can theoretically undergo malignant transformation. Scar cancer can be divided into five categories according to the type of cancerous cells: squamous cell carcinoma (accounting for 7–24%), melanoma (accounting for 0–6%), sarcoma (occupying 0–5%) and other rare cell types (accounting for 0–7%). According to the degree of differentiation of scar tissue, scar cancer can be divided into high, medium and poorly differentiated types.

20.5.4 Treatment

Most scar cancers are squamous cell carcinomas, which rarely metastasize to distant sites. Therefore, radical surgical resection is the main treatment for scar cancer. The tumor-free principle needs to be strictly followed during the operation to avoid direct seeding and dissemination of discrete cancer cells. The risk of recurrence is greater if the scope of surgical resection is too small. Standard surgery emphasizes that the safety margin should be 2–3 cm away from the wound edge. The depth of resection is determined by the level of tissue invasion, especially if it reaches the periosteum. When bone is eroded, the diseased bone must be removed. Penetrating scar cancer of the scalp often invades the skull, meninges, brain tissue, and falx cerebri, requiring multidisciplinary collaboration to complete tumor resection. Regional lymph node dissection is required when there is evidence of regional lymph node metastasis. There is still controversy as to whether prophylactic lymph node dissection is needed for patients with scar cancer without regional lymph node metastasis, but it is generally considered unnecessary. SLNB can provide a reference for the range of surgical approaches for treating scar cancer [67].

Nonsurgical treatment includes radiotherapy and chemotherapy. Reports in the literature show that other treatment methods for scar cancer include photodynamic therapy, laser therapy, cryotherapy, and topical medication. Due to the difficulty in determining the tumor boundary, these nonsurgical treatment methods have limited therapeutic effects and are associated with high recurrence rates; however, they can be used as alternative or supplementary treatment options for those patients who cannot tolerate or refuse surgery [61, 62].

20.6 Other Primary Malignant Tumors of the Scalp and Metastatic Carcinoma of the Scalp

In addition to squamous cell carcinoma, basal cell carcinoma, malignant melanoma, and scar cancer, primary malignant tumors of the scalp, such as angiosarcoma, pilomatrix carcinoma, eccrine pore carcinoma, sebaceous gland carcinoma, etc., have also been reported. These rare malignant tumors are mostly reported in case reports, and the patients range from newborns to elderly individuals.

Angiosarcoma is a malignant tumor derived from vascular endothelial cells. Most angiosarcomas are located in the skin and can become cutaneous angiosarcomas. The head and face are the most common sites of cutaneous angiosarcoma. Angiosarcoma is difficult to diagnose in its early stages, and its clinical manifestations are often nonspecific. The initial appearance of angiosarcoma is similar to bruising or raised purple-red papules. It is easily misdiagnosed as benign lesions such as hemangioma or trauma-related abrasions and abscesses, and the appearance of angiosarcomas can be delayed. Early diagnosis is crucial for optimal treatment. Tumor size, patient age, and clean margins are major determinants of patient prognosis. The treatment of cutaneous angiosarcoma is mainly comprehensive. Postoperative radiotherapy is the most common treatment modality, and chemotherapy is the main method for the treatment of metastatic angiosarcoma. Radical surgical resection should be considered an important option for treatment [68–71].

Pilomatrix carcinoma is a very rare low-grade cutaneous malignant tumor. It is considered to be the corresponding malignant tumor of pilomatricoma. It has low metastatic potential but has a high risk of recurrence after resection, especially in the case of incomplete resection, for which the recurrence rate is as high as 59%. Lesions are most common on the head, neck, and back in older adults, with a lower incidence in children and young adults and a male to female ratio of 3:1. Pilomatrix carcinoma often presents as a single asymptomatic dermal or subcutaneous mass that is firm, painless, and mobile. There is currently a lack of standard treatment options for pilomatrix carcinoma, and extensive resection is the preferred treatment. In view of the easy recurrence of pilomatrix carcinoma, adjuvant radiotherapy may be considered after surgery for patients with a wide range of lesions. However, due to the rarity of pilomatrix carcinoma, the roles of chemotherapy and radiotherapy are still controversial and require further clinical research [72].

Scalp sebaceous gland cancer is a rare malignant tumor of the head and face. The incidence rate is higher in elderly people, and 75% of cases occur around the orbit. Extraorbital sebaceous gland cancer is rare. Because of its low incidence and lack of specific clinical manifestations, it can easily be misdiagnosed before surgery, which will delay treatment. Therefore, we should be highly vigilant about the malignant source of new tumors in elderly patients and be prepared for extended resection. The scope of resection should be determined based on a frozen pathological examination of the resection margin. Sebaceous gland carcinoma can directly invade adjacent tissues and can also metastasize to lymph nodes and distant sites. Due to the rarity of the tumor, there is currently no standard treatment option for sebaceous gland carcinoma, and wide surgical resection is the first choice. It is still unclear whether postoperative radiotherapy and chemotherapy are necessary [73–75].

Scalp metastatic cancer ranks third among scalp malignant tumors (12.8%), second only to scalp basal cell carcinoma and squamous cell carcinoma. Scalp metastasis is common in lung cancer (23.53%), colon cancer (11.76%), liver cancer (7.84%), breast cancer (7.84%), etc. [76]. Skin metastases usually appear as solitary painless nodules with clinical manifestations similar to those of benign nodules and tend to occur near the primary tumor. The mechanism of primary cancer metastasis to the scalp has not been clearly elucidated. It is generally believed that skin metastasis of tumors indicates a high chance for malignancy, a late stage, and a poor prognosis. However, clinically, there are only a few reports of scalp metastasis of malignant tumors, with a scalp mass as the first symptom. Therefore, clinicians should remain vigilant, make comprehensive judgments, and carefully give accurate diagnoses to patients. When a patient with a confirmed malignant tumor develops a new scalp mass, the mass needs to be biopsied to confirm the pathology, and a comprehensive and systematic examination is needed. Giving reasonable antitumor treatments may extend patient survival and improve quality of life.

20.7 Surgical Treatment of Scalp Malignancies

How to repair scalp defects after resection of malignant scalp tumors requires the surgeon to formulate a plan before surgery. Comprehensive decisions are made based on the size and depth of the wound, the adjacent available tissue structure, and the patient's overall condition. Preoperative evaluation includes scalp mobility, hair growth, scalp surgery history, lesion extent and depth of infiltration, and patient comorbid diseases (cardiovascular disease, diabetes, smoking history, etc.). Before performing flap reconstruction, the resection margin needs to be clarified. If the nature of the resection margin cannot be immediately confirmed by an intraoperative frozen pathology examination, the wound can be left alone or temporarily covered, and complex flap reconstruction surgery can be considered after the pathology results are confirmed.

For defects involving only the scalp, direct suturing can be used for small areas, and scalp flaps or free skin grafts should be used for medium-sized areas. If the scalp defect is accompanied by exposed bone and if the conditions of the surrounding tissue around the defect are acceptable, then adjacent skin flaps or fascial flaps can be selected to cover it. If the tissue inflammation around the defect is severe, if the patient needs to undergo subsequent radiotherapy, or if the patient's systemic conditions can tolerate prolonged surgery, a free flap should be the first choice for surgical technique. If the tumor erodes the skull or even the intracranium, a skull defect repair needs to be considered. Generally, applicable materials include autologous bone flaps and artificial materials. With the development of technology, 3D-printed metal and polymer materials have been used for the personalized repair of skull defects.

For small-scale simple scalp defects, pulling together and suturing of the defect edges are preferred. The preoperative incision design should ensure that incision tension is minimized. Due to the limited mobility and elasticity of the scalp during the operation, subgaleal dissection is required around the scalp wound to increase the mobility of local tissues and reduce the incisional tension. If necessary, the galea aponeurosis can be scored in the vertical direction of scalp advancement to increase scalp extensibility and reduce tension. At this time, care should be taken to avoid damaging the rich blood supply area under the aponeurosis to reduce the impact of the damage on the blood supply and nerves of the scalp. The benefits placing sutures are obvious, but reliable and effective repair cannot be obtained for larger wounds with only suturing.

For large defects that cannot be closed and sutured, local flaps are preferred for repair. The advantage of the local skin flap is that it complies with the principle of "approximate repair" and uses the "scalp" technique to repair the "scalp." After wound repair, the local blood supply is good, the wear resistance is good, the appearance is good, and it does not have effects on postoperative radiotherapy. Local flaps usually need to be rotated and advanced to cover the wound. Due to the extensibility of the scalp, the length of the rotated flap needs to be five to six times greater than that of the wound to effectively reduce the tension on the sutures. If a rotated flap cannot cover the wound, two or even multiple flaps, such as the O–Z flap or the Orticochea multi-flap method, can be used to repair the wound. While making a flap incision design, the surgeon should pay attention to the direction of hair follicle growth, the hair flow direction should be considered as much as possible when determining the direction of flap rotation, and the flap lifting layer should be located under the galea aponeurosis. Small flaps can be selected as random flaps, and larger flaps are generally designed as axial flaps with an axial blood supply. In addition, island flaps with an axial blood supply, such as island flaps with superficial temporal vessels as pedicles and island scalp flaps with occipital vessels as vascular pedicles, are also used in scalp defect repair.

When a local flap cannot be used due to early radiotherapy or surgery and if the local flap tissue is insufficient, anastomotic free flap transplantation can be used to repair the scalp defect. This type of surgery is difficult and time-consuming, so it requires thorough preoperative assessment and preparation. The blood vessels in the donor site and the recipient site should be thoroughly inspected before surgery to clarify the details of flap selection and separation. During the selection of vessels in the recipient area, the proximity to the defect and the appropriate size of the lumen should be considered. The commonly selected vessels are superficial temporal vessels and occipital arteries. If necessary, facial vessels or other branches of the external carotid artery can be selected, among which superficial temporal vessels are the most widely used. During surgery, the recipient site blood vessels should first be explored to evaluate whether they can be used for vascular anastomosis. Otherwise, other blood vessels on the same side or the blood vessels closest to the wound surface should be preferred as the recipient site vessels, and vein bridging should be avoided as much as possible before consideration. Finally, the use of the contralateral neck vessel as the recipient vessel should be considered. The free flaps that can be selected include the latissimus dorsi free flap, serratus anterior free flap, rectus abdominis free flap, radial forearm free flap, anterolateral thigh free flap, etc. If the amount of skin tissue provided by the donor flap is insufficient, a free muscle flap combined with medium-thickness skin graft transplantation can also be performed. In addition, there are also reports of the use of free omentum transplantation combined with skin grafting to repair scalp defects. The advantages are that the omentum has long pedicles and strong anti-infection ability. The disadvantages are that it requires surgical entry into the abdominal cavity, and there may be long-term complications such as intestinal adhesion and intestinal obstruction. These symptoms are possible.

Some patients with large-area or full-thickness scalp defects cannot undergo local flap or free flap surgery due to poor systemic conditions or other factors. In this case, free skin grafts can be chosen to repair the wound. Skin grafting is suitable for the reconstruction of scalp defects with a rich blood supply and is not limited by the defect area. Skin grafts can be transplanted on the periosteum surface, and the periosteum provides blood supply support. When the periosteum is missing, the galea aponeurosis flap or skull periosteum flap adjacent to the scalp can be rotated and advanced to cover the exposed bone surface, and then skin grafting can be performed. In addition, holes can be drilled into the exposed bone surface to cultivate granulation tissue, and skin can be grafted after the granulation tissue grows. Alternatively, the outer plate can be removed, the plate barrier with a rich blood supply can be exposed, and a skin graft can be grafted on it. The disadvantages of skin grafting include an unsightly appearance, unstable skin grafts, and the inability to tolerate radiotherapy. The advantages are that the surgical procedure is relatively simple and requires limited patient conditions and operation time. Early wound repair is achieved through skin grafting, and in the long term, the wound can be repaired by means of skin flap transfer or tissue expansion.

References

1. Verdaguer-Faja J, et al. Management of cutaneous squamous cell carcinoma of the scalp: the role of imaging and therapeutic approaches. Cancers (Basel). 2024;16(3)
2. Deutsch J, Dippel E, Delank KW. Cutaneous squamous cell carcinoma of the head and neck. Laryngorhinootologie. 2023;102(3):186–93.
3. Bernardini N, et al. Face and scalp basal cell carcinoma treatment: a review of the literature. Acta Dermatovenerol Croat. 2019;27(1):22–7.
4. Faltaous AA, et al. A rare transformation of epidermoid cyst into squamous cell carcinoma: a case report with literature review. Am J Case Rep. 2019;20:1141–3.
5. Xu F, et al. A TP53-associated gene signature for prediction of prognosis and therapeutic responses in lung squamous cell carcinoma. Onco Targets Ther. 2020;9(1):1731943.
6. Corchado-Cobos R, et al. Cutaneous squamous cell carcinoma: from biology to therapy. Int J Mol Sci. 2020;21(8)
7. Wang Y, et al. Oxymatrine inhibits proliferation and migration of vulvar squamous cell carcinoma cells via attenuation of the RAS/RAF/MEK/ERK pathway. Cancer Manag Res. 2020;12:2057–67.
8. Schmults CD, et al. NCCN guidelines(R) insights: squamous cell skin cancer, version 1.2022. J Natl Compr Cancer Netw. 2021;19(12):1382–94.
9. Mittal A, Mittal BB. Comparative analysis of US guidelines for the management of cutaneous squamous cell and basal cell carcinoma. J Skin Cancer. 2024;2024:3859066.
10. Christensen RE, et al. Dermatopathologic features of cutaneous squamous cell carcinoma and actinic keratosis: consensus criteria and proposed reporting guidelines. J Am Acad Dermatol. 2023;88(6):1317–25.
11. Dreyfuss I, et al. Squamous cell carcinoma: 2021 updated review of treatment. Dermatol Ther. 2022;35(4):e15308.
12. Moreno-Ramírez D, et al. Surgery for cutaneous squamous cell carcinoma and its limits in advanced disease. Dermatol Pract Concept. 2021;11(Suppl 2):e2021167S.
13. Firnhaber JM. Basal cell and cutaneous squamous cell carcinomas: diagnosis and treatment. Am Fam Physician. 2020;102(6):339–46.
14. Leiter U, et al. Cutaneous squamous cell carcinoma. Hautarzt. 2020;71(8):597–606.
15. Breuninger H, et al. Local surgical treatment of cutaneous squamous cell carcinoma: deficits and controversies in the literature. J Dtsch Dermatol Ges. 2019;17(10):999–1004.
16. Fox M, et al. Nodal staging of high-risk cutaneous squamous cell carcinoma. J Am Acad Dermatol. 2019;81(2):548–57.

17. Hunt W, et al. A review of Mohs micrographic surgery for skin cancer. Part 3: squamous cell carcinoma. Clin Exp Dermatol. 2022;47(10):1765–73.
18. Chitwood K, Etzkorn J, Cohen G. Topical and intralesional treatment of nonmelanoma skin cancer: efficacy and cost comparisons. Dermatologic Surg. 2013;39(9):1306–16.
19. Zaar O, et al. Effectiveness of photodynamic therapy in Bowen's disease: a retrospective observational study in 423 lesions. J Eur Acad Dermatol Venereol. 2017;31(8):1289–94.
20. Ribero S, et al. Drug therapy of advanced cutaneous squamous cell carcinoma: is there any evidence? Curr Opin Oncol. 2017;29(2):129–35.
21. Amos-Arowoshegbe EO, et al. Basal cell cancer of the scalp. Cureus. 2022;14(6):e26469.
22. Winder G, Kawar M, Shalom A. Anatomical distribution of basal cell carcinoma in Israel using relative tumor density scores. Int J Dermatol. 2021;60(11):1373–5.
23. Kim M, et al. Basal cell carcinoma of the scalp shows distinct features from the face in Asians. Sci Rep. 2022;12(1):10183.
24. Peris K, et al. European consensus-based interdisciplinary guideline for diagnosis and treatment of basal cell carcinoma-update 2023. Eur J Cancer. 2023;192:113254.
25. Requena C, Serra-Guillén C, Sanmartín O. Histologically agressive basal cell carcinoma with particular emphasis on galeal infiltration of the scalp. Actas Dermosifiliogr. 2022;113(6):575–82.
26. Castanheira A, Soares P, Boaventura P. Scalp basal cell carcinoma: a different entity? Dermatol Ther. 2019;32(2):e12828.
27. Hernandez LE, et al. Basal cell carcinoma: an updated review of pathogenesis and treatment options. Dermatol Ther. 2022;35(6):e15501.
28. Basset-Seguin N, Herms F. Update in the management of basal cell carcinoma. Acta Derm Venereol. 2020;100(11):adv00140.
29. Queirolo P, et al. Guidelines for the diagnosis and treatment of basal cell carcinoma: a GRADE approach for evidence evaluation and recommendations by the Italian Association of Medical Oncology. ESMO Open. 2023;8(6):102037.
30. Peris K, et al. Diagnosis and treatment of basal cell carcinoma: European consensus-based interdisciplinary guidelines. Eur J Cancer. 2019;118:10–34.
31. Patel PV, et al. Recommendations for cost-conscious treatment of basal cell carcinoma. Dermatol Ther (Heidelb). 2023;13(9):1959–71.
32. Kuhlmann C, et al. Dermatofibrosarcoma protuberans of the scalp: surgical management in a multicentric series of 11 cases and systematic review of the literature. Surgery. 2023;173(6):1463–75.
33. Vitiello GA, Lee AY, Berman RS. Dermatofibrosarcoma protuberans: what is this? Surg Clin North Am. 2022;102(4):657–65.
34. Kibbi N, et al. Dermatofibrosarcoma protuberans in pregnancy: a case series and review of the literature. Int J Dermatol. 2021;60(9):1114–9.
35. Lyu A, Wang Q. Dermatofibrosarcoma protuberans: a clinical analysis. Oncol Lett. 2018;16(2):1855–62.
36. Mujtaba B, et al. Dermatofibrosarcoma protuberans: pathological and imaging review. Curr Probl Diagn Radiol. 2021;50(2):236–40.
37. Badhey AK, Tikhtman R, Tang AL. Management of dermatofibrosarcoma protuberans. Curr Opin Otolaryngol Head Neck Surg. 2021;29(4):278–82.
38. Grizzetti L, Gaide O, Kuonen F. Dermatofibrosarcoma protuberans: clinico-pathological aspects and management. Rev Med Suisse. 2020;16(688):640–5.
39. Rust DJ, et al. Surgical management of dermatofibrosarcoma protuberans. J Surg Oncol. 2023;128(1):87–96.
40. Houdek MT, et al. Surgical outcomes of primary dermatofibrosarcoma protuberans: a retrospective, multicenter study. Ann Surg Oncol. 2022;29(13):8632–8.
41. Zongo N, et al. Dermatofibrosarcoma protuberans surgery: experiences of four African surgical oncology units and literature review. J Surg Oncol. 2022;126(8):1512–9.
42. Allen A, Ahn C, Sangüeza OP. Dermatofibrosarcoma protuberans. Dermatol Clin. 2019;37(4):483–8.
43. Sangrador M, Olvera JG, Ortiz VM. Dermatofibrosarcoma of the scalp. Surg Neurol Int. 2019;10:221.
44. Kanesen D, et al. Dermatofibrosarcoma protuberans of the scalp: therapeutic challenges. ANZ J Surg. 2019;89(3):261–4.
45. Hongo T, et al. Evaluation of tumor cell infiltration to the skull in dermatofibrosarcoma protuberans of the scalp: case report and literature review. NMC Case Rep J. 2021;8(1):287–93.
46. Fezza R, et al. A rare presentation of dermatofibrosarcoma protuberans of the scalp treated with "Slow-Mohs" micrographic surgery. J Drugs Dermatol. 2022;21(5):534–5.
47. Ramirez-Fort MK, et al. Dermatofibrosarcoma protuberans: the current state of multidisciplinary management. Skinmed. 2020;18(5):288–93.
48. Hao X, et al. Dermatofibrosarcoma protuberans: update on the diagnosis and treatment. J Clin Med. 2020;9(6)
49. Saaiq M, et al. A brief synopsis on scalp melanoma. Dermatol Ther. 2020;33(4):e13795.
50. Licata G, et al. Diagnosis and management of melanoma of the scalp: a review of the literature. Clin Cosmet Investig Dermatol. 2021;14:1435–47.
51. Wood RP, et al. Association of known melanoma risk factors with primary melanoma of the scalp and neck. Cancer Epidemiol Biomarkers Prev. 2020;29(11):2203–10.
52. Garbe C, et al. European consensus-based interdisciplinary guideline for melanoma. Part 1: diagnostics: update 2022. Eur J Cancer. 2022;170:236–55.

53. Swetter SM, et al. NCCN Guidelines® insights: melanoma: cutaneous, version 2.2021. J Natl Compr Cancer Netw. 2021;19(4):364–76.
54. Chinese expert consensus on the surgical treatment of cutaneous/acral melanoma V1.0. Zhonghua Zhong Liu Za Zhi. 2020;42(2):81–93.
55. Pathak, S. and P.M. Zito, Clinical guidelines for the staging, diagnosis, and management of cutaneous malignant melanoma. 2024.
56. Coit DG, et al. Cutaneous melanoma, version 2.2019, NCCN clinical practice guidelines in oncology. J Natl Compr Cancer Netw. 2019;17(4):367–402.
57. Garbe C, et al. European consensus-based interdisciplinary guideline for melanoma. Part 2: treatment – update 2022. Eur J Cancer. 2022;170:256–84.
58. Seth R, et al. Systemic therapy for melanoma: ASCO guideline update. J Clin Oncol. 2023;41(30):4794–820.
59. Wright FC, et al. Primary excision margins, sentinel lymph node biopsy, and completion lymph node dissection in cutaneous melanoma: a clinical practice guideline. Curr Oncol. 2019;26(4):e541–50.
60. Michielin O, et al. Cutaneous melanoma: ESMO Clinical Practice Guidelines for diagnosis, treatment and follow-up†. Ann Oncol. 2019;30(12):1884–901.
61. Mousa AK, et al. Post-burn scar malignancy: 5-year management review and experience. Int Wound J. 2022;19(4):895–909.
62. Sun W, et al. New progress of tuberculosis scar carcinoma. Cancer Metastasis Rev. 2023;42(3):653–9.
63. Kowal-Vern A, Criswell BK. Burn scar neoplasms: a literature review and statistical analysis. Burns. 2005;31(4):403–13.
64. Chalya PL, et al. Marjolin's ulcers at a university teaching hospital in Northwestern Tanzania: a retrospective review of 56 cases. World J Surg Oncol. 2012;10:38.
65. Cangkrama M, Wietecha M, Werner S. Wound repair, scar formation, and cancer: converging on activin. Trends Mol Med. 2020;26(12):1107–17.
66. Nthumba PM. Marjolin's ulcers: theories, prognostic factors and their peculiarities in spina bifida patients. World J Surg Oncol. 2010;8:108.
67. Chirukandath R, et al. Squamous cell carcinoma scalp with intracranial extension: challenging case of multidisciplinary care. Cureus. 2023;15(2):e34975.
68. Katano A, Yamashita H, Nakagawa K. Radical radiotherapy for localized cutaneous angiosarcoma of the scalp. Mol Clin Oncol. 2021;15(3):195.
69. Messias H, et al. Multifocal cutaneous angiosarcoma of the scalp – a challenging reconstructive case managed with skin substitutes. Cancer Rep (Hoboken). 2022;5(10):e1659.
70. Li Y, et al. Scalp angiosarcoma with skull roof infiltration and metastasis to the lung. Indian J Dermatol. 2022;67(3):315.
71. Dunaeva ER, Orlova EV. Cutaneous angiosarcoma of the scalp. J Cutan Med Surg. 2024:12034754241235965.
72. Mlay K, et al. Giant pilomatrix carcinoma of the scalp with intracranial extension: a case report. Clin Case Reports. 2023;11(11):e8123.
73. Marnouche EA, et al. Sebaceous carcinoma of the parotid gland: a case report and review of the literature. J Med Case Rep. 2016;10:174.
74. Hamid RN, et al. Sebaceous carcinoma of the scalp masquerading as a Pilar cyst. Dermatologic Surg. 2022;48(9):1000–1.
75. Li G, et al. Aggressive sebaceous carcinoma of the scalp: a case report and literature review. Transl Cancer Res. 2021;10(9):4237–42.
76. Dai Y, et al. Cutaneous metastasis from cervical cancer to the scalp and trunk: a case report and review of the literature. J Med Case Rep. 2023;17(1):435.

21 Malignant Neoplasms and Secondary Neoplasms of the Calvarium

Cameron Shuman, Brody Hooper, and Timothy Beutler

21.1 Introduction and Epidemiology

Malignant neoplasms of the calvarium can be broadly classified into primary or secondary neoplasms. Primary calvarial neoplasms arise from cells of the skull. They possess the ability to invade nearby tissue and spread to other parts of the body. Secondary neoplasms are malignancies that have metastasized from primary tumors located elsewhere in the body [1]. Bony tumors of the skull account for approximately 1% of all bone tumors, whereas calvarial metastases are found in 15–25% of all cancer patients [2, 3]. The most common primary sites are the breasts, lungs, prostate, lymph nodes, kidneys, and thyroid, which account for over 90% of all lesions (Chart 21.1) [4–6].

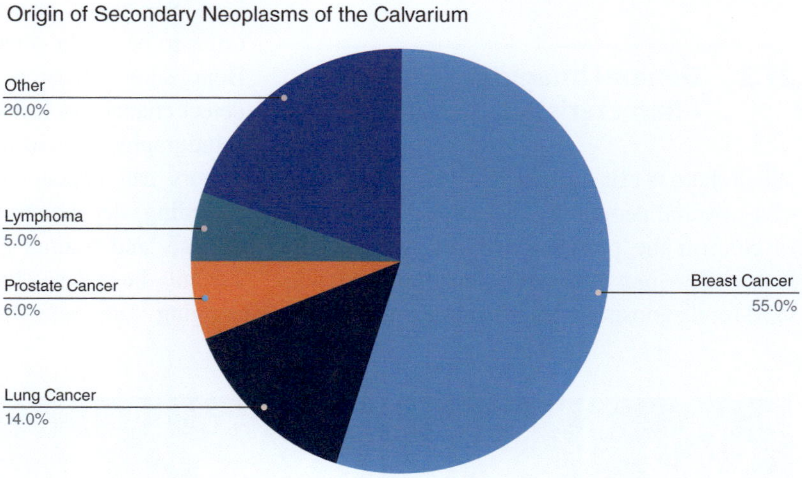

Chart 21.1 Most common areas of primary tumors that metastasize to the calvarium as a secondary neoplasm

C. Shuman · B. Hooper · T. Beutler (✉)
Department of Neurosurgery, State University of New York (SUNY) Upstate Medical University, Syracuse, NY, USA
e-mail: beutlert@upstate.edu

M. Turgut et al. (eds.), *Lesions of the Scalp and Cranial Vault*,
https://doi.org/10.1007/978-3-031-88244-9_21

21.2 Clinical Signs and Symptoms

The clinical signs and symptoms of a calvarial tumor are dependent on the location of the tumor and its degree of infiltration on adjacent structures. This may lead to a different combination of symptoms for each patient with varying tumor locations and sizes. When found in the epicranial region, lesions are commonly painless and can present as a mass [7]. Calvarial metastases can cause superficial focal pain as well as cosmetic deformity. When lesions erode through the calvarium and begin to exert mass effect on the brain parenchyma, patients can present with signs and symptoms of increased intracranial pressure, meningeal irritation, and focal neurological signs [5]. These symptoms include but are not limited to headaches, nausea, vomiting, confusion, lethargy, focal weakness or paralysis, difficulty with speech, and seizures. Neoplasms that arise or spread along the skull base can present with cranial nerve palsies and pain. Pain is the most common symptom for lesions in this location but patient also commonly report diplopia and sinusitis [7, 8].

21.3 General Imaging Characteristics

When there is clinical suspicion for the presence of a calvarial neoplasm, imaging is first obtained to confirm the presence and the extent of the tumor. The most common imaging modalities used for diagnosis are MRI and computed tomography (CT) imaging [5]. High-quality CT imaging is able to detect small skull lesions and determine the extent of bony involvement. Lesions on CT imaging are typically classified as lytic, blastic, or mixed. MRI is better suited to determine the extent of tumor infiltration into surrounding structures [4]. The standard approach for detecting skull metastases is T2- and T1-weighted MRI sequences before and after the administration of gadolinium contrast. Normal skull appears hyperintense on T1-weighted images and isointense on T2-weighted images. After administration of gadolinium, malignant neoplasms can show contrast enhancement [5]. Figure 21.1 depicts typical CT and MRI findings in a patient with a metastatic occipital metastasis. The lesion appears lytic on CT imaging and contrast enhances on MRI.

Other modalities that have been used in the diagnosis and management of calvarial neoplasms include plain X-rays, bone scintigraphy, and positron emission tomography (PET) imaging. Plain film X-rays are often used to screen for lesions but are nonspecific and are not sensitive to detect changes. A skull lesion would have to have changed in size by approximately 50% in order to be easily detected on plain film X-rays. Bone scintigraphy is more sensitive and can detect changes in lesions as small as 10%. Bone scintigraphy also has a high false-positive rate as tumors can appear similar to other processes including degeneration, inflammation, Paget's disease, and trauma [9]. PET imaging is more specific, however is much more expensive. PET imaging utilizes nonspecific tracers like

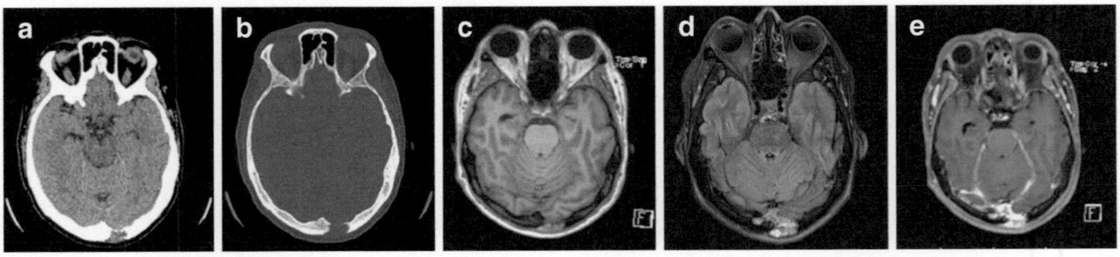

Fig. 21.1 Patient with history of thyroid papillary carcinoma presenting with left occipital metastasis. (**a**) CT head without contrast showing tumor isodense to the brain. (**b**) Bone window on CT imaging showing local invasion and lytic destruction of bone from metastasis. MRI showed that the lesion was isointense on T1-weighted imaging (**c**) and hyperintense on T2-weighted imaging (**d**). T1 with contrast showed avid enhancement (**e**)

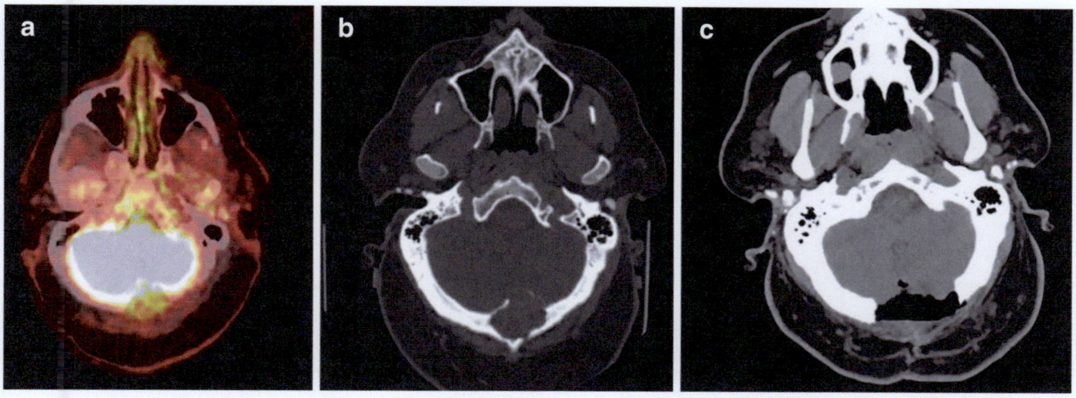

Fig. 21.2 Patient with history of renal cell carcinoma. (**a**) CT/PET imaging showed a lesion in the occipital region with increased uptake. (**b**) CT head without contrast showing an expansile lytic lesion. (**c**) CT head without contrast showing resection of the skull metastasis

^{18}F-fluorodeoxyglucose (^{18}FDG), an analog of glucose. PET scans show the increased glucose transport and glycolysis associated with tumors. The ^{18}FDG is phosphorylated inside the malignant cells by FDG-6-phosphate and is retained intracellularly. A standardized uptake value is then used to quantify the tissue activity in the region of interest [9]. Increased activity is associated with malignant cells. Figure 21.2a depicts an occipital calvarial lesion that was discovered incidentally on surveillance whole-body CT/PET imaging.

21.4 Principles of Treatment

After confirmation of the presence of a skull lesion on imaging, treatment options depend on the diagnosis. Imaging alone is often nonspecific and histologic diagnosis is often needed. A thorough history can be helpful in determining whether the lesion is likely a metastatic tumor. If history is negative for malignancy, sometimes a metastatic work-up may still be indicated to rule out the presence of a primary tumor and to assess the extent of additional skeletal involvement. General treatment options for primary and secondary malignancies are similar and include options for surgery, chemotherapy, radiation, and sometimes immunotherapy. Specific histologies may be more sensitive to different treatment modalities with tumor-specific mutations playing a larger role in the choice of targeted chemotherapy and immunotherapy agents. Malignant neoplasms may require multiple treatment modalities in order to obtain good local control [5, 10].

Lesions for which a diagnosis cannot be made on imaging and history alone often require surgery for biopsy and resection. Figure 21.2b and c show the preoperative and postoperative CT imaging for a simple resection of a metastatic calvarial tumor. Observation alone in cases of suspected malignant neoplasms is not recommended due to the invasive and progressive nature of the tumors. Due to the axial position of many tumors in the CNS, a complete surgical resection can sometimes be difficult and may result in increased morbidity or mortality. Therefore treatment needs to be customized in each individual case [11]. In cases that involve large portions of the scalp and skull, a multidisciplinary approach may be needed. Figure 21.3 shows imaging of a patient with extensive scalp and bony involvement who required a free-flap reconstruction of the scalp after resection of a large metastatic lesion.

Immunotherapy has begun to be shown as a promising emerging treatment for metastatic tumors. This is done through the manipulation of immune cells of cancer patients to combat metastatic spread and proliferation. The immune checkpoint inhibitors (ICIs), anti-CTLA-4 and

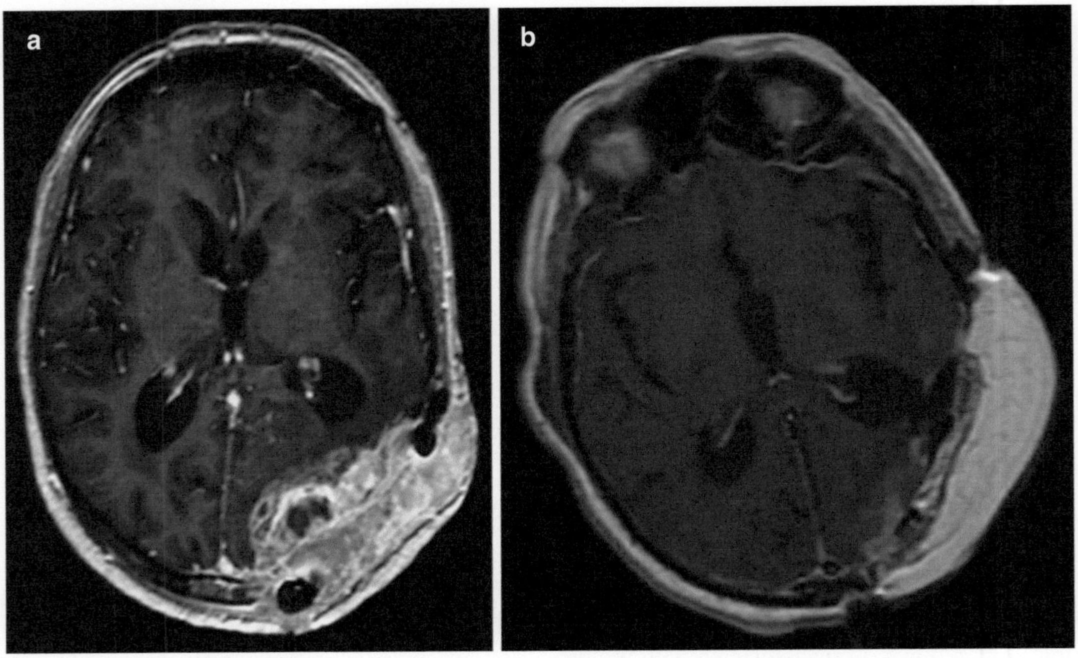

Fig. 21.3 Patient with metastatic lung cancer with extensive calvarial involvement with intracranial extension. (**a**) Preoperative T1 with contrast imaging showing an avidly enhancing mass involving the calvarium in the left parietal region. (**b**) Postoperative T1 with contrast imaging after tumor resection and free flap reconstruction of the scalp

anti-PD-1, have shown to be some of the most successful therapies, as they aim to keep anti-tumor T cells active [12]. However, resistance to ICIs is not uncommon, resulting in a need for new predictive immunotherapy biomarkers [13]. Other emerging modalities include the use of cell-based immunotherapy and inhibition of pro-tumor immune cells [12].

21.5 Primary Malignant Neoplasms of the Calvarium

21.5.1 Fibrosarcoma

Fibrosarcoma is a spindle cell malignancy originating from the fibroblast cell of connective fibrous tissue. These tumors comprise under 5% of all primary bone sarcomas [14]. While fibrosarcoma is most commonly found in the long bones of the extremities, it is also the second most common sarcoma of the head and neck and sometimes involves the skull base [5, 6]. The cause of fibrosarcoma is unknown, although genetic mutations may play a role and multiple other factors have shown to promote tumor proliferation. These include scar tissue, insertion of foreign material during surgery, and previously irradiated tissue [15]. The average age at time of diagnosis is 35 years of age, although fibrosarcomas can be found in children and elderly persons as well [16]. Patients typically present with a spherical, firm mass that measures 3–8 cm. Symptoms begin to arise as the mass compresses surrounding tissue and may include pain, sinusitis, nasal obstruction, epistaxis, and hypoesthesia [6, 14]. The primary imaging modality used for skull base fibrosarcomas is MRI. Lesions may be homogenous or heterogenous and show up isointense to muscle on T1-weighted imaging [14]. On CT imaging, this soft tissue tumor has been described as a mass exhibiting destruction and erosion of bone. On PET scans, fibrosarcomas experience increased glucose uptake [14]. Diagnosis should be confirmed with biopsy if possible [15].

The standard treatment is surgical excision or en bloc excision, depending on the location, size, and grade of the tumor. In addition to surgical removal, chemotherapy is also utilized to kill rapidly proliferating cells, allowing for disease control and prevention of tumor progression [15]. Prognosis of fibrosarcoma varies depending on tumor size, location, depth, involvement with adjacent structures, and metastatic potential. However, the most important prognostic indicator has shown to be histopathological grade [15]. The most commonly used grading scale was developed by the French Federation of Cancer Centers Sarcoma Group (FNCLCC). A histological assessment of the tumor's differentiation, mitotic activity, and necrosis is made and a higher score is associated with a worse prognosis. The 10-year survival rate is 60% for low-grade tumors and 30% for high-grade tumors. 80% of all adult fibrosarcomas are high-grade tumors. The average recurrence rate following resection is approximately 40–50% [15]. However, these tumors occur and are treated in children under 4 years of age; prognosis has shown to be significantly improved with lower rates of local recurrence and metastasis [14].

21.5.2 Osteosarcoma

Osteosarcoma is a malignant neoplasm arising from the osteoblast cells of bone, making places of rapid bone turnover the most commonly affected regions [17]. Osteosarcoma comprises approximately 35% of all malignant bone tumors, making it the most common bone sarcoma [17]. Primary osteosarcoma is present in the head and neck in roughly 6–13% of cases, while also accounting for 1.7–5% of total head and neck cancers [18]. Cases of the skull base normally occur in the third and fourth decades of life, affecting males and females at equal rates [18]. Certain contributory factors have been found to increase likelihood of development including prior chemotherapy or radiation, Paget disease, and fibrous dysplasia [2, 8, 9]. In cases of the skull base, patients may present with symptoms including proptosis, cranial nerve palsies, visual impairment, and headaches [18]. Both CT and MRI are used in order to assess the extent and invasiveness of the tumor, neurovascular involvement, and metastases [17]. Osteosarcoma may appear on radiographs demonstrating cortical destruction with a "moth-eaten" to permeative pattern with mineralized osteoid [19]. This presentation is very similar to that of Ewing sarcoma, so other factors must be taken into consideration for differentiation. This can also be accomplished with diffusion-weighted imaging using varying apparent diffusion coefficient values [19]. Chest CT scans should also be conducted, as osteosarcoma most often metastasizes in the lungs [20].

Treatment for high-grade osteosarcomas involves preoperative chemotherapy, surgical resection, and postoperative chemotherapy which is often performed with adjuvant radiotherapy [11, 12, 17]. Prognosis is classically dependent on tumor location and size, although osteosarcoma has a generally positive outlook. Craniofacial osteosarcomas, if entirely resected, have an 88% 5-year overall survival rate [20]. Cases of the skull have been shown to be more difficult to completely excise and have a 51% 5-year survival rate [21].

21.5.3 Chondrosarcoma

Chondrosarcoma is the second most common primary bone tumor following osteosarcoma. It can be present in both the appendicular and axial skeleton, affecting the head and neck region in 5% of cases and the skull base in 1% [8, 22]. Chondrosarcoma is classified as one of four different subtypes: conventional, dedifferentiated, clear cell, and mesenchymal. Over 90% of cases are classified as the primary conventional subtype, with almost all cases of chondrosarcoma in the skull base being the conventional subtype, as other subtypes rarely affect the axial skeleton [8]. Understanding of other subtypes remains essential, as optimal treatment may vary [22].

Conventional chondrosarcomas are composed of hyaline, myxoid, or a combination of hyaline and myxoid cartilage [8]. Chondrosarcomas of the skull base classically present de novo in the fourth decade of life [8]. Radiologically, tumors appear hypointense or isointense on T1-weighted imaging and hyperintense on T2-weighted imaging. They have an appearance of a lytic lesion with variable ring-like matrix mineralization [4]. Higher-grade lesions often appear more lytic and show less mineralization than less aggressive tumors [22]. Biopsy of the lesion is required for accurate diagnosis and histological grading of the tumor, as they are graded on cellularity, cytologic atypia, and mitotic activity [23]. It is important to distinguish chondrosarcoma from chordoma due to their similar presentation. This can be accomplished through immunohistochemistry using the markers of brachyury and cytokeratin, which are immunopositive in chordomas and negative in chondrosarcomas [2]. Symptoms are dependent on tumor location, but pain, headaches, cranial nerve palsies, hearing deficits, and gait disturbances are all commonly found [8].

Treatment involves surgical resection in conjunction with proton-beam irradiation, which has been shown to have 10-year recurrence control rates of 98% and a 10-year disease-specific survival rate of 99%. These rates are significantly lower if only surgical resection is performed, with a local recurrence rate of 53% [8]. Other treatment options may be explored if the tumor is unresectable after many recurrences or presentation of pulmonary metastases. Little evidence supports the use of conventional therapy [20].

21.5.4 Ewing Sarcoma

The histogenic cell of origin of Ewing sarcoma remains unknown even after 100 years since its discovery [24]. However, it is well understood genetically, with its primary cause being specific chromosomal translocations including those of the *EWSR1*, *FUS*, and *TAF15* genes [2, 24]. Ewing sarcoma mainly affects long bones (femur, tibia, pelvis) and is much less common in the skull than chordoma and chondrosarcoma. Primary Ewing sarcoma is only present in the skull 1% of the time in comparison to the rest of the body, making the extent of literature on the topic very limited [21]. It typically occurs in patients under 20 years of age, with a peak incidence at 15 years. There is still a possibility of manifestation in adulthood and males are more commonly affected than females. Interestingly, there is also a strong disparity in ethnicity of patients that are affected. There are approximately 1.5 cases of Ewing sarcoma per million children of European descent, whereas there are approximately 0.8 and 0.2 cases per million children in populations of Asian and African descent, respectively [24].

Patients can present with locoregional pain which increases in severity over time. This is usually followed by a palpable mass at the location. Given the genetic nature of Ewing sarcoma, a thorough family history is necessary during diagnostic work-up to discover any association with very rare germline mutations or cancer predispositions such as *TP53* [24]. There are no specific laboratory diagnostic measures for Ewing sarcoma, although nonspecific markers such as elevated alkaline phosphatase may indicate bony involvement. Radiographic imaging is useful for diagnosis and screening for metastases, which is important as 9% of cases result in secondary malignancies. Figure 21.4 shows typical MRI findings in a patient who presented with diffuse metastases from Ewing's sarcoma including calvarial and leptomeningeal involvement. Ewing sarcoma has an "onion skin" appearance, showing tumor-related osteolysis as a destructive mass arising from the bone [24].

Treatment once again varies based on the location and surgical resectability of the tumor. Most frequently, treatment involves a multimodal approach of surgical resection coupled with chemotherapy and radiotherapy [21, 25]. Prognosis is slightly better than other primary malignancies as Ewing sarcoma of the skull has a 68.5% 5-year survival rate, although older age is associated with worse survival. Recurrence is relatively infrequent but is also associated with lower survival rates [21].

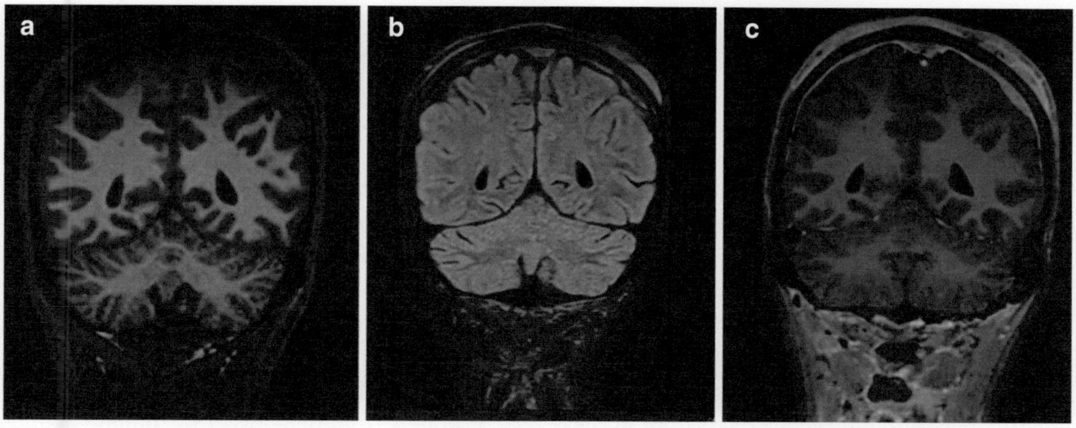

Fig. 21.4 Patient with Ewing's sarcoma presenting with diffuse spinal metastases and leptomeningeal disease with boney involvement. Tumor involvement seen over the bilateral parietal regions on MRI. (**a**) T1 without contrast showing tumor as hypointense. (**b**) T2 FLAIR showing tumor as isointense. (**c**) T1 with contrast showing diffuse contrast enhancement

21.5.5 Chordoma

A chordoma is a rare malignant tumor that manifests from remnants of the notochord, a structure present during embryonic development [4]. Chordomas are directly responsible for approximately 1–4% of all malignant bone tumors, with roughly 95% of all chordomas being intraosseous tumors affecting the axial skeleton [11]. Lesions of the skull base are equally as common as those of the vertebral bodies and sacrococcygeal bones and most commonly present between the ages of 40 and 60. Cases in the base of the skull have also been shown to arise approximately one decade earlier than those of the spine and sacrum. Gender distribution for the skull base is equal, and the majority of tumors arise in white patients according to the National Cancer Institute's Surveillance, Epidemiology, and End Results (SEER) program [8].

Patients may experience headaches, neck pain, diplopia, or cranial nerve palsies in cases involving the calvarium [11, 14]. A chordoma appears as an intraosseous lobulated mass that penetrates the boundary of the bone to invade adjacent tissues, which is often seen on CT scans [11]. Lesions vary in size, with an average size of 9 cm, but ranging from 4 to 22 cm according to one study of 99 patients [26]. Chordomas appear iso- or hypointense in T1-weighted images and appear inhomogeneous or hyperintense in T2-weighted images due to the lesion's myxoid matrix [4, 11].

The first-line treatment for chordomas is resection or en bloc resection; however, this is often complicated by the axial nature of the lesions. If a tumor is unable to be completely resected, radiation therapy is employed [11]. Prognosis is mostly dependent on tumor location, which correlates with resectability. In patients with all types of chordomas, the median survival length is 6.3 years [27].

21.6 Secondary Malignancies of the Calvarium

21.6.1 Breast Cancer

Breast cancer often results in bone metastases, although it is very rare that the metastases occur in the skull or skull base. However, breast cancer, lung cancer, and prostate cancer are the most common cancers to metastasize in this location [6]. The most common metastatic sites in this region include the maxillary, ethmoid, frontal, and sphenoid sinuses [28]. The mean time from primary breast cancer diagnosis to diagnosis of skull metastasis is 71 months according to prior retrospective studies [5].

Patients commonly present asymptomatically, making early diagnosis difficult, although varying clinical symptoms are also possible. These include pain, nausea, and cranial nerve palsies dependent on the structures impinged by the mass [5, 28]. When imaging the region, CT scan is sufficient for evaluating bony involvement, but MRI is also necessary for evaluating the extent of the metastases in both the skull and surrounding structures, including the brain. Metastases from breast cancer in the skull most frequently present as calvarial circumscribed intraosseous tumors, slightly more often than calvarial diffuse invasive metastases [5].

Treatment varies from case to case, but the most prevalent treatment option is radiation therapy, although surgical resection and chemotherapy are also utilized [5, 6]. Prognosis for skull base metastases is generally poor. One study found the overall average survival for skull base metastases from breast cancer to be 15 months. However, prognosis does vary based on tumor location, size, invasiveness, and dissemination of the primary tumor [5, 28].

21.6.2 Lung Cancer

The rate of lung cancer metastasizing in bone is relatively high, at 36%, but the rate of metastases in the skull or calvarium is very low, at a reported 3% [29, 30]. Still, lung cancer has been found to be the second most common primary tumor for skull metastases due to the relatively high frequency of lung cancer compared to other cancer types. Studies have found that the histological variations of lung cancer most likely to metastasize to the skull are adenocarcinoma (58%) and small cell carcinoma (18%). Like breast cancer, the mass most commonly forms as a calcarial circumscribed intraosseous lesion. The average time from initial diagnosis of lung cancer to the development of a skull metastasis is approximately 9 months. Patients most often have no symptoms, although if the metastases are invasive local pain and swelling can be present [5]. There have also been reports of intracerebral hemorrhages at the site of metastasis. Intracranial hemorrhage is associated with increased morbidity and mortality. Intracranial hemorrhage is likely due to the invasion of intracerebral vessels by skull metastasis [30].

For radiological examination of the calvarial tumor, CT scan and MRI are used to assess bony involvement and extent of the tumor and metastasis [5, 29]. Treatment of these tumors involves surgical biopsy vs excision if possible followed by aggressive chemotherapy and radiation [29]. Prognosis after a skull metastases from lung cancer is often unfavorable, with an overall survival of 5 months from diagnosis [5]. Immunotherapy has also shown to be an effective treatment for lung cancer. Immune checkpoint inhibitors are now being used as first-line therapy in metastatic disease for non-small cell lung cancer [13]. However, complications are still present as resistance to immune checkpoint inhibitors is common due to lack of response or disease progression following an initial response [13].

21.6.3 Prostate Cancer

Prostate cancer is the most common cancer in men and one of the most common causes of secondary bone tumors [31]. Even though only 2% of prostate cancer metastases form in the skull, some studies have found that prostate cancer is the most common primary tumor in skull base metastases (SBM) [5, 31]. This predilection may be due to Batson's venous plexus, which connects the prostate venous outflow to the axial skeleton and skull [31]. Due to the high rate of manifestation in the skull base in comparison to other metastases, patients are also more likely to experience symptoms such as cranial nerve palsies and pain [5, 32]. These symptoms occur when there is impingement on the neural foramina by tumor growth [32]. Confirmation of SBM diagnosis can be made by an isotope bone scan, CT, or MRI, which is also useful to assess soft tissue involvement [5, 32]. However, it is common that SBM from prostate cancer goes unnoticed without symptoms as patients may not undergo brain imaging during screening [5]. There should be deliberate screening for skull metastases in patients with prostate cancer [31]. The mean time from primary tumor diagnosis to secondary tumor diagnosis is 26 months for prostate cancer. Treatment is dependent on tumor location but often involves a primary surgical resection approach coupled with radiation therapy and chemotherapy. Overall survival from diagnosis of the secondary tumor for prostate cancer is approximately 23 months [5].

21.6.4 Melanoma

Melanoma is a malignant tumor arising from melanocytes, which are derived from neural crest cells. Approximately 10–25% of melanoma is found in the head and neck, with almost all of these cases affecting the face, scalp, neck, and ear. Major risk factors include ultraviolet (UV) light exposure, fair skin, and a family history of melanoma [33]. Mucosal melanoma is a rare subtype of melanoma accounting for only 1% of malignant melanomas that usually form in the nasal cavity and paranasal sinuses. However, according to the AJCC (American Joint Committee on Cancer) TNM staging for mucosal melanoma, a T4a- and T4b-rated tumor may impact the skull base, brain, dura, and lower cranial nerves [34]. These tumors are often found in later stages due to their often asymptomatic presentation, similar to other sinus tumors [35]. Figure 21.5 shows imaging from a patient with metastatic melanoma who presented with an symptomatic calvarial metastasis in the setting of hemorrhagic intracranial brain metastases. A metastatic work-up should be conducted in all cases including CT of the chest and abdomen, MRI of the brain, and PET CT. Diagnosis should be confirmed with a biopsy or resection of the lesion if possible.

The gold standard of treatment is a radical resection of the tumor with clear margins, although this can be difficult to accomplish without impacting aesthetics or neurologic function [34]. Surgical resection via a craniofacial approach has an overall mortality of 6% and a 26% complication rate, which is comparable to other craniofacial resections for skull base tumors. However, mucosal melanoma still has a poor prognosis, with 48% overall 5-year survival and 53% disease-specific 5-year survival [35].

Immunotherapy has started to play an increasingly large role in the treatment of metastatic melanoma. It has been shown to induce anti-tumor immunity through both cell-based immunotherapies and inhibition of pro-tumor

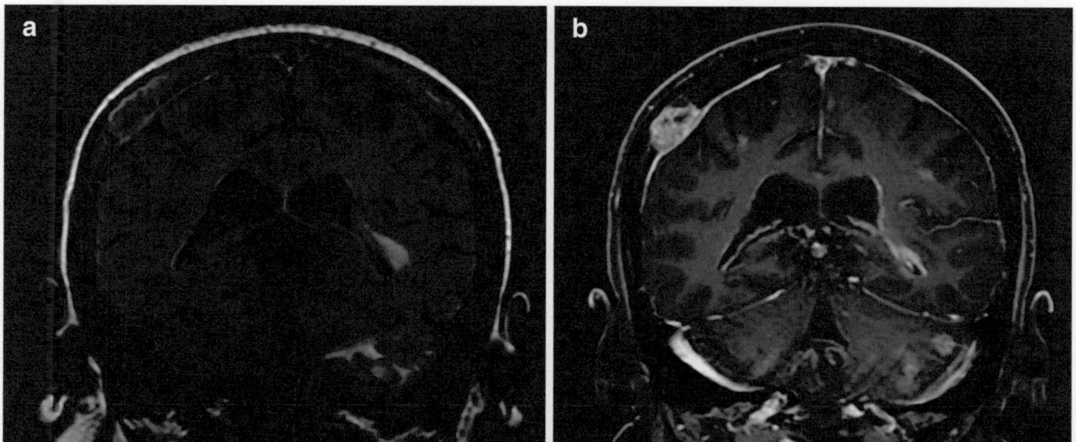

Fig. 21.5 Patient with history of melanoma presenting with calvarial and intracranial metastases. Coronal imaging showing a right parietal calvarial metastasis and left cerebellar metastasis. (**a**) T2 FLAIR imaging showing isointense lesions. (**b**) T1 with contrast showing avid contrast enhancement

immune cells [12]. In mouse models of metastatic melanoma, immunotherapy has been shown to significantly improve prognosis. Pembrolizumab and ONCOS-102 have been shown to have anti-tumor effects on primary melanoma tumors but are less effective on melanoma metastases. Other therapies using MICA α3 antibody have resulted in decreased lung and liver metastases. Utilization of IL-2 in mice has also been shown to eradicate metastatic growth in melanoma [36].

21.6.5 Thyroid Cancer (Usually Follicular)

Differentiated thyroid cancers, follicular and papillary subtypes, are generally curable when detected early [37]. However, follicular thyroid cancer is associated with distant metastases (including the skull) and increased mortality [38, 39]. Most cases begin asymptomatic and are diagnosed on physical exam with enlarged neck or lymph nodes [38]. The lungs and bone are the most common distant metastases locations, but metastases in the skull are very rare, with an occurrence of about 2.5% [37]. Distant metastases are most frequently present in older women. Thyroid cancer is also the second most common newly diagnosed cancer during pregnancy [38]. Research has shown that the most common presentation of skull metastases is soft hemispheric tumor, rich in vascularity, resting on the skull and contributing osteolytic changes [39]. A palpable mass is the most common symptom, although cranial nerve palsies, hemiparesis, and symptoms of intracranial hypertension are also possible [37]. The average period of time from diagnosis of thyroid cancer until the discovery of skull metastases is approximately 23.3 years [39]. Treatment can be a combination of different approaches, as surgical treatment, radioiodine therapy, and levothyroxine suppressive therapy have all been shown to prolong survival [37]. The prognosis is generally poor for skull metastases, as mean survival time from diagnosis is 4.5 years [39].

21.6.6 Renal Cell Cancer

Among renal tumors, renal cell carcinoma (RCC) is the most common malignancy, representing 85% of all malignant renal tumors. The median age of diagnosis is 66 years of age, with the highest incidence occurring between the sixth and seventh decades of life. RCC is also responsible for 2–3% of total adult malignancies [40]. However, renal cell cancer metastasizing to the skull and calvarium is very rare, with some studies documenting head and neck involvement in 8–15% of RCC cases [40, 41]. Of cases impacting the skull base, secondary tumors from the kidney arise most commonly in the frontal skull base, resulting in patient symptoms such as anosmia, facial pain, and diplopia [41]. Other tumor locations have also been documented with varying symptomatology. Standard treatment for metastatic renal cell cancer includes resection of the secondary skull tumor and a nephrectomy with chemotherapy [40]. Even after a nephrectomy, 20–50% of patients with RCC will still develop metastatic disease, resulting in a poor prognosis for RCC, with a median survival time of only 6–12 months [42].

21.6.7 Intrahepatic Cholangiocarcinoma (ICC)

ICC is the second most common type of primary liver cancer and is associated with a high rate of malignancy and poor prognosis. The incidence rate falls between 10 and 15%, but global rates have been rising [43]. The most common areas of metastases are the lungs and the liver, as ICC spreads lymphogenously, while metastatic disease in the skull is extremely rare [44]. Diagnosis is often challenging due to the lack of specific symptoms and very low incidence rate which leads to a delayed diagnosis when the cancer has reached an advanced stage [43]. Tumor location has been documented in the parietal and occipital regions of the calvarium but is not limited to these areas [43, 44]. One study examined four cases of skull tumors secondary to ICC and described the tumors as invasive to the skull barrier and internal and external cortical tables, forming a double convex shape. Tumors often invaded the epidural and subdural spaces, which resulted in patients exhibiting symptoms of scalp pain and swelling. ICC has shown to be resistant to chemoradiotherapy, which means therapeutic options are limited and surgical resection is usually the only viable treatment plan. Even so, ICC has a high rate of recurrence and prognosis is very poor, with a median survival time of 3 to 6 months [43].

21.6.8 Neuroblastoma

Following leukemia and primary CNS tumors, neuroblastoma is the third most common malignancy in children and frequently metastasizes [45]. In fact, it accounts for 10–15% of childhood malignancies and is the leading cause of calvarial metastases in children [7, 45]. The median age of diagnosis is 22 months, and 70% of children have metastatic disease at time of diagnosis. The most common primary tumor location is the adrenal gland which accounts for 48% of cases [46]. Among patients with neuroblastoma, 70% present with metastases, and this often manifests as an osseous tumor involving the calvaria, orbit, or skull base [45, 47]. These lesions may extend to the epidural and subdural spaces and produce deposits, as well as become diffuse and encompass multiple major skull bones [47, 48].

Radiologically, metastatic neuroblastoma of the skull can include lesions with thickened bone, lytic defects, and separation of sutures. The presentation of suture separation from neuroblastoma can be differentiated from generalized increased intracranial pressure by its nonuniform and indistinct margins [45]. Calvarial lesions from neuroblastoma have also shown a "hair-on-end" appearance on CT imaging. This is representative of the periosteal response to tumor cells extending from the lesion [47]. Early skull involvement may not be radiologically evident, but diagnosis can be confirmed with a radionuclide bone scan [48].

Patients may present with varying symptoms from primary and secondary lesions depending on location. The most common clinical presentation is a painless abdominal mass, as neuroblastoma can occur at any point along the sympathetic nervous system chain [46]. One of the most common clinical presentations is for secondary lesions to manifest symptoms before the primary tumor. When the orbital bone is affected by the metastases, patients can present with periorbital soft-tissue hematomas (black eyes), and this can be indicative of a primary metastatic neuroblastoma [46, 48]. The primary treatment option for neuroblastoma skull metastases is radiotherapy [47]. However, metastatic neuroblastoma is known for its high rate of recurrence and carries a poor prognosis [46].

21.7 Hematologic Malignancies

21.7.1 Lymphoma

Primary and secondary lymphomas of the skull and calvarium are rare [49, 50]. Primary bone lymphomas only account for 4% of all malignant non-Hodgkin's lymphomas and mainly affect the femur and pelvis. Only 0.2% of cases impact the cranial vault [49]. Primary non-Hodgkin's lymphoma generally affects teenagers and older patients. When affecting the skull base, the most common areas are the cavernous sinus and clivus. Common clinical symptoms include headaches and cranial nerve palsies. Diplopia is also common due to the paralysis of the abducens nerve [51]. Typically, lymphoma presents on MRI as isointense on T1-weighted and hyperintense on T2-weighted imaging. Cases typically exhibit evidence of bone destruction and thickened or enhanced dura mater. However, diagnosis of lymphoma cannot be made based on imaging and clinical findings alone, and a biopsy of the lesion is often required to make a pathological diagnosis [50, 52].

Lymphoma can also present as a large calvarial mass mimicking the appearance of a chronic subdural hematoma (Fig. 21.6). Surgical options for pathological diagnosis include open surgery, fine needle aspiration, ultrasound-guided needle

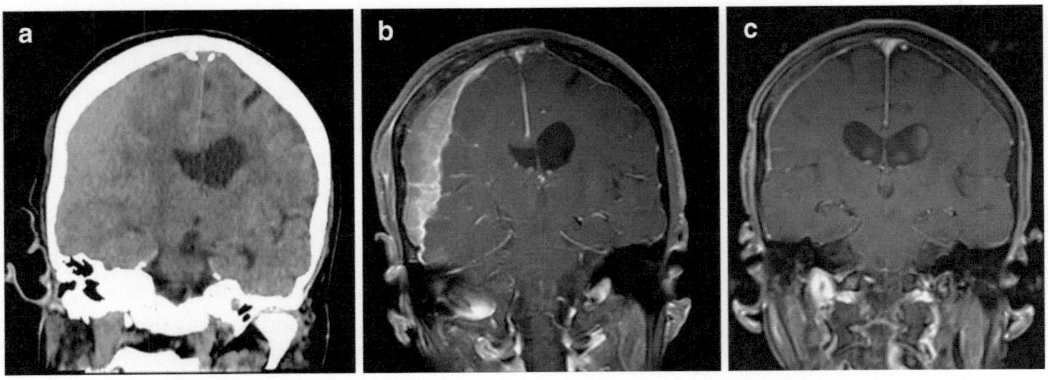

Fig. 21.6 Patient with marginal cell lymphoma presenting with left-sided weakness. (**a**) CT imaging showing large isodense extra-axial mass lesion resulting in midline shift mimicking appearance of a chronic subdural hematoma. (**b**) MRI with contrast imaging revealing diffuse enhancement of the dural-based mass as well as a periosteal enhancing mass. Patient underwent biopsy for diagnosis. (**c**) Repeat MRI with contrast imaging after treatment with chemotherapy

biopsy, and endoscopic skull base surgery [53]. The most common and favorable form of treatment is chemotherapy. For primary CNS lymphomas, a high-dose methotrexate is the recommended and often achievable of complete remission [51].

Malignant lymphoma has also been found responsible for secondary skull metastases. The average time from primary diagnosis to diagnosis of the skull metastases is 4 months [5]. One study of 175 patients found that malignant lymphoma was responsible for 5.1% of skull metastases, and another study of 279 patients found lymphoma responsible for 8% of metastases of the skull base [5, 54]. Lymphoma commonly metastasizes to the cavernous sinus, leading to cavernous sinus syndrome. This, coupled with early vision loss, may be indicative of systemic lymphoma [54]. Overall survival time for patients with a metastatic skull tumor from malignant lymphoma was 6 months [5].

21.7.2 Leukemia

Leukemia is the most common cancer among children, and acute lymphoblastic leukemia (ALL) is the most frequent subtype [55]. The second leading cause of death among childhood leukemia survivors is a secondary cancer later in life. The rates of secondary neoplasms from ALL for 10–15 years after treatment is 1.2–4.17% and 10.85% after 30 years past treatment. However, the likelihood of these metastases being located in the skull is very low [56]. In patients with ALL, it is possible to assess the infiltration of bone marrow in the skull using diffusion-weighted imaging, as infiltrations appear very hyperintense and are much more distinguishable than in T1 and T2-weighted imaging [55].

Acute myeloid leukemia (AML) has also been shown to metastasize to the skull and skull base [56]. This may be in the form of a myeloid sarcoma or, when in the cranium, an intracranial myeloid sarcoma (IMS). With an incidence rate of 0.4% in patients with AML, this is very rare and often misdiagnosed. Only 5% of IMS cases are found in the skull base. Clinical symptoms may include diplopia and vision loss, as well as headaches, nausea, and vomiting. Diagnosis via biopsy is the preferred method. Due to the rarity of this condition, there are no established treatment guidelines, but the standard approach includes radiotherapy or systemic chemotherapy. The overall 84-month survival rate is very mixed, sitting at 58.6% [57].

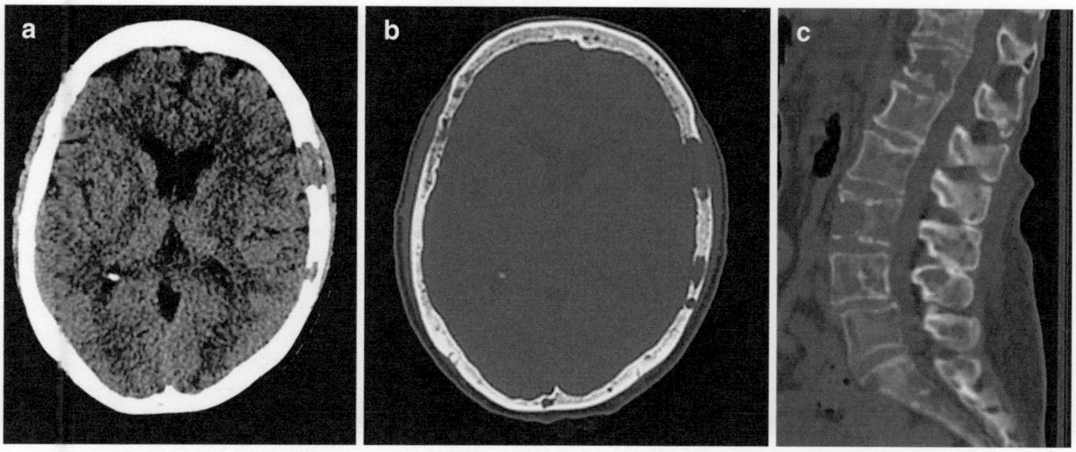

Fig. 21.7 Patient with history of multiple myeloma. CT imaging of the head showing multiple lytic lesions (**a**, **b**). CT of the lumbar spine showing similarly appearing lytic lesions (**c**)

21.7.3 Multiple Myeloma

Multiple myeloma (MM) is the most common primary malignancy of the skeleton and originates from the plasma cells of the bone marrow [58, 59]. This results in bone marrow infiltration and osteolytic lesions. These tumors are much more common in the elderly population, with peak presentation at 70 years old [58]. Multiple myeloma very rarely affects the calvarium, and intracranial myelomatosis is reported less than 1% of the time. This makes diagnosis increasingly difficult, and a confirmed diagnosis can only be made postoperatively [59]. Masses appear hyperintense to the brain on T1- and T2-weighted imaging and isointense to the brain on CT [58, 59]. Figure 21.7 shows CT imaging of typical calvarial and spinal lytic lesions seen in multiple myeloma. Patients typically experience bone pain and lassitude secondary to anemia or renal failure [58]. Due to its rarity, there is no standard treatment option, but cases have taken the approach of surgical resection if possible and then treatment with radiotherapy and chemotherapy postoperatively [58, 59]. Prognosis of multiple myeloma is mainly based on stage. There are a variety of staging systems in use which rely on laboratory markers in addition to imaging and cytogenetics. For example, the Durie-Salmon Staging System takes into account the degree of anemia, hypercalcemia, urine light chains, M-component production, renal failure, and number of bony lesions, while the Revised International Staging System looks at serum albumin, serum lactate dehydrogenase, serum beta-2-microglobulin, and presence of high-risk cytogenetics [58, 60]. Central intracranial myelomatosis only has a median survival time ≤1 year [59].

Bone pain is caused by the osteoclastic bone resorption that occurs due to the imbalance of osteoblastic and osteoclastic activity in multiple myeloma. Up to 70–95% of patients with MM develop bone metastases. This is known as myeloma bone disease (MBD) [61]. Subsequently, if the primary tumor does not impact the calvarium, MM has been shown to metastasize to the skull base and cause neurological deficiencies in some cases [62]. Bisphosphonate therapy (BPT) is the standard of care for treating MBD. BPT works through the inhibition of osteoclast formation and maturation, enhancement of osteoclast apoptosis, and reduction in osteoclast adherence to bone [61].

21.8 Conclusion

Primary and secondary malignant neoplasms of the calvarium present in many different histological forms and locations leading to a wide array of patient presentations. The overall occurrence of these tumors is rare across all types. However, understanding the characteristics of these tumors is essential for early diagnosis, appropriate management, and improved patient outcomes. The general diagnostic approach and principles of treatment follow similar patterns regardless of the tumor type. Multimodal imaging is employed in patients suspected of having calvarial lesions in order to identify and characterize the tumor. Obtaining a thorough history can also help to narrow the differential, but often surgery is needed to biopsy lesions in order to make a definitive diagnosis. Treatment strategies should be tailored to suspected tumor type and location. Multidisciplinary treatment with a combination of surgery, chemotherapy, radiation, and immunotherapy may be needed in order to maximize survival and minimize morbidity.

References

1. Goldbrunner R. Tumors of the skull. 2006:73–79.
2. Kakkar A, Nambirajan A, Suri V, Sarkar C, Kale SS, Singh M, Sharma MC. Primary bone tumors of the skull: spectrum of 125 cases, with review of literature. 2016;77:319–25.
3. Kotecha R, Angelov L, Barnett GH, Reddy CA, Suh JH, Murphy ES, Neyman G, Chao ST. Calvarial and skull base metastases: expanding the clinical utility of Gamma Knife surgery. 2014:91–101.
4. Gangadhar K, Santhosh D. Radiopathological evaluation of primary malignant skull tumors: a review. 2012;114:833–9.
5. Mitsuya K, Nakasu Y, Horiguchi S, Harada H, Nishimura T, Yuen S, Asakura K, Endo M. Metastatic skull tumors: MRI features and a new conventional classification. 2011;104:239–45.
6. Adachi K, Maeda Y, Hayama M, et al. Skull base metastasis of breast cancer with oculomotor and trochlear nerve palsy. 2022;101:NP270–2.
7. Gomez CK, Schiffman SR, Bhatt AA. Radiological review of skull lesions. 2018;9:857–82.
8. Harsh GR, Ojemann RE. Chordomas and chondrosarcomas of the skull base and spine. New York: Thieme; 2003.
9. Messiou C, Cook G, deSouza NM. Imaging metastatic bone disease from carcinoma of the prostate. 2009;101:1225–32.
10. Ozgiray E, Perumal K, Cinar C, Caliskan KE, Ertan Y, Yurtseven T, Oktar N, Ovul I, Oner K. Management of calvarial tumors: a retrospective analysis and literature review. 2016;26:690–8.
11. Ulici V, Hart J. Chordoma. 2022;146:386–95.
12. Edwards SC, Hoevenaar WHM, Coffelt SB. Emerging immunotherapies for metastasis. 2021;124:37–48.
13. Mamdani H, Matosevic S, Khalid AB, Durm G, Jalal SI. Immunotherapy in lung cancer: current landscape and future directions. 2022;13:823618.
14. Midyett FA, Mukherji SK. Skull base fibrosarcoma. 2020:329–332.
15. Augsburger D, Nelson PJ, Kalinski T, et al. Current diagnostics and treatment of fibrosarcoma -perspectives for future therapeutic targets and strategies. 2017;8:104638–53.
16. Mark RJ, Sercarz JA, Tran L, Selch M, Calcaterra TC. Fibrosarcoma of the head and neck: the UCLA experience. 1991;117:396–401.
17. Barnett S, Cable MG. Introductory chapter: integrating basic science with a multidisciplinary clinical approach for osteosarcoma. Ch. 1; 2019.
18. Ahrari A, Labib M, Gravel D, Macdonald KI. Primary osteosarcoma of the skull base treated with endoscopic endonasal approach: a case report and literature review. 2015;76:e270–4.
19. Şafak P, Bilge EF, Yüksel GY, Jale K, Burça AG, Kemal K, Üstün A. Diffusion-weighted imaging for the differentiation of Ewing sarcoma from osteosarcoma. 2021;50:2023–30.
20. Whelan JS, Davis LE. Osteosarcoma, chondrosarcoma, and chordoma. 2018;36:188–93.
21. Martin E, Senders JT, Ter Wengel PV, Smith TR, Broekman MLD. Treatment and survival of osteosarcoma and Ewing sarcoma of the skull: a SEER database analysis. 2019;161:317–25.
22. Weinschenk RC, Wang W-L, Lewis VO. Chondrosarcoma. 2021;29:553–62.
23. Davis KL LF, Sticco DD. Chondrosarcoma. 2023.
24. Thomas GPG, Cidre-Aranaz F, Surdez D, Tomazou EM, de Álava E, Kovar H, Sorensen PH, Delattre O, Dirksen U. Ewing sarcoma (Primer). 2018.
25. Hagihara R, Arishima H, Yamauchi T, Kawajiri S, Ito T, Fukushima M, Kikuta K. Ewing sarcoma with very late metastasis in the skull: a case report. 2022;16:1–419.
26. Radaelli S, Stacchiotti S, Ruggieri P, et al. Sacral chordoma: long-term outcome of a large series of patients surgically treated at two reference centers. 2016:41.
27. McMaster ML, Goldstein AM, Bromley CM, Ishibe N, Parry DM. Chordoma: incidence and survival patterns in the United States, 1973–1995. 2001;12:1–11.
28. Othman IA, Zahedi FD, Husain S. Base of skull metastatic adenocarcinoma from the breast 23 years after the primary diagnosis. 2020:2610597.
29. Turner RC, Lucke-Wold B, Hwang R, Underwood BD. Lung cancer metastasis presenting as a solitary skull mass. 2016;2016:rjw116.
30. Hiraki A, Tabata M, Ueoka H, Kiura K, Shibayama T, Yamane H, Harada M. Direct intracerebral invasion from skull metastasis of large cell lung cancer. 1997;36:720–3.
31. Brahima K, Fasnewindé Aristide K, Babagana Mustapha A, Mohamed S, Bienvenue Désiré K, Aïssata O. Skull metastasis in prostate cancer: a

compilation of four cases along with review of the literature. 2019.
32. Joe MO, Norman AR, McNair H, Dearnaley DP. Cranial nerve palsies in metastatic prostate cancer—results of base of skull radiotherapy. 2004;70:87–90.
33. Zito PM, Scharf R. Melanoma of the head and neck. Treasure Island (FL): StatPearls Publishing LLC; 2023.
34. Thierauf J, Glück A-M, Plinkert P, Veit JA, Hoffmann TK, Körber A, Bergmann C. Mucosal melanoma of the cranio-facial region: surgical challenges and therapeutic options. 2019;46:252–9.
35. Ganly I, Patel SG, Singh B, et al. Craniofacial resection for malignant melanoma of the skull base: report of an international collaborative study. 2006;132:73–8.
36. Kähkönen TE, Halleen JM, Bernoulli J. Immunotherapies and metastatic cancers: understanding utility and predictivity of human immune cell engrafted mice in preclinical drug development. 2020;12:1615. https://doi.org/10.3390/cancers12061615.
37. Chiofalo MG, Setola SV, Di Gennaro F, Fulciniti F, Catapano G, Losito NS, Sandomenico F, Catalano O, Pezzullo L. Follicular thyroid carcinoma with skull metastases. 2015;62:363–9.
38. Huang T-C, Cheng Y-K, Chen T-W, Hsu Y-C, Liu E-W, Chen H-H. A 'silent' skull metastatic follicular thyroid carcinoma mimicking as a benign scalp tumor in a pregnant woman. 2017;2017:1–6.
39. Nagamine Y, Suzuki J, Katakura R, Yoshimoto T, Matoba N, Takaya K. Skull metastasis of thyroid carcinoma. Study of 12 cases. 1985;63:526–31.
40. Badri M, Gader G, Bahri K, Zammel I. Skull metastasis revealing a renal tumor: A case report and review of the literature. 2018;43:56–60.
41. Kozak KJ, Valyi-Nagy T, Yu JW. Unusual head and neck presentation of metastatic renal cell carcinoma. 2023;26:100502.
42. Flanigan RC, Campbell SC, Clark JI, Picken MM. Metastatic renal cell carcinoma. 2003;4:385–90.
43. Wang D, He S, Chu L, Chao Q, Zhang Q, Shu H. A metastatic skull tumor from intrahepatic cholangiocarcinoma: a case report and literature review. 2019;98:e18291.
44. Fujimoto K, Kuroda J, Makino K, Hasegawa Y, Kuratsu J. Skull metastasis from intrahepatic cholangiocarcinoma: report of 3 cases and review of the literature. 2013;53:717–21.
45. D'Ambrosio N, Lyo JK, Young RJ, Haque SS, Karimi S. Imaging of metastatic CNS neuroblastoma. 2010;194:1223–9.
46. Chen AM, Trout AT, Towbin AJ. A review of neuroblastoma image-defined risk factors on magnetic resonance imaging. 2018;48:1337–47.
47. Wolden SL, Barker CA, Kushner BH, Bodduluri H, Della-Biancia C, Kramer K, Modak S, Cheung N-KV. Brain-sparing radiotherapy for neuroblastoma skull metastases. 2008;50:1163–8.
48. Zimmerman RA, Bilaniuk LT. CT of primary and secondary craniocerebral neuroblastoma. 1980;1:431–4.
49. Issara K, Yossi S, Caraivan I. Lymphome primitif de la voûte crânienne : cas clinique et revue de la littérature. 2016;20:811–4.
50. Jung CS, Zimmermann M, Seifert V. Clivus lymphoma. 2004;146:533–4.
51. Wang L, Lin S, Zhang J, Wang C. Primary non-Hodgkin's lymphoma of the skull base: a case report and literature review. 2013;115:237–40.
52. Xing Z, Huang H, Xiao Z, Yang X, Lin Y, Cao D. CT, conventional, and functional MRI features of skull lymphoma: a series of eight cases in a single institution. 2019;48:897–905.
53. Haruna M, Gupta P, Dhanasekar G. Skull base non-Hodgkin's lymphoma. 2017;4:4086–2090.
54. Laigle-Donadey F, Taillibert S, Martin-Duverneuil N, Hildebrand J, Delattre J-Y. Skull-base metastases. 2005;75:63–9.
55. Cao W, Liang C, Gen Y, Wang C, Zhao C, Sun L. Role of diffusion-weighted imaging for detecting bone marrow infiltration in skull in children with acute lymphoblastic leukemia. 2016;22:580–6.
56. Ohno M, Narita Y, Miyakita Y, Okita Y, Kayama T, Shibui S. Development of secondary skull sarcoma after treatment for childhood acute myeloid leukemia: skull sarcoma secondary to leukemia. 2012;8:e49–52.
57. Athukuri P, Khan AB, Gadot R, et al. Myeloid sarcoma of the skull base: a case report and systematic literature review. 2022;13:220.
58. Joshi A, Jiang D, Singh P, Moffat D. Skull base presentation of multiple myeloma. 2011;90:E6–9.
59. Yang W, Zheng J, Li R, et al. Multiple myeloma with pathologically proven skull plasmacytoma after a mild head injury: case report. 2018;97:e12327.
60. Durie BGM, Salmon SE. A clinical staging system for multiple myeloma correlation of measured myeloma cell mass with presenting clinical features, response to treatment, and survival. 1975;36:842–54.
61. Hameed A, Brady JJ, Dowling P, Clynes M, O'Gorman P. Bone disease in multiple myeloma: pathophysiology and management. 2014;7:33–42.
62. Roodman GD, Dougall WC. RANK ligand as a therapeutic target for bone metastases and multiple myeloma. 2008;34:92–101.

22 Hematologic Malignancies of the Scalp and Calvarium

Abad Cherif El Asri, Mohammed Benzagmout, and Ali Akhaddar

22.1 Introduction

Hematological malignancies represent a heterogeneous group of blood neoplasias commonly characterized by abnormal production of blood cells (hematopoiesis). The World Health Organization (WHO) categorized these malignancies according to the lineage of origin of the neoplastic cell (either myeloid or lymphoid), their acute or chronic development, their derivation from precursor or stem or differentiated or committed cells, and more specifically based on their clinical, morphological, and genetic features [1]. These malignancies, including disease categories such as Hodgkin and non-Hodgkin lymphoma (NHL), acute and chronic lymphocytic and myelogenous leukemia, and multiple myeloma (MM), comprise a set of prevalent yet clinically diverse diseases that can affect any organ system. Because blood components originate in the bone marrow, wherever the bone might be the site of primary or secondary hematologic neoplasm [2]. The clavarial localization of hematological malignancies is rare with only few cases and series have been reported in the literature [3]. Furthermore, the variability in imaging appearances and clinical behavior of these diseases make the primary diagnosis and monitoring of clinical progress a challenging deal that the imaging findings may be subtle, leading to missed diagnosis, or may be nonspecific and confused with infection or another benign disease, leading to incorrect diagnosis [2, 4].

The aim of this chapter is to analyze the clinical, radiological, and biological management and prognosis futures of these calvarial hematological malignancies either in their primary or secondary occurrence according to the WHO classification. We specifically study the behaviors of lymphoma, leukemia, and multiple myeloma involving the calvarium.

22.2 Lymphoma

Lymphoma represents a heterogeneous group of malignant neoplasms of B lymphocytes and less commonly T lymphocytes. The World Health Organization Classification of Disease recognizes more than 50 types of lymphoma [5, 6]. Bone involvement is a common finding in many

A. C. El Asri (✉)
Department of Neurosurgery, Mohamed V Military Hospital, University Mohammed V of Rabat, Rabat, Morocco
e-mail: abad20031@gmail.com

M. Benzagmout
Department of Neurosurgery, Hassan II Hospital, Sidi Mohamed Ben Abdellah University of Fès, Fes, Morocco

A. Akhaddar
Department of Neurosurgery, Avicenne Military Hospital of Marrakech, Mohammed V University in Rabat, Rabat, Morocco

M. Turgut et al. (eds.), *Lesions of the Scalp and Cranial Vault*,
https://doi.org/10.1007/978-3-031-88244-9_22

types of lymphoma with most cases secondary to metastatic spread from another primary site. However, primary and exclusive involvement of the skeletal system is rare, and it accounts for less than 5% of all bone malignancies, with diffuse large B-cell lymphoma (DLBCL) and follicular lymphoma being the most common types [7]. Synonyms for primary osseous lymphoma include reticulum cell sarcoma, malignant lymphoma of bone, and osteolymphoma [5, 7]. Cranial vault involvement is rare, and the majority of patients are found at staging to have concurrent disease in lymph nodes [5]. Otherwise, primary cranial vault lymphoma [PCVL] is extremely rare with very few reported cases in the literature. In fact, bone lymphoma is categorized as primary only if the bone is the only known site of disease for 6 months [5–7]. For instance, some authors may still consider calvarial lymphoma to be primary even in the presence of disseminated disease when it is the largest lesion and thus putatively the initially involved site. On the other hand, secondary calvarial lymphoma is often difficult to distinguish from primary disease, particularly when it originates from a contiguous site, as it often manifests with identical features [6].

The incidence of lymphomas increased progressively in the last decade, independently of the immunodeficiency compromise in the general population [5]. However, according to a systematic review, PCVL occurs in all ages but is much more common in older patients, with a mean age of 60.5 years and 60% of patients older than 60 years. The sex ratio was 1:1 M/F, showing no significant gender difference, and only 11.7% of patients were immunocompromised [5].

Skeletal disease may present with symptoms localized to the site of bone involvement, as an incidental finding on imaging for other reasons or as part of the staging of the disease. The most common presenting symptom was a progressively painless enlarging subcutaneous mass which was observed in 90% of patients; headache due to bone destruction or tumor infiltration of meninges was observed in 30% [5, 6]. Symptoms like seizures and focal neurological deficits resulting from intracranial extension with mass effect or infiltration of the cortex were also observed in patients with advanced tumors and were presented respectively in 10% and 20% of cases. Otherwise, the disease may primarily involve the skin, particularly in the head and neck region, and a rapidly growing, often painful mass can be seen to be of single nodal or extranodal size [5, 7]. Lymphoma cells spread along the emissary veins leading to the infiltration of the soft tissues on either side of the bone and resulting to typical pattern of lesions affecting all compartments of the cranial vault [5].

Radiological diagnosis of a PCVL is notoriously difficult to establish, as findings can be subtle, nonspecific, or even unapparent [2]. On CT scan, the majority of patients present with osteolytic changes which may be mild relative to the size of the lesion (Fig. 22.1). According to a review by El Asri et al., lesions were lytic in 75% of cases, hyperostosic in 5% of patients, and without apparent bone remodeling in 17.5% of cases. However, a mixed lytic lesion with sclerotic areas can be seen. Sclerotic to lytic transformation may herald disease progression, whereas lytic to sclerotic transformation may be related to tumor-directed therapy [5]. Early in the disease, sclerotic changes may occur before any frank bone destruction is observed, likely reflecting the permeative growth pattern of lymphoma whereby lymphoma cells invade the diploic space before traveling along emissary veins to infiltrate pericranial structures, leaving the overall bone structure intact [6]. In some cases, no bone destruction occurs because of the characteristic permeating growth pattern of lymphoma with a large soft-tissue component and very little bone destruction [5]. Furthermore, the absence of osteolytic changes does not exclude a diagnosis of calvarial lymphoma.

Cerebral infiltration of calvarial lymphoma is well studied by MRI. A trend toward hypointensity or isointensity on T1-weighted imaging and hyperintensity or isointensity on T2-weighted imaging with consistent T1 gadolinium enhancement has been observed by authors (Fig. 22.2). The fat saturation post-gadolinium T1-weighted sequences were useful to establish lesion extension and to show tumor enhancement in both the

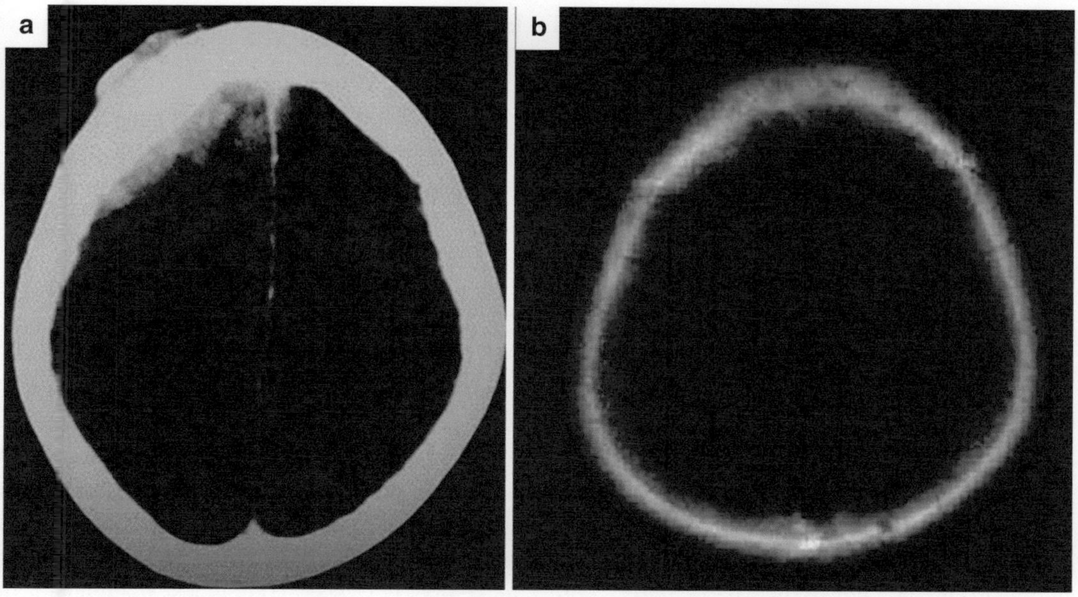

Fig. 22.1 Axial CT scan in parenchymal (**a**) window and bone window (**b**) revealing a right frontal calvarial lesion with both extra- and intracranial isodense soft tissue components with mild calvarial hyperostotic changes

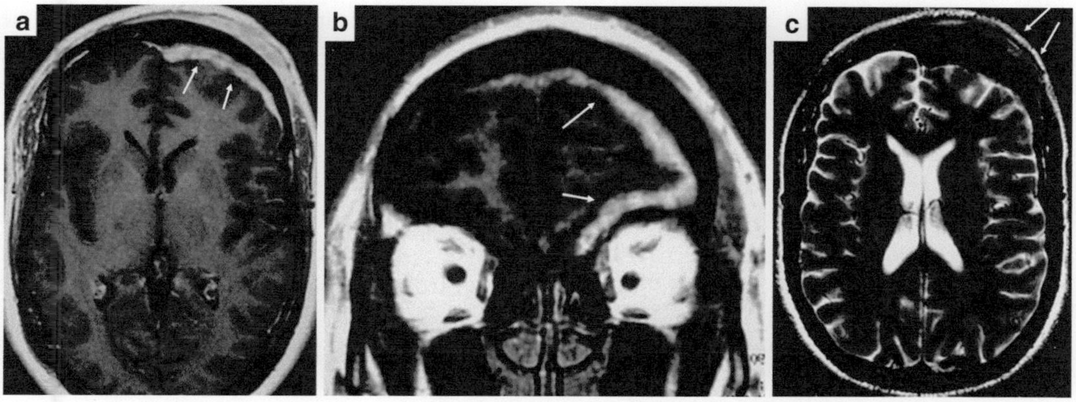

Fig. 22.2 T1-weighted with gadolinium on axial (**a**) and coronal (**b**) plan and axial T2 weighted (**c**) MR images showing a left frontal bone lesion invading the adjacent intracranial dura and subcutaneous tissue

intra- and extracranial compartments [5]. These findings, however, are highly nonspecific and may mimic other diseases, such as meningioma, hemangiopericytoma, metastatic carcinoma, subdural hematoma, and osteomyelitis.

The signal intensity on MRI is nonspecific; most reported cases of skull lymphomas report the signal intensity to be isointense on unenhanced MRI and to show marked enhancement on contrast-enhanced images [8]. In our review, on T1-weighted MRI, the lesion was isointense in 65% of cases and hypointense in 35% of cases. On T2-weighted MRI, 52% of lesions were isointense, 35% were hyperintense, and 9% were hypointense [5]. Imaging studies typically show intracranial and extracranial soft tissue components with involvement of the intervening bone, leading some authors to suggest that involvement of all three compartments of the cranial vault may be a better indicator of calvarial lymphoma than any specific bone changes [5, 6].

The management of patients with calvarial lymphomas should be interdisciplinary, as with other oncological diseases [4]. Owing to the aggressive nature of calvarial lymphoma, timely diagnosis and initiation of treatment will optimize prognosis. In 60–90% of cases, primary central nervous system lymphomas are predominantly diffuse large-cell, immunoblastic, lymphoblastic, or Burkitt's lymphomas. Only 20–30% of immunocompetent patients are affected by aggressive lymphomas [9]. According to the Kiel classification, centroblastic lymphoma, immunoblastic B-cell lymphoma, and large-cell anaplastic B-cell lymphoma are synonyms of diffuse large B-cell lymphoma [5, 9]. Due to the paucity of cases described in the literature, the optimal management of skeletal lymphoma remains uncertain, particularly with regard to the role of chemotherapy and radiotherapy. Historically, extranodal disease limited to a single site responds favorably to local treatments such as surgery or focal radiation [5, 8, 9]. Whenever the complete resection of calvarial lymphoma is achieved, one can consider clinical and radiological follow-up without any additional treatment [5, 9]. On the other hand, chemotherapy and radiation are used invariably with high remission rates, regardless of whether they are preceded by surgical intervention. Even in isolated disease, a simple biopsy followed by chemotherapy and/or radiation appears to achieve remission at comparable rates while avoiding the risks associated with open surgery [6, 10].

Limited studies exist on the role surgery, chemotherapy, and radiation therapy have on overall survival of patients. According to the study carried out by El Asri et al. which relieved the difficulty of the outcome analysis of the reported cases of skull vault lymphoma, where the follow-up was variable and incomplete, 91% of patients who received radiotherapy were free of disease at termination of follow-up, and one patient [HIV-positive] died at 18 months. Although the number of patients treated by the combined modality of chemotherapy and radiotherapy was small, the disease seems to have been well controlled [5]. Poor outcomes were independent of treatment modality, suggesting that overall prognosis is likely related to factors besides upfront surgery, such as early diagnosis, patient age, medical comorbidities, and treatment compliance [5, 6]. Thus, future retrospective studies must be done to assess the most efficacious management for patients with primary cranial vault lymphoma [10].

22.3 Leukemia

Leukemia, in its acute and chronic presentation, represents a malignant group of neoplastic proliferations of leukocytes that collect in the blood and bone marrow. Untreated, acute leukemias tend to be aggressive and rapidly fatal but also tend to respond better to treatment than chronic leukemias [11]. The commonest malignancy in children is acute leukemia and specifically the acute lymphocytic leukemia (ALL), which may be found primarily by the bony lesions and represents 30% of all childhood cancers. Whereas, the incidence of leukemia among adults is under 4%, with chronic lymphocytic leukemia (CLL) and acute myeloid leukemia (AML) being the most common subtypes [11, 12].

In acute lymphoblastic or myeloid leukemia, malignant myeloid and lymphoid precursors proliferate and replace the normal hematopoietic cells of the marrow, circulate in the blood, and invade other tissues of the body. Leukemic cells may also infiltrate the skin and the skull during the course of acute or chronic leukemia [12].

Furthermore, the presentation of leukemic infiltration is related to the suppression of hematopoiesis by leukemic cells, pallor, petechia, ecchymosis in the skin, and mucus membranes or infection due to neutropenia—the main symptoms [11–14]. On the other hand, growing skeleton is also an important site for the proliferation of leukemic cells and most of the cases with bony involvement presented with musculoskeletal pain, swelling, and joint effusion, and ended with functional impairment [13]. The skull has been an uncommon site of involvement with few reported cases. Calvarial localization's presentation may vary from asymptomatic to progressively painless enlarging subcutaneous mass, associated by headache or signs of neurological disabilities in advanced stage of tumor [11–13].

Due to the rarity of skull involvement, the radiological findings are modestly described [12]. Musculoskeletal imaging findings of leukemia are usually related to replacement of normal bone marrow with neoplastic monoclonal cell duplication. The most commonly reported radiographic finding of leukemic bone marrow infiltration is osteopenia. Osteolytic lesions occurred in 90% of children and almost half of adult patient and were by far the most common lesion in adults. These lesions varied considerably in size, though they were usually less than 5 mm in diameter. In the skull, the lytic defects were multiple, small, circular, and discrete [12–15]. The exact pathophysiology of osteolysis in ALL patients is unknown. However, serum from ALL patients with osteolysis can induce in vitro proliferation of osteoclasts, indicating the mechanism of lymphoblasts induces osteoclast activation in the body. Parathyroid hormone-related protein (PTHrP) secretion by lymphoblasts is the primary cause of osteolysis in ALL patients [16]. On the other hand, inflammatory cytokines excreted by lymphoblasts might be the contributing factors in a patient with normal serum PTHrP level [16, 17]. In children, these tended to remain discrete, whereas in adults they often coalesced and presented an appearance indistinguishable from that of metastases. Destructive cortical lesions, with or without periosteal elevation, were observed in 50% of children and in only 9% of adults [15].

Osteosclerotic lesions with periosteal reaction on CT scan may be seen in 7.4%–31% of the cases and are considered as bone marrow infarct or may be due to leukemic cell infiltration in the bone marrow [12, 13]. Magnetic resonance (MR) imaging findings of leukemia generally include signs of bone marrow infiltration, with decreased signal intensity on T1-weighted images, increased signal intensity on T2-weighted fat-saturated or Short Tau Inversion Recovery (STIR) images, and usually diffuse gadolinium enhancement. MR imaging has been shown to demonstrate leukemic infiltration of the bones even with a negative bone marrow biopsy in pediatric cases. A well-enhanced lesion invading both cortical of the calvarium and infiltrating the scalp and the dura is a classically presentation of solitary leukemia of the skull [12, 13, 15, 18].

Treatment options for leukemia include chemotherapy regimens, bone marrow or peripheral blood stem cell transplant, and antibody-mediated medications such as imatinib for chronic myeloid leukemia (CML) and ibrutinib or idelalisib for CLL [12, 13, 18]. The four major treatment components are induction phase, consolidation phase, maintenance phase, and therapy directed against the central nervous system involvement [13, 18, 19].

Pediatric patients with acute leukemia have an overall 5-year survival rate of 80% depending on their risk profile [19, 20]. A patient in the low-risk category has a 4-year event-free survival (EFS) rate of approximately 80%, whereas, a high-risk acute lymphoblastic lymphoma patient has a 4-year event-free survival rate of approximately 65% [13, 20]. However, in adults' population the prognosis is less favorable with only 30–40% of with ALL achieve long-term remission [12, 19].

22.4 Multiple Myeloma

Plasma cells represent 0.5–1% of all peripheral blood mononuclear cells in normal individuals. The etiopathogenesis of degeneration to malignant plasma cells is unknown. It is classified according to its biological behavior and histopathological features into a benign type, solitary plasmacytoma (SPC), and a malignant type, development of multiple myeloma (MM) [3]. Multiple myeloma is a malignant neoplastic clonal proliferation of plasma cells of B-cell origin with diffuse bone marrow infiltration and focal osteolytic lesions. This leads to overproduction of immunoglobulins and multiple systemic effects, including abnormalities on blood or urinary test [e.g., high erythrocyte sedimentation rate with normal C-reactive protein, anemia, or high total protein level with a monoclonal immunoglobulin on serum protein electrophoresis] pathologic fractures, and bone pain [21, 22].

Its prevalence is 5 in 100,000 population, and its peak age at presentation is 70 years, which makes it the most common primary malignancy of the skeleton and bone marrow. Lesions are usually disseminated throughout the axial skeleton, either multifocally or diffusely; solitary lesions, called plasmacytomas, are rare, particularly in the skull. Even if it's a classically finding in the course of the disease, plasma cell myeloma (PCM) of the skull is rarely encountered in neurosurgical practice. However solitary plasmacytoma of the skull without the development of MM is extremely rare; only few cases have been reported [3, 23, 24]. Plasmacytomas generally appear as a bone or soft tissue tumor with mass effect, pain, weakness, fatigue, fever, infection, and infiltrative behavior. In patients with primary brain tumors, the lesion itself generates direct focal cerebral dysfunction depending on tumor location and may therefore cause somatic symptoms such as fatigue, sleep disturbances, anorexia, etc.

Radiographs show multiple small, roundish osteolytic lesions that are relatively uniform in size with sharp and nonsclerotic margins (i.e., the classic "punched-out" lesions) (Fig. 22.3a). These may coalesce into larger osteolytic segments [21, 25]. Diffuse skull osteopenia is less frequently encountered. On CT scan (Fig. 22.3b), osteolytic lesions are better shown on bone windows when the skull is well mineralized and on soft-tissue windows when the skull is demineralized [21–24]. MR imaging of the bone marrow in multiple myeloma may show a diffuse or focal pattern of bone marrow involvement, with decreased signal intensity on T1-weighted images and elevated signal intensity on T2-weighted images; a "salt-and-pepper" appearance or diffuse bone marrow replacement may be noted [21]. Contrast-enhanced MR imaging can help detect diffuse involvement of bone marrow, the presence of which may be used by clinicians to make treatment decisions [24]. Because lesions in myeloma are exclusively osteolytic, they are usually not detected with 99mTc-based scintigraphy [21, 25]. Therefore, neuroradiological findings in solitary cranial vault plasmacytoma generally lack specificity and are often misdiagnosed preoperatively, and it may be confused with meningioma, metastasis, sarcoma, chordoma, and giant cell tumor (Fig. 22.4). The diagnosis is usually made when the lesions appear in the context of a previous MM or after pathological tissue is obtained after surgery.

The distinction between solitary plasmacytoma and MM is of paramount importance for the

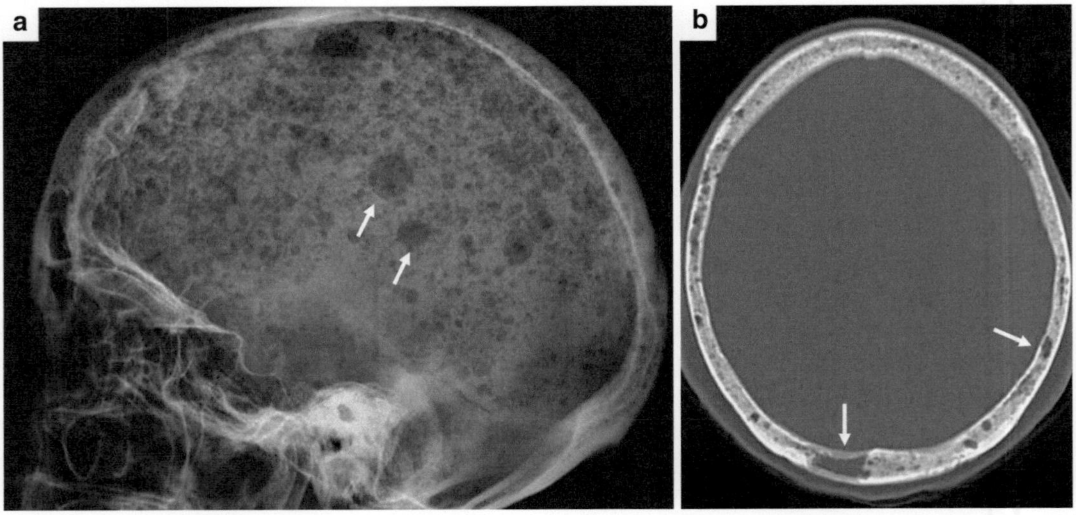

Fig. 22.3 Cranial X-ray (**a**) showing multiple small, roundish osteolytic lesions that are relatively uniform in size with sharp and nonsclerotic margins (the classic "punched-out" lesions). On CT scan (**b**), disseminated osteolytic lesions are better shown on bone windows

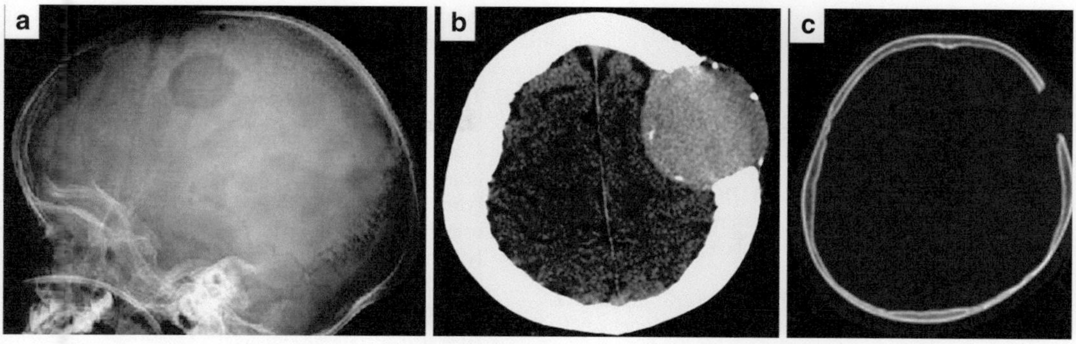

Fig. 22.4 Left frontal plasmacytoma as an osteolytic mass of the left frontal bone on X-ray (**a**) and axial CT scan in parenchymal (**b**) window and bone window (**c**)

management of calvarial myeloma. Treatment of multiple myeloma depends on the stage of the disease, and it is most commonly based on chemotherapy or grafting of hematopoietic cells [21, 24]. Even the radiation is the mainstay of therapy in solitary plasmacytoma, which is highly radiosensitive, surgical resection might be considered alone or in addition to radiation with ongoing monitoring to evaluate for progression to multiple myeloma [24, 26]. The high vascular feeding supply of this skull plasmacytoma will compromise hemostasis during surgery leading to excessive blood loss with reported cardiac arrest in the literature. Therefore, preoperative embolization in these cases is crucial. It is advisable to perform craniectomy and cranioplasty in all patients because of the high recurrence rate reported when leaving remnant cells of the tumor in the surrounding bone surface [27]. Otherwise, the local control rates can be achieved in 80–90% of cases with radiation therapy alone [19]. Furthermore, there are reports of complete cure after biopsy and radiotherapy [21, 26, 27]. Due to the limited available data, adjuvant chemotherapy is not recommended for patients with solitary plasmocytoma (SP). Adjuvant chemotherapy can be considered for patients with persistent disease, based on PET/CT, after initial radiotherapy [28].

Despite excellent local control rates, the majority of patients with solitary plasmacytoma will eventually progress to multiple myeloma of which the prognosis is not as good as solitary plasmacytoma [21, 28]. Regular radiological and biological follow-up are mandatory is very essential to do a thorough radiological evaluation and perform the required laboratory tests to make the correct diagnosis of solitary plasmacytoma and differentiate it from systemic myelomatosis, since their treatment and prognosis differs totally from each other. Long-term follow-up is required because tumor recurrence or progression to MM can occur [27].

22.5 Conclusion

Hematologic malignancies, including leukemia, lymphoma, and multiple myeloma, are a heterogeneous group of neoplasms that may affect the calvarium as a primary disease or secondarily as metastatic disease. Clinical presentation and radiological features are not specific in solitary lesion and make it as a diagnosis of exclusion. The radiologist must be aware and also be familiar with the standard imaging tools for assessment of these rare diseases, as well as with newer imaging tools that may become part of routine clinical practice, such as whole-body MR imaging using Diffusion-weighted Imaging (DWI) with background body signal suppression or dynamic contrast enhancement and fluorodeoxyglucose (FDG) PET/MR imaging. In any case, a surgical biopsy of a tissue sample is necessary to ensure the diagnosis, and whenever the risk of surgical procedure is without significant morbidity and mortality, the total excision with cranioplasty is the rule in solitary lesion. Radiotherapy and or chemotherapy are usually added as the standalone or as an adjuvant tool to surgery. Posttreatment radiological and biological monitoring is crucial to expect recurrence and toxicity of treatment.

References

1. Méndez-Ferrer S, Bonnet D, Steensma DP, Hasserjian RP, Ghobrial IM, Gribben JG, Andreeff M, Krause DS. Bone marrow niches in haematological malignancies. Nat Rev Cancer. 2020;20(5):285–98.
2. Navarro SM, Matcuk GR, Patel DB, Skalski M, White EA, Tomasian A, Schein AJ. Musculoskeletal imaging findings of hematologic malignancies. Radiographics. 2017;37(3):881–900.
3. Higurashi M, Yagishita S, Fujitsu K, Kitsuta Y, Takemoto Y, Osano S. Plasma cell myeloma of the skull base: report of two cases. Brain Tumor Pathol. 2004;21(3):135–41.
4. Nasi-Kordhishti I, Hempel JM, Ebner FH, Tatagiba M. Calvarial lesions: overview of imaging features and neurosurgical management. Neurosurg Rev. 2021;44(6):3459–69.
5. El Asri AC, Akhaddar A, Baallal H, Boulahroud O, Mandour C, Chahdi H, et al. Primary lymphoma of the cranial vault: case report and a systematic review of the literature. Acta Neurochir. 2012;154:257–65.
6. Toyota E, Taslimi S, Alkins R. Optimal management of calvarial lymphoma: a meta-analysis. World Neurosurg. 2021;151:e484–94.
7. Nitta N, Moritani S, Fukami T, Nozaki K. Characteristics of cranial vault lymphoma from a systematic review of the literature. Surg Neurol Int. 2022;13:231.
8. Kantarci M, Erdem T, Alper F. Imaging characteristics of diffuse primary cutaneous B-cell lymphoma of the cranial vault with orbital and brain invasion. Am J Neuroradiol. 2003;24:1324–6.
9. Evans LS, Hancock BW. Non-Hodgkin lymphoma. Lancet. 2003;362:139–46.
10. Ebinama U, Khan H, Akula V, Rios A. Primary cranial vault lymphoma misdiagnosed as atypical meningioma: a case report. Plasmatology. 2023;17.
11. Chennamadhavuni A, Lyengar V, Mukkamalla SKR, et al. Leukemia. In: StatPearls [Internet]. Treasure Island (FL): StatPearls Publishing; 2024.
12. Hunger SP, Mullighan CG. Acute lymphoblastic leukaemia in children. N Engl J Med. 2015;373:1541–52.
13. Al-Mashdali AF, Yassin MA. Osteolytic bone lesions as an initial presenting manifestation of acute lymphoblastic leukemia in adults. Blood. 2022;140(Suppl 1):11603–4.
14. Hanapi MS, Ghani S-I, Teo KSS, Wan-Embong W-Z, Ariffin N, Hitam W-HW. Extensive forehead swelling including the periorbital area in a child: a rare manifestation of acute lymphoblastic leukemia. Cureus. 2018;10(11):e3539.
15. Thomas LB, Forkner CEJR, Frei E, Besse BE, Stabenau JR. The skeletal lesions of acute leukemia. Cancer. 1961;14:608–21.
16. Shimonodan H, Nagayama J, Nagatoshi Y, et al. Acute lymphocytic leukemia in adolescence with multiple osteolytic lesions and hypercalcemia mediated by lymphoblast-producing parathyroid hormone-related peptide: a case report and review of the literature. Pediatr Blood Cancer. 2005;45:333–9.
17. Al-Mashdali AF, Al-Dubai HN, Yassin MA. Osteolytic bone lesions as an initial presenting manifestation of adult acute lymphoblastic leukemia: a mini review. Ann Med Surg (Lond). 2023;85(9):4404–9.
18. Cooper SL, Brown PA. Treatment of pediatric acute lymphoblastic leukemia. Pediatr Clin N Am. 2015;62:61–73.
19. Hutter J. Childhood leukemia. Pediatr Rev. 2010;31(6):234–41.
20. Jabbour E, O'Brien S, Konopleva M, Kantarjian H. New insights into the pathophysiology and therapy of adult acute lymphoblastic leukemia. Cancer. 2015;121(15):2517–28.
21. Pham A, Mahindra A. Solitary plasmacytoma: a review of diagnosis and management. Curr Hematol Malig Rep. 2019;14(2):63–9.
22. Colas L, Caron S, Cotten A. Skull vault lesions: a review. AJR Am J Roentgenol. 2015;205(4):840–7.
23. Gozzetti A, Cerase A, Defina M, Bocchia M. Plasmacytoma of the skull. Eur J Haematol. 2012;88:369.
24. Garfinkle J, Melançon D, Cortes M, Tampieri D. Imaging pattern of calvarial lesions in adults. Skeletal Radiol. 2011;40:1261–73.
25. Kuo Y, Huang W, Wu J. Surgical treatment for a giant solitary plasmacytoma with skull erosion. Cureus. 2018;10(11):e3535.
26. Castillejo LA, de Jesús Julian J, González P, Román R. Giant solitary extradural plasmacytoma of the skull: illustrative case. J Neurosurg. 2021;1(21):CASE21127.
27. Dong L, Zhang X, Zhang H, Song R, Gu X, He L. Solitary plasmacytoma of the skull: two case reports. Oncol Lett. 2013;5(2):479–82.
28. Joshi A, Jiang D, Singh P, Moffat D. Skull base presentation of multiple myeloma. Ear Nose Throat J. 2011;90(1):E6–9.

Intracranial Neoplasms with Involvement of the Scalp and Calvarium

23

Arya Nabavi and Bogdan-Marius Corbu

23.1 Overview

Anatomically the vault's layers are the skin, galea (periosteum/pericranial connective tissue), bone, and meninges covering the brain. Each layer can either be the origin or involved by a tumor, which accordingly determines the surgical strategy.

All intracranial lesions, either with metastatic, neuroepithelial, or most frequently meningeal origin, can transgress into the adjacent tissues. Whereas skull base lesions enjoy prominence due to their potential cranial nerve involvement with corresponding clinical findings, lesions of the calvarium often do not impress likewise. At the vault clinical presentation can range from headaches to neurological symptoms due to the local space-occupying effect to intra- and perilesional bleeding. However, lesions in this region can remain oligosymptomatic with a slowly growing bulge [1], which sometimes is only detected by the barber. Nevertheless, even with this unexceptional presentation, this can be the proverbial "tip of the iceberg," caused by underlying extensive disease. The treatment algorithm of intracranial lesions with involvement of dura and skull is directed at reducing mass effect, reconstructing the dura, and where necessary the skull and skin, either as definitive measure or the initial step of an integrated multimodal approach, which in turn is determined by the original lesion. Gross total resection of metastases can be achieved even in the vicinity of venous sinuses [2], according to the same principles as with solitary fibrous tumors (SFTs) (formerly known as hemangiopericytoma) and meningiomas.

A. Nabavi (✉) · B.-M. Corbu
Department of Neurosurgery, Nordstadt Hospital KRH, Hannover, Germany
e-mail: arya.nabavi@krh.de

23.2 Specific Neoplasms

23.2.1 Metastases

Neurosurgical treatment of metastatic disease has gained importance. Sophisticated treatment modalities and algorithms have increased overall survival and improved the clinical status at presentation of patients [3] even with multiple cerebral metastasis, presenting a surgical option. Computer-assisted navigation systems as well as intraoperative imaging, particularly intraoperative ultrasound (ioUS), facilitate the removal of smaller and even multiple lesions during one operation. Skull vault metastases are more common than skull base metastasis. In a single-center study spanning 13 years [4], they were as frequent as meningiomas involving the bone (19 and 20/133, respectively). Breast, lung, and prostate carcinomas (Fig. 23.1), which also have a preponderance for bone involvement, represent the main entities [5]. About 25% of patients with

M. Turgut et al. (eds.), *Lesions of the Scalp and Cranial Vault*,
https://doi.org/10.1007/978-3-031-88244-9_23

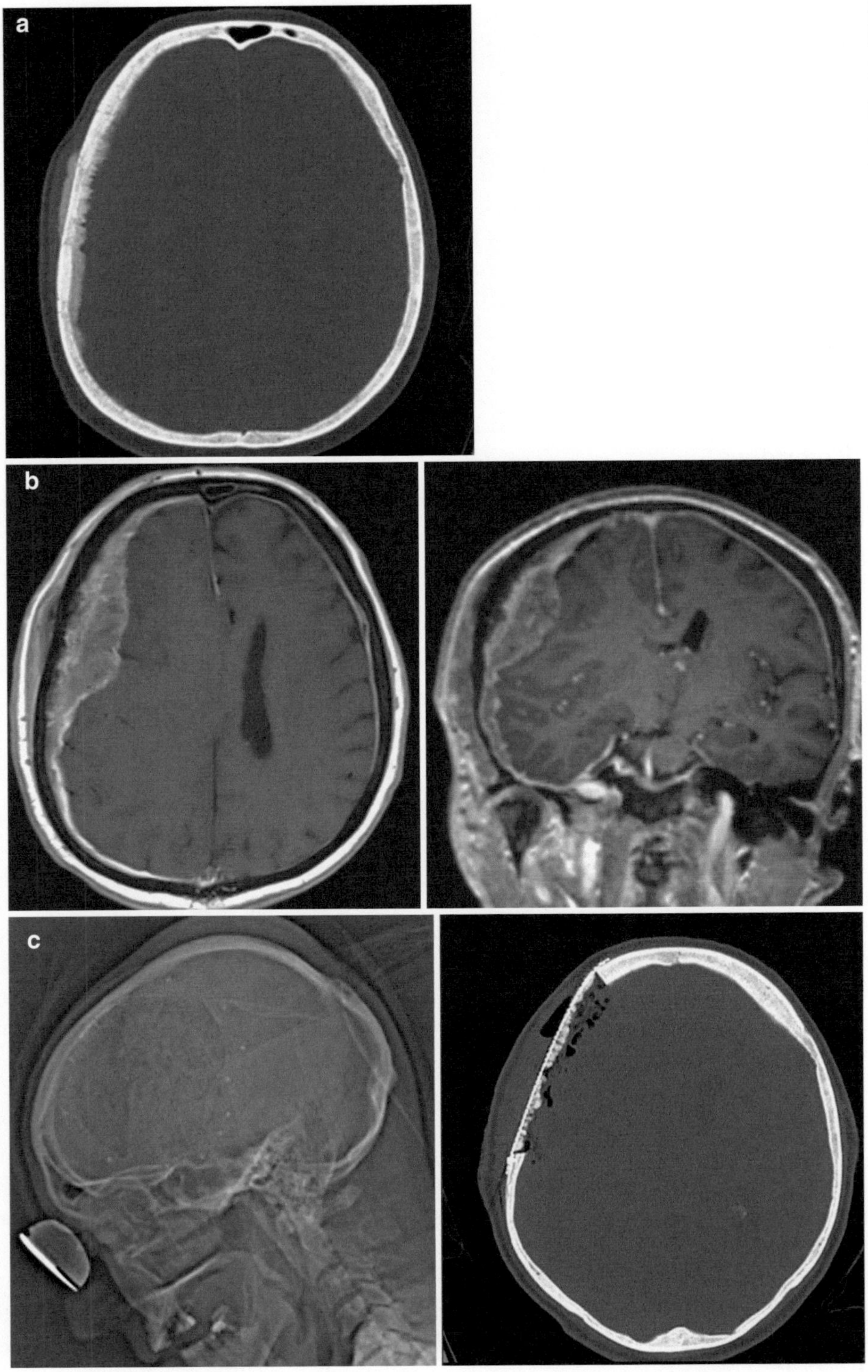

Fig. 23.1 (**a**) Prostate carcinoma: in CT hyperostosis and piculae, which are generally considered to be the indicator of a malignancy. (**b**) Preoperative MRI with holohemispheric tumor and mass effect. The surgical goal was to relieve the mass effect. (**c**) Prostate carcinoma: postoperative CT after titanium mesh reconstruction. After fixing multiple central tack sutures, we use the mesh matrix to apply PMMA as a sealant to complete the closure. Scout (left) shows the extend of the cranioplasty

metastatic disease have involvement of the brain [6]. Whether a metastatic lesion originating by hematogenic spread implanted within the brain, dura, or bone [7] can only be deduced by the level of involvement. Surgical resection provides histological verification, which is important, since it is not infrequent for metastases to the skull to represent the first manifestation of the disease [7]. Surgical resection provides the basis for pressure relieve, local control, avoidance of secondary complications (e.g. intralesional hemorrhage, skin infiltration), and reestablishment of neuroprotection through cranioplasty. Improvement in surgical techniques and presurgical planning have lowered morbidity significantly, even in higher-risk areas. Michael et al. [2] showed that 14 patients with sinus involvement had the same outcome parameters as 14 matched patients with calvarial involvement without. They resected the affected sinus portion in 10/14 patients and repaired the sinus in 4/14. This documents, that metastasis involving the sinus should not be excluded from surgical consideration.

In lymphoma [8, 9] and the rarer primary central nervous sytem (CNS) lymphoma [10, 11], involvement of the skull and meninges has been reported. However, this is the exception where surgery is not the initial treatment of choice. In lymphoma imaging may provide more clues than in many other entities [12, 13]. In this case biopsy may open additional therapeutic avenues [14, 15]. However, in large lymphomas and other secondary neoplasms with destruction of the bone the surgical removal and reconstruction of the layers remains the mainstay of therapy, followed by tailored adjuvant treatment [3].

23.2.2 Neuroepithelial Tumors

Rarely hemispheric gliomas, even when located on the convexity, show growth beyond the dura. With slow-growing tumors like oligodendroglioma and low-grade astrocytoma, it is conceivable and was reported that the calvarium was eroded by local pressure [16–18], which is corroborated in pediatric cases where swiftly expanding masses result in calvarial erosion [19–21]. Infiltration and destruction however involve more aggressive mechanisms. Such effects have been reported for oligodendroglioma [22], astrocytomas [23, 24], and even glioblastomas [25]. With the ongoing molecular redefinition, it may well be, that previously separated lesions with such aggressive behavior may be reclassified [26].

At present these lesions have to be resected adhering to principles as with other lesions involving dura and bone.

23.2.3 Solitary Fibrous Tumor (SFT) (WHO 5th ed)

Hemangiopericytomas do not appear as a separate entity in the 5th Edition of the WHO classification. They are subsumed as solitary fibrous tumors (SFT) [27] characterized by their distinct genetic signature (inversion of 12q13, fusion of NAB2, and STAT6 genes [28]). In the previous literature, the incidence of hemangiopericytoma was given at 0.06/100.000 [29, 30], with cranial manifestation of 40 cases over 21 years [31]. Mostly with meningeal origin, this mesenchymal tumors originating from pericytes show a more aggressive clinical course. It is commonly accepted that the radicality of the resection correlates with the longer recurrence-free survival [32]. Radiotherapy and the timing thereof have been discussed controversially. Rutkowski et al. [33] found no benefit and warn against the unjudicial application, whereas Kim et al. argue strongly in favor [34]. Patel et al. [32] discuss the timing of radiotherapy according to the achieved extent of resection. In gross total resection, they suggest observation and in case of recurrent tumor reoperation and subsequent radiation. In subtotal resection immediate irradiation is recommended [32]. Stereotactic radiation also repeatedly administered has been advocated to obtain local control [35]. In a recent Korean multicenter study, Lee et al. [36] reason that local tumor control is improved by postoperative radiotherapy. However, based on the data it is generally agreed that the extent of resection remains the main predictor. During follow-up the capacity of this lesion for distant metastasis [37] should be borne in mind.

As the lesion is based on the meninges, local involvement of the bone has been described in multiple cases (19/34 [38]) and is well documented [39]. As these lesions present with a very pronounced vascularization, presurgical embolization should be considered.

23.2.4 Convexity and Parasagittal Meningiomas

Surgical excision of meningiomas can be extremely challenging, as their inconspicuous clinical path may lend them undetected until reaching rather huge sizes as well as envelopment and compromise of critical structures (i.e. venous sinuses) and the necessity for complex bony reconstruction of the vault.

Convexity (20.8%) and parasagittal (16.1%) meningiomas account for more than a third of meningiomas [40]. WHO grade I (80.5%) and II (17.7%) are the majority, with grade III remaining rare (1.7%) [27, 41–43]. When clinically feasible, which may be easier at the cranial vault, gross total resection [44], preferably with a safety margin of excised dura, is the common basis of surgical treatment. The probability of recurrence and necessity for adjuvant treatment is linked to the extent of resection and the grading [42]. In contrast to the skull base, bone involvement can be addressed with the possibility of gross total resection of the afflicted skull. Sinus involvement represents a major surgical challenge. Subsequent sections will address these technical issues in detail. The depicted surgical principles for meningiomas are based on a solid data base and allow generalization to the less frequent intracranial neoplasms with involvement of the skull.

Parasagittal meningiomas are defined by their relation to the sagittal sinus [45], and the level of difficulty in their surgical treatment is related to their involvement thereof [46]. Abutting the sinus, protruding into it with partial conclusion and total occlusion, holds specific surgical tasks and challenges. If only the outer wall of the lesion is attached to the sinus, removal with coagulation of the origin is possible. Partial sinus obstruction has been deemed an indication for reconstruction with patches or venous grafts. DiMeco et al. reported their series on 108 reconstructions of the superior sagittal sinus [47]. Mortality was at 1.8%, and overall morbidity was very accurately reported at 28.7%. Raza et al. [48] suggest a more conservative approach, which implies a most complete resection of the tumor with preservation of the draining cortical veins, without reconstructing the sinus. Residual tumor is left within the sinus. If required, as determined by grade and growth of the residual, nonsurgical treatment modalities (radiation and focussed radiation: e.g. Gamma-Knife Surgery (GKS)) [48–50] show good results in regard to tumor control. Also, with progressive obstruction and final occlusion of the sinus rerouting and formation of collateral channels occurs [51, 52]. As MR venography improves, the noninvasive evaluation of venous collaterals has gained potential [53]. Usually angiography is not required to analyze the vascular supply, as most meningiomas of the convexity are served by branches of the external carotid artery, which will be occluded during the approach. However, if embolization is contemplated, the angiography should also be used for the analyses of the venous system with particular focus on collaterals including the skin. Then excision of the nonfunctional sinus segment can be planned. It is compulsory to be aware of these channels and investigate their location to ensure their preservation [54].

23.3 Operative Treatment

23.3.1 Bone Involvement and Cranioplasty

Bone involvement may affect the inner table only or extent through the diploe beyond the outer table. Accordingly, resection has to be tailored and the skull bone reconstructed where the integrity of inner and outer table could not be preserved. Calvarial vault restoration is not only necessary to restore cosmesis but also for protection and prevention of cognitive decline (however rare outside of cases with emergency craniectomy: syndrome of the trephined) [55].

Occasionally this implies rather elaborate planning and finishing with more extensive lesions.

Particularly in elderly patients local hyperostotic changes of the inner table can be dealt with reasonably by drilling off the affected area and replacing the bone. Lau et al. [56] reported tumor invasion in hyperostotic flaps in 35% of patients (12/34) and replaced the bone after drilling off these areas. However, their mean follow-up is too short (63.5 months) to provide a final analysis. Fathalla et al. [57] studied the extent of bone invasion in 14 patients. The visible border of the hyperostosis was indicated and four biopsies taken at 2 cm distance in four separate areas. In all, 14 patient's biopsies from the hyperostotic site were positive, while in WHO I ($n = 7$) and WHO II ($n = 5$) cases, the distant biopsies were tumor-free. Only in WHO III ($n = 2$) all biopsies were positive. In our clinical practice, we drill the affected portions of the inner table generously while preserving the outer table and replace the flap. (On a personal note: It is impressive that infiltrated bone "sounds and feels" different when drilling. Using these characteristics judiciously can be a good additional guide for the extent of resection).

Furthermore, the extent of bone resection has always been considered against the patient's age, biography, clinical status, and the probability of subsequent therapeutic avenues, as postoperative radiation [49], and—apart from meningioma—medical therapy.

Where bone cannot be preserved, various materials [58, 59] and techniques have been employed to reconstruct the cranial vault. The materials include titanium, ceramics (hydroxyapatite/HA), polyetheretherketone (PEEK), and prefabricated and intraoperatively modeled polymethyl methacrylate (PMMA). When cranioplasty, irrespective of the underlying entity, is required, its reconstruction can be during the same or in a second operation. In the latter custom-made 3D model is generated (e.g., titanium, PEEK, PMMA) based on the extent of the defect and implanted in the subsequent procedure. However, in neoplastic disease, the goal is to resect and reconstruct in the same surgery. In order to use prefabricated models, the craniotomy has to be adjusted to accommodate these implants. Neuronavigation is a major adjunct for this technique [60]. Oishi et al. [61] use the outlines of the prefabricated polyethylene plate to determine the size of the slightly smaller craniotomy. The outer table is removed further than the inner table, to prevent sinking.

Barros et al. [60] use a prefabricated computer-designed resection template to ensure a tailored craniotomy. Broeckx et al. [62] register the dimensions of the prefabricated implant into their navigation system to guide the craniotomy. All these approaches rely on a precise definition of the desired craniectomy on preoperative imaging. As imaging findings can be diverse [63], adjusting to different intraoperative discoveries may render the elaborate presurgical effort superfluous. Intraoperative extensive reconstruction of the convexity bears the difficulty to capture the curvature. While smaller lesions are easily reconstructed by hand-formed PMMA or a small titanium mesh (as, for instance, in intraosseous vascular lesions Chap. 17), other techniques are needed to handle larger lesions. Marbacher et al. [64] resect the lesion and cut out a surrounding outer ring into which PMMA is fashioned. Subsequently the hardened implant is fixed and the composite bone-PMMA replaced. Bloch et al. [65] describe their technique, where initially the hyperostotic area is leveled to the curvature of the bone and a titanium mesh fashioned to capture the curvature. Subsequently the affected bone is removed and an outer ring is cut. The mesh is reattached to the ring of normal bone and delimits the external margin of the PMMA modeled within the surrounding ring. Both techniques are certain to remodel the vault but demand the craniotomy size to be substantially beyond the necessary margins. This can be inadequate particularly in more extended lesions (Fig. 23.2). For this task we have suggested a novel technique for reconstructing large defects with a cast-mold technique [66] (Fig. 23.3). After exposure of the bone, we take a PMMA cast of the area overlapping the planned craniotomy. Hyperostosis is drilled to the level of the curvature (Fig. 23.4). In cases with potentially tight tumor adherence to the bone, fragmented craniotomies have been

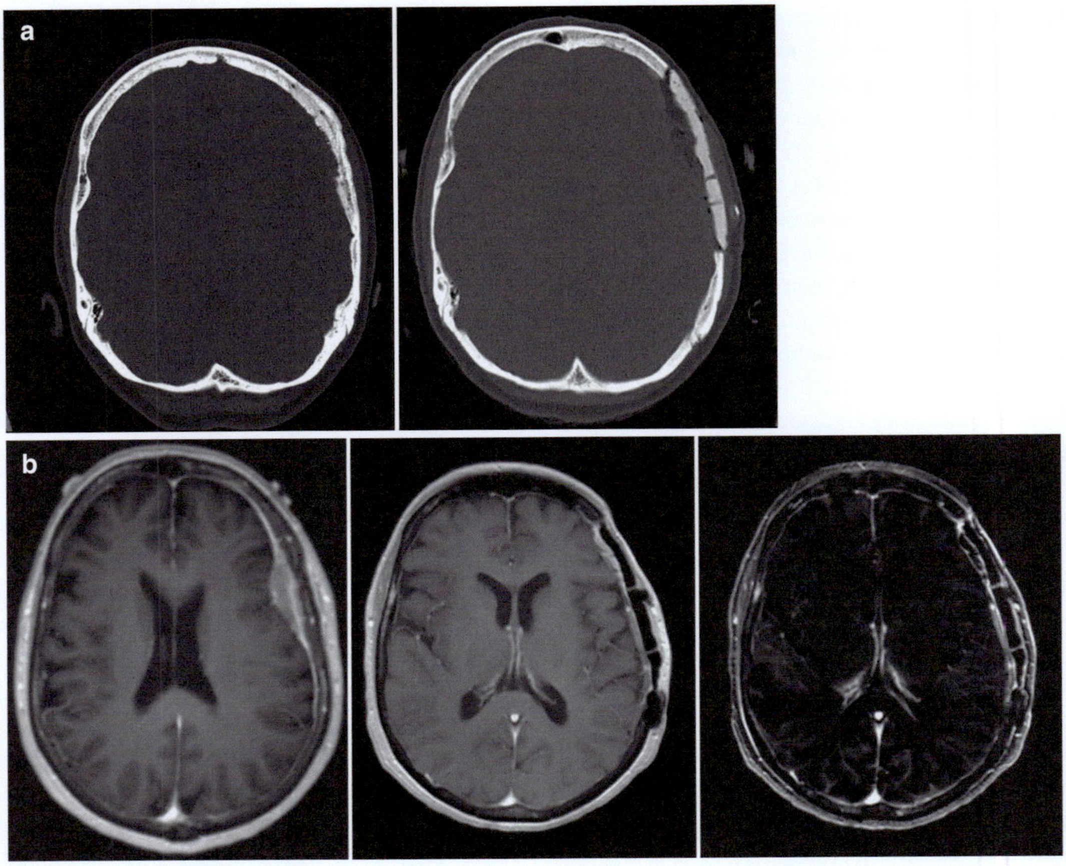

Fig. 23.2 (**a**) En plaque meningioma note spiculae on preoperative CT. Cranioplasty with PMMA-mold technique. (**b**) En plaque meningioma pre- and postoperative MRI: left pre with en plaque meningioma note dural tail. Middle and right: 6 months postoperative: dural graft with galea shows contrast enhancement, which will decrease further. Frontal area additional fat-graft shows of T1WI (middle) but not on T1W-subtraction image. Dural graft was with fascia lata due to the involvement of galea. Skin was unaffected

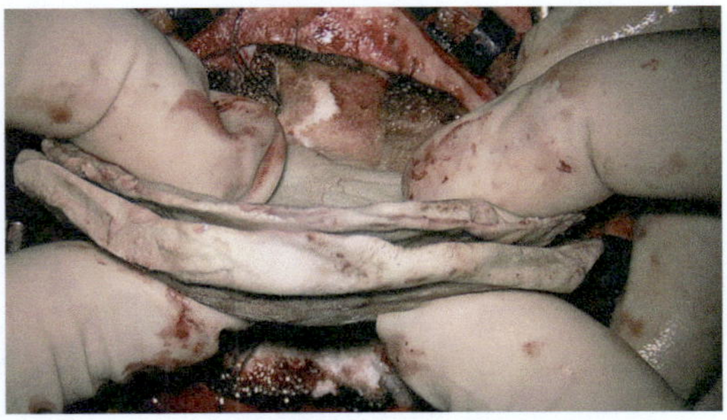

Fig. 23.3 Cast-mold technique (shown in a case with smaller implant): Before craniotomy a cast was taken, by modeling PMMA on the area of the craniotomy, before removing the bone but after drilling down the hyperostosis. This the larger PMMA piece, which is taken as a mold to form the upper, smaller piece, to retain the curvature of the skull

described in various manners. I use separate bone flaps (Fig. 23.5) to prevent lifting the tumor with the afflicted bone without control at the brain tumor interface. This is also a good technique, when the sinuses have to be traversed by the craniotomy. The lesion is resected and dura reconstructed with either galea or fascia lata and occasionally with additional abdominal fat (mostly in skull base lesions). Subsequently the initial cast is used as a mold to form the final PMMA implant, which is fixed with plates (Figs. 23.3 and 23.4).

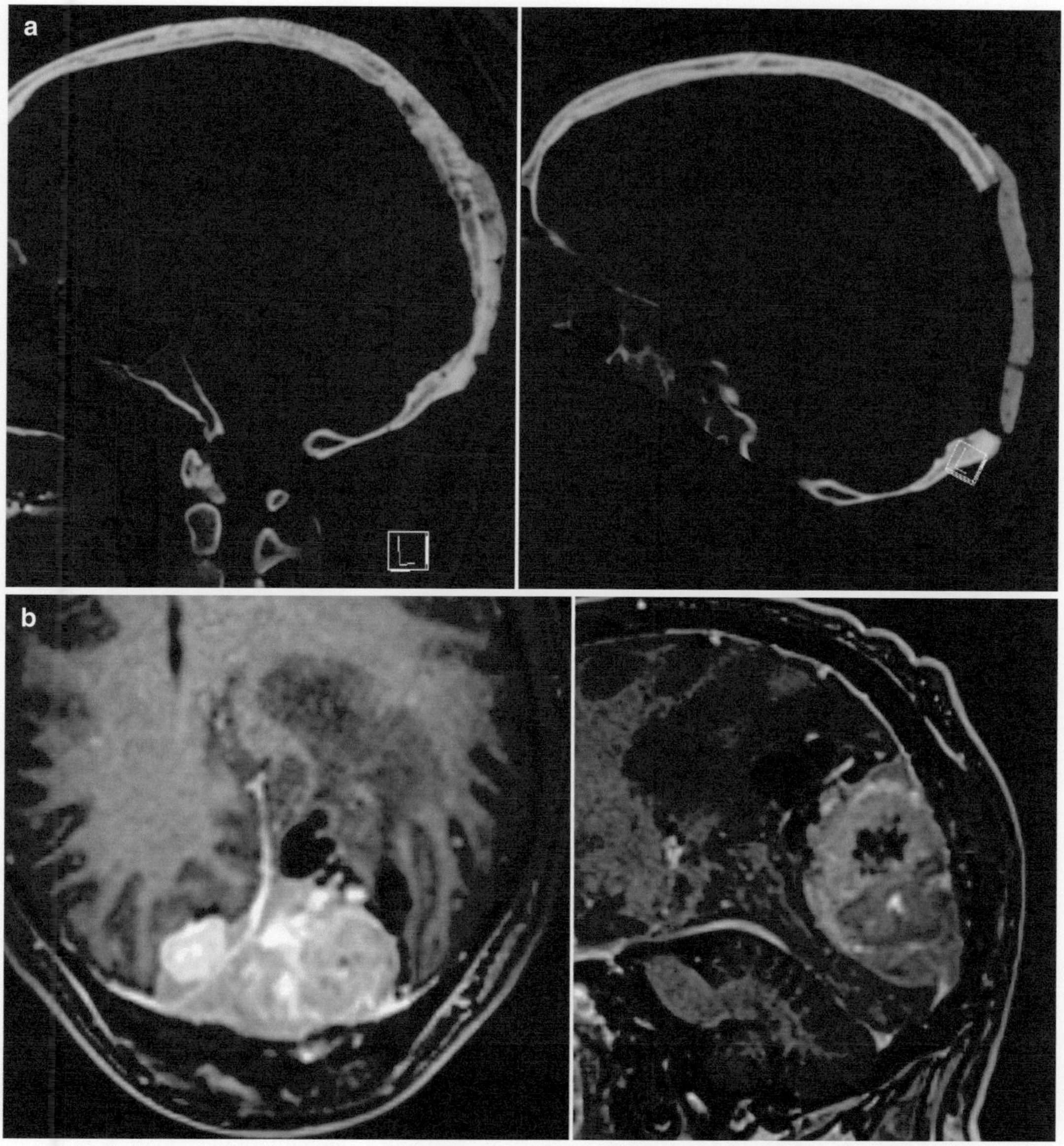

Fig. 23.4 (**a**) Hyperostotic, transosseous meningioma with bilateral growth an occlusion of the posterior third of the superior sagittal sinus. Both transvers sinuses were intact. The hyperostosis was drilled down; a PMMA cast was taken, as described above, the tumor and the tumor removed, including the occluded sinus, almost up to the open portion toward the middle third, although a small remnant of tumor was intentionally left to ensure that the residual sinus is not compromised. On postoperative MRI no residual tumor was identified. While presurgical MRI had not shown any additional venous channels, a midline incision was chosen, to conserve potential venous channels parallel to the occluded sinus. (**b**) Pre-op axial and sagittal enhanced T1WI demonstrating the obvious sinus occlusion. Not altered bone signal and subcutaneous pathological tissue. (**c**) Postoperative enhanced T1WI MRI. Note intact SSS distal of the resected area and reasonable reconstruction of a normal curvature with the PMMA fashion with the mold technique intraoperatively

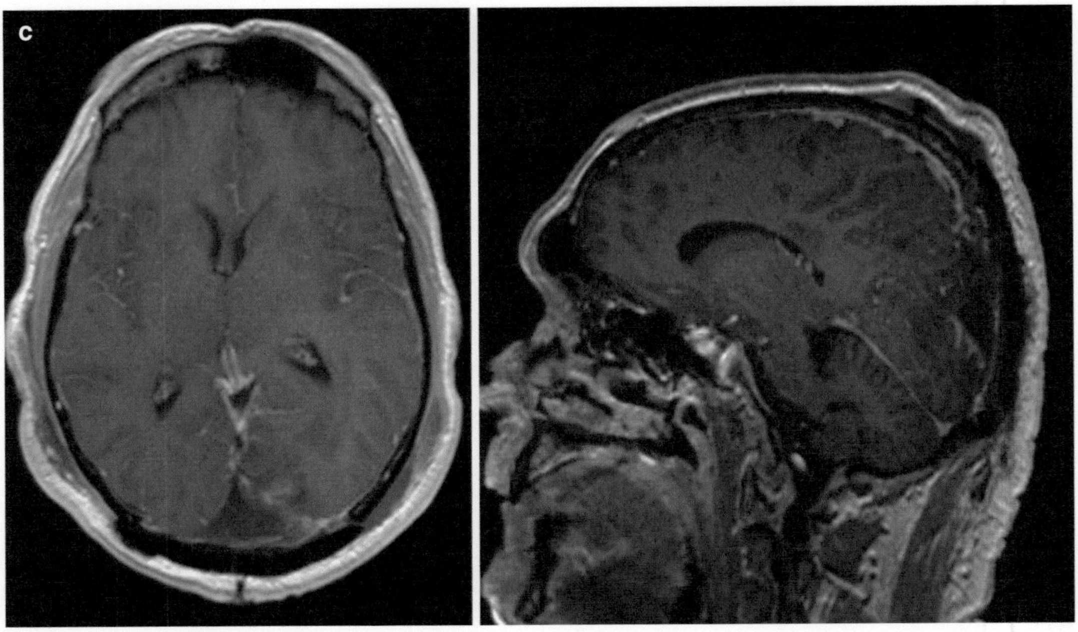

Fig. 23.4 (continued)

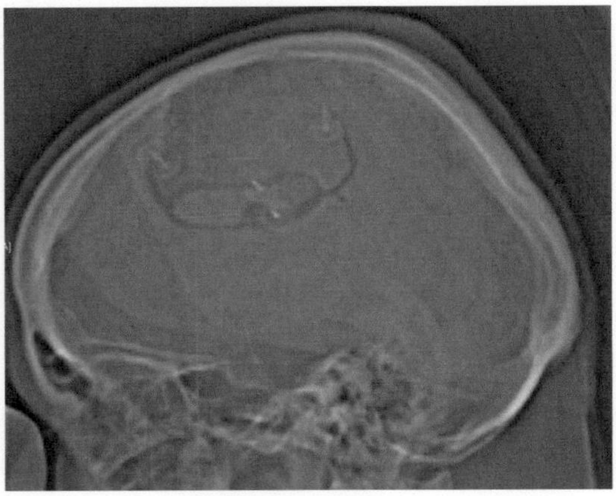

Fig. 23.5 Fragmented Craniotomy: With tightly adherent tumors, it is advisable to perform a fragmented craniotomy. Whether it is a double circular, as has been described or a fragmented, as in this case seems unimportant. I prefer such fragmented bone flaps. Lifting the smaller flap gives access to the epidural space to separate the bone from the underlying tumor before lifting the flap. Lifting the flap without such precautions may result in an inadvertent avulsion of vessels attached to the tumor, to which access is denied through the narrow space, with catastrophic sequelae. On closure this provides additional space for tack sutures in larger bone flaps. Fixing half of the bone flap, sutures at the medial flap border are placed, before implanting the second fragment

23.3.2 Surgical Lessons Learned

The lessons learned in Meningioma Surgery can and should be extended to all lesions adherent to the dura or transgressing it with infiltration and destruction of the adjacent bone and skin. Skin involvement is remarkably rare, even in malignancies. Nevertheless, tension-free skin closure is imperative to prevent graft infection and allow the timely initiation of further treatment of the primary tumor, particularly in malignancies. Rarely skin flaps are needed. If major skin involvement is encountered in a malignant tumor, which requires swift further treatment, it may be contemplated to perform a craniectomy to gain space. In this case it is also advisable to drill down the outer table of the surrounding bone, which may gain additional mm to cm needed for the tension-free skin adaptation. Sometimes it is also possible to implant a titanium mesh, without recreating the curvature. However, in doubt, whether the skin can be attached without strain, I would choose to not reconstruct the bone. Fortunately, these situations are rare and mostly occur on follow-up surgeries, i.e., recurrencies, where the skin is vulnerable in particular after radiation therapy or multiple GKS treatments.

This immediately leads to the point of planning the initial skin incision. Applying the principle of keyhole surgery, that the further remote the lesion is, the smaller the bone opening may be, holds true in the other direction as well: the more superficial a lesion is, the wider the opening needs to be, to enable a gross total resection including cranioplasty. Also, this provides enough galea to reconstruct the resected dura. Naturally all patients should be prepped for fascia lata harvesting, although I try to avoid it. Patient mobilization often is impaired by pain at the donor site.

Moreover, recurrent surgery should be borne in mind. Many problems with incorporating the old incision could be thus avoided. Particularly since the recurrence will be outside the dural reconstruction, extension of the approach will most likely be needed.

Also important for the initial step is the establishment of venous collaterals, when operating in the parasagittal area (see above). The safest incision is always the straight incision above the sinus because transgressing skin collaterals between the sides are rare. Nevertheless, particularly in recurrent disease, transgressing collaterals should be ruled out. Bone removal and cranioplasty have been described above.

In sinus involvement the improvement in radiation oncology and stereotactic radiosurgery has opened new avenues. Therefore, resection as close as possible to the sinus, without reconstruction, is intended. However, if precise imaging shows only a small tumor portion in the sinus, I incise the falx cerebri below the tumor attachment to form a flap, which can be reflected upward above the potential sinus opening. The sides are sutured in a running fashion and left attached. If there is venous bleeding, the flap is reflected further, and the sutures are finished to the convexity sinus portion. In small incidental openings, muscle patches suffice.

Generally, the tactic of leaving a residue to be irradiated or controlled, rather than risking morbidity through elaborate sinus reconstruction, is discussed with the patient. Also, the tumor-bearing sinus can be removed safely, once slow tumor growth led to the occlusion. In malignancies, which will be irradiated, gross total removal remains the basis for further treatment. Still, attempts at sinus repair are unnecessary. The potential of adjunct radiation modalities and the efficacy of modern chemo- and the growing field of immunotherapy [3, 6, 7] accentuate the necessity of a sinus-conserving surgical approach.

23.4 Conclusion

Driven by the refinement of meningioma surgery of the convexity including the parasagittal sinus, techniques have been established, which permit the resection of other varieties of intracerebral lesions involving the dura and skull. Principles of plastic surgery apply to the skin incisions. These should be planned to accommodate repeat surgery and possible larger fields of exposure. Involvement of the sinuses are not a contraindication to surgery. However, with adjunct therapeutic options, potential morbidity has to be carefully weight in. Modern neuronavigation and evolved techniques and materials for cranioplasty enable more elaborate skull reconstruction in one operation.

Interdisciplinary cooperation broadened the scope as well as improved the overall outcome and prognosis of our patients harboring these challenging tumors.

Acknowledgement The authors thank L. Helmbold, D. Yildirim, M. Lalk, K. Kniese, and C. Hartmann (Hannover) for support and assistance. AN thanks his friend and Mentor in Anatomy M. Schünke (Kiel) for providing invaluable advice.

References

1. Karatas D, Uygur S, Karabag H, Sayar H, Barut IT, Dagtekin A, Avci E. Calvarial tumors: a retrospective analysis and clinical experience. Turk Neurosurg. 2023;33(2):244–51.
2. Michael CB, Gokaslan ZL, DeMonte F, McCutcheon IE, Sawaya R, Lang FF. Surgical resection of calvarial metastases overlying dural sinuses. Neurosurgery. 2001;48(4):745–54. discussion 54–5
3. Mitchell DK, Kwon HJ, Kubica PA, Huff WX, O'Regan R, Dey M. Brain metastases: an update on the multi-disciplinary approach of clinical management. Neurochirurgie. 2022;68(1):69–85.
4. Nasi-Kordhishti I, Hempel JM, Ebner FH, Tatagiba M. Calvarial lesions: overview of imaging features and neurosurgical management. Neurosurg Rev. 2021;44(6):3459–69.
5. St. Clair EG, McCutcheon IE. Skull Tumors. In: Winn HR, editor. Youman's and Winn Neurological Surgery. 2. 7th ed: Elsevier; 2016. p. 5227–70.
6. Ostrom QT, Wright CH, Barnholtz-Sloan JS. Brain metastases: epidemiology. Handb Clin Neurol. 2018;149:27–42.
7. Harrison RA, Nam JY, Weathers SP, DeMonte F. Intracranial dural, calvarial, and skull base metastases. Handb Clin Neurol. 2018;149:205–25.
8. Ko MJ, Hwang SN, Park YS, Nam TK. Primary malignant lymphoma of the cranial vault with extra- and intracranial extension. Brain Tumor Res Treat. 2013;1(1):32–5.
9. Scott TF, Hogan EL, Carter TD, Garen PD, Brillman J, Kurent JE. Primary intracranial meningeal lymphoma. Am J Med. 1990;89(4):536–8.
10. D'Angelo CR. Diagnostic, pathologic, and therapeutic considerations for primary CNS lymphoma. JCO Oncol Pract. 2024;20(2):195–202.
11. Ouyang T, Wang L, Zhang N, Zhang Z, Xiong Y, Li M, Hong T. Clinical characteristics, surgical outcomes, and prognostic factors of intracranial primary central nervous system lymphoma. World Neurosurg. 2020;139:e508–e16.
12. Colas L, Caron S, Cotten A. Skull vault lesions: a review. AJR Am J Roentgenol. 2015;205(4):840–7.
13. Pons Escoda A, Naval Baudin P, Mora P, Cos M, Hernandez Ganan J, Narvaez JA, et al. Imaging of skull vault tumors in adults. Insights Imaging. 2020;11(1):23.
14. Hubel K. Lymphoma: new diagnosis and current treatment strategies. J Clin Med. 2022;11(6)
15. Toyota E, Taslimi S, Alkins R. Optimal management of calvarial lymphoma: a meta-analysis. World Neurosurg. 2021;151:e484–e94.
16. Barrer SJ, Simeone FA, Han SS. An unusual presentation of an oligodendroglioma. Case report. J Neurosurg. 1980;53(4):560–1.
17. Khan MA, Hashmi S. Low-grade astrocytoma causing calvarial scalloping. Pediatr Neurosurg. 2007;43(2):155–7.
18. Osborn RE, Ley CE. Astrocytoma with calvarial erosion. AJNR Am J Neuroradiol. 1986;7(1):178.
19. Satyarthee GD, Mahapatra AK. Giant pediatric glioblastoma multiforme causing primary calvarial erosion and sutural diastasis presenting with enlarged head. J Pediatr Neurosci. 2015;10(3):290–3.
20. Takaki Y, Tsutsumi S, Teramoto S, Nonaka S, Okura H, Suzuki T, Ishii H. Supratentorial extraventricular ependymoma presenting calvarial erosion: a report of 3 cases. Radiol Case Rep. 2021;16(10):3003–6.
21. Yang R, Yan H, Dewan MC, Tailor JK, Santisukwongchote S, Hawkins C, Ibrahim GM. Giant choroid plexus cysts with calvarial erosion: a case report and literature review. Childs Nerv Syst. 2021;37(7):2381–5.
22. Bajaj A. Multicystic oligodendroglioma with calvarial destruction. Asian J Neurosurg. 2014;9(2):93–5.
23. Belfquih H, Slioui B, Azami MA, Akhaddar A. Low-grade astrocytoma causing dural and calvarial destruction. Asian J Neurosurg. 2023;18(1):223–7.
24. Handzhiev DD, Kalevski SK, Handzhieva SV, Dzhenkov DL, Salieva-Badi S. Low grade astrocytoma causing dural and calvarial destruction. J Clin Neurosci. 2017;40:84–9.
25. Gheyi V, Hui FK, Doppenberg EM, Todd W, Broaddus WC. Glioblastoma multiforme causing calvarial destruction: an unusual manifestation revisited. AJNR Am J Neuroradiol. 2004;25(9):1533–7.
26. Capper D, Jones DTW, Sill M, Hovestadt V, Schrimpf D, Sturm D, et al. DNA methylation-based classification of central nervous system tumours. Nature. 2018;555(7697):469–74.
27. Louis DN, Perry A, Wesseling P, Brat DJ, Cree IA, Figarella-Branger D, et al. The 2021 WHO classification of tumors of the central nervous system: a summary. Neuro-Oncology. 2021;23(8):1231–51.
28. Schweizer L, Koelsche C, Sahm F, Piro RM, Capper D, Reuss DE, et al. Meningeal hemangiopericytoma and solitary fibrous tumors carry the NAB2-STAT6 fusion and can be diagnosed by nuclear expression of STAT6 protein. Acta Neuropathol. 2013;125(5):651–8.
29. Wang K, Mei F, Wu S, Tan Z. Hemangiopericytoma: incidence, treatment, and prognosis analysis based on SEER database. Biomed Res Int. 2020;2020:2468320.
30. Kinslow CJ, Bruce SS, Rae AI, Sheth SA, McKhann GM, Sisti MB, et al. Solitary-fibrous tumor/hemangiopericytoma of the central nervous system: a population-based study. J Neuro-Oncol. 2018;138(1):173–82.
31. Rutkowski MJ, Jian BJ, Bloch O, Chen C, Sughrue ME, Tihan T, et al. Intracranial hemangiopericytoma: clinical experience and treatment considerations in a modern series of 40 adult patients. Cancer. 2012;118(6):1628–36.
32. Patel AR, Flores BC, Ban VS, Hatanpaa KJ, Mickey BE, Barnett SL. Intracranial hemangiopericytomas: recurrence, metastasis, and radiotherapy. J Neurol Surg B Skull Base. 2017;78(4):324–30.

33. Rutkowski MJ, Sughrue ME, Kane AJ, Aranda D, Mills SA, Barani IJ, Parsa AT. Predictors of mortality following treatment of intracranial hemangiopericytoma. J Neurosurg. 2010;113(2):333–9.
34. Kim YJ, Park JH, Kim YI, Jeun SS. Treatment strategy of intracranial Hemangiopericytoma. Brain Tumor Res Treat. 2015;3(2):68–74.
35. Golub D, McBriar JD, Donaldson H, Wong T, Unadkat P, White TG, et al. Postoperative stereotactic radiosurgery for intracranial solitary fibrous tumors: systematic review and pooled quantitative analysis. J Neuro-Oncol. 2023;165(2):229–39.
36. Lee JH, Jeon SH, Park CK, Park SH, Yoon HI, Chang JH, et al. The role of postoperative radiotherapy in intracranial solitary fibrous tumor/hemangiopericytoma: a multi-institutional retrospective study (KROG 18-11). Cancer Res Treat. 2022;54(1):65–74.
37. Kinslow CJ, Rajpara RS, Wu CC, Bruce SS, Canoll PD, Wang SH, et al. Invasiveness is associated with metastasis and decreased survival in hemangiopericytoma of the central nervous system. J Neuro-Oncol. 2017;133(2):409–17.
38. Chiechi MV, Smirniotopoulos JG, Mena H. Intracranial hemangiopericytomas: MR and CT features. AJNR Am J Neuroradiol. 1996;17(7):1365–71.
39. Nishioka K, Tsutsumi S, Teramoto S, Nonaka S, Okura H, Suzuki T, et al. Atypical meningeal hemangiopericytoma presenting with punched-out calvarial erosion. Radiol Case Rep. 2020;15(11):2129–35.
40. Sun C, Dou Z, Wu J, Jiang B, Iranmanesh Y, Yu X, et al. The preferred locations of meningioma according to different biological characteristics based on voxel-wise analysis. Front Oncol. 2020;10:1412.
41. Champeaux C, Jecko V, Houston D, Thorne L, Dunn L, Fersht N, et al. Malignant meningioma: an international multicentre retrospective study. Neurosurgery. 2019;85(3):E461–E9.
42. Ogasawara C, Philbrick BD, Adamson DC. Meningioma: a review of epidemiology, pathology, diagnosis, treatment, and future directions. Biomedicines. 2021;9(3)
43. Ostrom QT, Cioffi G, Gittleman H, Patil N, Waite K, Kruchko C, Barnholtz-Sloan JS. CBTRUS statistical report: primary brain and other central nervous system tumors diagnosed in the United States in 2012-2016. Neuro-Oncology. 2019;21(Suppl 5):v1–v100.
44. Behling F, Fodi C, Hoffmann E, Renovanz M, Skardelly M, Tabatabai G, et al. The role of Simpson grading in meningiomas after integration of the updated WHO classification and adjuvant radiotherapy. Neurosurg Rev. 2021;44(4):2329–36.
45. Cushing H, Eisenhardt L. Meningiomas, their classification, regional behaviour, life history, and surgical end results. Springfield, IL: Charles C Thomas; 1938.
46. Sindou MP, Alvernia JE. Results of attempted radical tumor removal and venous repair in 100 consecutive meningiomas involving the major dural sinuses. J Neurosurg. 2006;105(4):514–25.
47. DiMeco F, Li KW, Casali C, Ciceri E, Giombini S, Filippini G, et al. Meningiomas invading the superior sagittal sinus: surgical experience in 108 cases. Neurosurgery. 2004;55(6):1263–72. discussion 72–4
48. Raza SM, Gallia GL, Brem H, Weingart JD, Long DM, Olivi A. Perioperative and long-term outcomes from the management of parasagittal meningiomas invading the superior sagittal sinus. Neurosurgery. 2010;67(4):885–93. discussion 93
49. Gatterbauer B, Gevsek S, Hoftberger R, Lutgendorf-Caucig C, Ertl A, Mallouhi A, et al. Multimodal treatment of parasagittal meningiomas: a single-center experience. J Neurosurg. 2017;127(6):1249–56.
50. Munich SA, Eddelman D, Byrne RW. Retrospective review of a venous sparing approach to resection of parasagittal meningiomas. J Clin Neurosci. 2019;64:194–200.
51. Marc JA, Schechter MM. Cortical venous rerouting in parasagittal meningiomas. Radiology. 1974;112(1):85–92.
52. Oka K, Go Y, Kimura H, Tomonaga M. Obstruction of the superior sagittal sinus caused by parasagittal meningiomas: the role of collateral venous pathways. J Neurosurg. 1994;81(4):520–4.
53. Du YP, Jin Z, Hu Y, Tanabe J. Multi-echo acquisition of MR angiography and venography of the brain at 3 Tesla. J Magn Reson Imaging. 2009;30(2):449–54.
54. Mathiesen T. Parasagittal meningiomas. Handb Clin Neurol. 2020;170:93–100.
55. Clynch AL, Norrington M, Mustafa MA, Richardson GE, Doherty JA, Humphries TJ, et al. Cranial meningioma with bone involvement: surgical strategies and clinical considerations. Acta Neurochir. 2023;165(5):1355–63.
56. Lau BL, Che Othman MI, Fathil M, Liew DNS, Lim SS, Bujang MA, Wong ASH. Does putting Back hyperostotic bone flap in meningioma surgery cause tumor recurrence? An observational prospective study. World Neurosurg. 2019;127:e497–502.
57. Fathalla H, Tawab MGA, El-Fiki A. Extent of Hyperostotic bone resection in convexity meningioma to achieve pathologically free margins. J Korean Neurosurg Soc. 2020;63(6):821–6.
58. Siracusa V, Maimone G, Antonelli V. State-of-art of standard and innovative materials used in cranioplasty. Polymers (Basel). 2021;13(9)
59. Zanotti B, Zingaretti N, Verlicchi A, Robiony M, Alfieri A, Parodi PC. Cranioplasty: review of materials. J Craniofac Surg. 2016;27(8):2061–72.
60. Barros A, Brauge D, QuEhan R, Cavallier Z, Roux FE, Moyse E. One-step customized PEEK cranioplasty after 3D printed resection template assisted surgery for a frontal intraosseous meningioma: a case report. Turk Neurosurg. 2021;31(1):142–7.
61. Oishi T, Sameshima T, Totsuka T, Yamasaki T, Koizumi S, Namba H. Cosmetic and neuroprotective placement of custom-made ultra-high-molecular-weight polyethylene cranial plate (SKULPIO) in

single-step surgery: technical note and case report. World Neurosurg. 2019;130:187–91.
62. Broeckx CE, Maal TJJ, Vreeken RD, Bos RRM, Ter Laan M. Single-step resection of an intraosseous meningioma and cranial reconstruction: technical note. World Neurosurg. 2017;108:225–9.
63. Huang RY, Bi WL, Griffith B, Kaufmann TJ, la Fougere C, Schmidt NO, et al. Imaging and diagnostic advances for intracranial meningiomas. Neuro-Oncology. 2019;21(Suppl 1):i44–61.
64. Marbacher S, Coluccia D, Fathi AR, Andereggen L, Beck J, Fandino J. Intraoperative patient-specific reconstruction of partial bone flap defects after convexity meningioma resection. World Neurosurg. 2013;79(1):124–30.
65. Bloch O, McDermott MW. In situ cranioplasty for hyperostosing meningiomas of the cranial vault. Can J Neurol Sci. 2011;38(1):59–64.
66. Nabavi A, Henneck N, Helmbold L, Corbu BM. Cast and Mold technique for single step cranioplasty in large bone defects in oncologic surgery: a novel technique. submitted for publication. 2024.

Part VI

Treatment and Outcome for Lesions of the Scalp and Calvarium

Editor's Summary

In this "Part VI: Treatment and Outcome for Lesions of the Scalp and Calvarium," there are six chapters that are pertinent to the management of calvarial lesions that is not always surgical in nature. The first of these chapters is Chap. 24 which covers the nonsurgical treatment of these lesions that involve the scalp and calvarium. Other important topics that are contained in this section include a discussion of the principles of surgery and reconstructive procedures for lesions of the scalp and calvarium which is found in Chap. 25. Obviously, the use of anesthesia for any of the scalp or calvarial lesions that requires surgery is essential and necessitates the inclusion of Chap. 26 which provides anesthetic guidance. Unfortunately, postoperative complications can occur which warrants the need for Chap. 27 to add further information for the management of such events. The overall prognosis for scalp and calvarial lesions is generally favorable and is summarized in Chap. 28. And in today's medical environment where patient expectations can often be challenging, a discussion on the medicolegal aspects of lesions of the scalp and calvarium in Chap. 29 is both timely and warranted.

Nonsurgical Treatment of the Scalp and Calvarium Lesions

24

Mohammed Benzagmout, Kossi Kouma Félix Segbedgi, Brahim Abdenbaoui, and Meryem Himmiche

24.1 Introduction

Scalp and calvarium lesions are characterized by heterogeneous clinical and radiological features. The diagnostic approach is primordial, and the treatment choice may constitute a serious challenge due to the patient's conditions and comorbidities (newborn versus elderly patients), the clinical and radiological landscapes of the lesion, and the desired or expected cosmetic result.

Surgery constitutes the cornerstone of treatment in most cases. However, nonsurgical treatment might be indicated in many lesions, providing cautious follow-up and good outcomes. The choice of surgical versus nonsurgical management of these lesions depends on the origin of the lesion "scalp versus calvarium," the extension of the lesion "from scalp to calvarium or the opposite," the clinical status of the patient, the unicity/multiplicity of the lesion, and other radiological features [1].

The objective of this chapter is to shed light on the nonsurgical treatment of scalp and calvarial lesions. Conservative management can involve observational supervision, medical treatment, and/or local noninvasive treatment.

24.2 Wait-and-See Approach

Scalp and calvarium lesions can be classified as congenital, traumatic, inflammatory, metabolic, and neoplastic. Malignant neoplasms and locally aggressive tumors are frequent and require surgery. However, incidentally discovered lesions and some benign tumors are not rare. Therefore, the strategy of a wait-and-see approach to scalp and calvarium lesions might be one of many treatment modalities applied to these lesions.

Observation as a first treatment option (follow-up strategy) depends strongly on the patient history, physical examination, radiological findings, and local invasion. It seems obvious to observe only presumed benign tumors and discuss other treatments if we suspect malignancy [2], or in cases of clinical/radiological evolution.

Indeed, a small skull lesion, sclerotic juxtacortical calvarium lesion as osteoma and meningioma, and lesion with trabeculations or sunburst pattern images as hemangiomas can be controlled

M. Benzagmout (✉)
Department of Neurosurgery, Hassan II Hospital, Sidi Mohamed Ben Abdellah University of Fès, Fes, Morocco
e-mail: benzagmout@hotmail.fr

K. K. F. Segbedgi
Department of Neurosurgery, Hôpital DOGTA LAFIE, Lomé, Togo

B. Abdenbaoui
Department of Neurosurgery, University Hospital of Fez, Fez, Morocco

M. Himmiche
Department of Neurosurgery, University Hospital of Tangiers, Tangier, Morocco

M. Turgut et al. (eds.), *Lesions of the Scalp and Cranial Vault*,
https://doi.org/10.1007/978-3-031-88244-9_24

radiologically, especially when asymptomatic [3]. Conservative management for some primary benign cone tumors has been discussed in the literature such as "osteoid osteoma" with long-term nonsteroidal anti-inflammatory drugs [4]. Calvarial hemangiomas are usually small, unifocal, and asymptomatic. Therefore, the follow-up is clinical and radiological. In some aggressive cases, surgical treatment can be proposed to the patient [5]. Some primary skull lesions as a solitary eosinophilic granuloma of the calvarium, the most common form of histiocytosis, can be also treated conservatively. Some series reported that unifocal calvarial forms of eosinophilic granulomas undergo spontaneous remission and need nonsurgical interventions [6, 7].

Hyperostosis frontalis interna is a morphological frontal vault aspect with an overgrowth of the inner table. It's an idiopathic calvarial lesion related to an endocrine imbalance, usually asymptomatic and mostly treated conservatively. Surgery is indicated when the lesion becomes symptomatic and leads to frontal lobe compression [8].

Scalp lesions are usually benign and frequently seen in dermatological practice. The clinical exam is important to predict the nature of the lesion. Cystic lesions such as trichilemmal cysts, sebaceoma, dermoid, and epidermoid cysts can be managed conservatively with a regular clinical follow-up. However, patients are usually seeking surgical management due to cosmetic impairment caused by these lesions. Congenital scalp lesions such as aplasia cutis congenita with small skin defects can be managed conservatively with topical ointment while larger lesions that involve the skull and adjacent structures should be treated surgically [9].

24.3 Negative-Pressure Wound Therapy

Negative-pressure wound therapy (NPWT) is a well-established treatment that uses negative pressure to promote wound healing by removing excess fluid, improving blood flow, reducing bacterial colonization, and promoting granulation tissue formation [10–15]. The sponge and adjacent skin are covered by an adhesive semipermeable membrane such as a V.A.C. (vacuum-assisted closure) drape. Shaving, cleaning the skin, placing adhesive film around the wound circumference, and layering smaller strips to adapt the film to varied head topography are all techniques used for the successful application of NPWT [16]. The pad and connection tubing attach the suction apparatus to the wound via perforation created in the film.

Important considerations in the NPWT application include the size and shape of the perforation created, the potential space needed for two pads if intermittent pressure therapy is used, and the placement of the pad in a location that will maximize the patient's comfort [17]. Indeed, a too-small perforation can impair adequate suction, and too large may cause debris to accumulate in and clog the suction tubing. One alternative that can be used is to create a ring of small perforations in the film. Typically, a suction device allows the provider to select low-, medium-, or high-intensity therapy as well as a specific negative pressure level (mmHg). The intensity and/or pressure level can be lowered to improve the patient's comfort because there are instances in which a patient may be poorly tolerant to NPWT due to pain [18, 19].

Most devices are equipped with alarms to detect a loss in pressure or a leak, and most have some battery life to allow patient transport or mobilization. Moreover, some models are designed for outpatient use and are purely battery-powered.

NPWT can be routinely maintained for at least 1 week. However, for complicated, active, or infected wounds, it is more common to change the NPWT dressing every 2–3 days. Depending on the location of the wound or the tolerance level of the patient, the dressing changes can be performed in the operating room or at the bedside. To improve the patient's tolerance of dressing changes at the bedside, it is recommended to soak the sponge in a dilute solution containing lidocaine or hydrogen peroxide [19, 20].

24.4 Cryotherapy

Cryotherapy or cryosurgery is a minimally invasive technique using an extremely local cold liquid (liquefied nitrogen gas) or instruments for a short period. It is a promising nonsurgical technique to treat scalp lesions, even some malignant scalp tumors. Cryotherapy or cryoablation is considered a destructive procedure to destroy normal and/or abnormal skin tissue [21]. The destructive effect of cryotherapy is immediate and remains effective due to delayed host immune response. Indeed, superficial cryotherapy alters the immunological processes of the tissue, increases blood flow, and improves microcirculation by reactive vasodilation [22, 23].

This technique is normally performed in outpatient care to treat a variety of benign, premalignant, and malignant skin lesions. It's considered as a first-line treatment for scalp actinic keratosis [24], seborrheic keratosis, and alopecia areata [25]. In addition, superficial basal cell carcinoma with definite margins can be treated solely with cryosurgery and lead to better results [26].

24.5 Dynamic Phototherapy

Dynamic phototherapy (DPT) is a form of phototherapy involving light and a photosensitizing chemical substance to create a photochemical reaction that destroys cancer cells. The photosensitizer agents are methyl aminolevulinic acid cream, aminolevulinic acid hydrochloride topical cream, BF-200 ALA (which is a combination of a nanoscale-lipid vesicle formulation and the prodrug 5-aminolevulinic acid), and intravenous porfimer sodium, and the light source include laser, non-laser, and ambient daylight [27]. This technique is widely used to treat large skin conditions even skin cancer [28]. It is used to treat scalp actinic keratosis, scalp psoriasis, in situ squamous cell carcinomas, and superficial basal cell carcinoma [29]. Another promoting luminous therapy is photobiomodulation AKA also known as low-level laser therapy. This technique can be used exclusively to treat some scalp chronic inflammatory diseases or in association with DPT to treat hidradenitis suppurativa [30].

24.6 Chemotherapy

As the first treatment for skull multiple myelomas, chemotherapy followed by autologous stem cell transplantation constitutes the main treatment. The current regimen includes variant chemotherapeutic agents to improve the outcome [31]. Besides, electrochemotherapy (ECT) represents an alternative technique to treat some skin and subcutaneous metastasis. It's a minimally invasive oncologic treatment, using the pulses of electric current to render the cell membranes permeable to impermeant or poorly permeant anticancer drugs to potentiate the toxicity of such cytostatic agents. In addition, ECT is an effective method of local tumor ablation that may help to relieve pain, minimize bleeding, and improve the quality of life [32].

24.7 Radiotherapy

Palliative radiotherapy is used to relieve bone pain, shrink the tumor, relieve intracranial pressure, improve symptoms, and stop bleeding. Radiotherapy is considered as the first treatment choice for some radiosensitive scalp malignant tumors. For instance, scalp squamous carcinoma is a radio-responsive tumor that can be treated by radiotherapy alone using a high dose of radiation and achieving a long-term efficient outcome in patients who are not candidates for surgical intervention [33, 34].

The use of radiotherapy alone to treat some musculoskeletal neoplasms had been established to be a definitive local treatment for bone unresectable tumors and/or when surgery can't be a reasonable therapeutic option [35]. Primary bone neoplasms, like bone aneurysmal cysts or giant cell tumors, can be treated by radiotherapy alone and lead to good tumoral response [36]. In addition, bone solitary plasmacytoma can be treated by low-dose radiotherapy without requiring surgery [37].

Moreover, radiotherapy can be used as a single modality treatment for some scalp lesions which tend to be multiple and extensive. It has been reported as a single treatment for aggressive scalp angiosarcoma using mixed proton and electron beam technique [38]. Conventional radiotherapy is the treatment of choice for calvarial metastasis. However, Gamma knife surgery has been widely used in the last decades and seems to be effective in the treatment of calvarial and skull base metastasis [39]. Furthermore, radiosurgery was reported to be an alternative treatment for recurrent head and neck malignancies, especially recurrent squamous cell carcinomas [40].

24.8 Hyperbaric Oxygen Therapy

Hyperbaric oxygen therapy (HBOT) exposes the body to 100% of pure oxygen in a hyperbaric chamber. It is a well-established treatment considered to treat life-threatening conditions such as carbon monoxide poisoning, decompression illness, and gas embolism. Moreover, the utility of HBOT tends to remedy some tissue problems. The partial increase in blood oxygen pressure improves cellular oxygenation, prevents ischemia, and reduces tissue inflammation [41].

Nowadays, the use of oxygen therapy is extended to a large spectrum of pathologies including scalp infections, inflammatory/systemic diseases, and posttraumatic wound healing related to vascular complications [42, 43]. For calvarium, hyperbaric treatment has shown its efficacy in treating osteomyelitis and chronic osteomyelitis [44].

24.9 Low-Temperature Plasma Therapy

Low-temperature plasma therapy (LTPT) is a novel treatment modality that promotes wound healing by inducing angiogenesis, cell proliferation, and migration via intracellular signaling pathways [15]. It is a nonthermal, noninvasive treatment that uses positive and negative ion gases to promote tissue healing through ion-catalyzed peroxidation. Moreover, it has been shown to reduce inflammation and exhibit antimicrobial properties via lipid peroxidation [45–48]. LTPT represents a potential wound care option for patients with nonhealing wounds, such as pressure ulcers, diabetic ulcers, and chronic wounds [48]. The treatment uses different systems and devices powered by carrier gas argon or helium and is referred to as "cold atmospheric plasma" (CAP). CAP stimulates keratinocytes and fibroblasts, resulting in faster cell proliferation and migration which can shorten the wound healing process [49]. This is produced through the activation of cytokines and growth factors synthesis like transforming growth factors (TGF-ß1/2), alpha-smooth muscle actin (α-SMA), and type I collagen [50]. The interaction of particles at the argon/helium plasma interface with the atmosphere is a known feature of CAP. Indeed, CAP application generates a surge of highly reactive species including reactive oxygen species (ROS) such as singlet oxygen (O_2), ozone (O_3), superoxide (O_2 −), and hydroxyl radicals (OH−), as well as reactive nitrogen species (RNS) such as nitric oxide (NO), peroxynitrite (ONOO−), and nitrogen dioxide (NO_2) [25]. These species contribute considerably to inducing angiogenesis, promote cell proliferation, reducing inflammation, and exert an antimicrobial effect [45, 47, 48]. In fact, ROS has the ability to regulate angiogenesis at the wound site and increase local microcirculation. Besides, they act as a secondary messenger to many cells involved in the repair process and appear to be important in coordinating the recruitment of immune cells to the wound site and ensuring effective tissue repair.

24.10 Conclusion

Scalp defects and calvarium lesions are rare and can present as various diseases. The treatment is challenging and reconstructive surgery is usually indicated. However, nonsurgical treatment can be discussed in a wide range of situations. Multiple options are available in the non-operative management of scalp and calvarium lesions. The treatment choice depends on the patient's conditions and comorbidities, the clinical and radiological scenes of the lesion, the expected functional result, and the treatment cost.

References

1. Khodarahmi I, Alizai H, Chalian M, et al. Imaging spectrum of calvarial abnormalities. Radiographics. 2021;41(4):1144–63.
2. Ozgiray E, Perumal K, Cinar C, et al. Management of calvarial tumors: a retrospective analysis and literature review. Turk Neurosurg. 2016;26(5):690–8.
3. Nasi-Kordhishti I, Hempel JM, Ebner FH, Tatagiba M. Calvarial lesions: overview of imaging features and neurosurgical management. Neurosurg Rev. 2021;44(6):3459–69.
4. Feletar M, Hall S. Osteoid osteoma: a case for conservative management. Rheumatology. 2002;41(5):585–6.
5. Ilyas M, Shah SA, Gojwari T, Rafiq S, Ellahi I, Ganaie KH. Classic imaging features of calvarial hemangioma-a case report. Egyptian J Radiol Nucl Med. 2018;49:663–5.
6. Benato A, Riva G, Raneri F. Eosinophilic granuloma of the calvarium: is conservative management a valid option? Illustrative case and systematic review of the literature. Childs Nerv Syst. 2023;39(8):2221–7.
7. De Angulo G, Nair S, Lee V, Khatib Z, Ragheb J, Sandberg DI. Nonoperative management of solitary eosinophilic granulomas of the calvaria. J Neurosurg Pediatr. 2013;12(1):1–5.
8. Zukovitsj D, Allard M, Djekic J. Hyperostosis frontalis interna: etiology and differential diagnosis. Rev Med Liege. 2022;77(12):701–5.
9. Maillet-Declerck M, Vinchon M, Guerreschi P, et al. Aplasia cutis congenita: review of 29 cases and proposal of a therapeutic strategy. Eur J Pediatr Surg. 2013;23(2):89–93.
10. Aldabagh B, Cook JL. Reconstruction of scalp wounds with exposed calvarium using a local flap and a split-thickness skin graft: case series of 20 patients. Dermatologic Surg. 2014;40(3):257–65.
11. Desai SC, Sand JP, Sharon JD, Branham G, Nussenbaum B. Scalp reconstruction: an algorithmic approach and systematic review. JAMA Facial Plastic Surg. 2015;17:56–66.
12. Furlanetti LL, de Oliveira RS, Santos MV, Farina JA, Machado HR. Multiple cranial burr holes as an alternative treatment for total scalp avulsion. Childs Nerv Syst. 2010;26:745–9.
13. Colpanian S, Kassira W, Habal MB, Thaller SR. Treatment options for exposed calvarium due to trauma and burns. J Craniofac Surg. 2017;28:318–24.
14. Mühlstädt M, Thomé C, Kunte C. Rapid wound healing of scalp wounds devoid of periosteum with milling of the outer table and split-thickness skin grafting. Br J Dermatol. 2012;167:343–7.
15. Ongkasuwan P. A novel treatment approach for traumatic scalp defects with exposed calvaria denuded of pericranium by combined application of low-temperature plasma and negative pressure wound therapy: a case series. Health Sci Rep. 2023;6:e1578.
16. Andrews BT, Smith RB, Goldstein DP, Funk GF. Management of complicated head and neck wounds with vacuum-assisted closure system. Head Neck. 2006;28:974–81.
17. Liebman RM, Hanubal KS, Dziegielewski PT. Negative pressure wound therapy in the head and neck: a summary of uses and application techniques. Semin Plast Surg. 2022;37(1):9–18.
18. Kadry HM. Negative pressure wound therapy in head and face trauma, can it change the reconstruction ladder? Egypt J Plastic Reconstr Surg. 2022;46(1):89–96.
19. Witty J, Banatkiewicz P, Pruska-Pich MW, Mitura S, Gisterek I. Angiosarcoma of the scalp: a case report. J Contemp Brachytherapy. 2014;6(2):208–12.
20. Hershcovitch MD, Hom DB. Update in wound healing in facial plastic surgery. Arch Facial Plast Surg. 2012;14(6):387–93.
21. Weshahy AH, Abdel Hay RM, Metwally D, Weshahy OA, Gad Z. The efficacy of intralesional cryosurgery in the treatment of small- and medium-sized basal cell carcinoma: a pilot study. J Dermatolog Treat. 2015;26:147–50.
22. Kim TH, Kim DS, Kim SW. Effect of cryotherapy with liquid nitrogen on alopecia areata. Korean J Dermatol. 1994;32:421–6.
23. Lei Y, Nie Y, Zhang JM, Liao DY, Li HY, Man MQ. Effect of superficial hypothermic cryotherapy with liquid nitrogen on alopecia areata. Arch Dermatol. 1991;127:1851–2.
24. Arisi M, Guasco Pisani E, Calzavara-Pinton P, Zane C. Cryotherapy for actinic keratosis: basic principles and literature review. Clin Cosmet Investig Dermatol. 2022;15:357–65.
25. Jablonowski H, von Woedtke T. Research on plasma medicine-relevant plasma–liquid interaction: what happened in the past five years? Clin Plasma Med. 2015;3(2):42–52.
26. Tchanque-Fossuo CN, Eisen DB. A systematic review on the use of cryotherapy versus other treatments for basal cell carcinoma. Dermatol Online J. 2018;24(11):13030.
27. Rkein AM, Ozog DM. Photodynamic therapy. Dermatol Clin. 2014;32(3):415–25.
28. Zhang Q, Li L. Photodynamic combinational therapy in cancer treatment. J Balcan Union Oncol. 2018;23(3):561–7.
29. Neves DR, Gontijo DR, Magalhães GM, Da Costa RR, Alves B, de Souza J. Photodynamic therapy for treatment of multiple lesions on the scalp in nevoid basal cell carcinoma syndrome: case report. An Bras Dermatol. 2010;85(4):545–8.
30. Tricarico PM, Zupin L, Ottaviani G, et al. Photobiomodulation as potential novel third line tool for non-invasive treatment of hidradenitis suppurativa. G Ital Dermatol Venereol. 2020;155(1):88–98.
31. Cowan AJ, Green DJ, Kwok M, et al. Diagnosis and management of multiple myeloma: a review. JAMA. 2022;327(5):464–77.

32. Cavaco D, Carvalhal S, Leite V. Palliative electrochemotherapy treatment of cutaneous metastases in a patient with advanced thyroid papillary carcinoma. Eur Thyroid J. 2020;9(4):221–4.
33. Ostheimer C, Janich M, Hübsch P, Gerlach R, Vordermark D. The treatment of extensive scalp lesions using coplanar and non-coplanar photon IMRT: a single institution experience. Radiat Oncol. 2014;9:82.
34. Xing D, Hettige S, Yan Shan Chee L, Nair R, Rajendra Hegde R. Curative radiotherapy for locally advanced scalp squamous cell carcinoma. Cureus. 2021;13(10):e18514.
35. Hristov B, Shokek O, Frassica DA. The role of radiation treatment in the contemporary management of bone tumors. J Natl Compr Cancer Netw. 2007;5(4):456–66.
36. Zhu S, Hitchcock KE, Mendenhall WM. Radiation therapy for aneurysmal bone cysts. Am J Clin Oncol. 2017;40(6):621–4.
37. Alghisi A, Borghetti P, Maddalo M, et al. Radiotherapy for the treatment of solitary plasmacytoma: 7-year outcomes by a mono-institutional experience. J Cancer Res Clin Oncol. 2021;147(6):1773–9.
38. Willy C, Anagnostakos K. The theory and practice of vacuum therapy: scientific basis, indications for use, case reports, practical advice. Altusried-Krugzell: Lindqvist; 2005.
39. Kotecha R, Angelov A, Barnett GH, et al. Calvarial and skull base metastases: expanding the clinical utility of gamma knife surgery. J Neurosurg. 2014;121(Suppl):91–101.
40. Kawaguchi K, Sato K, Horie A, et al. Stereotactic radiosurgery may contribute to overall survival for patients with recurrent head and neck carcinoma. Radiat Oncol. 2010;5:51.
41. Hajhosseini B, Kuehlmann BA, Bonham CA, Kamperman KJ, Gurtner GC. Hyperbaric oxygen therapy: descriptive review of the technology and current application in chronic wounds. Plast Reconstr Surg Glob Open. 2020;8(9):e3136.
42. Gill AL, Bell CN. Hyperbaric oxygen: its uses, mechanisms of action and outcomes. QJM. 2004;97(7):385–95.
43. Ortega MA, Fraile-Martinez O, García-Montero C, et al. A general overview on the hyperbaric oxygen therapy: applications, mechanisms and translational opportunities. Medicina. 2021;57(9):864.
44. Hanley ME, Hendriksen S, Cooper JS. Hyperbaric treatment of chronic refractory osteomyelitis. StatPearls publishing LLC; 2024.
45. Al Okla SM, Al Nazwani NS, Al-Mudarris FA. Overview of cold atmospheric plasma in wound treatment. Med Clin Res. 2020;5:280–9.
46. Chuangsuwanich A, Assadamongkol T, Boonyawan D. The healing effect of low-temperature atmospheric-pressure plasma in pressure ulcer: a randomized controlled trial. Int J Low Extrem Wounds. 2016;15:313–9.
47. Chutsirimongkol C, Boonyawan D, Polnikorn N, Techawatthanawisan W, Kundilokchai T. Non-thermal plasma for acne and aesthetic skin improvement. Plasma Med. 2014;4:79–88.
48. Chutsirimongkol C, Boonyawan D, Polnikorn N, et al. Non-thermal atmospheric dielectric barrier discharge plasma, medical application studies in Thailand. Plasma Med. 2016;6:429–46.
49. Schmidt A, Bekeschus S, Wende K, Vollmar B, von Woedtke TA. Cold plasma jet accelerates wound healing in a murine model of full-thickness skin wounds. Exp Dermatol. 2017;26:156–62.
50. Gan L, Zhang S, Poorun D, et al. Medical applications of nonthermal atmospheric pressure plasma in dermatology. J Dtsch Dermatol Ges. 2018;16(1):7–13.

25 Principles of Surgery and Reconstructive Procedures for Lesions of the Scalp and Calvarium

Ali Akhaddar

25.1 Introduction

Various lesions should be considered in the scalp and cranial vault regions. The clinical diagnosis is often obvious on physical examination for some large masses; however, other small lesions may be hidden by hair and consequently overlooked for a long time. Furthermore, atypical forms may present a true diagnosis challenge. However, the introduction of the needle biopsy and its occasional application for scalp and skull masses has shown comparable efficacy to the excision biopsy, which might allow the avoidance of unnecessary surgery.

In this perspective, better knowledge of the various types of lesions of these regions and their natural history along with familiarity with different therapeutic options, will help the neurosurgeon in preparation for the surgical planning. Indeed, different courses can be proposed for action:

- Patient reassurance.
- Simple survey.
- Biopsy for pathologic confirmation.
- Conservative treatment.
- Complete surgical resection with reconstructive procedures if feasible.

Surgical experience with these relatively uncommon lesions is thus limited in any given practice. As reported in the neurosurgical literature, it appears that most case reports of scalp and/or cranial vault lesions are still managed on an individual decision basis depending on the results of appropriate clinical presentation, nature of the lesion, and treatment objective [1]. Some items should always be considered for surgical treatment of scalp and cranial vault lesions (Table 25.1).

In this chapter, various surgical therapy options for lesions of the scalp and the cranial

A. Akhaddar (✉)
Department of Neurosurgery, Avicenne Military Hospital of Marrakech, Mohammed V University in Rabat, Rabat, Morocco
e-mail: akhaddar@hotmail.fr

M. Turgut et al. (eds.), *Lesions of the Scalp and Cranial Vault*,
https://doi.org/10.1007/978-3-031-88244-9_25

Table 25.1 The main principles for surgical treatment of scalp and cranial vault lesions

– Establishing correct diagnosis, especially for histopathologic studies
– Lesion resection as much as possible (curative or palliative)
– Decompression of neural structures
– Relief of pain
– Treatment of any concomitant lesions
– Preventing further complications (e.g. recurrence, malignant transformation…)
– Restoration of durable scalp, cranial, and meningeal coverage (reconstructive procedures)
– Esthetic concerns

vault as described. However, surgical treatment of cutaneous and subcutaneous lesions will not be discussed here.

25.2 Surgical Principles

Some superficial and limited scalp lesions can be managed with local anesthesia. On the other hand, large and deep scalp lesions as well as bone lesions are surgically treated using general anesthesia in the operating room.

Although the majority of authors state that resection of the scalp and calvarial lesions is safe, the decision for surgery should be made under the stated circumstances with a multidisciplinary approach for better results and fewer complications [1–5].

Many techniques may be applied for surgical management of lesions involving these regions [2, 6–11]:

- Biopsy.
- Curettage (the contents debrided).
- Lesion excision/resection.
- Tissue expansion.
- Scalp restoration.
- Cranial bone reconstruction (autologous bone graft, …).

The initial scalp incision should always consider vascular supplies and the potential need for secondary reconstructive procedures.

Sometimes, patients with highly vascular lesions underwent acute normovolemic hemodilution to decrease intraoperative blood loss. When needed, angiography was found to be *diagnostic* by delineating the major arterial vessels and draining veins as well as *therapeutic* by embolization of the major vessels [12–16]. After the embolization procedure, most tumoral and vascular lesions require complete resection followed by primary reconstruction.

Most scalp approaches can be performed via a linear incision or a "U" shaped scalp flap based inferiorly on the superficial temporal vessels or other scalp vessels depending on localization. To ensure lesion resection, a one-centimeter margin of macroscopically healthy scalp and/or cranial bone should be done and all scalp and/or bony irregularities may be corrected. Solitary calvarial neoplasms not involving the dural sinus require simple en-bloc resection. Lesions adherent to the dura should not be removed too vigorously in order not to weaken this meningeal layer. Bleeding from dural vessels may be encountered and these can be controlled with bipolar cautery. If needed, dural and/or intradural components may be resected. The lesions that were close to adjacent dural venous sinuses underwent maximal safe resection. The intraparenchymal extension was managed as per micro neurosurgical techniques (Figs. 25.1, 25.2, 25.3, 25.4, 25.5, 25.6, 25.7, 25.8, 25.9, 25.10, 25.11, 25.12, 25.13, 25.14, 25.15, 25.16, and 25.17).

If a dural defect exists, it should be closed using pericranial graft, fascia-lata graft, or dural substitutes (e.g. collagen-based or bovine origin) then the dura should be closed hermetically to avoid cerebrospinal fluid (CSF) leaks (Figs. 25.9 and 25.14). At the end of the procedure, a closed drainage system can be used for a few days to minimize any bleeding collection. Lastly, the wound should be closed without further tension. Usually, scalp closures require two-layer closure using absorbable sutures for the epicranium.

Post-operatively, close clinical, radiologic, and sometimes biologic surveillance is recommended [1].

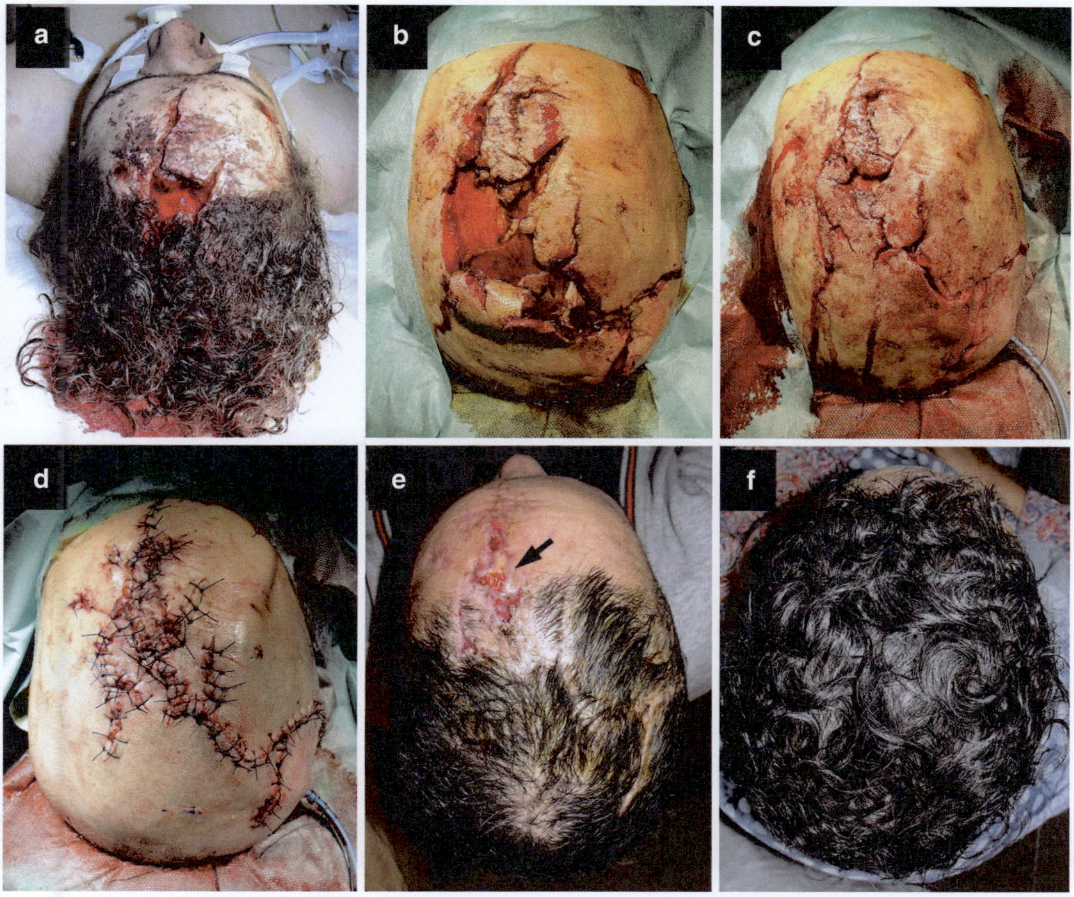

Fig. 25.1 Patient A. Post-traumatic extensive scalp laceration (**a**). Operative view after shaving and cleaning (**b**). Closing subcutaneous plane after placing a surgical drain (**c**). Superficial wound closure (**d**). Wound inflammation 5 weeks later (**e**). Complete healing (head photograph 4 months later) (**f**) (Reproduced from Akhaddar, A. (2017). Surgical Site Infections in Cranial Surgery. In: Atlas of Infections in Neurosurgery and Spinal Surgery. Springer, Cham. https://doi.org/10.1007/978-3-319-60086-4_21.; with permission)

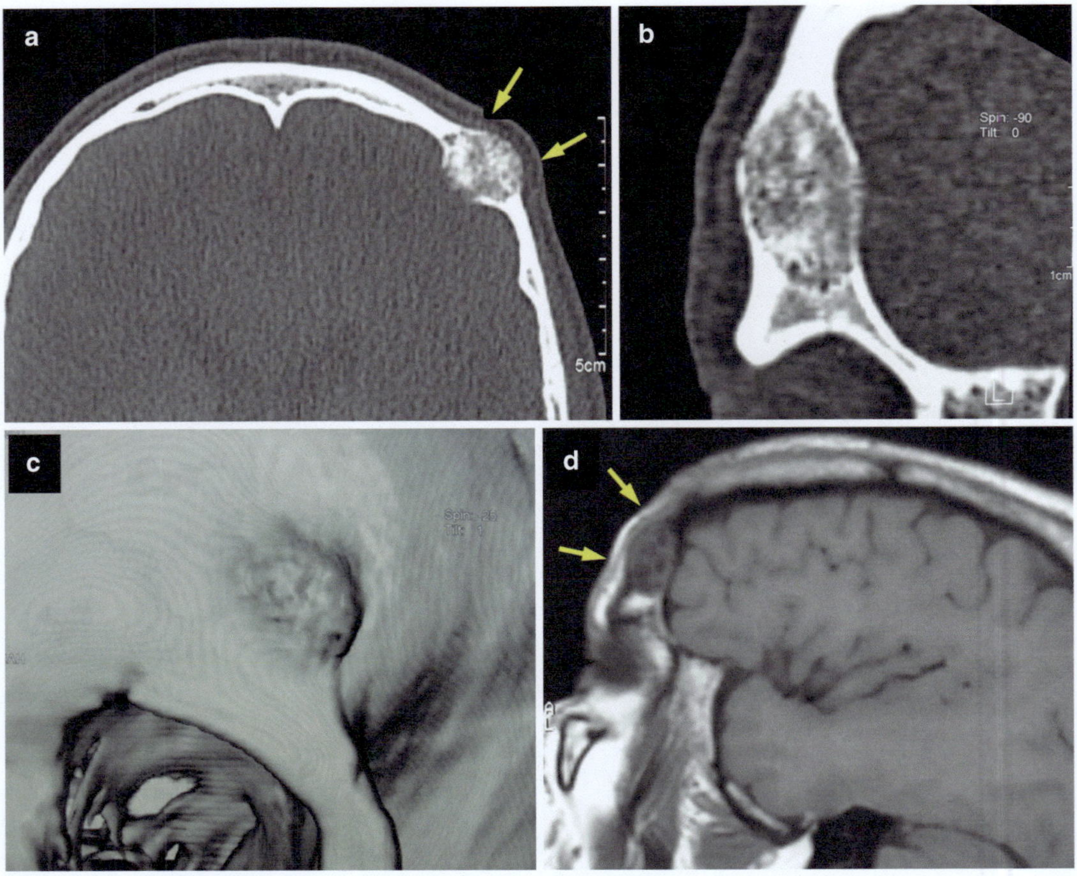

Fig. 25.2 Patient B. Frontal intraosseous hemangioma as seen on axial (**a**) and sagittal reconstruction (**b**) CT-scan as well as on 3D CT-scan (reformatted volume-rendered) (**c**) and sagittal T1-weighted MRI (**d**)

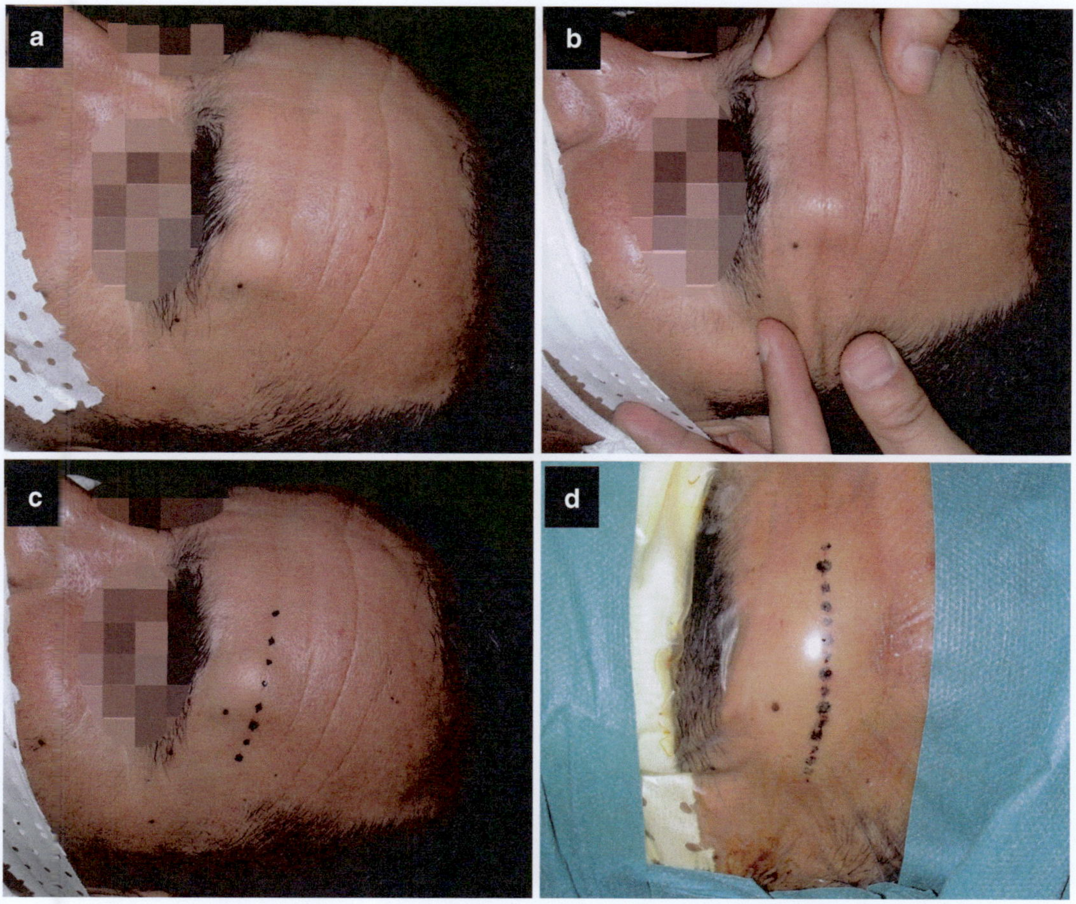

Fig. 25.3 Patient B. Clinical pictures showing the outline of the surgical incision in a frontal crease of the frontal scalp (**a**–**d**)

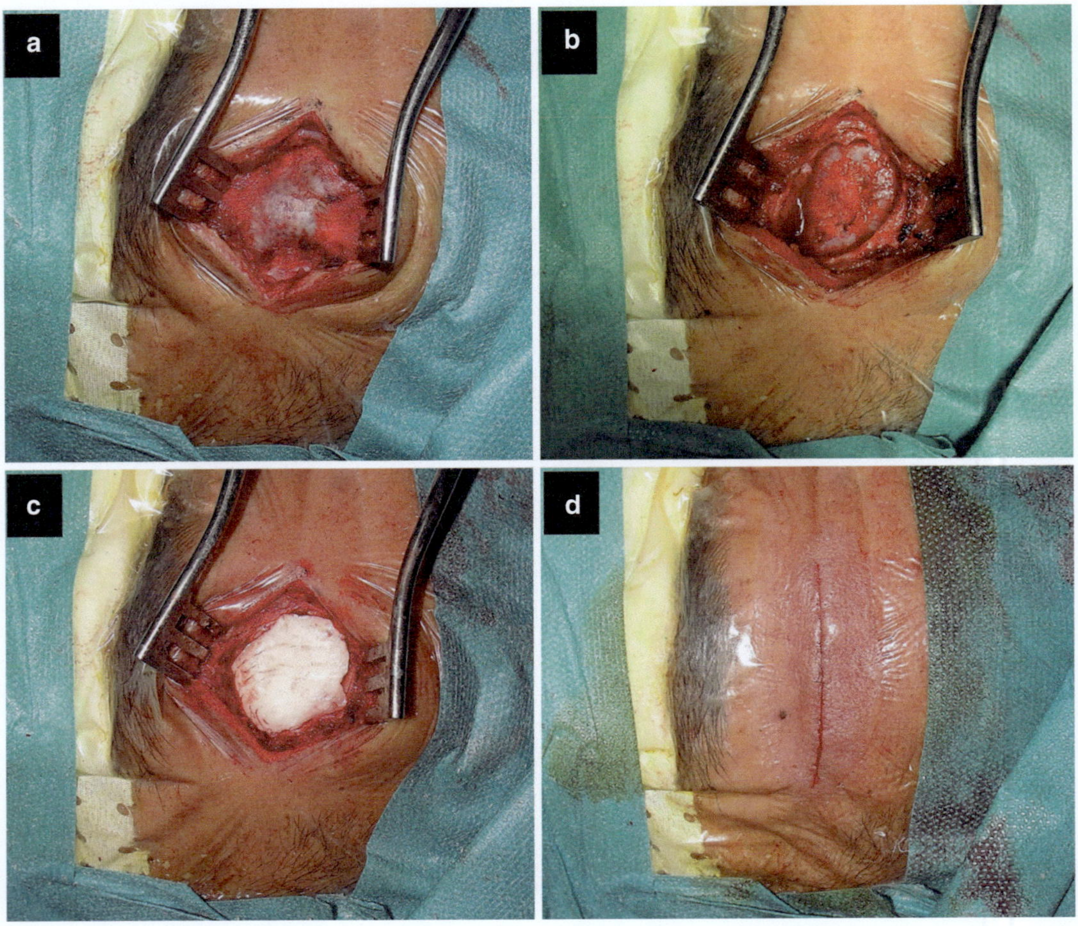

Fig. 25.4 Patient B. Per-operative views showing the lesion exposure (**a**), complete surgical resection (**b**), small methylmethacrylate cranioplasty (**c**), and closure of the scalp at the end of the surgical procedure (**d**)

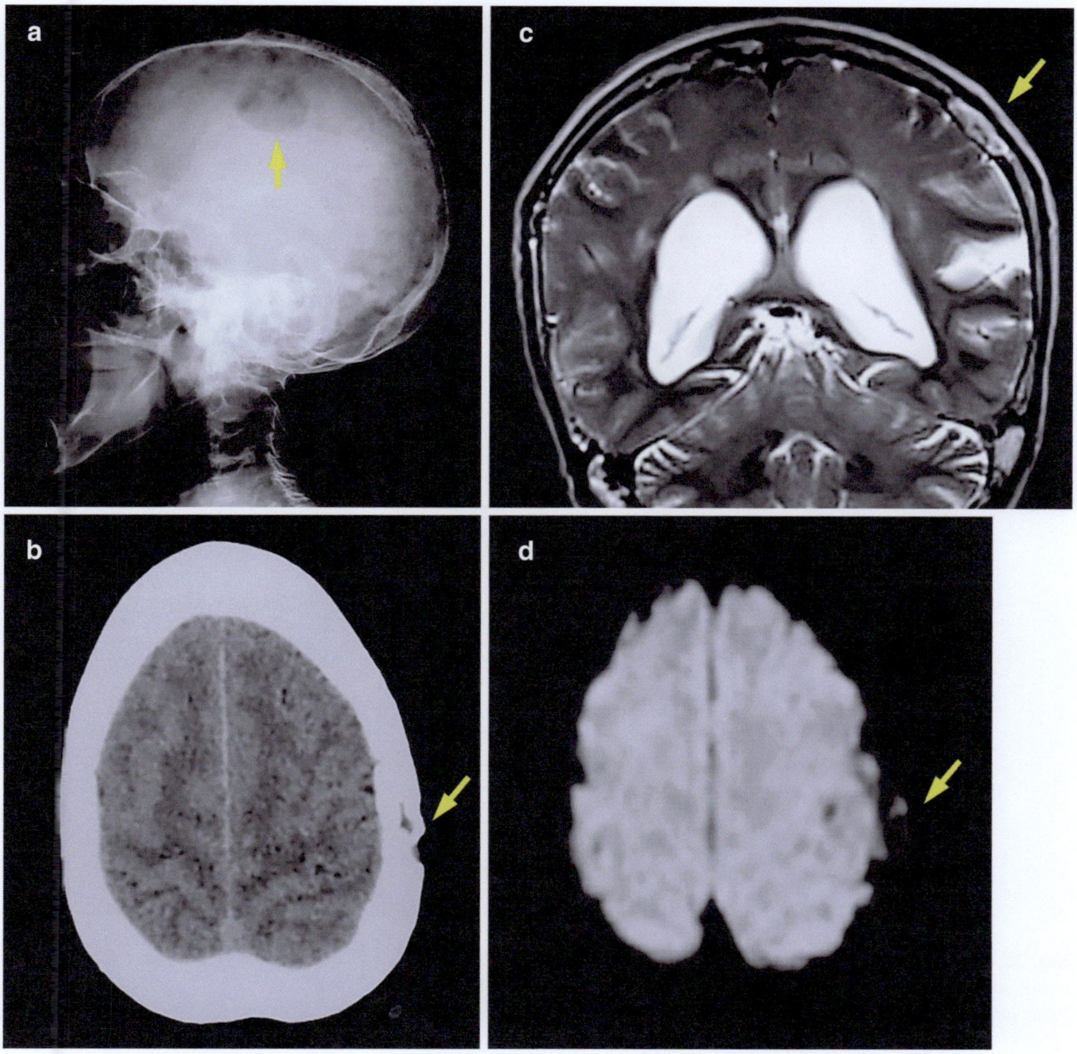

Fig. 25.5 Patient C. Solitary plasmacytoma of the parietal vault (arrows) as seen on lateral plain radiography (**a**), axial CT-scan (**b**), coronal T2-weighted MRI (**c**), and on diffusion weighted-sequences DWI (**d**)

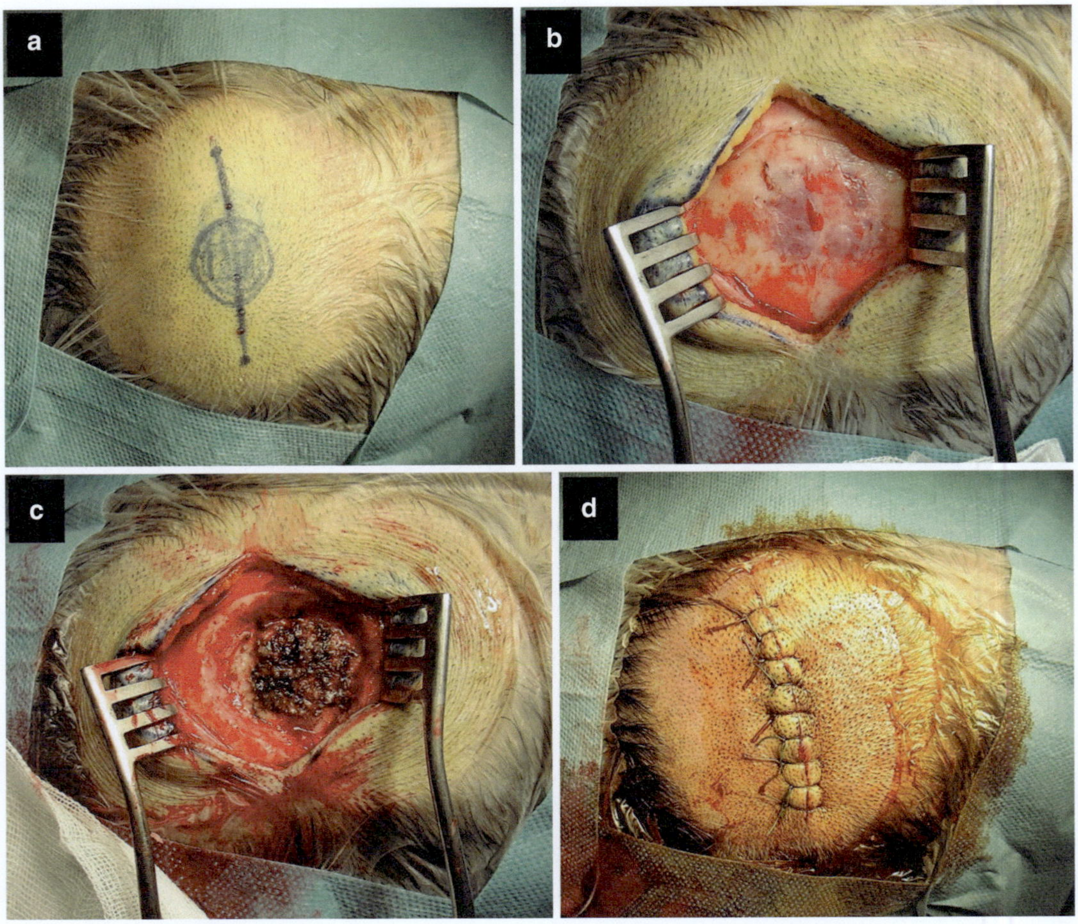

Fig. 25.6 Patient C. Per-operative views showing cutaneous location of the lesion (**a**), tumor exposure (**b**), complete surgical resection of the tumor (**c**), and closure of the scalp at the end of the surgical procedure without cranial reconstructive technique (**d**)

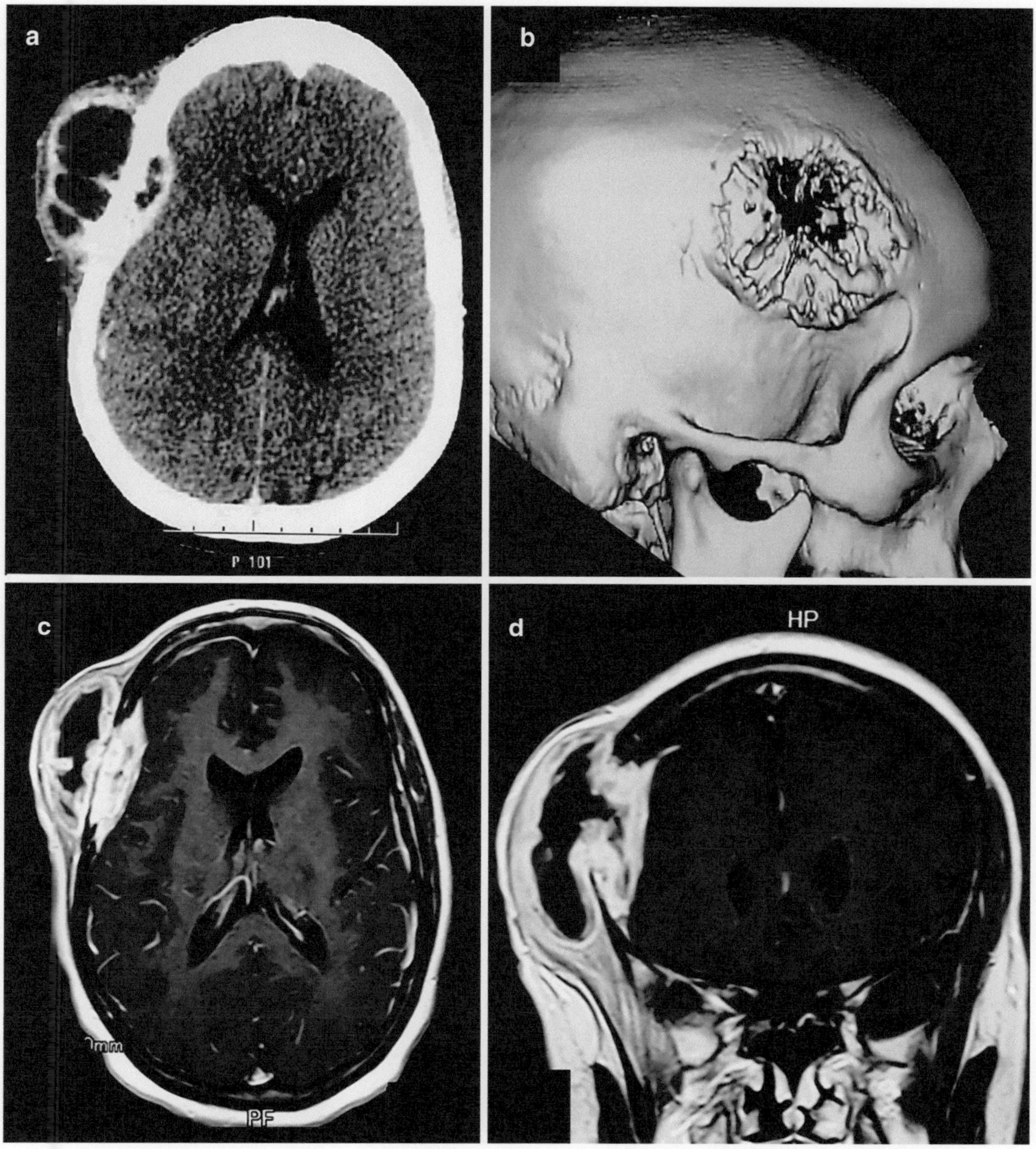

Fig. 25.7 Patient D. Frontal transdiploic thyroid metastasis with intracranial and extracranial extension as seen on axial CT-scan (**a**), 3D CT-scan (reformatted volume-rendered) (**b**), as well as on axial (**c**) and coronal (**d**) post-gadolinium T1-weighted MRI

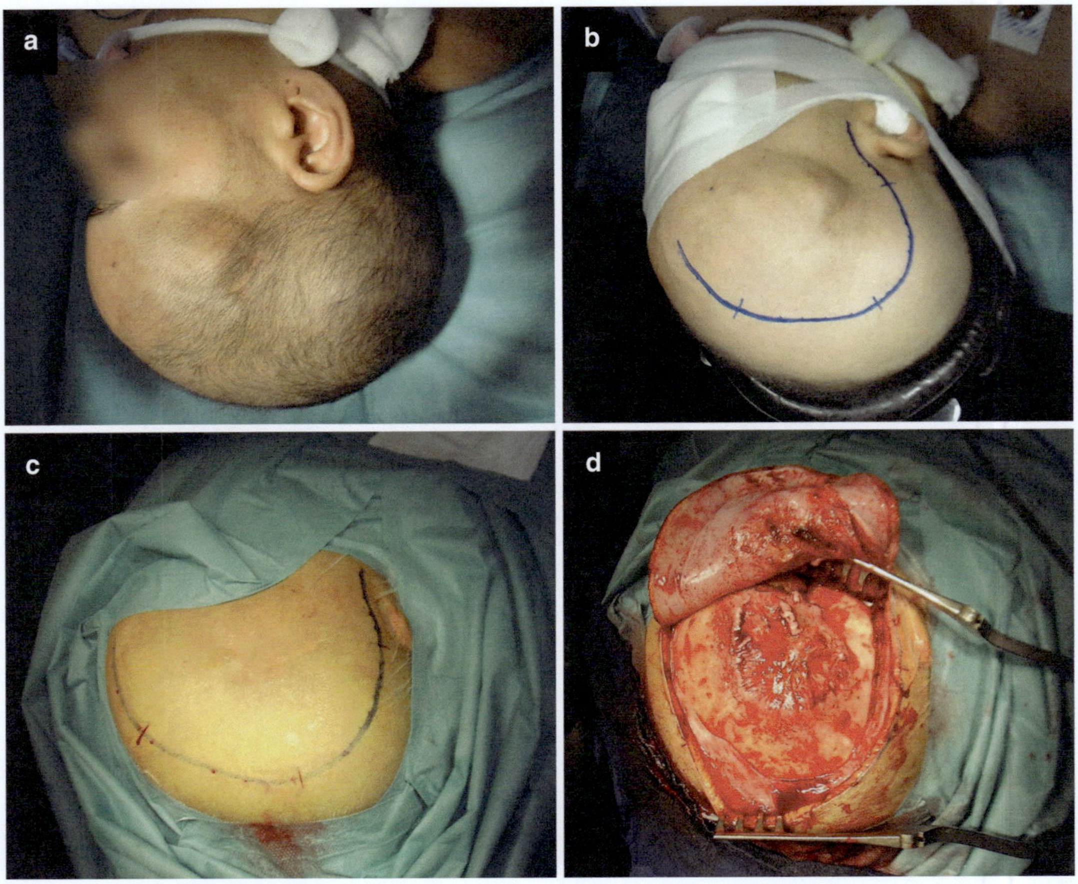

Fig. 25.8 Patient D. Operative view of the extracranial part of the lesion (**a**), the outline of the surgical incision before (**b**) and after setting up the operating fields (**c**). Tumor appearance after lifting the scalp (**d**)

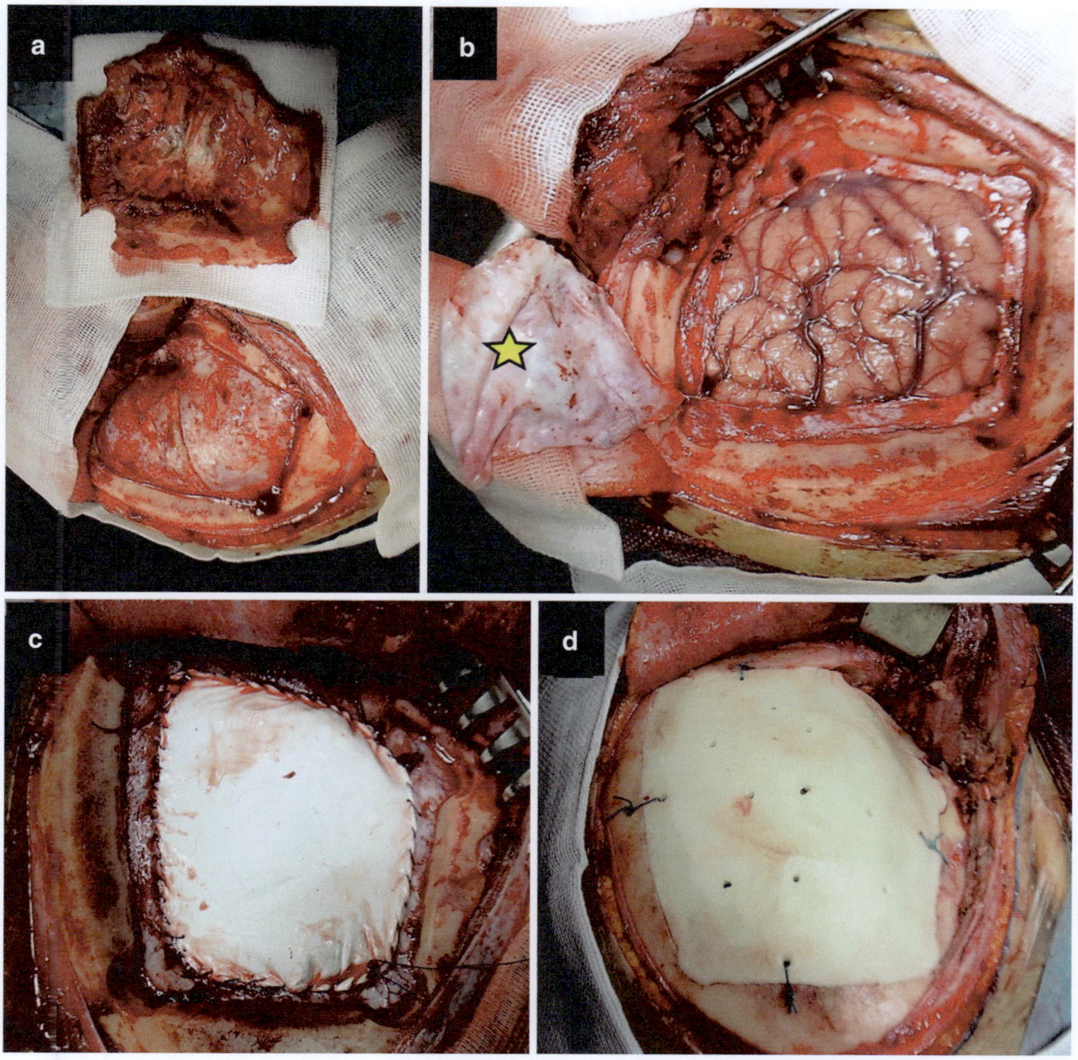

Fig. 25.9 Patient D. Intraoperative views after frontal cranial vault removal (**a**), dural component resection (**b**) (star) and dural substitute graft (**c**). The cranial bone defect was restored using polymethylmethacrylate implantable cranioplasty (**d**)

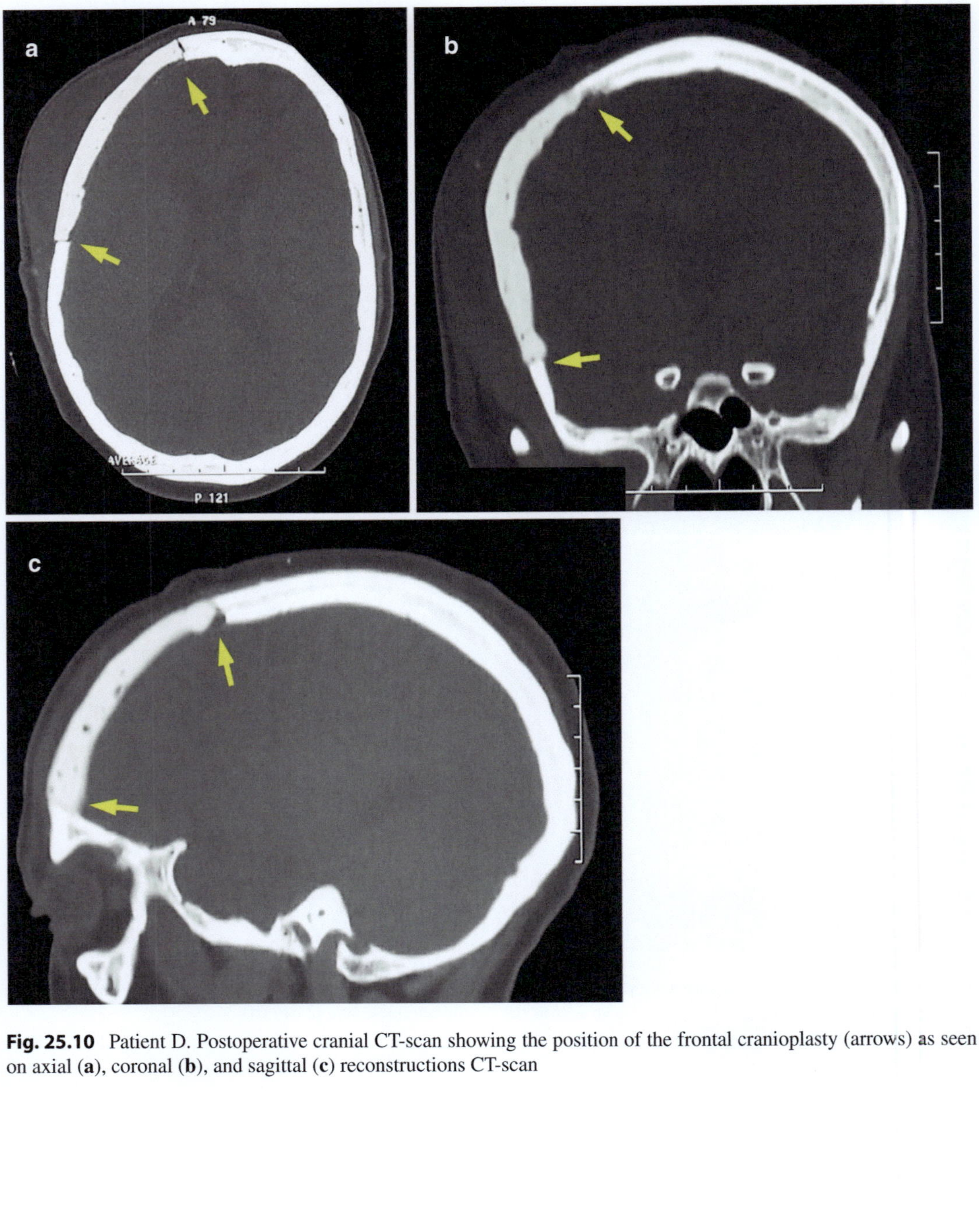

Fig. 25.10 Patient D. Postoperative cranial CT-scan showing the position of the frontal cranioplasty (arrows) as seen on axial (**a**), coronal (**b**), and sagittal (**c**) reconstructions CT-scan

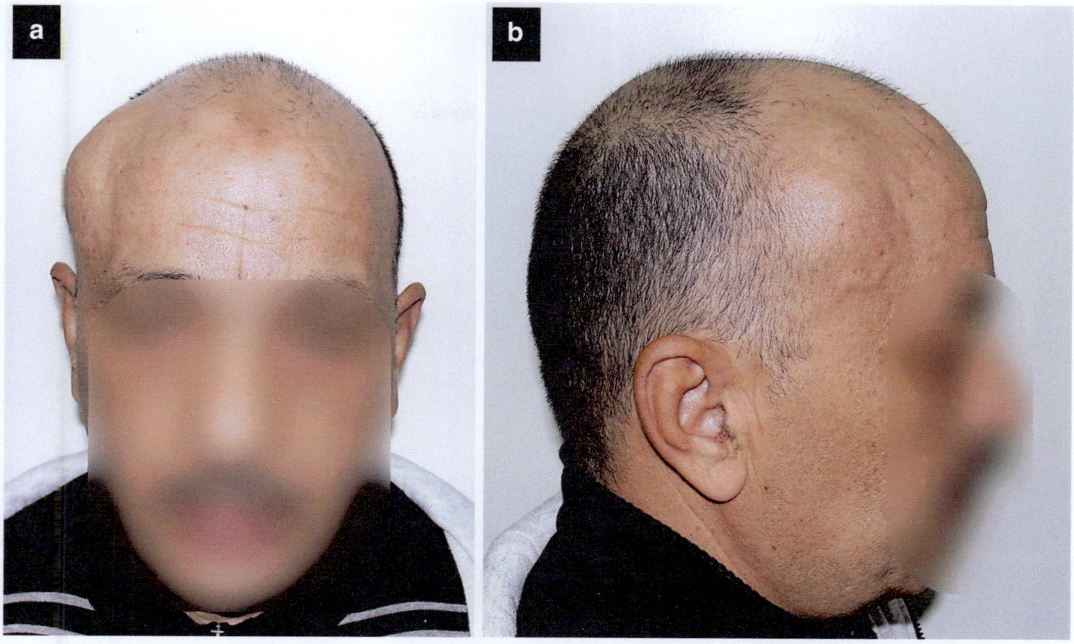

Fig. 25.11 Patient E. Clinical pictures of a patient with a fronto-temporal anaplastic meningioma (**a**, **b**)

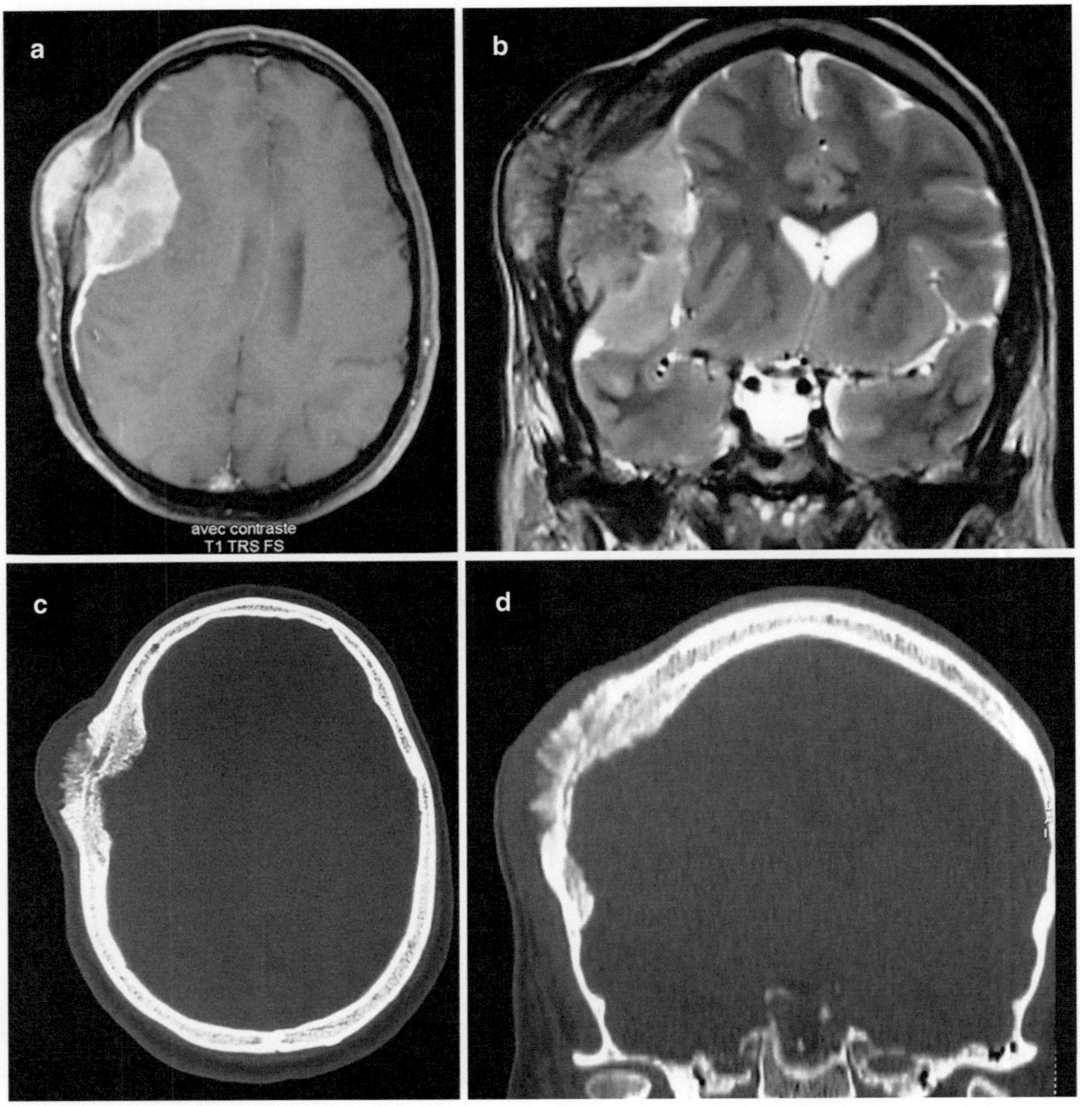

Fig. 25.12 Patient E. Intracranial anaplastic fronto-temporal meningioma with transdiploic involvement and extracranial extension as seen on axial post-gadolinium T1- (**a**) and coronal T2- weighted MRI (**b**). The same lesion on axial (**c**) and coronal (**d**) CT-scan on bone windows. Note the aggressive cranial bone involvement

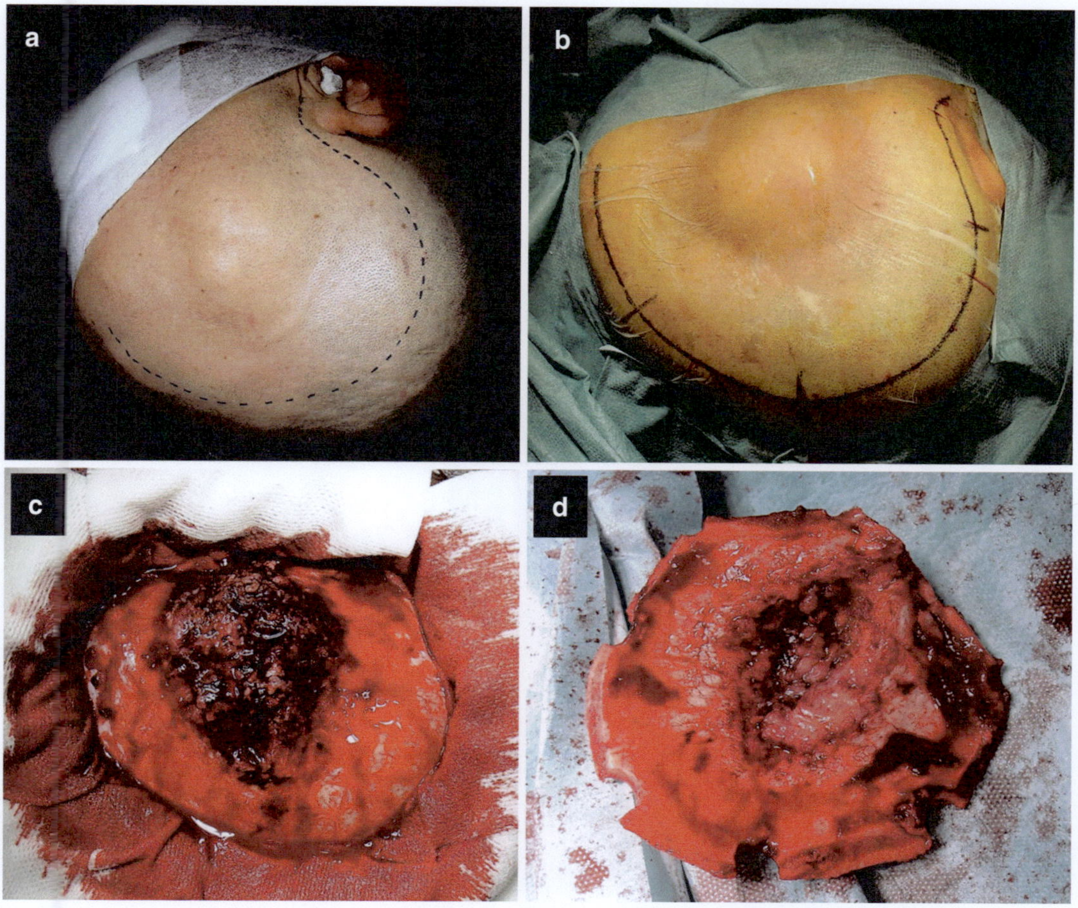

Fig. 25.13 Patient E. Operative views of the extracranial part of the lesion and the outline of the surgical incision before (**a**) and after setting up the operating fields (**b**). Extradural tumor appearance after removing the cranial vault flap (**c**). Endocranial view of the cranial tumor bone flap (**d**)

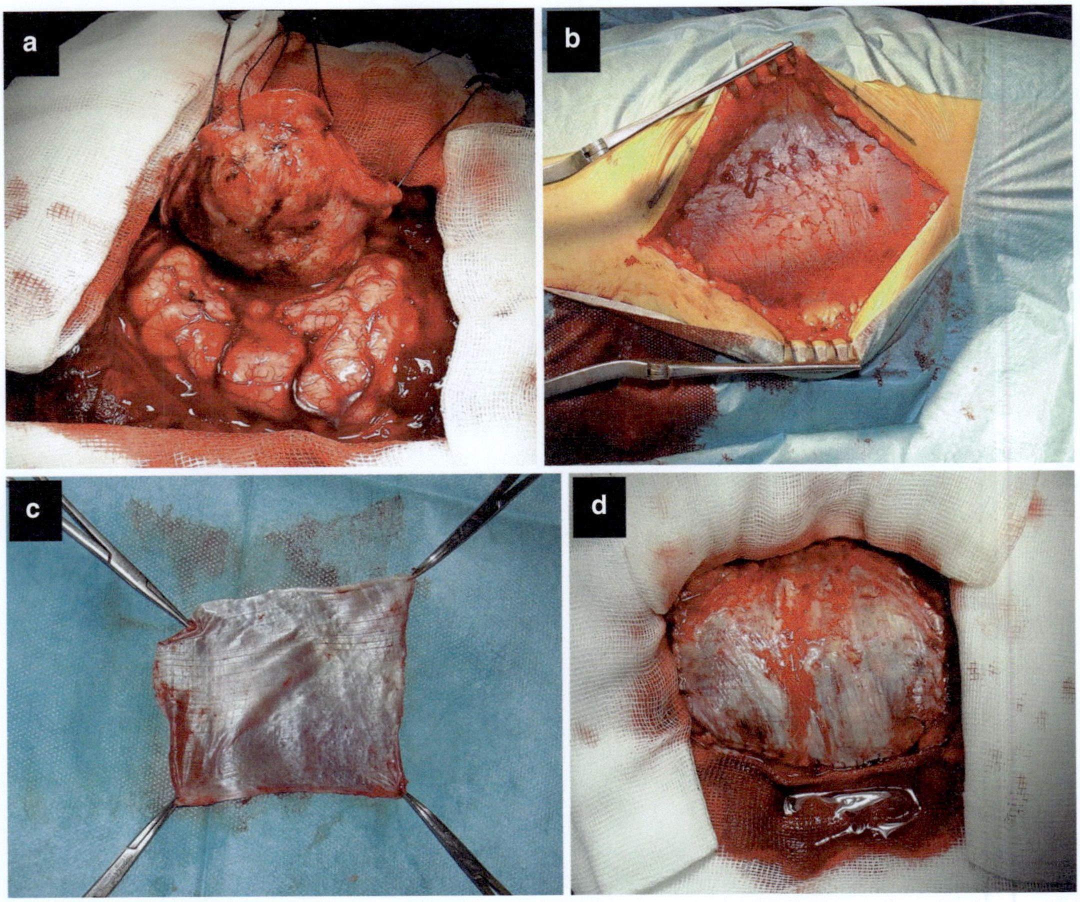

Fig. 25.14 Patient E. Intraoperative view of the dural and intradural tumoral component (**a**). Preparation of the fascia-lata graft for reconstruction of the dural defect (**b**, **c**). The dural defect was closed hermetically using the fascia-lata graft (**d**)

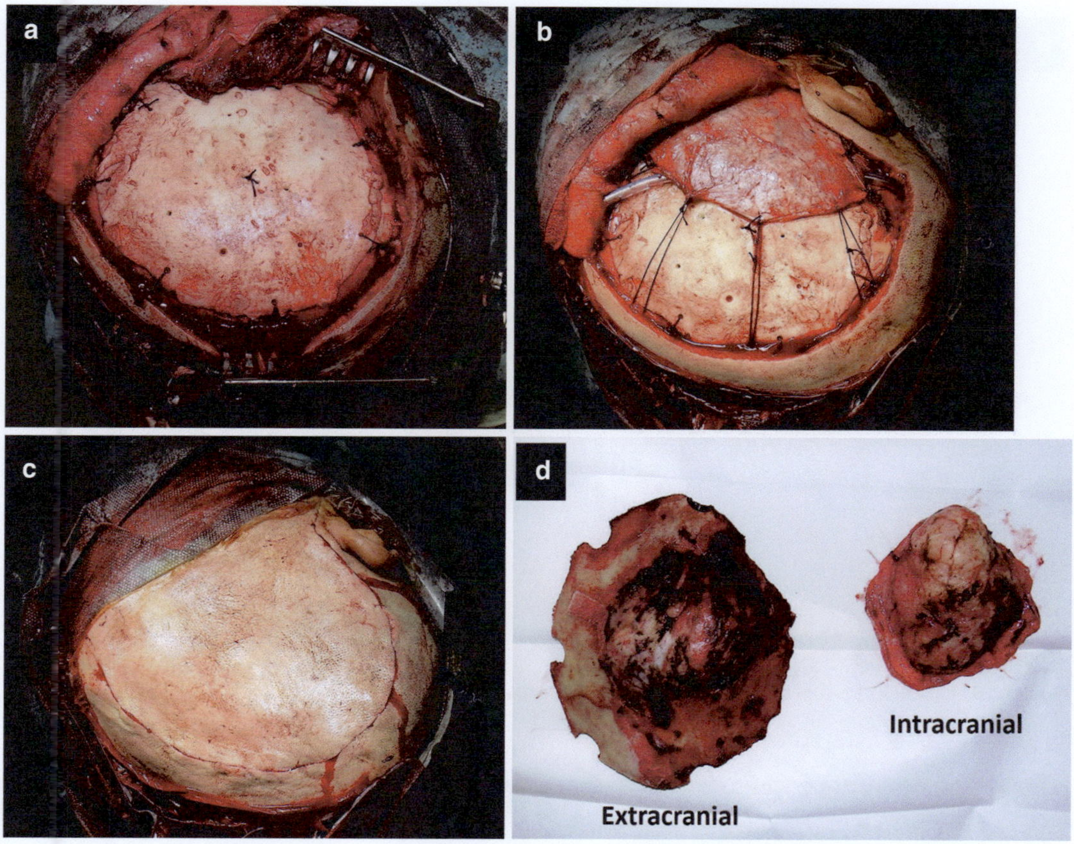

Fig. 25.15 Patient E. Operative views. The cranial bone defect was restored using polymethylmethacrylate implantable cranioplasty (**a**). At the end of the procedure, the temporalis muscle was repositioned and a closed drainage system was used extracranially to minimize any bleeding collection (**b**). Lastly, the wound was closed without further tension (**c**). Extracranial view of the cranial tumor bone flap and the intracranial intradural component of the meningioma (**d**)

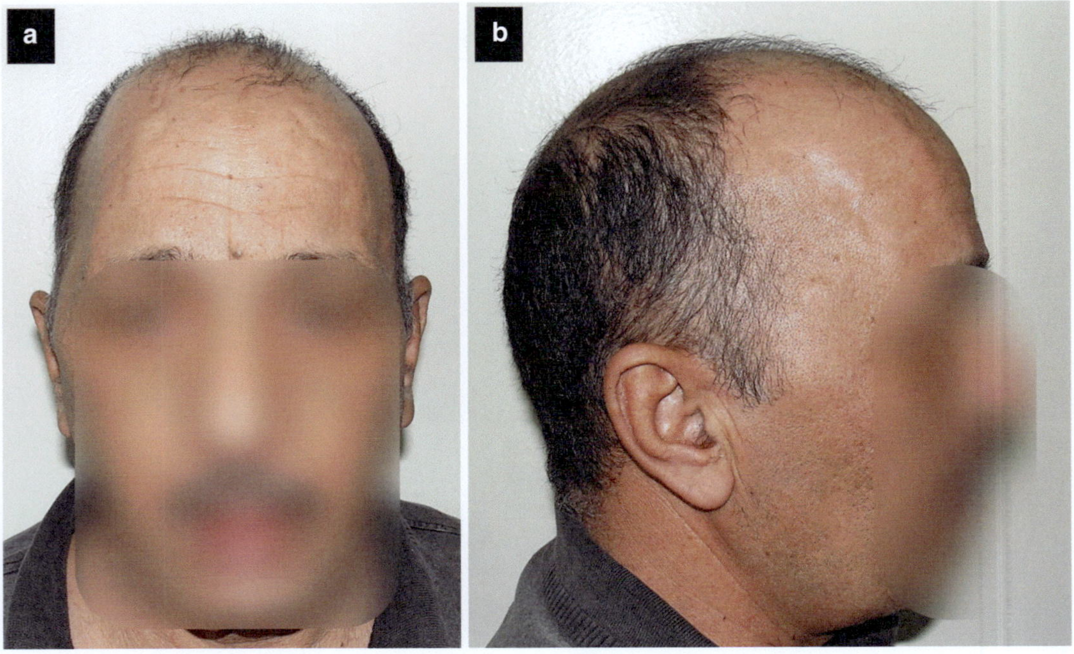

Fig. 25.16 Patient E. Postoperative clinical pictures of the patient (control) (**a**, **b**)

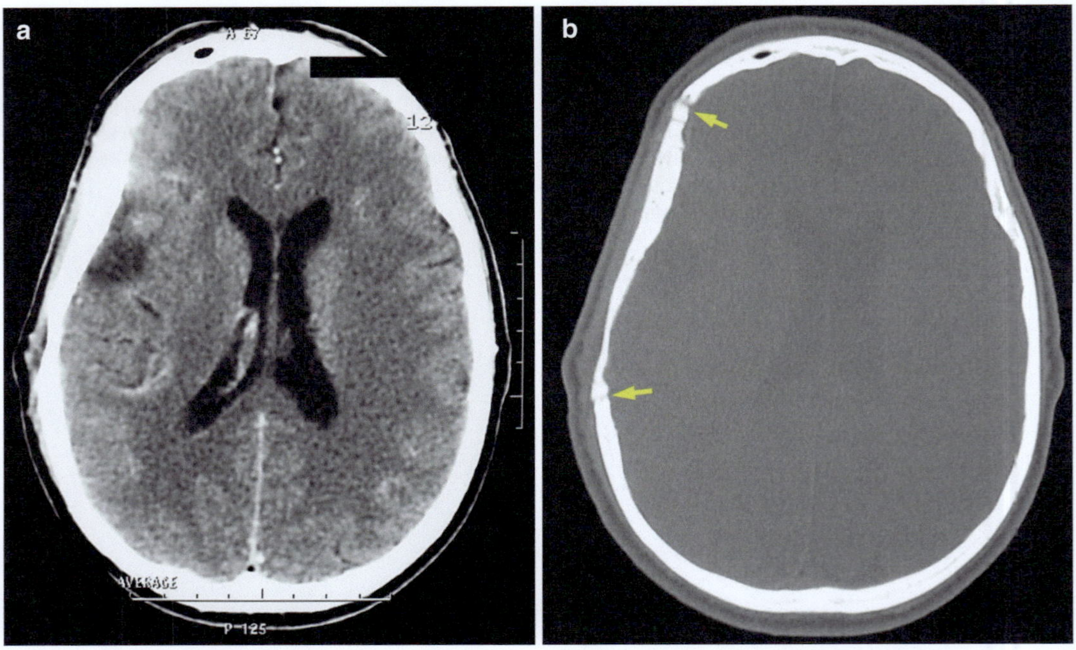

Fig. 25.17 Patient E. Postoperative axial CT-scan (control) on parenchymal (**a**) and bone (**b**) windows. Note the position of the cranioplasty (arrows)

25.3 Reconstructive Procedures

25.3.1 Scalp Defect Reconstructions

Scalp defect reconstructions can be treated in various ways. The particular surgical technique that is chosen depends on the type of lesion, its exact anatomic location and extension, and the surface scalp area that is lost [17–24]. Some general principles are recommended:

- Esthetic considerations must not be overlooked.
- Favor the use of a hair-bearing scalp in the repair.
- If a flap is rotated, the rotation must be from pericranium to pericranium.
- Preservation of vascular supplies is critically important.
- Closure without tension.
- Avoid using the electrocautery that heats or burns the wound edges.
- Proper wound care is essential.

The most used reconstructive procedures for scalp defects are as follows:

(a) *Granulation* (healing by secondary intention). This technique requires moist wound care. The healing process may take from 2 weeks to 2 months to occur depending on the depth of the wound (Figs. 25.18 and 25.19).
(b) *Side-to-side closure* (primary closure). Layered closure with proper wound tension. The wound should be elliptical with a length-to-width ratio of 3:1. Sutures should be removed at 7–10 days if using non-resorbable sutures.
(c) *Advancement flap*. It consists of elevating a flap of full-thickness scalp adjacent to the scalp defect and then making radial cuts in the aponeurosis, which will allow the scalp to be stretched to cover the defect.
(d) *Rotation flap*. The principle is that the primary movement is to rotate nearby redundant skin into the skin defect.
(e) *Transposition flap*. The movement is the mobilization of non-adjacent skin and the transposition of the skin over intervening skin into the defect.
(f) *Split-thickness skin graft*. This variety is a graft of the epidermis or partial thickness dermis.
(g) *Full-thickness skin graft*. It is a graft of the epidermis and complete dermis with or without subcutaneous fat (Fig. 25.18).
(h) *Microvascular free tissue transfer*. Using fascio-cutaneous, muscular, or omental flaps. Usually, the donor site is sutured directly or covered with split-thickness skin.
(i) *Tissue expansion techniques*. Using a tissue expander, which is a silicone prosthesis placed into a pocket of tissue following the subgaleal plane, the prosthesis is expanded weekly for 6 to 8 weeks through an injection port (Fig. 25.20).
(j) *Vaccum-assisted closure therapy*. The principle of this procedure is to expose the wound bed to negative pressure, resulting in the elimination of edema fluid, enhancement of blood supply, and stimulation of cellular proliferation of reparative granulation tissue.

Overall, when a scalp defect is small, side-to-side closure may be used. But, if the scalp defect is too large, a flap or thickness skin graft is recommended. The tissue expansion procedure is an attractive technique to have available a larger quantity of scalp for coverage [21].

25.3.2 Cranioplasties

Cranioplasty is a reconstructive surgical procedure for restoring a cranial bone defect. The main goal of this technique is to restore the normal barriers protecting the intracranial structures combined with an adequate cosmetic result [1, 18, 25–27].

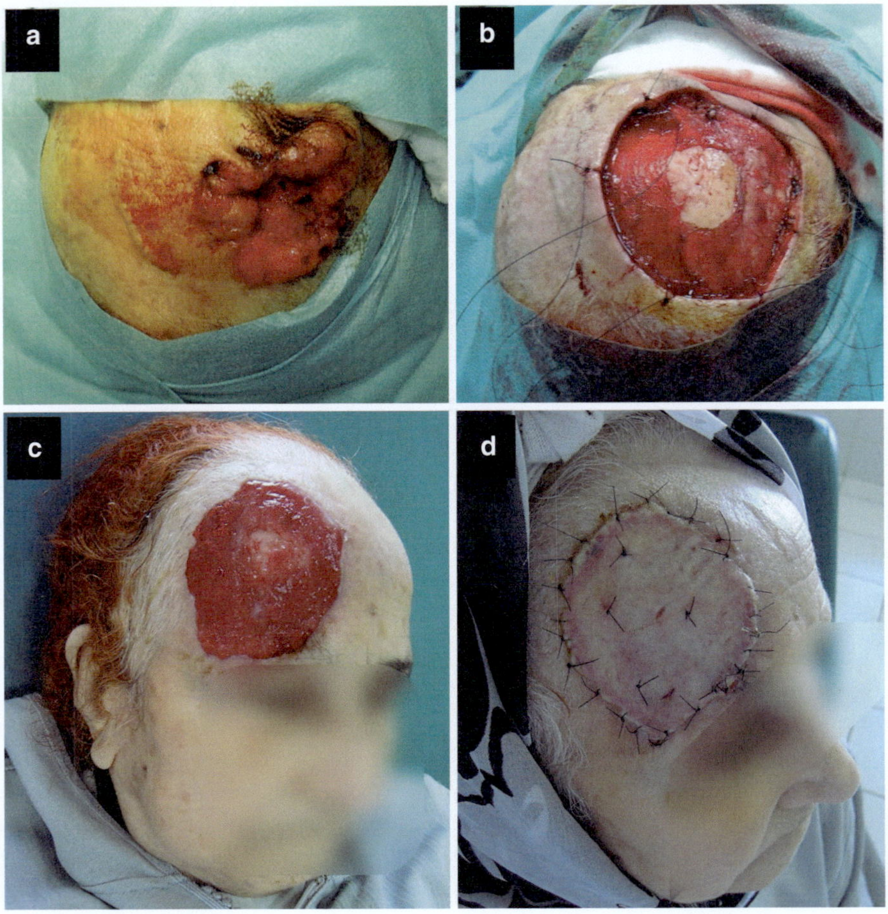

Fig. 25.18 Patient F. Clinical picture of a frontal squamous cell carcinoma (**a**). Operative view of the complete tumoral excision (**b**). Local granulation (**c**). Split-thickness skin graft taken from the inner side of the thigh (**d**) (Courtesy of Professor Adil Arrob, M.D)

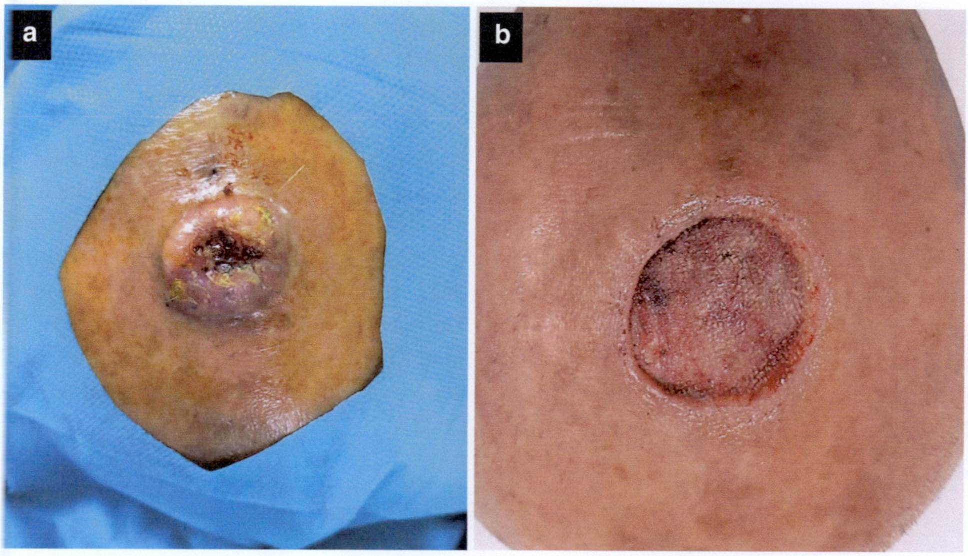

Fig. 25.19 Patient G. Clinical picture of a basal cell carcinoma at the vertex (**a**). Postoperative Clinical control following the complete tumoral excision (**b**). A full-thickness skin graft taken from the supraclavicular region will be carried out secondarily (Courtesy of Professor Adil Arrob, M.D., and Professor Khalid Tourabi, M.D)

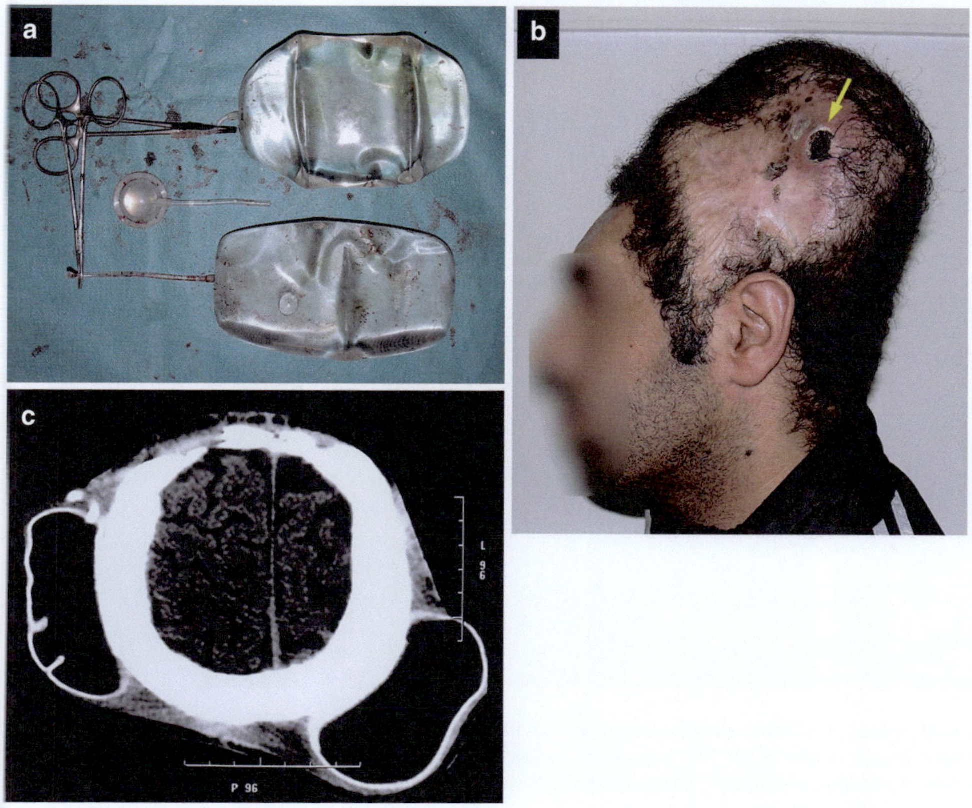

Fig. 25.20 Patient H. Tissue expansion technique using "tissue expander devices", which is silicone prostheses (**a**) placed into a pocket of tissue following the subgaleal plane. Clinical picture of a patient with local scalp necrosis (arrow) in whom a tissue expansion technique was used (**b**). Axial CT-scan in the same patient showing the expander prostheses implanted bilaterally in the subgaleal plane (**c**)

This bone replacement can be performed using various techniques including:

A. *Autologous bone grafts* which can be taken from the adjacent cranial vault, the ribs, or the iliac crest.
B. *Cadaver bone.*
C. *Implantable cranioplasty materials* such as polymethylmethacrylate, hydroxyapatite, polylactic/polyglycolic acid, silicone and silastic implants, polyetheretherketone (PEEK), and titanium mesh implants (Figs. 25.9d, 25.15a, b, 25.21, 25.22, 25.23, 25.24, 25.25 and 25.26).

In recent years, the development of 3D reconstructs has made it possible to obtain tailored implants using "Additive Manufacturing Technology" and "3D Printed Cranioplasties".

Technically and first, the cranial defect should be prepared. The surgical bed must be cleaned and well vascularized. According to many surgeons, it is important to minimize the use foreign materials (e.g. bone wax, Gelfoam…) when replacing bone flaps. Foreign materials reduce bone healing and can be the source of potential infectious complications [9, 26–28].

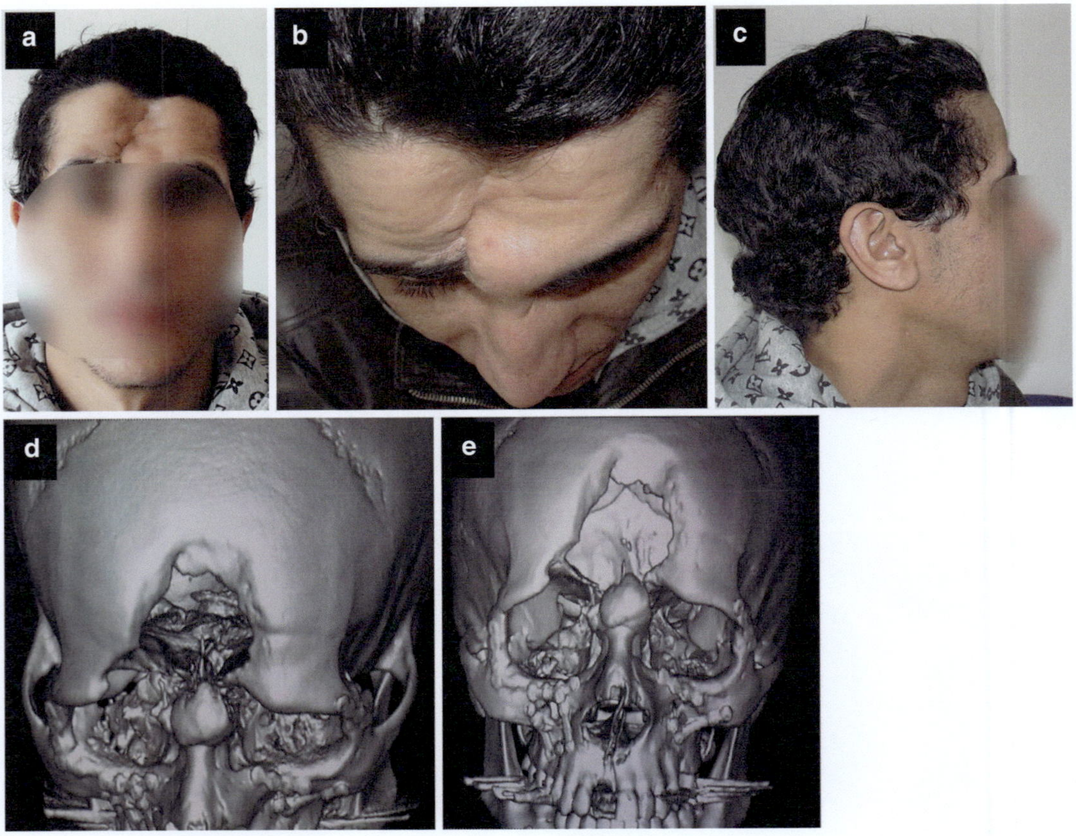

Fig. 25.21 Patient I. Clinical pictures of a patient with nasofrontal cranial defect (**a–c**). This patient was the victim of a severe craniofacial injury. The nasofrontal craniofacial defect as seen on 3D CT-scan (reformatted volume-rendered) (**d**, **e**) (Courtesy of Professor Mohamed Lakouichmi, M.D)

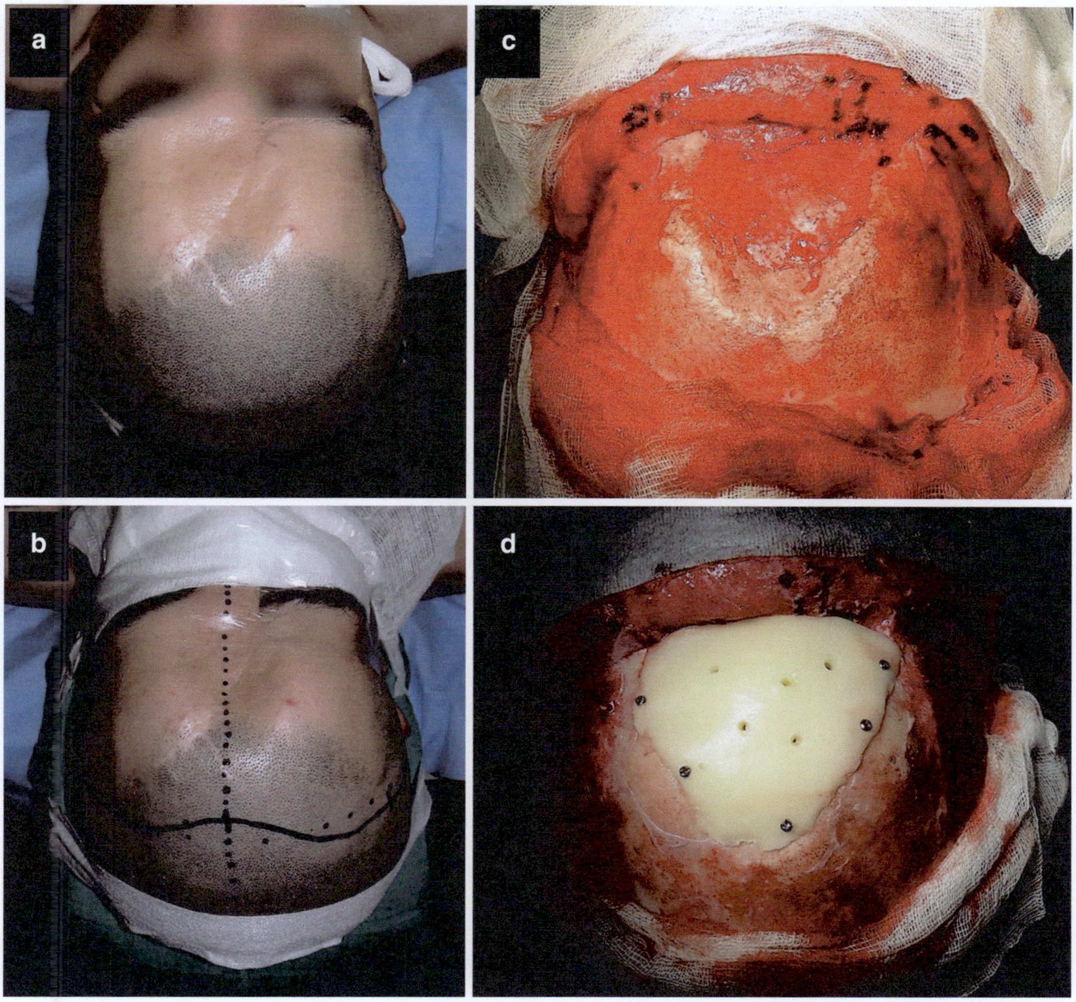

Fig. 25.22 Patient I. Intraoperative views of different steps for the nasofrontal cranioplasty procedure (**a**–**d**): the head positioning (**a**), the outline of the surgical incision before setting up the operating fields (**b**), the skull bone defect after lifting the scalp (**c**), and the cranioplasty fixation (**d**)

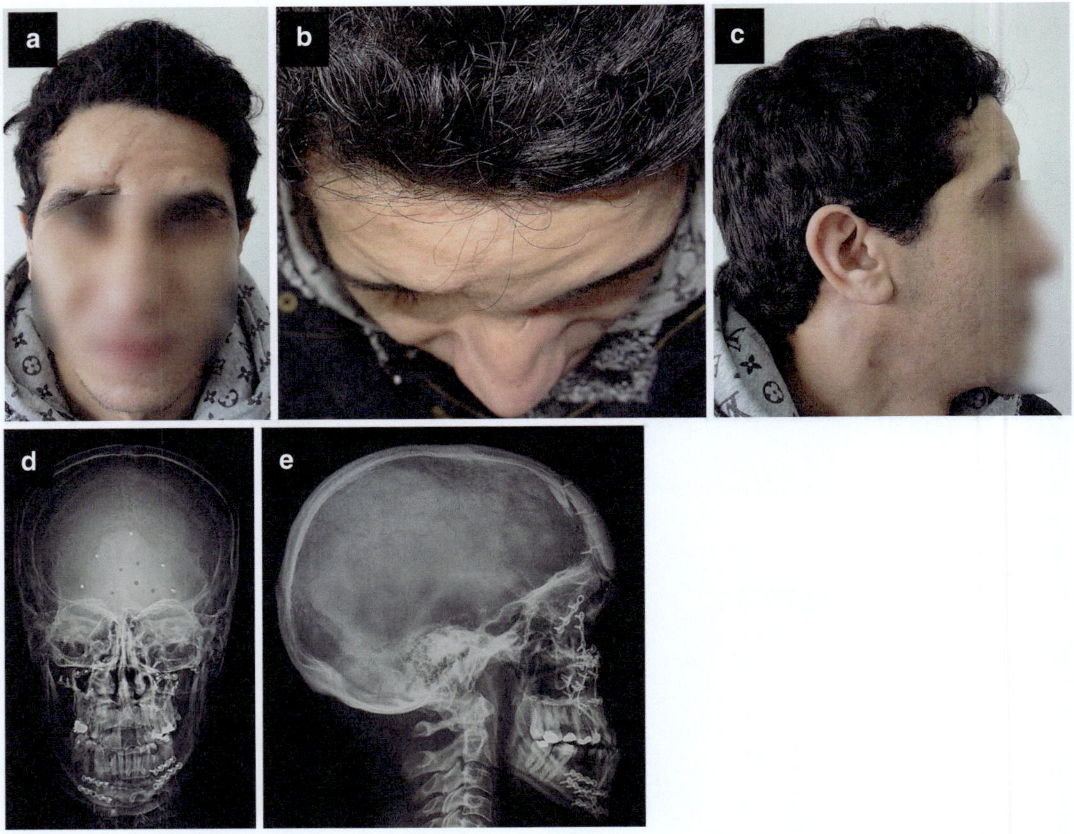

Fig. 25.23 Patient I. Postoperative clinical pictures of the patient (control) (**a**–**c**). Postoperative plain radiographies (control) showing the position of the bifrontal cranioplasty (**d**, **e**)

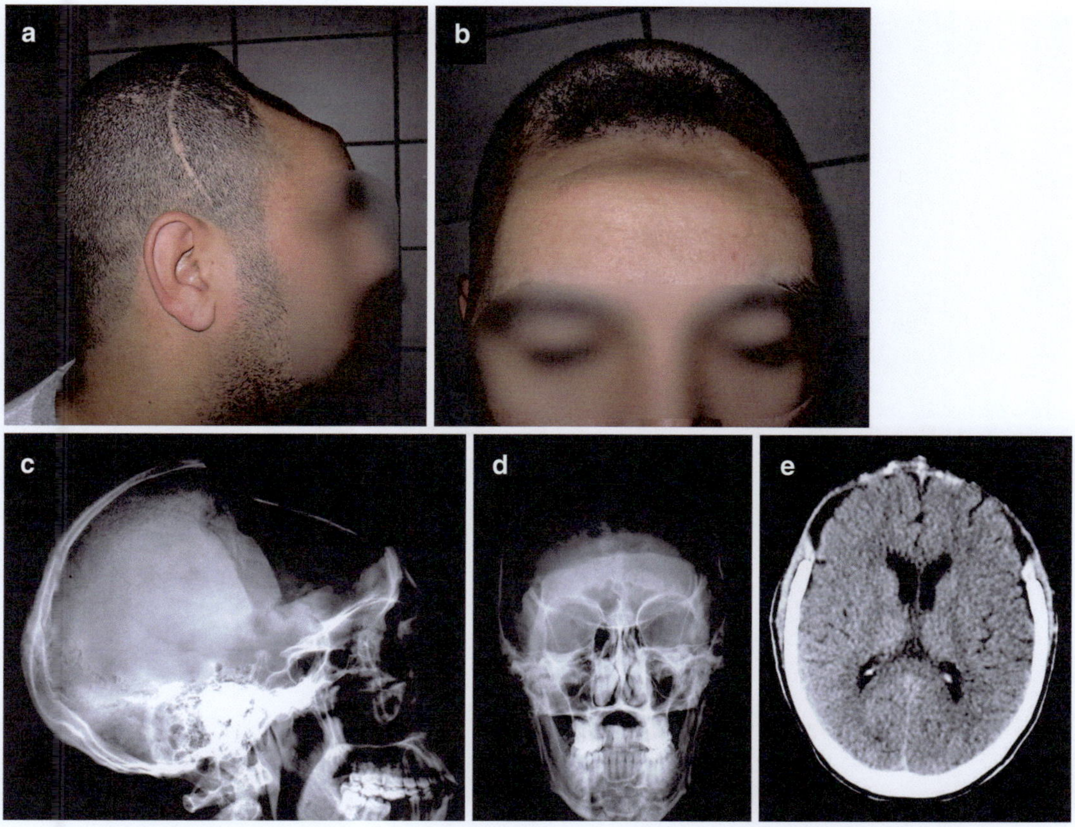

Fig. 25.24 Patient J. Clinical pictures of a patient with bifrontal cranial defect (**a**, **b**). This patient had undergone a decompressive craniectomy following a severe cranio-cerebral injury. The bifrontal skull defect as seen on plain radiographies (**c**, **d**) and on axial CT-scan (**e**)

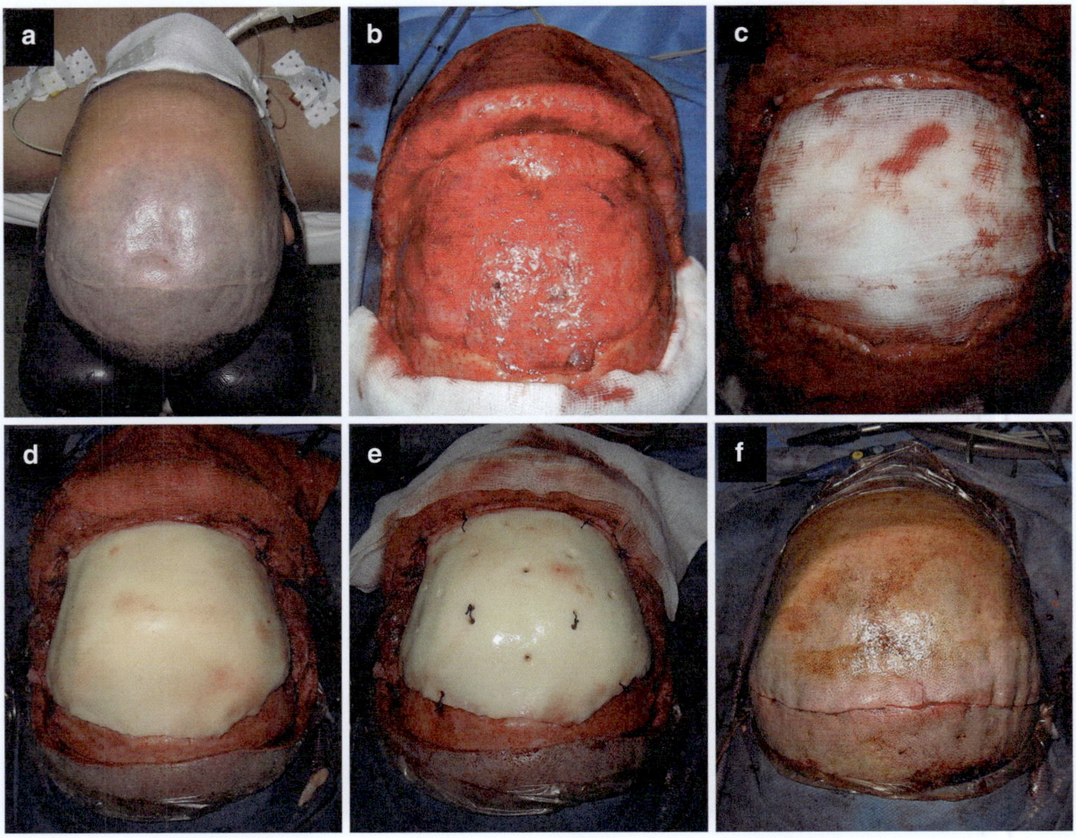

Fig. 25.25 Patient J. Intraoperative views of different steps for the bifrontal cranioplasty procedure (**a**–**f**): the head positioning (**a**), the skull bone defect after lifting the scalp (**b**, **c**), preparation and placing of the paste (polymethylmethacrylate) (**d**), the cranioplasty fixation (**e**), and the scalp closure after putting a closed drainage system extracranially (**f**)

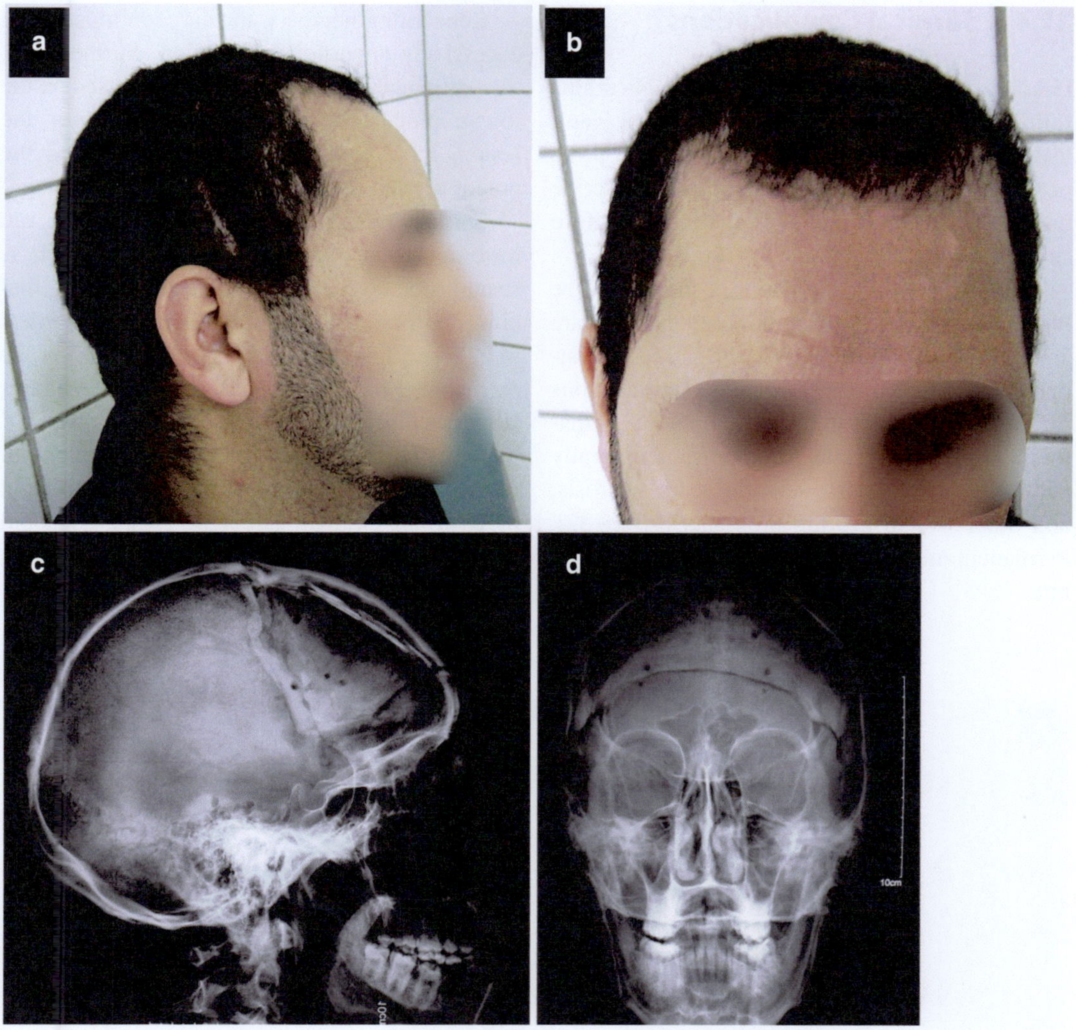

Fig. 25.26 Patient J. Postoperative clinical pictures of the patient (control) (**a, b**). Postoperative plain radiographies (control) showing the position of the bifrontal cranioplasty (**c, d**)

25.4 Surgical Complications

Despite a low rate of postoperative complications following surgery for scalp and cranial vault lesions, neurosurgeons should know about these potential problems, prevent them, and describe them to the patients and/or their families before surgery.

During surgical resection, intraoperative bleeding and accidental opening of the dura are among the most important difficulties. Postoperatively, the most frequent complications include surgical site infections, epidural hematoma, CSF fistula, sinus thrombosis, temporally neurological disorders, seizure, scalp necrosis, and other wound healing problems [9, 29–32]. Permanent neurological deficits or deaths are rare.

Concerning necrosis: the surgeon must avoid excessively superficial dissection. Furthermore, the scalp incision should be planned based on the topographic localization and extension of the lesion, its vascular supplies as well as on the potential need for secondary scalp flap coverage.

Furthermore, reconstructive procedures can have additional potential complications such as scars, poor cosmetics, wound breakdown, specific flap or graft failure, cranioplasty disorders (e.g. resorption, fracture, infection, erosion, or extrusion (Fig. 25.27)), and the need for further surgeries [29, 32].

Many options exist for the management of these problems, but none of them can be thought of as a standard of care (*c.f.* Chap. 26 about Postoperative complications of surgery for lesions of the scalp and calvarium).

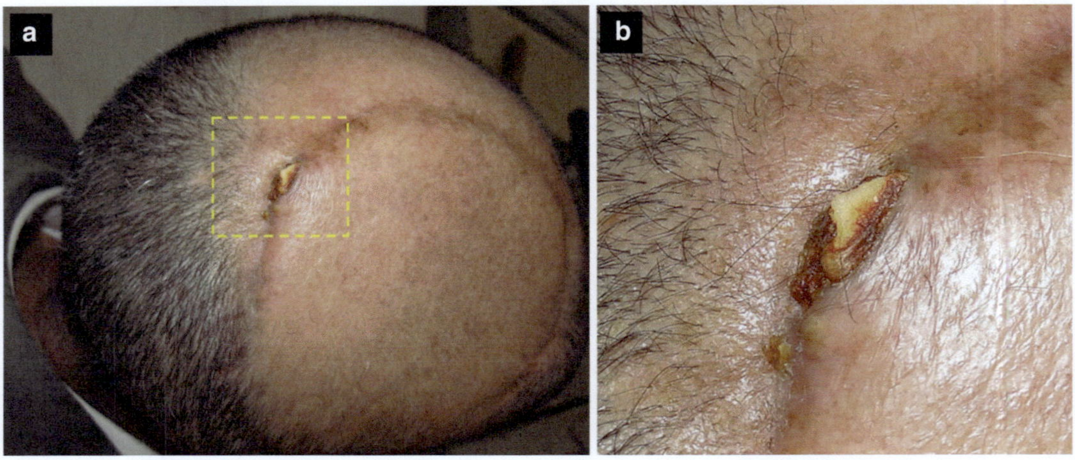

Fig. 25.27 Patient K. Clinical pictures (**a**, **b**) showing an exposed cranial acrylic plate. This patient has also contiguous cranial osteomyelitis. He was operated on eleven years before for an acute subdural hematoma with methylmethacrylate cranioplasty (Reproduced from Akhaddar, A. (2017). Surgical Site Infections in Cranial Surgery. In: Atlas of Infections in Neurosurgery and Spinal Surgery. Springer, Cham. https://doi.org/10.1007/978-3-319-60086-4_21.; with permission)

25.5 Conclusion

There is no standard protocol for the management of scalp and/or cranial vault lesions. Many lesions are amenable to surgical resection by means of variable operative techniques with or without additional reconstructive procedures.

The decision for surgery should depend on the operative team's experience, the nature and topographic location of the lesion, the relationship between the lesion and the adjacent anatomic structures, clinical symptoms and signs, the patient's age and comorbidities, and any other concomitant lesion or disease. Moreover, precaution and prudence should be taken in the course of surgical planning, during the surgical procedure, and in the postoperative period to reduce potential morbidity and mortality.

Collaboration with craniofacial and plastic surgeons has markedly improved reconstruction surgery in the treatment of these lesions.

References

1. Akhaddar A. General considerations and surgical therapy. In: Cranial osteomyelitis. 1st ed. Cham: Springer International Publishing; 2016. https://doi.org/10.1007/978-3-319-30268-3_10.
2. Barnett RR, Piazza MG, Elton SW. Pediatric neurosurgery in primary care: masses of the scalp and skull in children. Pediatr Clin N Am. 2021;68(4):743–57. https://doi.org/10.1016/j.pcl.2021.04.003.
3. Karki M, Roka YB. Surgical excision of cirsoid aneurysm of the scalp: case series and review of the literature. World Neurosurg. 2021;155:e600–4. https://doi.org/10.1016/j.wneu.2021.08.102.
4. Liu Y, Wang H, Shao H, Wang C. Primary extradural meningiomas in head: a report of 19 cases and review of literature. Int J Clin Exp Pathol. 2015;8(5):5624–32.
5. Umana GE, Scalia G, Vats A, Pompili G, Barone F, Passanisi M, et al. Primary extracranial meningiomas of the head and neck. Life (Basel). 2021;11(9):942. https://doi.org/10.3390/life11090942.
6. Bernardini N, Skroza N, Zuber S, Tolino E, Balduzzi V, Mambrin A, et al. Face and scalp basal cell carcinoma treatment: a review of the literature. Acta Dermatovenerol Croat. 2019;27(1):22–7.
7. El Asri AC, Akhaddar A, Baallal H, Boulahroud O, Mandour C, Chahdi H, et al. Primary lymphoma of the cranial vault: case report and a systematic review of the literature. Acta Neurochir. 2012;154(2):257–65. https://doi.org/10.1007/s00701-011-1124-0.
8. Lim EJ, Leong N, McAdory LE, Ho CL. Multimodality imaging and treatment strategy for malignant scalp neoplasms in adults. Clin Imaging. 2021;77:48–57. https://doi.org/10.1016/j.clinimag.2021.02.036.
9. Malcolm JG, Mahmooth Z, Rindler RS, Allen JW, Grossberg JA, Pradilla G, et al. Autologous cranioplasty is associated with increased reoperation rate: a systematic review and meta-analysis. World Neurosurg. 2018;116:60–8. https://doi.org/10.1016/j.wneu.2018.05.009.
10. Nasi-Kordhishti I, Hempel JM, Ebner FH, Tatagiba M. Calvarial lesions: overview of imaging features and neurosurgical management. Neurosurg Rev. 2021;44(6):3459–69. https://doi.org/10.1007/s10143-021-01521-5.
11. Wong CH, Foo CL, Seow WT. Calcified cephalohematoma: classification, indications for surgery and techniques. J Craniofac Surg. 2006;17(5):970–9. https://doi.org/10.1097/01.scs.0000229552.82081.de.
12. Matsoukas S, Feng R, Gilligan J, Gutzwiller EM, De Leacy R, Shrivastava R, et al. Combined transarterial and percutaneous preoperative embolization of transosseous meningioma. Interv Neuroradiol. 2022;4:15910199221095982. https://doi.org/10.1177/15910199221095982.
13. Prasad GL, Pai K. Pediatric cranial intraosseous hemangiomas: a review. Neurosurg Rev. 2018;41(1):109–17. https://doi.org/10.1007/s10143-016-0779-7.
14. Punchak MA, Hollawell ML, Viaene AN, Cahill AM, Storm PB, Madsen PJ, et al. Large scalp venous malformation in a pediatric patient managed with sclerotherapy and surgery: a case report and review of literature. Childs Nerv Syst. 2023;39(1):295–9. https://doi.org/10.1007/s00381-022-05608-2.
15. Yuan SM, Guo Y, Cui L, Wang J, Hu XB, Zhou JH, et al. Surgical management of giant scalp neurofibroma after ultra-selective embolization of nutrient artery. J Craniofac Surg. 2015;26(5):e405–7. https://doi.org/10.1097/SCS.0000000000001873.
16. Zhou MH, Dunn GP, Osbun JW, Cross DT 3rd, Moran CJ, Dacey RG Jr, et al. Direct puncture onyx embolization of a large calvarial metastasis with intracranial extension: case report. Interv Neuroradiol. 2018;24(2):220–4. https://doi.org/10.1177/1591019917740353.
17. Alvi S, Jenzer AC. Scalp Reconstruction. 2023 Jan 20. In: StatPearls [Internet]. Treasure Island (FL): StatPearls Publishing; 2023 Jan–.
18. Bradford BD, Lee JW. Reconstruction of the forehead and scalp. Facial Plast Surg Clin North Am. 2019;27(1):85–94. https://doi.org/10.1016/j.fsc.2018.08.009.
19. Dedhia R, Luu Q. Scalp reconstruction. Curr Opin Otolaryngol Head Neck Surg. 2015;23(5):407–14. https://doi.org/10.1097/MOO.0000000000000191.
20. Gishen K, Yoo J, Plotsker E, Thaller SR. Revisiting the pericranial flap for scalp reconstruction. J Craniofac Surg. 2021;32(Suppl 3):1275–80. https://doi.org/10.1097/SCS.0000000000007033.

21. Mangubat EA. Scalp repair using tissue expanders. Facial Plast Surg Clin North Am. 2013;21(3):487–96. https://doi.org/10.1016/j.fsc.2013.05.006.
22. Messias H, Martins M, Zagalo C, Gomes P. Multifocal cutaneous angiosarcoma of the scalp-A challenging reconstructive case managed with skin substitutes. Cancer Rep (Hoboken). 2022;5(10):e1659. https://doi.org/10.1002/cnr2.1659.
23. Prior A, Anania P, Pacetti M, Secci F, Ravegnani M, Pavanello M, et al. Dermoid and epidermoid cysts of scalp: case series of 234 consecutive patients. World Neurosurg. 2018;120:119–24. https://doi.org/10.1016/j.wneu.2018.08.197.
24. Song P, Pu LLQ. Microsurgical scalp reconstruction: an overview of the contemporary approach. J Reconstr Microsurg. 2022;38(7):530–8. https://doi.org/10.1055/s-0041-1740131.
25. Akhaddar A, Gazzaz M, Kadiri B, Lrhezzioui J, Boucetta M. Giant epidermoid cyst of the skull with extra and intracranial extension. A case report. J Neuroradiol. 2002;29(3):193–9.
26. Alkhaibary A, Alharbi A, Alnefaie N, Oqalaa Almubarak A, Aloraidi A, et al. Cranioplasty: a comprehensive review of the history, materials, surgical aspects, and complications. World Neurosurg. 2020;139:445–52. https://doi.org/10.1016/j.wneu.2020.04.211.
27. Lane C, Lin A, Goyal N. Scalp and Calvarium reconstruction. Otolaryngol Clin N Am. 2023;56(4):741–55. https://doi.org/10.1016/j.otc.2023.04.003.
28. Chang KW, Zhong LM, Lee DS, Puram SV, Jackson RS, Yaeger LH, et al. Outcomes of mesh cranioplasty in scalp-free tissue reconstruction: a systematic review and meta-analysis. Otolaryngol Head Neck Surg. 2023;168(5):970–8. https://doi.org/10.1002/ohn.199.
29. Cerveau T, Rossmann T, Clusmann H, Veldeman M. Infection-related failure of autologous *versus* allogenic cranioplasty after decompressive hemicraniectomy - a systematic review and meta-analysis. Brain Spine. 2023;3:101760. https://doi.org/10.1016/j.bas.2023.101760.
30. Frassanito P, Fraschetti F, Bianchi F, Giovannenze F, Caldarelli M, Scoppettuolo G. Management and prevention of cranioplasty infections. Childs Nerv Syst. 2019;35(9):1499–506. https://doi.org/10.1007/s00381-019-04251-8.
31. Sadhwani N, Garg K, Kumar A, Agrawal D, Singh M, Chandra PS, et al. Comparison of infection rates following immediate and delayed cranioplasty for postcraniotomy surgical site infections: results of a meta-analysis. World Neurosurg. 2023;173:167–175.e2. https://doi.org/10.1016/j.wneu.2023.01.084.
32. Sahoo NK, Tomar K, Thakral A, Kumar S. Failures in cranioplasty - a clinical audit & review. J Oral Biol Craniofac Res. 2021;11(1):66–70. https://doi.org/10.1016/j.jobcr.2020.11.013.

Anesthesia for Lesions Involving the Scalp and Calvarium

26

Ferdi Gülaştı and Sinem Sarı

26.1 Introduction

Several diseases may be hidden behind intraosseous lesions of the calvarium and can be a primary bone lesion or lesions invading the bone. Although most benign lesions (e.g., osteomas, meningiomas, or intraosseous hemangiomas) can usually be completely resected, malignant lesions such as plasmacytoma, metastasis, or osteolysis require adjuvant therapy [1]. Although scalp lesions mostly consist of congenital lesions, trauma sequelae, and vascular anomalies in pediatric patients, they mostly include neoplastic lesions in the elderly. Depending on size and etiology, scalp lesions may involve a large surgical area and may require simple resection or grafting. Depending on the surgical procedure and the age of the patients, local anesthesia, sedation, regional anesthesia, and general anesthesia may be required [2, 3]. In the current literature, scalp and calvarial lesions were reported in the form of a limited number of case reports. It is possible to explain anesthesia management with these case reports and up-to-date anesthesia information.

F. Gülaştı · S. Sarı (✉)
Department of Anesthesiology and Reanimation, Aydın Adnan Menderes University Faculty of Medicine, Aydın, Türkiye
e-mail: sarisinem@yahoo.com

26.2 Preoperative Evaluation

The state of consciousness of patients who have intracranial lesions, the presence of focal neurological deficits, and symptoms of increased intracranial pressure (IICP) must be evaluated and recorded before any surgery. The symptoms and signs of increased ICP are pupillary edema, unilateral pupil dilation, headache, nausea, vomiting, n. oculomotorius and n. abducens paralysis in patients. Patients who have IICP are at risk of herniation after respiratory depression with benzodiazepines and opioids. For this reason, routine premedication is not recommended in patients who have IICP.

26.3 Anesthetic Agents

In cranial surgeries, agents used for general and sedation have different effects on brain physiology. The effects of these anesthetic agents must be known to maintain brain functions.

26.3.1 Intravenous Anesthetics

26.3.1.1 Barbiturates

Thiobarbiturates are preferred frequently as hypnotic agents in anesthesia induction for patients scheduled to undergo surgery because of intracranial lesions. They show their effects by

M. Turgut et al. (eds.), *Lesions of the Scalp and Cranial Vault*,
https://doi.org/10.1007/978-3-031-88244-9_26

prolonging the open time of GABA-A receptors in chloride ion channels and inhibiting the reticular activating system [4]. Thiopental sodium induction dose is 3–5 mg/kg for adults, 5–6 mg/kg for children, and 6–8 mg/kg for infants, which reduces cerebral metabolic rate of oxygen ($CMRO_2$) significantly. They have a cerebral vasoconstrictor effect and cause a decrease in cerebral blood flow (CBF) and IICP and show the "Robin Hood effect" because the vasoconstrictor effect does not occur in the ischemic lesion. They are also used in status epilepticus because of their strong anticonvulsant effect.

26.3.1.2 Benzodiazepines

They have hypnotic, sedative, anxiolytic, anterograde amnesia, anticonvulsant, and centrally acting muscle relaxant characteristics. Midazolam, diazepam, and lorazepam are the most commonly used benzodiazepines. They bind to the GABA-A receptor, increasing the opening frequency of chloride ion channels. Benzodiazepines reduce $CMRO_2$, IICP, and inracerebral blood flow (IBF). Although they do not cause complete suppression on electroencephalography (EEG), they are used in grand mal seizures.

26.3.1.3 Propofol

Propofol is a hypnotic agent with a 1.5–2.5 mg/kg recommended induction dose. The maintenance infusion dose is 50–200 μ kg^{-1} min^{-1} and usually causes apnea following the administration at an induction dose [5]. The frequency and duration of the apnea depend on the dose administered, the rate of administration, and other drugs administered concomitantly [5, 6]. Its vasodilatation and myocardial depressant characteristics may cause severe hypotension. For this reason, caution should be exercised in hypovolemic and catecholamine-depleted patients. It also causes a dose-dependent decrease in CBF, IICP, and $CMRO_2$. It has an important place in the total intravenous anesthesia (TIVA) in intracranial surgery as well as being used for sedation purposes. Propofol-remifentanil combination is recommended for TIVA in craniotomies.

26.3.1.4 Etomidate

Etomidate is a hypnotic agent with a 02–0.6 mg/kg induction dose. It reduces $CMRO_2$, IBF, and IICP and also has neuroprotective effects.

26.3.1.5 Ketamine

It is an N-methyl-D-aspartate (NMDA) receptor antagonist with an intravenous induction dose of 1–2 mg/kg. It has the effect of IICP. However, no IICP is detected with controlled normocapnic ventilation.

26.3.1.6 Opioids

Opioids are synthetic or natural drugs with morphine-like effects on the brain, spinal cord, and peripheral nerves. $CMRO_2$ minimally reduces CBF and IICP.

26.3.1.7 Dexmedetomidine

Alpha-2 agonist is a new-generation drug. The stimulation of receptors in the presynaptic forehead in the "locus coeruleus" creates inhibition of sympathetic activity and sedation, which reduces pain transmission by stimulating the receptors in the spinal cord. It is administered intravenously for sedation at a dose of 0.3–0.7 mcg/kg.

26.3.2 Halogenated Inhalation Agents

Anesthetic gases increase CBF and decrease $CMRO_2$, which is most evident in isoflurane, making it preferred in craniotomic surgeries. Desflurane causes an increase in cerebrospinal fluid and reduces its absorption. Isoflurane, desflurane, and sevoflurane increase latency in dose-dependent neuromonitoring, depress synaptic transmission in the cerebral cortex, and cause a decrease in amplitude, impairing the interpretation of the cortical region more significantly than the subcortical region. Motor evoked potential (MEP) is impaired at gas release greater than 0.5 MAC. For this reason, if possible, inhalation anesthetics should not be used in MEP monitoring.

26.4 Intraoperative Positions

Different patient positions can be used for different surgical procedures. Ventilation, hemodynamic changes, and nerve compression may occur as complications in patient positions. Aside from these, cerebral edema, bleeding, vision loss, venous air embolism, pneumocephalus, and macroglossia are serious positional problems.

26.5 Anesthesia Management

The surgery of tumoral masses originating from the skull (bony form) and dura mater (boneless form) is preferably performed under general anesthesia [7]. The cases that require bone and scalp reconstruction will also need general anesthesia because of the need for transplanted tissue from other parts of the body [8]. Also, regional methods and pharmacological preferences used for pain management can be considered together as part of multimodal analgesia. The purpose of anesthesia is to provide unconsciousness, amnesia, and analgesia in scalp and calvarium surgeries. Propofol-based total intravenous anesthesia is preferred for anesthesia instead of general anesthesia with a volatile agent. In case of craniopagus of conjoined twins, airway management and endotracheal intubation may be difficult. If the venous sinuses are junctions, these patients are inoperable or cause excessive blooding. This vascular access can sometimes only be done via the femoral route [9].

Neuromonitoring can be used incalvarial surgeries of the lesions penetrating the brain to alert the surgeon in terms of potential neurological damage and critical structures. Monitoring of evoked potentials, electroencephalography (EEG), electromyography (EMG), and cerebral oximetry are neuromonitoring methods [10]. The reaction of the cerebral vascular system to the changes in partial pressure of carbon dioxide ($PaCO_2$) is fast. A large decrease in $PaCO_2$ might pose a risk of secondary ischemic damage. It is usually adequate to stabilize $PaCO_2$ in the range of 30–35 mmHg.

Propofol is a frequently used agent in TIVA for induction and maintenance of anesthesia in craniotomy surgeries for tumor resection. The hypotensive effect of propofol may impair cerebral perfusion and require intervention. In cranial trauma surgery, mannitol or hypertonic saline is employed to reduce brain swelling and IICP. Mannitol has decreasing effects on serum sodium concentration and increasing effects on serum osmolality and serum potassium concentration. Previous studies tried to use mannitol in doses of 0.25–0.5–0.751 g/kg, and it has been shown that the use of 1 g/kg is the most appropriate dose for brain relaxation. It does not reduce cerebral edema and causes electrolyte abnormalities at higher doses. Dexmedetomidine is preferred frequently for analgesic and sedation purposes in neurosurgeries because it reduces pain without causing respiratory depression [11].

In-vehicle traffic accidents and gunshot wounds are the main causes of traumatic brain injuries. For this reason, the prognosis of head injuries is poor. IICP, brain perfusion pressure, and autoregulation are negatively affected in a brain exposed to a trauma, and hemodynamics remains unstable in these patients. It is recommended to apply it only for short periods because hyperventilation may cause vasoconstriction and impair perfusion in these patients. Propofol and thiopental should be administered slowly because the patient may experience a serious hypotensive attack after their administration during anesthesia induction. Although ketamine basically IICP, it has been shown to be neuroprotective and does not affect normocapnia and IICP [12]. It should not be forgotten that cervical damage might occur in these patients, and caution should be exercised during the intubation.

26.6 Pain Management

A total of 90% of patients face pain problems after craniotomy. Half of them suffer from moderate and severe pain [13, 14]. Infratentorial surgery causes more intense pain than supratentorial surgery. The pain is usually superficial and origi-

Table 26.1 Timings of analgesics for craniotomy

Preoperative/intraoperative medication	Postoperative medication
Paracetamol NSAIDs Scalp block or incision-site infiltration Intravenous dexmedetomidine infusion	Paracetamol Opioids as rescue

nates from a somatic origin, involving the scalp, pericranial muscles, soft tissue, and the dura mater. Poorly managed pain might cause agitation, vomiting, hypertension, and IICP. This may initiate and increase postoperative bleeding. In other words, failure to control the pain after craniotomy is among the causes of morbidity and mortality. Although the most effective methods for controlling postoperative pain in craniotomy are still not known, different methods such as pharmacological methods, regional anesthesia, and acupuncture are used (Table 26.1). In recent years, efforts have been made to develop recommendations for post-craniotomy pain treatment with current practices under the name of PROSPECT methodology [15].

26.6.1 Pharmacological Methods

Paracetamol, opioids, nonsteroidal anti-inflammatory drugs (NSAIDs), dexmedetomidine, gabapentinoids, flupirtine, methimazole, magnesium sulfate, and vitamin D are among the drugs administered and investigated. Although paracetamol is a reliable analgesic, it has not been found adequate alone to control the pain after craniotomy, and it needs to be used in combination with drugs such as NSAIDs and opioids or with regional methods [16–19]. Although NSAIDs reduce pain, their opioid-sparing effectiveness is low [18]. NSAIDs used in addition to paracetamol are useful in the early postoperative period, but, although it has been argued that they may increase the risk of bleeding, this is not clear. PROSPECT is recommended for use in the treatment of postoperative pain. Opioid drugs are successful in post-craniotomy pain management, especially if used with patient-controlled analgesia. However, they both impair neurological evaluation and may cause an IICP with their sedative and respiratory depression effects [20–24]. For this reason, its use only in rescue pain comes to the forefront. Intraoperative dexmedetomidine infusion reduces postoperative pain scores and opioid consumption [25, 26].

26.6.2 Regional Methods

Regional analgesia techniques are recommended strongly as an indispensable part of multimodal analgesia management because they reduce opioid consumption and pain scores. Usually, these blocks can be performed before the surgical incision or before waking the patient.

26.6.2.1 Scalp Block

Scalp nerve block was introduced and applied in various neurosurgeries to stabilize surgical procedures, manage postoperative pain, and reduce opioid consumption. The ERAS protocol and PROSPECT recommend the use of a scalp block for elective craniotomy in addition to NSAIDs, but evidence on this subject is still lacking [27–32]. During a craniotomy, noxious stimulants (e.g., skull-pin fixation) are a serious cause of pain and can increase blood pressure even during deep general anesthesia and cause increased intracranial pressure and/or bleeding in the injured parenchyma. The modern scalp block consists of local anesthesia injections that target the supraorbital, supratrochlear, zygomaticotemporal, auriculotemporal, and greater and lesser occipital nerves [33] (Fig. 26.1). Adding dexmedetomidine to the scalp block provides better perioperative hemodynamic stability with no effect on the duration of the block [34].

26.6.2.2 Local Anesthesia Infiltration

Local anesthetic infiltration to the scalp can be used to reduce intraoperative hemodynamic responses caused by craniotomy. However, local anesthetic is recommended for the treatment of acute pain after brain surgery, but its effectiveness is considered to be less compared to scalp block. it is necessary to be careful about the toxicity of local anesthesia because of the vascularization of the skin tissue.

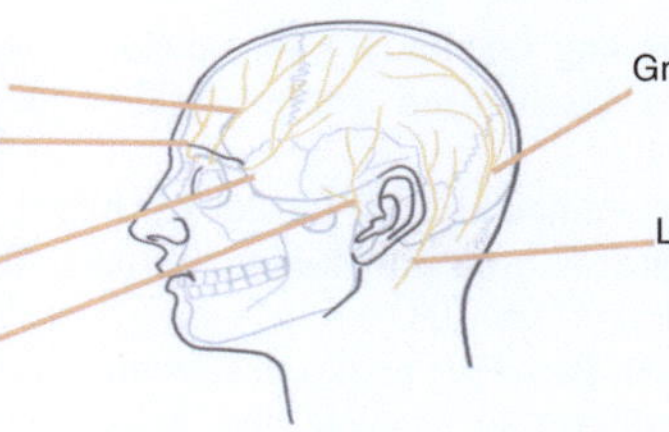

Fig. 26.1 Target of nerves scalp block

26.7 Conclusion

Patients might undergo surgical procedures that may require from local anesthesia to general anesthesia in the resection of the scalp lesions. This might also include anesthesia management to control the spread of calvarial and scalp lesions to the brain, advanced monitoring needed by neuroanesthesia, and preservation of brain functions.

Acknowledgments The authors declare that no funds, grants, or other support were received during the preparation of this manuscript. We express our gratitude to Dr. Kağan Buğra Şeker for their significant contributions to Fig. 26.1, enhancing the visual representation in this article.

References

1. Ozgiray E, Perumal K, Cinar C, Caliskan KE, Ertan Y Yurtseven T, Oktar N, Ovul I, Oner K. Management of calvarial tumors: a retrospective analysis and literature review. Turk Neurosurg. 2016;26:690–8.
2. Mandikiyana Chirimuta LA, Ndowa FJ, Pascoe MJ. Cutaneous squamous cell carcinoma in vertically acquired HIV and epidermodysplasia verruciformis. South Afr J HIV Med. 2022;23(1):1368.
3. Rizvi MM, Singh RB, Sarkar A, Choubey S Anaesthesia for a "Scalped" patient. J Clin Diagn Res. 2015;9(6):UD03–4. https://doi.org/10.7860/JCDR/2015/12863.6038. [Epub 2015 Jun 1.].
4. Zhu H, Cottrell JE, Kass IS. The effect of thiopental and propofol on NMDA- and AMPA-mediated glutamate excitotoxicity. Anesthesiology. 1997;87(4):944–51.
5. Butterworth JF, Mackey DCWJ. Morgan&Mikhail's clinical anesthesiology. 5th ed; 2013.
6. Y. Keçik. Nonopioid İntravenöz Anestezikler. In: Temel Anestezi 2.Ed.; 2016:99–118.
7. Salvati M, Cervoni L, Ciappetta P, Artico M, Raco A. Solitary plasmacytoma of the skull: report of two cases. Clin Neurol Neurosurg. 1994;96(1):66–70.
8. Harada K, Uozumi T, Kuwabara S, Kiya K, Arita K, Ogasawara H, Fujimura K. Plasma cell tumor of the parieto-occipital bone; a case report. No Shinkei Geka. 1991;19(11):1067–71. Japanese
9. Thomas JM. Anaesthesia for conjoined twins. Childs Nerv Syst. 2004;20:538–46.
10. Thomas B, Guo D. The diagnostic accuracy of evoked potential monitoring techniques during intracranial aneurysm surgery for predicting postoperative ischemic damage: a systematic review and meta-analysis. World Neurosurg. 2017;103:829–840.e3. https://doi.org/10.1016/j.wneu.2017.04.071. Epub 2017 Apr 20
11. Rajan S, Hutcherson MT, Sessler DI, Kurz A, Yang D, Ghobrial M, Liu J, Avitsian R. The effects of dexmedetomidine and remifentanil on hemodynamic stability and analgesic requirement after craniotomy: a randomized controlled trial. J Neurosurg Anesthesiol. 2016;28(4):282–90.
12. Bell JD. In vogue: ketamine for neuroprotection in acute neurologic injury. Anesth Analg. 2017;124(4):1237–43.
13. Vacas S, Van de Wiele B. Designing a pain management protocol for craniotomy: a narrative review and consideration of promising practices. Surg Neurol Int. 2017;8:291–1291.
14. Chowdhury T, Garg R, Sheshadri V, et al. Perioperative factors contributing the post-craniotomy pain: a synthesis of concepts. Front Med (Lausanne). 2017;4:23.
15. Mestdagh FP, Lavand'homme PM, Pirard G, Joshi GP, Sauter AR, Van de Velde M, PROSPECT Working Group* of the European Society of Regional Anaesthesia and Pain Therapy (ESRA). Pain management after elective craniotomy: a systematic review with procedure-specific postoperative pain management (PROSPECT) recommendations. Eur J Anaesthesiol. 2023;40(10):747–57.
16. Greenberg S, Murphy GS, Avram MJ, et al. Postoperative intravenous acetaminophen for craniotomy patients: a randomized controlled trial. World Neurosurg. 2018;109:e554–62.
17. Artime CA, Aijazi H, Zhang H, et al. Scheduled intravenous acetaminophen improves patient satisfaction with postcraniotomy pain management: a prospective, randomized, placebo-controlled, double-blind study. J Neurosurg Anesthesiol. 2018;30:231–6.
18. Sivakumar W, Jensen M, Martinez J, et al. Intravenous acetaminophen for postoperative supratentorial craniotomy pain: a prospective, randomized, double-blinded, placebo-controlled trial. J Neurosurg. 2019;130:722–66.
19. Burbridge MA, Stone SA, Jaffe RA. Acetaminophen does not reduce postoperative opiate consumption in

patients undergoing craniotomy for cerebral revascularization: a randomized control trial. Cureus. 2019;11:e3863.
20. Williams DL, Pemberton E, Leslie K. Effect of intravenous parecoxib on postcraniotomy pain. Br J Anaesth. 2011;107:398–403.
21. Na H-S, An S-B, Park H-P, et al. Intravenous patient-controlled analgesia to manage the postoperative pain in patients undergoing craniotomy. Korean J Anesthesiol. 2011;60:30–5.
22. Morad A, Winters B, Stevens R, et al. The efficacy of intravenous patient-controlled analgesia after intracranial surgery of the posterior fossa: a prospective, randomized controlled trial. Anesth Analg. 2012;114:416–23.
23. Hassani E, Mahoori A, Sane S, Tolumehr A. Comparison the effects of paracetamol with sufentanil infusion on postoperative pain control after craniotomy in patients who have brain tumor. Adv Biomed Res. 2015;4:64.
24. Akcil EF, Dilmen OK, Vehid HE, et al. The role of 'integrated pulmonary index' monitoring during morphine-based intravenous patient-controlled analgesia administration following supratentorial craniotomies: a prospective, randomized, double-blind controlled study. Curr Med Res Opin. 2018;34:2009–14.
25. Rahimi SY, Alleyne CH, Vernier E, et al. Postoperative pain management with tramadol after craniotomy: evaluation and cost analysis: clinical article. J Neurosurg. 2010;112:268–72.
26. Song J, Ji Q, Sun Q, et al. The opioid-sparing effect of intraoperative dexmedetomidine infusion after craniotomy. J Neurosurg Anesthesiol. 2016;28:14–20.
27. Rajan S, Hutcherson MT, Sessler DI, et al. The effects of dexmedetomidine and remifentanil on hemodynamic stability and analgesic requirement after craniotomy: a randomized controlled trial. J Neurosurg Anesthesiol. 2016;28:282–90.
28. Stumpo V, Staartjes VE, Quddusi A, Corniola MV, Tessitore E, Schroder ML, Anderer EG, Stienen MN, Serra C, Regli L. Enhanced recovery after surgery strategies for elective craniotomy: a systematic review. J Neurosurg. 2021;135:1857–81.
29. Elayat A, Jena SS, Nayak S, Sahu RN, Tripathy S. Enhanced recovery after surgery—ERAS in elective craniotomies-a non-randomized controlled trial. BMC Neurol. 2021;21:127.
30. Galvin IM, Levy R, Day AG, Gilron I. Pharmacological interventions for the prevention of acute postoperative pain in adults following brain surgery. Cochrane Database Syst Rev. 2019;2019:CD011931.
31. Ahn HJ, Kim JA, Lee JJ, Kim HS, Shin HJ, Chung IS, Kim JK, Gwak MS, Choi SJ. Effect of preoperative skull block on pediatric moyamoya disease. J Neurosurg Pediatr. 2008;2:37–41.
32. Wang D, Fang J, Liu J, Hao Q, Ding H, Liu B, Liu Z, Song H, Ouyang J, Liu R. Improving recovery after microvascular decompression surgery for hemifacial spasm: experience from 530 cases with enhanced recovery after surgery (ERAS) protocol. Br J Neurosurg. 2021;35:486–91.
33. Harbell MW, Bolton PB, Koyyalamudi V, Seamans DP, Langley NR. Evaluating the anatomic spread of selective nerve scalp blocks using methylene blue: a cadaveric analysis. J Neurosurg Anesthesiol. 2023;35(2):248–52.
34. Stachtari C, Stergiouda Z, Koraki E, Sifaki F, Bagntasarian S, Chatzopoulos S. Dexmedetomidine as an adjuvant to scalp block in patients undergoing elective craniotomy: a prospective randomized controlled trial. Clin Neurol Neurosurg. 2023;227:107669.

27 Postoperative Complications of Surgery for Lesions of the Scalp and Calvarium

Mohammed Benzagmout, Josué Kazayi Ilunga, Marouane El Ouahabi, and Mohammed Amine Houssa

27.1 Introduction

Lesions of the scalp and calvarium are diverse and come in a wide range. The treatment is basically surgical and often challenging given the complexity of reconstruction especially in the presence of cranial defects and complications. Such lesions fall within the remit of neurosurgery and require early diagnosis, proper neurosurgical management, and rigorous postoperative follow-up to reduce the risk of complications.

The management of postoperative complications is a complex collaborative work of general practitioners, radiologists, intensive care anesthetists, plastic surgeons, and neurosurgeons, in other terms, qualified human resources and appropriate equipment.

Postoperative complications vary from cutaneous to infectious, hemorrhagic, nervous, or aesthetic issues. Understanding their mechanisms, chronology of onset, and the effectiveness of their management is crucial to ensure prevention and effective treatment.

In the present work, we aim to provide a comprehensive review of postoperative complications of surgery for lesions of the scalp and calvarium, as well as to identify the associated risk factors and to suggest the management techniques that can reduce the risk of such complications.

27.2 Scalp Complications

The incidence of scalp complications following craniofacial surgery is variable [1]. Butenschoen et al. reported an incidence of 12.8% of skin wound healing problems after reconstructions of large combined scalp and skull defects [2]. Similarly, the incidence of temporal hollowing varies between 30 and 75% in surgeries involving the temporal area [3–5].

Scalp complications increase morbidity, mortality, and healthcare costs [6]. Risk factors include age, poor nutrition, underlying diseases such as diabetes mellitus, immunosuppressive treatment, active smoking, previous surgical interventions, and preoperative irradiation [1, 7].

In surgical planning, it is essential to decide beforehand which surgical incision to undertake

M. Benzagmout (✉)
Department of Neurosurgery, Hassan II Hospital, Sidi Mohamed Ben Abdellah University of Fès, Fes, Morocco
e-mail: benzagmout@hotmail.fr

J. K. Ilunga · M. El Ouahabi
Department of Neurosurgery, University Hospital of Fez, Fez, Morocco

M. A. Houssa
Department of Plastic Surgery, El Hassani Hospital, Nador, Morocco

M. Turgut et al. (eds.), *Lesions of the Scalp and Cranial Vault*,
https://doi.org/10.1007/978-3-031-88244-9_27

to guarantee the best surgical exposure and a perfect reliable closure, so as to prevent scalp complications, avoid unnecessary reinterventions, and improve aesthetic results. The skin incisions should generally parallel the Langer lines [8], which are defined as the tension lines parallel to the fibers of the dermis and perpendicular to the underlying muscle fibers. These lines are directed anteroposteriorly in the vertex and circumferentially in the temporal and posterior regions [7]. In addition, the incision scheme and route should avoid the main arteries supplying the scalp, especially the superficial temporal artery and occipital arteries to ensure adequate flap perfusion [9].

Careful attention should also be given to the closure step of surgery to achieve a layered tension-free closure and to guarantee good wound healing [9].

However, and despite preventive efforts, various scalp complications could occur. Wound dehiscence remains the most common and happens more in thinner than in thicker parts of the scalp [10, 11]. Multiple soft tissue defects can also develop after craniofacial surgeries due to several factors altering the integrity of the scalp layers, particularly ischemia, denervation, muscle atrophy or injury, and inadequate repositioning or resuspension of a muscle [12] (Fig. 27.1). In addition, Matic et al. reported weight loss as a preoperative risk factor for temporal hollowing complication [3].

Finally, flap necrosis incidence varies between 0.7 and 5.5% in the literature. Its risk factors include iatrogenic injuries of the supplying arteries, an insufficient skin pedicle, inadequate venous drainage, long-time lasting traction of the skin flap, and excessive tension in scalp closure [13] (Fig. 27.2). Some authors advocate increasing the width of the pedicle as a good technique to prevent flap necrosis since it increases both collateral circulation and venous drainage. The recommended scalp flap length/width ratio is 3:1 [14].

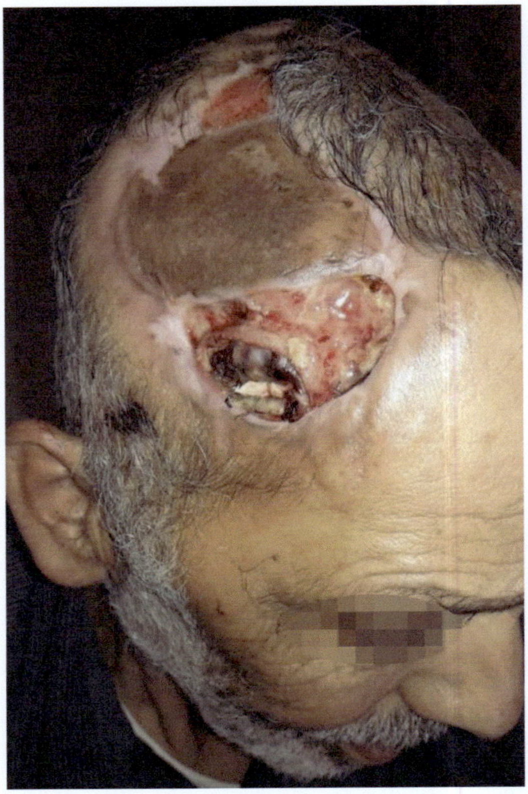

Fig. 27.1 Anteroposterior view demonstrating a large right frontotemporal defect involving the skin, the temporal muscle, and the dura and revealing the brain parenchyma below

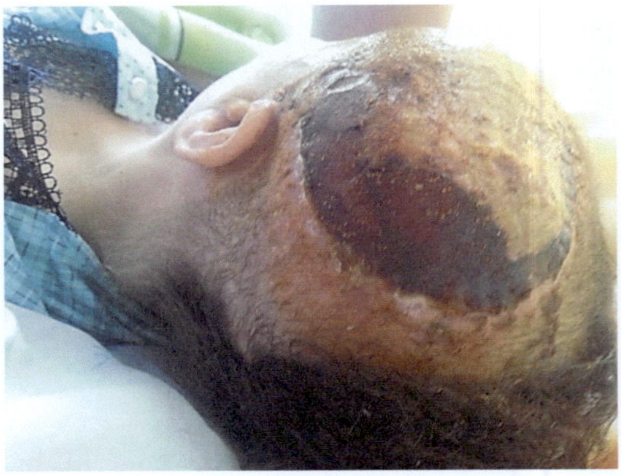

Fig. 27.2 Left lateral view demonstrating a large necrosis of the skin flap

27.3 Infectious Complications (Fig. 27.3)

The incidence of infection is extremely variable and depends strongly on the type of surgery performed. In nontraumatic scalp reconstructive surgeries, the percentage of infection ranged between 0.7 and 10% [10, 11, 15–18]. Leedy et al. reported that 25% of their cases developed infection of tissue expanders that usually require explantation and reinsertion after healing and infection resolution [19].

These complications make the management of scalp and calvarial defects even more difficult, thus leading to increased healthcare costs and usually to other large defects of greater complexity.

Risk factors of surgical site infections are divided into factors intrinsically related to the type of surgery performed and those that are patient-related. The first category includes surgical time, the extension of the tissue exposure, the use of foreign material, and the type of surgery.

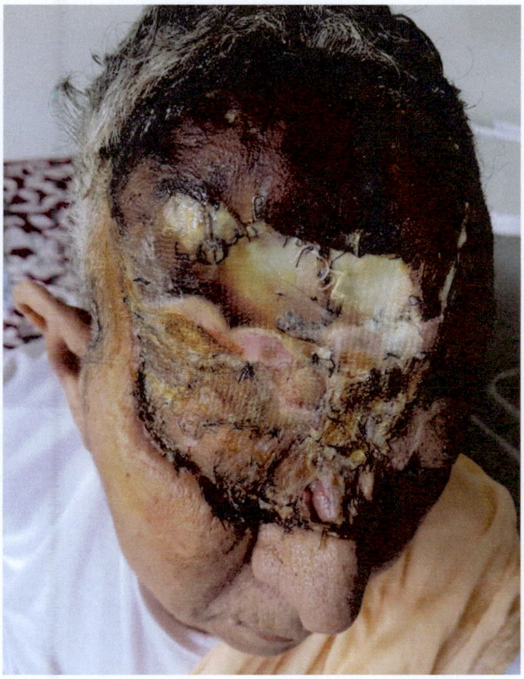

Fig. 27.3 Anteroposterior view demonstrating ischemia of the skin flap associated to signs of infection

The second comprises the patient's own risk factors, namely, age, comorbidities like diabetes mellitus, smoking, or corticosteroid use, previous surgeries, radiotherapy, previous infections, and functional status [20, 21].

Preoperative measures are crucial as well as drastic compliance with aseptic measures including proper surgical handwashing, use of chlorhexidine or other alcohol-based solutions for skin preparation, draping the scalp, and using sterile gloves and changing them every 2 h and before contact with any implantable material [21]. Regarding showering with antiseptic solutions and shaving the scalp before surgery, the evidence supporting infection prevention is unsettled. However, several studies reported a possible increase in infection rate following shaving due to epidermal injury [21].

In the postoperative stage, the patient's head is generally 45 degrees elevated in cases of scalp replantation or microvascular free-flap scalp reconstruction for adequate perfusion. The patient is also positioned to prevent pressure on the vascular pedicle or the flap. Low-pressure or negative-pressure dressings should be used over skin grafts. Broad-spectrum antibiotics are usually prescribed for several days, and drains are often inserted following wide undermining of the scalp for local flaps [22].

Calvarial reconstruction is performed to provide protective coverage of the intracranial contents, to restore cranial contour, and to prevent infections. Reconstruction should be delayed if infection is already present awaiting recovery [22]. Furthermore, it is important to underline that cerebrospinal fluid leaks may contribute to wound healing complications by adding fluid accumulation and potentially lethal infections [22].

Whenever possible, autologous cranioplasty is always preferred to alloplastic materials [22]. Exposure and infection of autologous bone can sometimes be managed without complete graft loss, whereas infection of alloplastic materials always require removal of the foreign material to ensure healing [22].

27.4 Hemorrhagic Complications

The vascular supply of the scalp is rich and comprises bilaterally the supratrochlear, supraorbital, superficial temporal, posterior auricular, and occipital arteries, as well as their accompanying veins. The supratrochlear and supraorbital arteries arise from the ophthalmic artery, whereas the remaining arteries arise from the external carotid artery.

Surgical treatment of scalp and calvarial lesions can result in various hemorrhagic complications including excessive intraoperative bleeding and postoperative hematomas [1]. The latter remains a major life-threatening complication of cranial surgery. Its exact incidence is unknown with only partly identified risk factors [23]. One study found that extradural hematoma following craniotomy of various indications occurred in 0.8% of cases, usually within 24 h of surgery [24]; other authors reported 1% [25].

As a rare surgical complication of scalp and calvarial lesions, the exact mechanisms of development of postoperative extradural hematoma are not well-known. An easier separation of the dura in a large craniotomy area, as well as considerable intraoperative blood loss, and a sudden drop of intracranial pressure from the abrupt loss of cerebrospinal fluid are all believed as major causes of postoperative extradural hematoma formation [26]. Other causes might be due to inadequate hemostasis, coagulopathy, and hypertension [27]. Furthermore, intraoperative blood loss probably contributes to the development of an extradural hematoma through the loss of coagulation factors or platelet dysfunction. Kim et al. found that 800 ml or more of intraoperative blood loss to be an independent risk factor for postoperative extradural hematoma [27].

Overall, extradural hematoma, albeit extremely rare, should be emphasized as a possible serious complication to be prevented before and during surgery by performing complete hemostasis assessment, considering preoperative embolization of highly vascularized lesions, and ensuring good hemostasis at the end of surgery. For such, dural tack-up sutures should be used for large-sized craniotomy as well as small craniotomy in which tamponade effects were expected to prevent the development of hematoma.

The management depends on the size and rate of seroma/hematoma formation. Small collections that are not expanding are generally treated conservatively with pressure and observation and usually abate. However, large or expanding lesions may need drainage [22].

27.5 Nervous Complications

These complications are generally caused by direct nerve damage. Therefore, their prevention lies principally in the proper planning of the incision and the surgical technique for adequate protection of the nerves, especially the motor nerves.

For instance, temporoparietal and pterional approaches are known as risky in terms of the potential damage they may incur to the temporal branch of the facial nerve, causing paralysis of the orbicularis, frontalis, and corrugator supercilii muscles [28]. Two techniques have been described to provide better surgical exposure with optimal nerve protection: subpericranial and interfascial subfascial dissection [5].

For posterior lesions, postsurgical occipital neuropathy should be considered as a possible complication related to the excision of scalp and/or calvarial mass [29]. This complication is common because of the anatomical configuration of the occipital nerves, which are formed of three nerves: the greater occipital nerve (GON), the lesser occipital nerve (LON), and the third occipital nerve. The GON is the largest of the three nerves and arises as the medial branch of the posterior (dorsal) ramus of C2; the LON arises from the anterior (ventral) rami of C2 and C3, whereas the third occipital nerve, also known as the least occipital nerve, emerges from the medial subdivision of the posterior (dorsal) ramus of C3.

The anatomical superficial course of the LON makes it highly vulnerable, especially for occipital lesions located below the superior nuchal line and external to the lateral margin of trapezius muscle [19]. Thus, surgeons should be aware of this potential complication to understand the appropriate treatment and clinical prognosis. In case of mild sensory symptoms, the patient usually recovers within few months. However, if occipital neuropathy is troublesome, a range of pain treatments are available including medications, chemical neurolysis [30], pulsed radiofrequency neuromodulation [31], neurectomy [32], and surgical neurolysis [33].

27.6 Aesthetic Complications

The appearance of the healed surgical site varies considerably depending on the type of the lesion, the extent of surgery and its site, and the possible occurrence of the aforementioned complications. Some scar tissue always forms after surgery because the dermis (deep skin layer) was damaged. Small calvarial defects can be left especially in scalp regions covered by a muscle or by a flap. However, larger partial-thickness defects, especially in aesthetically visible areas such as the forehead, usually require repair [22].

Alopecia constitutes the most classical cosmetic complication. Besides, the hair-bearing quality of the scalp in most patients makes aesthetically pleasing reconstruction a real challenge [34].

27.7 Conclusion

Lesions of the scalp and calvarium are common and multiple. They can be caused by trauma, thermal or electrical burns, infections, and tumors. Surgery is the cornerstone of treatment in most cases. However, it remains challenging because of the wide variety of complications that can occur and the usual complexity of reconstruction. Overall, reconstruction of composite defects presents a unique challenge given the relative tissue inelasticity of the scalp, the need for tension-free closure, and the convex shape of the cranium.

The management of postoperative complications of scalp and calvarial lesions is difficult and must be tailored to the particularities of each patient. The appropriate flap and the suture technique used for closure are crucial. Reconstruction in patients with scalp and/or calvarial defects can be simple or complex.

However, the main treatment of these complications is prevention. The main goals of surgery need to be established, and the surgical technique clearly planned and surely accomplished to allow better exposure of the lesion and good performance of the primary surgery in order to prevent neurovascular complications and to reduce the incidence of secondary reconstruction, which often lead to more complications [35]. This requires a detailed knowledge of the anatomy of scalp and calvaria, skin biomechanics, hair physiology, and a perfect collaboration of a multidisciplinary specialized team completely dedicated to this kind of surgery.

References

1. Pedroza Gómez S, Gómez Ortega V, Tovar-Spinoza Z, Ghotme KA. Scalp complications of craniofacial surgery: classification, prevention, and initial approach: an updated review. Eur J Plast Surg. 2023;46:315–25.
2. Butenschoen VM, Weitz J, Ritschl LM, et al. CSF disturbances and other neurosurgical complications after interdisciplinary reconstructions of large combined scalp and skull deficiencies. Neurosurg Rev. 2021;44:1583–9.
3. Matic DB, Kim S. Temporal hollowing following coronal incision: a prospective, randomized, controlled trial. Plast Reconstr Surg. 2008;121:379–85.
4. Santiago GF, Terner J, Wolf A, et al. Post-neurosurgical temporal deformities: various techniques for correction and associated complications. J Craniofacial Surg. 2018;29:1723–9.
5. Sriamornrattanakul K, Akharathammachote N, Wongsuriyanan S. Suprafascial dissection for pterional craniotomy to preserve the frontotemporal branch of the facial nerve with less temporal hollowing. Surg Neurol Int. 2021;12:559.
6. Engstrand T. Biomaterials and biologics in craniofacial reconstruction. J Craniofac Surg. 2012;23:239–42.
7. Persing SM, Persing JS, Cabrejo R, et al. Incisions and closures. 8th ed. Elsevier Inc; 2022.
8. Murphy J, Goodhall W, Patterson A. Langer's lines—what are they and do they matter? Br J Oral Maxillofac Surg. 2017;55:e86–7.
9. Quiñones-Hinojosa A. Schmidek and sweet: operative neurosurgical techniques 2-volume set: indications, methods and results. 7th ed. Elsevier; 2021.
10. Chung J, Lee S, Park JC, et al. Scalp thickness as a predictor of wound complications after cerebral revascularization using the superficial temporal artery: a risk factor analysis. Acta Neurochir. 2020;162:2557–63.

11. Jang HU, Choi YW. Scalp reconstruction: a 10-year experience. Arch Craniofac Surg. 2020;21:237–43.
12. Thiensri T, Limpoka A, Burusapat C. Analysis of factors associated with temporal hollowing after pterional craniotomy. Indian J Plastic Surg. 2020;53:71–82.
13. Belmahi A. The secondary surgeries after unfavorable results in scalp defects treatment. Ann Chir Plast Esthet. 2019;64:540–51.
14. Sittitavornwong S, Morlandt ABP. Reconstruction of the scalp, calvarium, and frontal sinus. Oral Maxillofac Surg Clin North Am. 2013;25:105–29.
15. Chang V, Hartzfeld P, Langlois M, et al. Outcomes of cranial repair after craniectomy: clinical article. J Neurosurg. 2010;112:1120–4.
16. Fialkov JA, Holy C, Forrest CR, et al. Postoperative infections in craniofacial reconstructive procedures. J Craniofac Surg. 2001;12:362–8.
17. Janus JR, Peck BW, Tombers NM, et al. Complications after oncologic scalp reconstruction: a 139-patient series and treatment algorithm. Laryngoscope. 2015;125:582–8.
18. Moreira-Gonzalez A, Jackson IT, Miyawaki T, et al. Clinical outcome in cranioplasty: critical review in long-term follow-up. J Craniofacial Surg. 2003;14:144–53.
19. Leedy JE, Janis JE, Rohrich RJ. Reconstruction of acquired scalp defects: an algorithmic approach. Plast Reconstr Surg. 2005;116(4):54e–72e.
20. Bruce JN, Bruce SS. Preservation of bone faps in patients with postcraniotomy infections. J Neurosurg. 2003;98:1203–7.
21. Paredes I, Lagares A, San-Juan R, et al. Reduction in the infection rate of cranioplasty with a tailored antibiotic prophylaxis: a non-randomized study. Acta Neurochir. 2020;162:2857–66.
22. Lin SJ, Hanasono MM, Skoracki RJ. Scalp and calvarial reconstruction. Semin Plast Surg. 2008;22(4):281–93.
23. Di Rienzo A, Pangrazi PP, Riccio M, Colasanti R, Ghetti I, Iacoangeli M. Skin flap complications after decompressive craniectomy and cranioplasty: proposal of classification and treatment options. Surg Neurol Int. 2016;7:S737–45.
24. De Bonis P, Sturiale CL, Anile C, et al. Decompressive craniectomy, interhemispheric hygroma and hydrocephalus: a timeline of events? Clin Neurol Neurosurg. 2013;115:1308–12.
25. Honeybul S, Ho KM. Decompressive craniectomy for severe traumatic brain injury: the relationship between surgical complications and the prediction of an unfavorable outcome. Injury. 2014;45:1332–9.
26. Yang NR, Song J, Yoon K-W, Seo EK. How early can we perform cranioplasty for traumatic brain injury after decompressive craniectomy? A retrospective multicenter study. World Neurosurg. 2018;110:e160–7.
27. Malcolm JG, Rindler RS, Chu JK, Chokshi F, Grossberg JA, Pradilla G, et al. Early cranioplasty is associated with greater neurological improvement: a systematic review and meta-analysis. Neurosurgery. 2018;82:278–88.
28. Poblete T, Jiang X, Komune N, Matsushima K. Rhoton - preserving nerves to frontalis. J Neurosurg. 2015;122:1274–82.
29. Yang JS, Choi HJ, Cho YJ, Kang SH. Sensory complications in patients after scalp mass excision and its anatomical considerations. J Korean Neurosurg Soc. 2014;55(4):200–4.
30. Jürgens TP, Müller P, Seedorf H, Regelsberger J, May A. Occipital nerve block is effective in craniofacial neuralgias but not in idiopathic persistent facial pain. J Headache Pain. 2012;13(3):199–213.
31. Choi HJ, Oh IH, Choi SK, Lim YJ. Clinical outcomes of pulsed radiofrequency neuromodulation for the treatment of occipital neuralgia. J Korean Neurosurg Soc. 2012;51(5):281–5.
32. Jung SJ, Moon SK, Kim TY, Eom KS. A case of occipital neuralgia in the greater and lesser occipital nerves treated with neurectomy by using transcranial Doppler sonography: technical aspects. Korean J Pain. 2011;24(1):48–52.
33. Gille O, Lavignolle B, Vital JM. Surgical treatment of greater occipital neuralgia by neurolysis of the greater occipital nerve and sectioning of the inferior oblique muscle. Spine. 2004;29(7):828–32.
34. Tolhurst DE, Carstens MH, Greco RS, et al. The surgical anatomy of the scalp. Plast Reconstr Surg. 1991;87:603–12.
35. Shay T, Belzberg M, Asemota AO, et al. Risk of complications in primary versus revision-type cranioplasty. J Craniofac Surg. 2020;31:423–7.

28 Prognosis of Lesions of the Scalp and Calvarium

Abad Cherif El Asri, Mohammed Benzagmout, and Ali Akhaddar

28.1 Introduction

Skull vault lesions are rare and represent 1–2% of all bone masses. They are commonly an incidental finding or may be discovered during staging work-up for other diseases [1, 2]. The neurosurgical literature lacks large series highlighting calvarial tumors. Lesions of the calvarium may originate from the bony structures or may be secondary to invasion of scalp-based lesions or brain-based lesions into the skull vault [1]. For many of these lesions, the clinical and radiological features are often nonspecific making the diagnosis cumbersome. Recognition of benign and malignant imaging features is important for the radiological diagnosis, management, and also monitoring and follow-up [1]. Different classification systems can be employed in order to categorize such lesions: primary (benign and malignant) or secondary as well as neoplastic and non-neoplastic (inflammatory and proliferative). In this chapter, we classify calvarial masses into three groups: (1) benign lesions (2) tumor-like lesions, and (3) malignant lesions. Another category might be distinguished like traumatic and congenital lesions. Infectious lesions are excluded in this article.

The management of patients with calvarial lesions should be interdisciplinary, as with other oncological diseases. The therapeutic strategy is dictated by the risk of progression, aesthetic issue, or compromising of the adjacent structure. Most benign lesions, such as osteomas, meningiomas, or intraosseous hemangiomas, can usually be completely resected and do not need further treatment [1–3]. However, malignant lesions, such as metastasis or osteolysis in plasmacytoma, potentially require an adjuvant therapy such as chemotherapy, immunotherapy, or radiation [4]. Rare diseases such as histiocytosis require individual diagnostic and therapeutic evaluations [1, 4].

The aim of this chapter is to define the outcomes and prognosis factors for scalp and calvarial lesions according to their origin and behavior.

A. C. El Asri (✉)
Department of Neurosurgery, Mohamed V Military Hospital, University Mohammed V of Rabat, Rabat, Morocco
e-mail: abad20031@gmail.com

M. Benzagmout
Department of Neurosurgery, Hassan II Hospital, Sidi Mohamed Ben Abdellah University of Fès, Fes, Morocco

A. Akhaddar
Department of Neurosurgery, Avicenne Military Hospital of Marrakech, Mohammed V University in Rabat, Rabat, Morocco

M. Turgut et al. (eds.), *Lesions of the Scalp and Cranial Vault*,
https://doi.org/10.1007/978-3-031-88244-9_28

28.2 Lesions of the Cranial Vault

28.2.1 Malignant Tumors

28.2.1.1 Metastasis

Cranial vault is most often involved by metastases from extracranial primary neoplasms, with more than half of cases are represented by breast and lung carcinomas [4]. In adult, other primary tumors that can metastasize to the skull are carcinomas of the prostate, kidney, uterus, colon, liver, ovary, and thyroid as well as other nonepithelial and bone tumors. However, in children the most common primary causes are sarcoma and neuroblastoma [5].

The prevalence of skull metastases (SM) is higher during the sixth and seventh decades of life. SM may be located in any layer of the skull and appear as lytic, usually solitary and destroying either the inner or the outer table of the skull with invasion of the intra- or extracranial tissues. SM though not rare is often diagnosed incidentally; and when they are symptomatic (neurologic deficit or increased intracranial pressure due to dural sinus involvement), the patient almost always has disseminated disease [3, 5].

Treatment and prognosis are dictated by the nature and the clinical course of the primary tumor. Although SM is usually seen in the late stages of the primary tumor with a secondary deposit in other bones in 90% of cases and with brain metastasis in 30% of cases, removing the calvarial lesion and diagnosing the pathology earlier are very important for the treatment of primary lesions [5]. Karatas et al. reported that 72.2% of calvarial metastases were detected before the primary tumor was diagnosed. Whenever surgery is indicated, the aim should always be total excision of the mass followed by cranioplasty with autologous grafts or synthetic materials, such as titanium mesh, porous polyethylene implants, and methyl methacrylate [2]. The difficulty of surgery depends on the involvement of vital structures such as the dural sinuses. Thus, radiotherapy is another option for treatment. Radiosurgery can provide good tumor control in selected cases, while bisphosphonates can be used in the palliative treatment of painful lesions [5]. Systemic chemotherapy with cytotoxic agents didn't show a success and induced a modest reduction in tumor mass and will likely have a role in the management of CNS metastases alongside surgery and radiation. Overall prognosis is poor for patients with skull base involvement as these metastases appear late during the course of the disease [3].

28.2.1.2 Ewing's Sarcoma

Primary Ewing's sarcoma (ES) is the second most common osseous malignancy in children, specifically after osteosarcoma. The skull is uncommonly the primary localization of ES (less than 4% of all cases), while the secondary hematogenous spread from other localizations is far more frequent [6]. The distinction of primary from secondary is vital as primary cranial ES does respond to chemotherapy and radiotherapy, with better prognosis [7].

The management of primary ES involves a multimodal treatment protocol. Radical surgical resection followed by radiation and chemotherapy has improved the overall results with a 2- to 5-year progression-free survival of 50–80% [8]. Where the lesion's primary surgery may not be possible, neoadjuvant chemotherapy will try to downstage the tumor and will allow the wide local excision and postoperative radiotherapy [15]. Recently, proton beam therapy has been associated with favorable results in children with excellent local control of disease [9]. The prognosis for patients with local recurrent disease is poor, with a 5-year survival following recurrence of 10–15% [6]. Primary calvarial ES has a lesser propensity for distant metastases compared with ES of other sites, suggestive of a better overall prognosis. Older age at presentation and raised lactate dehydrogenase levels in ES have been associated with poor prognosis except for the primary calvarial ES [7].

28.2.1.3 Osteogenic Sarcoma

Osteogenic sarcoma is a non-meningotheliomatous malignant mesenchymal neoplasm arising from multipotent mesenchymal cells of perivascular sheaths. Osteosarcoma accounts for approximately 20% of all primary bone malignancies with only 5–10% are located in the craniofacial bones. It is exceedingly rare in the skull with less than 1% are found in the cranial vault, despite being the second most common overall primary bone malignancy after multiple myeloma (MM) [10].

Treatment of craniofacial osteosarcomas follows the same principles as those in the extremities, consisting of gross total resection with wide margins to achieve local control of disease. In order to decrease local recurrence and metastatic spread, the surgery must be supplemented by chemotherapy and radiotherapy in incomplete resection, aggressive, or recurrent cases [11]. Consensus on optimal regimen does not exist, and no regimen has been found prognostically superior [8]. Despite treatment, the prognosis is poor with only a minority of patients achieving long-term survival, whereas, osteosarcomas of calvarium tend to have a better prognosis than those arising elsewhere in the body [11, 12]. Local recurrence is the main cause of treatment failure in head and neck osteosarcomas and is seen in 25–50% cases, usually in the first year posttreatment [11]. Distant metastasis can be seen occasionally as a late event [11, 12].

28.2.1.4 Fibrosarcoma

A fibrosarcoma is an uncommon malignant tumor derived from deep fibrous tissue. It is characterized by the presence of immature fibroblasts with variable amounts of collagen formation. Adult-type fibrosarcoma is a rare and highly aggressive type of soft tissue tumor that mostly occurs secondary to a Paget's disease of the bone, prior irradiation, fibrous dysplasia, giant cell tumor, bone infarction, or chronic osteomyelitis and usually affects middle-aged adults [13, 14]. Adult-type fibrosarcoma occurs in the area around the thighs and knees [15]. Skull involvement is seen in 1.5–3.5% of all fibrosarcoma and is often the consequence of the invasion from a nearby primary site (paranasal sinuses, face, scalp, dura). No standard treatment has been established. Gross total resection with wide margins is the most effective but difficult for the skull lesion as to the critical organ nearby [13–15]. However, a multidisciplinary approach is mandatory. Radiotherapy should be administrated for the case of high-grade (G2–3), deep, larger than 5 cm lesions with the best technique available, to a total dose of 50 Gy in 1.8–2 Gy fractions, possibly with a boost up to 66 Gy [16].

The highly aggressive character of this tumor, its low response rate to radio- and chemotherapy, and the high rate of tumor recurrences and distant metastasis contribute to its poor prognosis. In general, recurrences occur in 10–20% of patients after adequately resected tumor, within 5 years [13, 14, 16]. In addition, hematologically spread metastases to the lungs and bones of the axial skeleton have been reported in 9–63% of patients with an adult-type fibrosarcoma. The prognosis of adult fibrosarcoma is closely related to histologic grade, as determined by the degree of cytologic atypia and the amount and character of the stroma. The 5-year survival rate is about a 30% for high-grade fibrosarcomas while 60% for low-grade fibrosarcomas. Furthermore, quality of excision and use of adjuvant radiation therapy will have a major impact on prognosis [14, 15].

28.2.1.5 Neuroblastoma

Neuroblastoma is derived from the neural crest cells, aimed to develop into the sympathetic system. This explains its tendency to metastasize, in 70% of patients at the time of diagnosis, to the craniofacial skeleton, which shares the same neuroectodermal origin [16]. As the most common extracranial solid tumor of childhood, neuroblastoma accounts for 10% of childhood malignancies and 15% of malignancy-related deaths [16, 17]. Calvarial/dural metastases occur in 25% of patients and may sometimes precede the diagnosis of the main primary tumor [16, 17].

Radiation therapy is the mainstay of treatment, given the radiosensitive nature of the disease, and is used in combination with chemotherapy and surgery, if focal compression of the neurovascular structures is present. New chemotherapeutic regimens have improved the survival rate of the patients, which makes it more probable for us to face with new appearances of neuroblastoma metastases [17].

28.2.1.6 Multiple Myeloma

Multiple myeloma (MM) is a malignant disseminated disease of the bone marrow, characterized by a monoclonal proliferation of terminally differentiated plasma cells, replacing the normal marrow, and producing monoclonal immunoglobulins [4]. MM is the most common primary malignant bone lesion with a peak of incidence falling on the eighth decade.

Lesions are usually disseminated throughout the axial skeleton, and multiple skull lesions are found in about 2/3 of patients with multiple myeloma. They usually arise in the diploe, sparing the inner table and deforming the periosteum, with a macroscopic appearance of a gelatinous red-brown tissue replacing the bone marrow [18, 19].

The mainstay of treatment is medical, through the combination of chemotherapy and focal radiation therapy. The reported rate of 5-year survival is 20%, with a median survival of 3 years with conventional treatment protocols and 6 months if left untreated. Chromosome 13 or 11q deletions are predictors of poor prognosis. However, solitary plasmacytomas may be treated with surgical excision alone or followed by radiation therapy [4, 18, 19].

The development of MM is strongly predicted by the location of the plasmacytoma of the skull base. However, within a median of 2 years, despite excellent local control rates, 50–60% of patients with SP will eventually progress to multiple myeloma of which the prognosis is not as good as solitary plasmacytoma with a 10-year survival rate of only 16% [18, 19]. Therefore, surveillance must be closely continued after treatment, based on clinical examination, X-ray, SPEP, and the medullogram to detect any progression to MM.

28.2.1.7 Lymphoma

Surgical excision is considered adequate for the treatment of the disease, regardless of whether postoperative local radiotherapy is performed [20]. The prognosis of a lymphoma appearing in the skull vault is uncertain, but any involvement of the cerebral structures by direct invasion or by leptomeningeal seeding indicates a less favorable prognosis. According to the study carried out by El Asri et al. which relieved the difficulty of the outcome analysis of the reported cases of skull vault lymphoma, where the follow-up was variable and incomplete, 91% of patients who received radiotherapy were free of disease at termination of follow-up, and one patient (HIV-positive) died at 18 months [21]. By contrast, the survival time of non-Hodgkin's central nervous system tumor patients was observed to be 12–18 months, with only 8% of patients surviving for >3 years [20]. Poor outcomes were independent of treatment modality, suggesting that overall prognosis is likely related to factors besides upfront surgery, such as early diagnosis, patient age, medical comorbidities, and treatment compliance [20, 21].

28.2.2 Benign Tumors

28.2.2.1 Hemangioma

Hemangiomas are a benign mesenchymal and slow-growing neoplasm with predominantly vascular components that rarely requires treatment. Hemangioma is the second most common primary calvarial neoplasm, accounting for approximately 7–10% of primary skull tumors. It is three times as common in women as in men and usually presents in the fourth decade of life. It is typically a solitary lesion but can be multiple in up to 15% of cases [22, 23].

Indications for surgery include correction of mass effect, cosmesis, and hemorrhage control. Whenever indicated, surgery with en bloc removal together with a rim of normal bone and autolog or synthetic reconstruction (cranioplasty) is the recommended treatment and is determinant of a definitive diagnosis. Curettage may lead to excessive bleeding and recurrence [22, 23]. Unresectable lesions, deeply invading and permeating the surrounding tissues, may be treated with doses of radiotherapy up to 30 Gy (3000 rads), in 3 weeks [24]. The risk of recurrence after surgical removal is very low where the malignant sarcomatous transformation is exceedingly rare.

28.2.2.2 Osteoclastoma (Giant Cell Tumor)

Giant cell tumor (GCT), believed to originate from mononuclear cells of macrophage origin, typically arises at the epiphyses of long bones. It is a very rare tumor of the calvarium, with a hundred of cases reported in the literature and are most often centered in temporal bone [25, 26]. In the literature, radical surgical resection is the gold standard, but it is not always achievable because of the location and infiltrative pattern. Recurrence seems to be directly related to the extent of resection and rates decrease with complete tumor resection. When partially resected these tumors have a tendency to recur within a relatively short time frame (1–2 years). While the local recurrence rate for intralesional surgical approach is 27%, marginal excision recurrence rate is reported to be approximately 8% [9]. However, wide local excision of the tumor is generally inconvenient in the skull base and temporal bone due to the neighboring vital structures and the morbidity associated with surgery. Giant cell tumors are generally radio-resistant and may undergo malignant transformation when irradiated [26]. The role of adjuvant radiotherapy in treatment is still controversial and has been advocated only for inaccessible nonresectable recurrence and when a clearly malignant behavior is displayed. When radiotherapy is used as a single-modality treatment, recurrence rates up to 60%–70% are seen [10]. GCT may have pulmonary metastases in addition to causing local bone destruction [25, 26] promising therapeutic targeting the receptor activator of NF-KB ligand (RANKL) which has recently been shown to play a key role in the pathogenesis giant cell tumors by a signaling pathway that regulates osteoclast differentiation a, when surgical intervention is not feasible [25, 26]

28.2.2.3 Aneurysmal Bone Cyst (ABCs)

Aneurysmal bone cysts (ABCs) are benign, expansile vascular lesions consisting of blood-filled channels. They typically occur in the tibia and femur and are rarely seen in the calvaria. ABCs are generally solitary lesions that account for 9% of benign bone tumors [27]. It is also evenly distributed along the skull vault bones, involving symmetrically both inner and outer tables. ABCs primarily occur in individuals less than 20 years old, although they may occur at any age. ABCs are often associated with other tumors such as giant cell tumors, fibrous dysplastic tumors, chondroblastomas, chondromyxoid fibromas, and non-ossifying fibromas [28].

The neoplastic nature of an ABC is debated, and its progression is often unpredictable and variable. Because of its benign nature, the optimal treatment of ABCs is total excision of the lesion with extensive or radical surgery. However, large lesion and skull base involvement may be treated by partial excision or intralesional curettage preceded by arterial embolization because of its huge vascularity [29]. Recently, denosumab has been used for lesions in the spine or pelvis to inhibit bone resorption, when the ABC cannot be treated surgically [11]. Although resection is typically curative, there is a 10–50% recurrence rate [28].

If deemed nonresectable because of location or risk of hemorrhage, radiation therapy has been recommended. Cryosurgery and alcohol embolization have also been suggested to decrease recurrence rates of partially resected lesions. In secondary ABCs, treatment depends of the primary lesion identified. Although complete surgical excision is considered as curative, recent studies have indicated a local recurrence rate from 10% to 20% in primitive ABCs treated by total excision in referral centers, depending of the patient's age, the lesion's size, the presence of mitosis, and the completeness of the resection [29].

28.2.2.4 Intraosseous Lipoma

Intradiploic lipoma is one of the rarest bone tumors known, with only few case reports in the literature. In fact, osseous lipoma has been considered either a neoplasm or a degenerative phenomenon related to trauma, infection, or vascular compromise [30]. It is a benign lesion, consisting of mature adipocytes in a matrix of thin bony trabeculae, originating from errors in the differentiation of mesenchymal stem cells covering the mature brain [31]. They present clinically as a slowly growing lesion that spares the periosteum.

In view of benign clinical history, radical resection is probably unjustified, and in asymptomatic cases continued observation is acceptable [31]. Recurrence has not been reported and malignant transformation is exceptional.

28.2.2.5 Intradiploic Epidermoid and Dermoid Cysts

These are benign calvarial lesions, which histologically represent inclusion cysts that result from entrapment of ectodermal or dermal elements during neural tube closure in embryonic development or rarely as a result of traumatic implantation. Epidermoid cysts contain only epidermal tissue and keratinized debris, whereas dermoids may contain dermal elements, such as hair follicles, skin glands, and teeth [32, 33].

Surgical treatment often considered for cosmetic reasons and to prevent the potential but rare complication of intracranial rupture of rapidly growing cysts involving the inner table. Complete removal of the tumor with its capsule should be done before it reaches a large size. Operative options include open and endoscopic resection and curettage [33]. Incomplete removal of the tumor wall is usually followed by recurrence. Total removal of tumor is associated with a good long-term prognosis with permanent cure and minimal operative mortality. Overall prognosis is excellent, and spontaneous regression can occur even with nonoperative management. Rarely, these cysts may undergo malignant degeneration, and the recurrence rates of 8.3–25.0% have been reported [32].

28.2.2.6 Intraosseous Meningioma

The subset of extradural meningiomas arising from bone is called primary intraosseous meningioma, and it accounts for <2% of all meningiomas. The frontoparietal and orbital regions are the most common locations [34].

In a symptomatic primary intraosseous meningioma, a total wide surgical removal with resection of the involved dura and any intradural tumor followed by cranial reconstruction is the treatment of choice. The location of the tumor determines the approach and the amount of resection, keeping in mind preservation of function. When the resection is subtotal due to involvement of critical structures within the orbit, paranasal sinuses, or skull base, the residual tumor should be followed radiologically [35].

The use of adjuvant therapy is reserved for cases of tumor recurrence after incomplete resection or cases in which histology reveals atypical meningioma. The rate of recurrence depends on multiple factors, including tumor grade; tumor location; radiological type, with osteolytic being worse; and extent of surgical excision [34, 35]. In their systematic review, Omofoye et al. [8] reported a recurrence rate of 12.6%. Other authors demonstrated that the recurrence rate will be higher for skull base intraosseous meningiomas compared with convexity intraosseous meningiomas [36–38].

28.2.2.7 Osteoma

Osteoma is a benign mesenchymal tumor, macroscopically resembling mature lamellar bone. It's the most common primary benign bone tumors of the skull and facial structures and account for 0.43% of tumor in the general population with an incidental finding on 1% of plain radiographs and on 3% of computed tomography (CT) scans [1]. They can be subdivided into bone surface tumors (or exostoses) and the more common sino-orbital (or paranasal sinus) osteomas [39]. Tumor size, location, and extension determine the clinical manifestations [3].

The surgical decision or clinical follow-up are mainly undertaken for cosmetic reasons. If the lesion is small and arising from the outer table, it can be removed sparing the inner table by drilling or curettage. Formal craniotomy might be required for larger lesions or for those arising from the inner table, with subsequent simultaneous cranial reconstruction [40].

The growth rate of an osteoma is very slow, from 12 to 30 years according to reported series, even though after incomplete excision, relapse may occur after 2–8 years [39].

28.2.2.8 Chondroma and Chondrosarcoma

Chondroma is a benign cartilaginous tumor which can be presented in solitary or multiple forms. It is the most common benign skeletal osseocartilaginous tumor, accounting for 9–10% of all bone tumors. It is very rare in the neurocranium, representing less than 0.5% of intracranial tumors. It therefore mainly arises in the skull base in the sphenoid (spheno-occipital synchondrosis), occipital (petro-occipital synchondrosis), and ethmoid (spheno-ethmoidal synchondrosis) areas [41].

The mainstay of treatment is surgical, with complete, excision. When not completely resectable, decompression of the neural structures should be the primary aim. Transformation into chondrosarcoma is rare (1%) but more likely in the context of syndromic enchondromatosis (25–30%) and responds well to surgical excision [41, 42]. Recurrence is observed in 5–18% of cases. But the metastasis to respiratory system secondary to chondrosarcoma is a common finding [41, 43].

28.2.2.9 Hyperostosis Frontalis Interna

Hyperostosis frontalis interna is a boney overgrowth of the inner side of the frontal bone of the skull caused by overgrowth of the endocranial surface. It is most often found in women after menopause. It is also associated with hormonal imbalance, being overweight, history of headaches, and neurocognitive degenerative conditions [44]. This condition consists of an irregular thickening of the inner table, diploe, and frontal squama, due to idiopathic deposition of new bone, typically in a nodular pattern. It tends to be bilateral, sparing the midline at the insertion of the falx. The incidence in the general population is 1.4–5% and is most common in elderly white females, with a F/M ratio as high as 9:1 [45]. Its pathologic significance is debated, and it is almost always asymptomatic.

There is little evidence in the literature regarding the surgical treatment of this condition, with lack of significant case series.

28.2.3 Tumor-Like Lesions

28.2.3.1 Langerhans Cell Histiocytosis

Langerhans cell histiocytosis (LCH) is a multisystemic, idiopathic granuloma-forming proliferative disorder characterized by a spectrum of abnormal proliferation of Langerhans cells in various tissues and comprises a related group of three histiocytic disorders: eosinophilic granuloma (70%), the localized benign form, characterized by a focal infiltration of histiocytes, with the calvarium involved in most cases; Hand–Schüller–Christian syndrome (20%), which is the multifocal chronic disseminated form; and Letterer–Siwe syndrome (10%), the acute, malignant, disseminated type [4, 46, 47].

The natural history is variable, depending on factors such as age of onset, extent of involvement, presence of multiorgan dysfunction, and relapse. Mortality reaches 18% in multifocal disease. Treatment depends on the extent of disease. Surgical resection or curettage is the commonly recommended treatment for solitary calvarial Langerhans cell histiocytosis (LCH) in children [1]; however, prospectives and retrospective case series have shown spontaneous regression of these lesions which may avoid the risks associated with invasive treatments, particularly surgery [48]. But recurrence is reported in 30% of cases, often in a different site, mostly in children. Simple observation, local surgical resection, radiotherapy to treat recurrences, and combined irradiation and chemotherapy in case of multifocal calvarial involvement have been described [47, 48].

28.2.3.2 Paget's Disease of Bone

Paget disease is a focal disorder of bone turnover in which there is excessive bone resorption coupled with abnormal new bone formation, resulting in architecturally disorganized and mechanically weak bone [4]. Incidence increases with age, reaching a prevalence of 3% in adults older than 40 years of age, and 10% in older than 80 years. Skull involvement is present in 30–65% of cases, mostly in the frontal and occipital bone.

It's most often localized to a single bone or extending to the contiguous segments. It entails abnormal osteoclast activation, causing increased rate of bone resorption, with reactive osteoblastic hyperactivity and production of weaker, woven bone. Paget's disease ranges from active lytic phases to reparative/quiescent ones; these may or may not coexist, with individual sites progressing at variable rates [49].

Treatment depends on the location and activity of the disease. Asymptomatic patients usually do not require treatment, and pain is the only symptom for which there is proven benefit from treatment. The mainstay of treatment is medical, with the goal of pain control, mainly achieved with osteoclast inhibitors [50]. Close monitoring of the disease phases and imaging follow-up to detect malignant degeneration are warranted. Surgical treatment may be challenging because of the hypervascular nature of the disease, and profuse bleeding is common [49, 50].

28.2.3.3 Fibrous Dysplasia

Fibrous dysplasia is a congenital non-hereditary benign disorder of the mesenchymal precursor of bone. It is a consequence of the mutation of Gs alpha protein—encoded by GNAS gene—in osteoblastic progenitors' cells, resulting in an abnormal osteoblastic differentiation and maturation, with progressive replacement of normal bone by immature woven bone mixed with fibrous connective tissue [4]. It represents 2.5% of all bone tumors.

Malignant degeneration is rare, seen in less than 1% of cases. The risk is greater in monoostotic locations, especially of the maxilla and mandible as well as following radiation therapy [51]. Osteosarcoma is the most common associated malignancy followed by fibrosarcoma and chondrosarcoma. Lesions usually grow during childhood and do not progress beyond puberty (Colas et al., 2015), with the end of skeletal maturation (Wu et al., 2014). The polyostotic form of the disease can be part of McCune-Albright syndrome, characterized by the triad: polyostotic disease, café au lait spots, and multiple endocrine dysfunctions [52].

Surgical indications depend on the presence of progressive neurological impairment, the extent of the disease, and the age of the patient. When indicated, complete surgical resection is the goal of treatment. If not feasible, the aim is to achieve decompression of the neural structures. The lesions are radio- and chemo-resistant, and radiotherapy has been reported to increase the risk of sarcomatous transformation [4, 51, 52].

28.2.4 Traumatic and Congenital Lesions

28.2.4.1 Sinus Pericranii

Sinus pericranii (SP) is a rare cranial venous anomaly in which there is an abnormal communication between intracranial dural sinuses and extracranial venous structures, usually via an emissary transosseous vein. It is a very rare finding, usually diagnosed from childhood to the third decade. Sinus pericranii is mainly located along the sagittal sinus, in the midline frontal region, but can occur also more laterally. Two types are described: "closed" type, where the flow comes from and drains into a dural sinus, and "drainer" type, where blood drains transdiploe [53].

There is little available evidence with regard to available guidelines and recommendations concerning the management of this condition. Surgical correction is indicated mainly for cosmesis, prevention of massive intracranial hemorrhage, and risk of air embolism and is achieved mainly through craniotomy/craniectomy, closure of the communication between the extracranial veins and the intracranial venous sinus, and excision of the extracranial component with subsequent cranioplasty [53, 54], whereas, the surgery should be avoided in cases of dominant SP due to the high risks associated with it. Endovascular approach to treatment has proven to be safe and effective when treated for cosmetic reasons in accessory SP but still carries the risk of causing skin necrosis and embolic events [54]. The prognosis of this condition is generally good even with conservative management.

28.2.4.2 Cephalohematoma

A cephalohematoma is an accumulation of subperiosteal blood, typically located in the occipital or parietal region of the calvarium. This consists of a subperiosteal hemorrhage, by definition stopping at the sutures. It occurs as a result of birth trauma, in 1% of live births, but can be also nontraumatic, if coagulopathy coexists. It may become apparent 24–48 h after birth, or progresses over a few days [55].

Treatment and management of cephalohematoma are primarily observational. The mass from a cephalohematoma takes weeks to resolve as the clotted blood is slowly absorbed. If it does not resolve after a month, calcification may occur in the site where the periosteum was lifted, with remodeling of the outer table. There is an ongoing debate regarding conservative management versus early surgical intervention for cephalohematoma, as there are no randomized controlled trials for reference. Head wrapping has been described and may promote resorption. Needle aspiration of the fluid prior to wrapping is debated, since it may introduce infection. Surgical removal by drilling may be required if calcification occurs, mainly for cosmetic reasons [56]. The surgical technique involves resection of the overlying newly formed bone, the soft tissue mass, as well as the underlying original bone. Following removal, the underlying depressed region is often sectioned into multiple pieces and is remodeled as a bone graft [55, 56].

28.2.4.3 Leptomeningeal Cyst

Leptomeningeal cysts are scalp swelling occurring primarily in infants and children under 3 years of age associated with a skull fracture. Post-traumatic intradiploic leptomeningeal cysts are a variant in which the fracture involves the inner table with the dural tear. This leads to cerebrospinal fluid (CSF) accumulation in a sac lined by the arachnoid membrane and located within the diploic space [57].

The leptomeningeal cyst is benign and carries a good prognosis. The cyst can remain asymptomatic in some individuals; however, it still requires repair, given the risk of progressive enlargement and irreversible neurological complications. Early diagnosis and surgical intervention are crucial to avoid progressive and potentially permanent neurological sequelae. The surgical intervention of the leptomeningeal cyst involves a craniotomy, resection of the mass, repair of the dural defect with a pericranial patch, and repair with a bone graft [58].

Recurrence of the cyst remains possible and occurs in 2% of cases. Risk factors of recurrence are syndromic craniosynostosis, hydrocephalus, elevated intracranial pressure, repeated surgical interventions, endoscopic repair, and incomplete duraplasty/cranioplasty [59].

However, timely diagnosis and prompt surgical repair are crucial to avoiding long-term complications. In addition, epilepsy, brain herniation with neurological deficit, and mental retardation can be associated with poor quality of life and significant morbidity.

Good-to-excellent outcomes, even in the delayed presentation, are observed in most cases. However, large bony defect (>7 cm), initial severe head injury, calvarial defects crossing the midline, and delayed repair (>8 months) have been associated to poor prognosis [57, 58].

28.3 Scalp Malignancies

Scalp tumors are heterogeneous in their clinical profiles. A total of 1–2% of scalp tumors are malignant, and they comprise up to 13% of all malignant cutaneous neoplasms [60]. Even though scalp neoplasms are generally benign, malignant ones deserve special attention due to their aggressive nature, high recurrence rates, and metastasis potential based on histologic subtype [61]. High suspicion, histological diagnosis, and clear surgical margins are all requirements in successfully treating scalp tumors.

The majority of primary malignant tumors of the scalp arise from epithelium, the most common of which are BCCs and SCCs. Melanoma accounted for only 2% of malignant scalp tumors, whereas metastatic malignancies were the third most common malignancy, representing 12.8% of the total [60, 61]. Other more rare tumors of the scalp include Merkel cell carcinoma (MCC), dermatofibrosarcoma protuberans, atypical fibroxanthoma, microcystic adnexal carcinoma, syringocystadenocarcinoma papilliferum, trichoblastoma, clear cell acanthoma, keratoacanthoma, apocrine gland carcinoma, sebaceous gland carcinoma, cutaneous angiosarcoma, and others [60–62].

28.3.1 Melanoma

Cutaneous melanoma is a public health issue. The head and neck region is of particular interest, despite accounting for only 9.0% of the total body surface; it harbors 20% of melanoma cases. Scalp melanomas (SMs) represent between 24.9 and 35% of cutaneous head and neck melanoma (CHNM) [63]. Thus, melanomas arising in the scalp might be a high-risk subset of CHNM. Moreover, SMs are more common in the elderly than in young population, and they occur six times more frequently in men than in women. Management follows the same principles as for non-head and neck melanoma. Breslow thickness of the SM gives instructions for the excision margins. Surgery should be performed with resection margins, as for other cutaneous melanomas [64]. The behavior of SM is different from melanomas arising at other body sites, and the overall survival compared with other head and neck melanomas is lower [64]. The complex lymphatic drainage of this area may lead to an unpredictable risk of distant or local recurrence. Furthermore, recurrence rate for scalp melanoma is 13% compared to 5% for melanoma of the face neck and ear according to Shaw et al. [65]. Therefore, it is important to make a diagnosis as early as possible [66]. Unfortunately, scalp melanomas commonly have predominant CCND1 and CDK4 oncogenes and therefore are less likely to respond to target therapy. Data from the literature show that scalp melanomas (SMs) carry high mortality rates, with a 10-year survival rate of 60% which lead them to be named as the "invisible killer" [67].

28.3.2 Nonmelanoma Scalp Malignant Tumors

Nonmelanoma skin cancers, predominantly basal cell carcinoma (BCC) and squamous cell carcinoma and SCCs, are the most common primary malignant scalp tumors from the epithelium [68]. As a result of thick hair and the difficulty of self-inspecting certain areas, early detection is often difficult. Even rare, melanoma is one of the most commonly detected scalp malignancies. Relatively frequently are scalp tumors diagnosed only at an advanced stage when they present as visible/palpable masses. Stratified scalp structures significantly influence tumor growth patterns due to resistance to infiltration, as only 4.5% of patients in this study had bone infiltration. As a result of the vertical limitations created by the cranial bones, tumors typically grow horizontally. In this particular location, both tumors are clinically characterized by a greater tendency for ulceration. Thus, they more frequently present as chronic, nonhealing ulcer, compared to elsewhere on the skin [69].

28.3.2.1 Basal Cell Carcinoma (BCC)

Once confirmed through biopsy, treatment of BCC would depend on the location, type, and size. In the majority of cases, surgical excision is the standard of treatment. Histology plays a key role in determining the margins of resection and lymph node dissection, so it is always good to obtain a preoperative histological diagnosis. Reconstruction of the scalp after tumor removal requires more attention. Primary repair is used in small defects without tension; however, in large defects, local/regional flaps or free flaps are necessary [60, 69].

The 5-year recurrence rate using the Mohs surgery technique is 1.4% [70]. Other treatments include radiation therapy using high-energy beams such as X-rays and protons to treat any remaining remnant of the cancer cells. Electrodesiccation and curettage (E&D) are also commonly done, which involves surgical removal of the affected tissue with a curette with maximal margins [71]. A side effect of E&D is the development of a hypopigmented scar. Topical treatment includes imiquimod 5% cream five times/week for 6 weeks, approved by the Food and Drug Administration (FDA) for treatment of superficial BCC in low-risk zones, resulting in a histologic clearance rate of 82% 12 weeks after the treatment [72].

28.3.2.2 Cutaneous Squamous Cell Carcinoma (cSCC)

Cutaneous squamous cell carcinoma (cSCC) is the second most common nonmelanoma skin cancer, and its incidence is increasing globally. Surgical treatment, for which several options are available, is the standard of care for cSCC, and securing a sufficient surgical resection margin is always important. Squamous cell carcinoma is most curable in the early stages before it spreads. If it's diagnosed early, the 5-year survival rate is approximately 99%. Due to their slow progression, scalp SCC is usually diagnosed before extension into the skull. Invasion into the bone, cortex, and dura mater is rare [5]. But once there is dural or brain invasion, the patient may develop neurological deficits, and the lesion may become inoperable. Dural involvement significantly reduces 3-year survival from 83% to 22% [73]. Hence, the depth of invasion is a significant prognostic factor, and cranial involvement is associated with a poorer prognosis [74].

Although the majority of cSCCs are successfully eradicated by surgical excision, advanced cSCC poses a significant risk in terms of morbidity, impact on quality of life, and risk of death. cSCC of the scalp sometimes exhibits unusually aggressive behavior [75]. While, unlike melanoma, a tumor thickness of less than 10 mm correlates only slightly with clinical stage and rate of metastasis, the primary location on the scalp is a distinct risk factor for larger MCCs associated with distant metastasis (8.7%), which reduces the median survival to 9 months [74, 75].

The prognostic factors for head and neck cutaneous squamous cell carcinoma that were most consistently reported as significant in the literature are a state of immunosuppression, tumor depth, margins involved, number of lymph nodes affected by carcinoma, parotideal disease, and age [73, 75].

28.3.3 Metastatic Carcinoma

Internal malignancies can metastasize through different routes, including the hematogenous route, lymphatics, or via direct extension from the primary tumor [60]. The most common sites of metastasis in breast cancer are the lungs, bone, liver, and brain [75].

Cutaneous metastases are commonly found in the late stages of lung, gastric, and breast cancers [75]. Scalp metastases are rare and account for only 2% of all skin tumors. However, the scalp region accounts for 4–6.9% of all cutaneous metastases, as this region has an abundant blood supply [4, 60]. Scalp metastases indicate a sign of progression and unfavorable prognosis [75].

References

1. Gomez CK, Schiffman SR, Bhatt AA. Radiological review of skull lesions. Insights Imaging. 2018;9(5):857–82.
2. Karatas D, Uygur S, Karabag H, Sayar H, Barut IT, Dagtekin A, Avci E. Calvarial tumors: a retrospective analysis and clinical experience. Turk Neurosurg. 2023;33(2):244–51.
3. Gupta S, Sharma G, Sajeevan S, Raut SN, Ahuja R, Joseph D, Gupta A, Gupta M. Varied clinical presentation and management of calvarial metastases. Asian J Neurosurg. 2022;17(4):631–4.
4. Colas L, Caron S, Cotten A. Skull vault lesions: a review. AJR Am J Roentgenol. 2015;205(4):840–7.
5. Mitsuya K, Nakasu Y, Horiguchi S, et al. Metastatic skull tumors: MRI features and a new conventional classification. J Neuro-Oncol. 2011;104:239–45.
6. Salunke PS, Gupta K, Malik V, et al. Primary Ewing's sarcoma of cranial bones: analysis of ten patients. Acta Neurochir (Case Rep). 2011;153:1477–85.
7. Mohindra S, Tripathi M, Batish A, Kapoor A, Patil NR, Mahendru S, Ahuja C, Chatterjee D. Primary Calvarial Ewing sarcoma: a case series. J Neurol Surg B Skull Base. 2021;83(Suppl 2):e181–90.
8. Krishnamani K, Kumar TN, Gandhi LV, Raghunadharao D, Sadashivudu G, Megha U. Primary Ewing's sarcoma of the cranium: case series and review of literature. J Cancer Res Ther. 2014;10(02):377–80.

9. Kharod SM, Indelicato DJ, Rotondo RL. Outcomes following proton therapy for Ewing sarcoma of the cranium and skull base. Pediatr Blood Cancer. 2020;67(02):e28080.
10. Fernandes GL, Natal MRC, da Cruz CLP, Nascif RL, Tsuno NSG, Tsuno MY. Primary osteosarcoma of the cranial vault. Radiol Bras. 2017;50(4):263–5.
11. Singh R, Jha K, Pant I, Satti D. Primary osteogenic sarcoma of the skull: report of two cases with review of literature. J Postgrad Med. 2018;64(4):232–6.
12. Mathkour M, Garces J, Beard B, Bartholomew A, Sulaiman OA, Ware ML, et al. Primary high-grade osteosarcoma of the clivus: a case report and literature review. World Neurosurg. 2016;89:730.e9–7.3E+15.
13. Kaur H, Gupta V, Mishra D, Yadav VS. Fibrosarcoma: origin, differential diagnosis, and report of a case in the mandible. J Indian Soc Periodontol. 2022;26(2):169–77.
14. Elmi SM, Mouhssani M, Obame FLO, Imbunhe N, El Asri AC, Gazzaz M. Primary Ewing's sarcoma of the occipital bone: a case report and review of the literature. Surg Neurol Int. 2023;14:309.
15. Bahrami A, Folpe AL. Adult-type fibrosarcoma: a reevaluation of 163 putative cases diagnosed at a single institution over a 48-year period. AJNR. 2010;34:1504–13.
16. D'Ambrosio N, Lyo JK, Young RJ, Haque SS, Karimi S. Imaging of metastatic CNS neuroblastoma. AJR Am J Roentgenol. 2010;194(5):1223–9.
17. Khoei S, Boustani MR, Pak N. An atypical imaging characteristic of calvarial metastasis of neuroblastoma as multiple multi-loculated cystic masses with internal blood-fluid levels: a case report. BMC Neurol. 2022;22:471.
18. Pham A, Mahindra A. Solitary plasmacytoma: a review of diagnosis and management. Curr Hematol Malig Rep. 2019;14(2):63–9.
19. Joshi A, Jiang D, Singh P, Moffat D. Skull base presentation of multiple myeloma. Ear Nose Throat J. 2011;90(1):E6–9.
20. El Asri AC, Akhaddar A, Baallal H, Boulahroud O, Mandour C, Chahdi H, et al. Primary lymphoma of the cranial vault: case report and a systematic review of the literature. Acta Neurochir. 2012;154:257–65.
21. Parekh HC, Sharma RR, Keogh AJ, Prabhu SS. Primary malignant non-Hodgkin's lymphoma of cranial vault: a case report. Surg Neurol. 1993;39:286–9.
22. Yang Y, Guan J, Ma W, Li Y, Xing B, Ren Z, Su C, Wang R. Primary intraosseous cavernous hemangioma in the skull. Medicine (Baltimore). 2016 Mar;95(11):e3069.
23. Alexiou GA, Lampros M, Gavra MM, Vlachos N, Ydreos J, Boviatsis EJ. Primary intraosseous cavernous hemangioma of the cranium: a systematic review of the literature. World Neurosurg. 2022;164:323–9.
24. Salunke P, Sinha R, Khandelwal NK, et al. Primary intraosseus cavernous hemangioma of the skull base. Br J Neurosurg. 2010;24:84–5.
25. Kaya İ, Benzer M, Turhal G, Sercan G, Bilgen C, Kirazlı T. Giant cell tumor of the temporal bone and skull base: a case report. J Int Adv otol. 2018;14:151–4.
26. Harris AE, Beckner ME, Barnes L, Kassam A, Horowitz M. Giant cell tumor of the skull: a case report and review of the literature. Surg Neurol. 2004;61:274–7.
27. Woldow A, Foy VM. Aneurysmal bone cyst of the skull: a case report. SAGE Open Med Case Rep. 2022;10:2050313X221117727.
28. Jayakumar N, Ismail HMB, Mulay S, et al. Aneurysmal bone cyst in the cervical spine. BMJ Case Rep. 2019;12:e231870.
29. Hermann AL, Polivka M, Loit MP, Guichard JP, Bousson V. Aneurysmal bone cyst of the frontal bone - a radiologic-pathologic correlation. J Radiol Case Rep. 2018;12(7):16–24.
30. Arslan G, Karaali K, Cubuk M, Senol U, Luleci E. Intraosseous lipoma of the frontal bone. Acta Radiol. 2000;41:320–1.
31. Kaneko Y, Hokao K, Ogasawara N, Nakano S, Masuda T. A case of intraosseous lipoma in the frontal bone. No Shinkei Geka. 2011;39(10):975–80.
32. Han GY, Won YS, Yang JY, Choi CS. Intradiploic epidermoid cyst of the skull. J Korean Neurosurg Soc. 2005;38:68–70.
33. Khalid S, Khan SA, Aurangzeb A, Muhammad G, Khan Afridi EA, Muhammad D. Intradiploic epidermoid cyst of the skull. J Ayub Med Coll Abbottabad. 2021;33(2):349–51.
34. Tokgoz N, Oner YA, Kaymaz M, Ucar M, Yilmaz G, Tali TE. Primary intraosseous meningioma: CT and MRI appearance. AJNR Am J Neuroradiol. 2005;26(8):2053–6.
35. Harary M, Tung JK, Sood S, Corrales CE, Smith T, Iorgulescu JB. Benign purely intraosseous meningioma of the skull: diagnosis and surgical outcomes. J Clin Neurosci. 2020;82(Pt A):36–42.
36. Lang FF, Macdonald OK, Fuller GN, DeMonte F. Primary extradural meningiomas: a report on nine cases and review of the literature from the era of computerized tomography scanning. J Neurosurg. 2000;93(6):940–50.
37. Elwatidy S, Alanazi A, Alanazi RF, Alraddadi KK. Intraosseous meningioma, a rare presentation of a common brain tumor: illustrative case. J Neurosurg Case Lessons. 2022;4(15):CASE22331.
38. Omofoye OA, Huynh T, Jhun R, Ashfaque H, Cronk K. Primary intraosseous meningioma of the calvarium: a systematic review. Clin Neurol Neurosurg. 2020;199:106283.
39. Yudoyono F, Sidabutar R, Dahlan RH, Gill AS, Ompusunggu SE, Arifin MZ. Surgical management of giant skull osteomas. Asian J Neurosurg. 2017;12(3):408–11.
40. Secer HI, Gonul E, Izci Y. Surgical management and outcome of large orbitocranial osteomas. J Neurosurg. 2008;109:472–7.

41. Feuvret L, Bracci S, Calugaru V, et al. Efficacy and safety of adjuvant proton therapy combined with surgery for chondrosarcoma of the skull base: a retrospective, population-based study. Int J Radiat Oncol Biol Phys. 2016;95:312–21.
42. Nazar E, Ghanadan A. Cutaneous metastasis of chondrosarcoma: a case report with literature review. Case Rep Clin Pract. 2019;4(3):73–7.
43. Konovalov A, Shekhtman O, Shekhtman AP, Bezborodova T. Chondrosarcoma of the skull base: a case study and literature review. Cureus. 2020;12(12):e12412. https://doi.org/10.7759/cureus.12412.
44. Vuković M, Vujanić M, Nosek I, Stojić I, Jakobsen W, Kozić D. Hyperostosis frontalis interna and frontal bone thickness among various age groups - differences between males and females. Arch Ital Biol. 2020;158(2):57–63.
45. She R, Szakacs J. Hyperostosis frontalis interna: case report and review of literature. Ann Clin Lab Sci. 2004;34:206–8.
46. Chen HC, Shen WC, Chou DY, Chiang IP. Langerhans cell histiocytosis of the skull complicated with an epidural hematoma. AJNR Am J Neuroradiol. 2002;23(3):493–5.
47. Satter EK, High WA. Langerhans cell histiocytosis: a review of the current recommendations of the histiocyte society. Pediatr Dermatol. 2008;25(3):291–5.
48. Steinbok P, Cheong A, Dix DB, Bhatia S, Handler MH, Limbrick DD Jr, Niazi T, Price AV, Ragheb J, Souweidane M, Tamber MS, Sandberg DI. Nonoperative management of childhood calvarial langerhans-cell histiocytosis. N Engl J Med. 2022;386(26):2532–4.
49. Corral-Gudino L, Borao-Cengotita-Bengos M, Del Pino-Montes J, Ralston S. Epidemiology of Paget's disease of bone: a systemic review and meta-analysis of secular changes. Bone. 2013;55:347–52.
50. Reid IR, Lyles K, Su G, Brown JP, Walsh JP, del Pino-Montes J, Miller PD, Fraser WD, Cafoncelli S, Bucci-Rechtweg C, Hosking DJ. A single infusion of zoledronic acid produces sustained remissions in Paget disease: data to 6.5 years. J Bone Miner Res. 2011;26:2261–70.
51. Kim DY. Current concepts of craniofacial fibrous dysplasia: pathophysiology and treatment. Arch Craniofac Surg. 2023;24(2):41–51.
52. DiCaprio MR, Enneking WF. Fibrous dysplasia: pathophysiology, evaluation, and treatment. J Bone Joint Surg Am. 2005;87:1848–64.
53. Kessler IM, Esmanhoto B, Riva R, et al. Endovascular transvenous embolization combined with direct puncture of the sinus pericranii. A case report. Interv Neuroradiol. 2009;15:429–34.
54. Goffin J, MacKenzie SA, Tallur KK, Kaliaperumal C. Sinus pericranii: long-term outcome in a 10-year-old boy with a review of literature. BMJ Case Rep. 2018;2018:bcr2017223631.
55. Wong CH, Foo CL, Seow WT. Calcified cephalohematoma: classification, indications for surgery and techniques. J Craniofac Surg. 2006;17(5):970–9.
56. Chung HY, Chung JY, Lee DG, Yang JD, Baik BS, Hwang SG, Cho BC. Surgical treatment of ossified cephalhematoma. J Craniofac Surg. 2004;15(5):774–9.
57. Açikgöz B, Tekkök IH. Post-traumatic intradiploic leptomeningeal fistula and cyst. J Clin Neurosci. 2002;9(4):468–73.
58. Kim H, Jo KW. Treatment of a traumatic leptomeningeal cyst in an adult with fibrinogen-based collagen. J Korean Neurosurg Soc. 2013;53(5):300–2.
59. Seo BR, Lee JK, Jeong IH, Moon SJ, Joo SP, Kim TS, et al. Post-traumatic intradiploic leptomeningeal cyst of the posterior fossa in an adult. J Clin Neurosci. 2009;16:1367–9.
60. Prodinger CM, Koller J, Laimer M. Scalp tumors. J Dtsch Dermatol Ges. 2018;16(6):730–53.
61. Anrade P, et al. Epidemiology of basal cell carcinomas and squamous cell carcinomas in a Department of Dermatology: a 5 year review. An Bras Dermatol. 2012;87(2):212–9.
62. Chiu CS, Lin CY, Kuo TT, et al. Malignant cutaneous tumors of the scalp: a study of demographic characteristics and histologic distributions of 398 Taiwanese patients. J Am Acad Dermatol. 2007;56(3):448–52.
63. Ross MI, Balch CM. Excision margins of melanoma make a difference: new data support an old paradigm. Ann Surg Oncol. 2016;23(4):1053–6.
64. Ng AK, Jones WO, Shaw JH. Analysis of local recurrence and optimizing excision margins for cutaneous melanoma. Br J Surg. 2001;88(1):137–42.
65. Shaw HM, McCarthy WH, McCarthy SW, Milton GW. Thin malignant melanomas and recurrence potential. Arch Surg. 1987;122(10):1147–50.
66. Licata G, Scharf C, Ronchi A, Pellerone S, Argenziano G, Verolino P, Moscarella E. Diagnosis and management of melanoma of the scalp: a review of the literature. Clin Cosmet Investig Dermatol. 2021;14:1435–47.
67. Palacios-Diaz RD, de Unamuno-Bustos B, Pozuelo-Ruiz M, Morales-Tedone EG, Ballester-Sánchez R, Botella-Estrada R. Scalp melanoma: a high-risk subset of cutaneous head and neck melanomas with distinctive clinicopathological features. J Clin Med. 2023;12:7643.
68. Ghanadan A, Abdollahi P, Rabet M, et al. Different anatomical distribution of basal cell carcinoma subtypes in Iranian population: association between site and subtype. Ann Dermatol. 2014;26(5):559–63.
69. Youl PH, Janda M, Aitken JF, et al. Body-site distribution of skin cancer, pre-malignant and common benign pigmented lesions excised in general practice. Br J Dermatol. 2011;165(1):35–43.
70. Marzuka AG. Basal cell carcinoma: pathogenesis, epidemiology, clinical features, diagnosis, histopathology, and management. Yale J Biol Med. 2015;88:167–79.

71. Amos-Arowoshegbe EO, Varghese R, Joseph AB, Kanu-Ivi C, Sadi N, Sadana S, Latif F, Abdul A, Ratra R, Blume K, Tiesenga F. Basal cell cancer of the scalp. Cureus. 2022;14(6):e26469.
72. Geisse J, Caro I, Lindholm J, Golitz L, Stampone P, Owens M. Imiquimod 5% cream for the treatment of superficial basal cell carcinoma: results from two phase III, randomized, vehicle-controlled studies. J Am Acad Dermatol. 2004;50:722–33.
73. Dahal A, Neupane D, Lageju N, et al. Invasive cutaneous squamous cell carcinoma of scalp: a case report. Ann Med Surg (Lond). 2022;82:104702.
74. Karia PS, Morgan FC, Ruiz ES, Schmults CD. Clinical and incidental perineural invasion of cutaneous squamous cell carcinoma: a systematic review and pooled analysis of outcomes data. JAMA Dermatol. 2017;153:781–8.
75. Ryu HR, Lee DW, Choi HJ, Kim JH, Ahn H. Scalp metastasis of advanced gastric cancer. Arch Craniofac Surg. 2021;22(3):157–60.

Medicolegal Aspects of Scalp and Calvarial Lesions

29

Mehmet Turgut

29.1 Introduction

Head injuries, especially those that occur during childbirth, and pediatric age group pathologies such as craniosynostosis are among the clinical conditions that are quite common today and have the potential to lead to various medicolegal problems. These conditions can be diagnosed by neuroimaging studies such as X-ray, ultrasound (US) computed tomography (CT), or magnetic resonance imaging (MRI) [1–6]. Therefore, it is apparent that these lesions should be carefully evaluated by a team of healthcare personnel that include a midwife, nurse, and physicians such as an obstetrician, neurosurgeon, radiologist, pediatrician, and plastic surgeon.

A review of the literature revealed that case reports and small case series have provided various conclusions regarding the appropriate management of patients with different lesions involving the scalp and calvarium, such as various forms of head injuries that occur during childbirth and craniosynostosis. This chapter will focus on these fascinating but complex issues, while also addressing positional plagiocephaly and hair transplantation pathologies that may be subject to malpractice claims due to a delayed or inaccurate diagnosis and/or inappropriate clinical management. In comparison, hypoxic-ischemic birth injuries, such as hypoxic-ischemic encephalopathy, cerebral palsy, and cranial nerve injuries will be excluded from the scope of this chapter because the scalp and calvarium are not primarily affected in these pathologies.

Considering basic legal concepts such as medical negligence, medical malpractice, patient interviewing, informed consent, and the parents' right to information, common medical conditions involving the scalp and calvarium as a potential source of medicolegal problems and their medicolegal aspects are discussed in detail below. Medicolegally, it is highly important that every healthcare provider including physicians recognize and appreciate that any negligent act or lack of care in such a clinical situation can lead to an allegation of malpractice regarding the management of patients with various lesions involving the scalp and calvarium.

M. Turgut (✉)
Department of Neurosurgery, Aydın Adnan Menderes University Faculty of Medicine, Aydın, Türkiye

Department of Histology and Embryology, Aydın Adnan Menderes University Institute of Health Sciences, Aydın, Türkiye
e-mail: drmturgut@yahoo.com

M. Turgut et al. (eds.), *Lesions of the Scalp and Cranial Vault*,
https://doi.org/10.1007/978-3-031-88244-9_29

29.2 Common Medical Conditions Involving the Scalp and Calvarium as a Potential Source of Medicolegal Problems

Even today, there is still controversy surrounding various aspects of the management of lesions involving the scalp and calvarium. Three common medical conditions that are a source of potential medicolegal problems, head injury during childbirth, craniosynostosis and positional plagiocephaly, and hair transplantation will be discussed in detail below before considering their medicolegal aspects in subsequent sections.

29.2.1 Head Injury During Childbirth

29.2.1.1 Birth Injury Involving the Scalp

29.2.1.1.1 Accidental Fetal Scalp Laceration

In recent years, as a defensive medical behavior, malpractice has caused a decrease in vaginal birth rates because of the possible risks in obstetrical practice, in contrast to that of caesarean section (CS) delivery [7]. Nevertheless, accidental fetal incisional wounds, called "fetal lacerations," involving superficial surface structures of the fetus such as the scalp, are well-recognized complications of CS deliveries, mostly in the form of scalpel-related lacerations [8–10]. Based on their experience from 14926 deliveries in 3108 women delivered by CS birth, Dessole et al. reported an incidence of about 3.0% for accidental fetal lacerations (mild, moderate, or severe) for CS delivery [8]. As a result of their review, regardless of the CS type, Wiener et al. reported that fetal lacerations occurred in nearly 1.5% of CS deliveries performed in their hospital, and they concluded that this complication should be addressed in the preoperative evaluation of patients undergoing CS delivery [11]. Importantly, Dessole et al. reported that the risk of accidental fetal scalp lacerations was higher in fetuses undergoing an urgent CS birth and lower for urgent and elective CS deliveries [8]. Therefore, a signed informed consent stating that the patient was informed about the risk of fetal scalp laceration and other complications during CS delivery should be obtained to avoid any potential for litigation [9].

29.2.1.1.2 Caput Succedaneum

"Caput succedaneum," a kind of birth injury characterized by swelling of the scalp, may occur during a difficult labor and vaginal delivery with the use of some instruments, such as forceps or a vacuum extractor [2]. The injury is characterized by a noticeable lump on the head, due to a hematoma located in the subcutaneous layer of the scalp, which may extend beyond the suture lines of the cranium and midline [2]. Currently, it is one of the most frequent birth injuries that develop from pressure on the scalp of the baby during a prolonged, difficult, or head-first delivery, and in particular in those cases requiring instrumental deliveries using vacuum extraction or forceps. It is well-known that the risk factors for such a birth injury are the early rupture of the membranes or diminished amniotic fluid, resulting in an absence of the protective effect of the amniotic sac for the head of the baby. Thus, in such conditions, the child can be born with caput succedaneum, even in CS births where this state can be diagnosed with a prenatal US examination, providing a chance to take the necessary precautions [2].

Clinically, a soft swelling involving the scalp, either unilateral or bilateral extending beyond the midline, indicates the presence of caput succedaneum of the scalp area that traveled through the birth canal early during the delivery. This process leads to an over-molding of the skull bones of the infant caused by pressure during the childbirth. As a rule, this result is self-limited, and the swelling of the scalp resolves within several days after the delivery; as such, there is no specific treatment required for caput succedaneum [2]. However, this occurrence should not be ignored because of the risk of jaundice (excessive amounts of bilirubin) in a newborn. Jaundice usually resolves within several days, but it should be closely monitored by healthcare personnel including the physician of the child, because it could lead to a rare condition called "kernicterus," which can cause permanent brain damage and even death in cases where it progresses. From a medicolegal point of view, this injury may or may not have been avoidable, but careful prenatal care and appropriate management of the labor and delivery should be applied to prevent the development of such an injury. In such unfortunate cases, the family might sustain a substantial financial burden, and healthcare personnel including the physician will be faced with a medical malpractice claim for compensation, if a physician fails to consider this risk. In such cases, it is expected that impartial and competent medical experts will provide objective and fair opinions regarding the malpractice claim.

29.2.1.1.3 Subgaleal Hematoma

"Subgaleal hematoma," resulting from an injury to an emissary vein during birth, occurs within the loose areolar tissue between the galea aponeurosis and the periosteum; therefore it can extend beyond the suture lines of the skull and progressively expand over time [2]. This hematoma occurs in about 30 cases per 100000 patients with an uncomplicated elective normal vaginal delivery, while about 60 cases per 100000 patients occur in the presence of vacuum usage [2]. It has been reported that 90% (70% vaginal delivery and the remaining 20% CS delivery) of cases with subgaleal hematoma are related with instrument-assisted deliveries [2, 12]. About 40% of patients with a subgaleal hematoma have a concurrent skull fracture, intracranial hemorrhage, or brain edema [12]. Clinically, visual inspection and palpation of the scalp are adequate for the early detection of a diffuse, soft, and fluctuant mass [2]. It has been reported that monitoring the head circumference, vital signs, and laboratory tests (cell blood count, coagulation test, etc.) is important because the hemorrhage may be life-threatening in some cases [2]. Radiologically, cranial US, CT, and MRI are useful for the appropriate evaluation of these cases [2]. Management involves a conservative approach, consisting of correction of hypovolemia, anemia, hyperbilirubinemia, and metabolic acidosis, and surgical evacuation in rare cases with increased intracranial pressure (IICP) [2].

29.2.1.1.4 Cephalohematoma

"Cephalohematoma" is a collection of blood in the subperiosteal space of the scalp covering the calvarium, often over the parietal bone, which occurs in about 1% of all deliveries, in particular those with the use of certain assistive devices such as the forceps or vacuum extractor [2, 13]. In some rare cases, however, a cephalohematoma develops naturally without any external iatrogenic influence related to the pressure to the head of the fetus from the pelvis of the mother during delivery. It is well-known that there are several risk factors for the development of a cephalohematoma that include macrosomia, small maternal pelvic dimensions, preterm birth, breech birth, and multiple births (twin, triplet, quadruplet, and other multiples). Typically, cephalohematoma is usually self-limited because it does not cross the suture lines of the calvarium or extend past the midline [2]. Clinically, a child with a cephalohematoma may present with various signs or symptoms, including swelling and a painful head, feeding difficulty, loud crying, vomiting, fatigue, and seizures. It has been reported that the erythrocyte count may be low in newborns with cephalohematoma; therefore monitoring of the erythrocyte count in their blood is very important for diagnosis and follow-up [2]. Furthermore, radiological studies, such as X-rays, MRI scans, and CT scans, will be necessary for the confirmation of the cephalohematoma in such cases [2]. Fortunately, the prognosis for children with cephalohematoma is usually favorable, and observation until resorption of the hematoma within several days or weeks is adequate in most of the cases. Although it is possible to encounter any complication such as calcification of the hematoma, anemia, jaundice, and scalp infection with osteomyelitis or meningitis, close observation of the child is necessary [2]. Medical (antibiotics or blood transfusion) and/or surgical treatment may be necessary in some complex children with infections and anemia [2]. Moreover, jaundice characterized by yellow skin and eyes may develop due to an excessive accumulation of bilirubin, and light therapy may be necessary in some children. Fatal brain damage due to kernicterus may occur in some children with jaundice. In such children, timing is critical, and the physician should recognize the condition promptly and treat it appropriately because permanent brain injury is unavoidable in the existence of neglect of the signs and symptoms of the condition and its possible complications. In those children, it is highly likely that you will be faced with a medical malpractice claim for compensation for the preventable complications of a cephalohematoma.

29.2.1.2 Birth Injury Involving the Calvarium

29.2.1.2.1 Skull Fractures

The skull of the newborn is soft and not easily affected by a fracture as a result of the decreased bone mineralization and the presence of cranial sutures which allow for the delivery of the fetus through the birth canal; it is more susceptible to fracture during delivery with an incidence of 3 per 100000 births or immediately following delivery resulting in cerebral damage, in contrast to the skull of an adolescent or an adult [2, 4, 14]. As a rule, birth injury involving the scalp is generally observed in association with calvarial fractures, but birth injury involving the brain is rare [2].

29.2.1.2.1.1 Causes

One of the potential causes of brain trauma during the delivery is a skull fracture, most often of the parietal bone [2]. The most frequent cause of infant skull fractures is external pressure from surgical instruments, such as forceps or vacuum extractors, used during childbirth to grip or pull the head of the baby out of the uterus [14]. Unfortunately, these surgical tools can fracture the skull during delivery when used excessively and improperly where about 50% of calvarial fractures in infants are associated with vacuum extractor- or forceps-assisted vaginal delivery which are called "instrumental births" [14]. Calvarial fractures are more common with: (a) extraction difficulty during childbirth; (b) greatest molding forces in utero caused by prolonged labor, breech presentation, or macrosomia; or (c) accidental fall after childbirth in the hospital [4]. The bones of the skull of the newborn can easily be fractured because of excessive force during labor and childbirth particularly if a midwife, nurse, or physician improperly uses the instruments such as forceps or vacuum extractor, in the presence of macrosomia or a long and difficult labor, or a traumatic event caused by being "mishandled" (e.g., accidental drop of the baby or "abused" (e.g., shaking or striking of crying baby)) [15, 16]. In such circumstances or when he or she should have performed an emergency CS delivery but failed to do so, there is no doubt that healthcare personnel might be liable for malpractice. Fortunately, however, the vast majority of in-hospital falls do not result in calvarial fractures, and therefore imaging is not necessary, but documentation of the presence of any kind of the skull fracture (given below in detail) following an accidental fall is important from a legal point of view [4]. On the other hand, some calvarial fractures can also occur spontaneously because of the pressure placed on the head of the baby while going through the birth canal; therefore it is not the result of malpractice [4].

29.2.1.2.1.2 Types

In clinical practice, there are five major types of infant skull fractures: (a) linear skull fractures, (b) depressed skull fractures, (c) diastatic skull fractures, (d) spontaneous skull fractures, and (e) basilar skull fractures. There is no doubt that each of these skull fractures can affect an infant differently and may require a unique, individualized plan for monitoring and treatment.

(a) *Linear skull fracture:* A linear skull fracture can occur when too much force is used with forceps or vacuum extractors during delivery. A fracture can also result after an infant is dropped after delivery or by another similar incident. Unfortunately, it is difficult to diagnose approximately one quarter of the skull fractures by X-rays because of the decreased mineralization of the skull and the presence of widened cranial sutures [2, 4]. In general, linear fractures may not require surgery and pose only modest risks to the infant [2, 5]. In most cases, further imaging with CT is not recommended to avoid the risks of radiation exposure despite the presence of CT with low-dose and three-dimensional (3D) reformat features. Observation alone is adequate for these cases because they will heal on their own over time [4, 5]. However, there is a risk of development of a "growing skull fracture" in the presence of a dural laceration associated with a previous fracture [4]. CT or MRI is indicated in such cases with a calvarial defect and a protruding pulsatile cystic scalp mass that requires surgical intervention for repair of the dural defect [4].

(b) *Depressed skull fracture:* A depressed skull fracture, also known as "ping-pong fracture," can be due to a penetrating injury that breaks the skull and pushes it into the brain, causing a depression of the skull, or it can be from a sharp blow to the head that causes the skull to fracture and impacts the brain. The presence of pressure on the brain, in contrast with a simple linear fracture of the skull, may require surgery to repair the fracture [1, 2, 17]. The severity of the brain damage depends on the area in which the injury occurred, and it is difficult to predict the lasting damage or long-term prognosis after developing a depressed skull fracture. In contrast to those patients with a linear skull fracture, an additional imaging study which is most often a low-dose CT with 3D reconstruction is necessary to define the fracture with a minimal radiation risk [2, 6].

A depressed skull fracture is an inward collapse of the skull (calvarium) bones and is called a "ping-pong" fracture [16, 18]. In clinical practice, those cases after vaginal delivery or CS delivery without use of medical instruments are classified as "spontaneous," while cases after a childbirth with the use of forceps or vacuum extractors are classified as "instrument-associated" (application of forceps or vacuum extractors) [1, 16]. As expected, the incidences of a depressed skull fracture and an associated intracranial lesion are higher in cases with instrumental deliveries [16].

(c) *Diastatic skull fracture:* A diastatic skull fracture in infants and newborns, located along the suture lines of the skull, will generally cause a wider separation between the bones of the skull [4]. Therefore, this type of fracture may lead to a potentially devastating condition known as a "growing skull fracture" [4]. In these cases, close follow-up of the child is necessary for the detection of a growing fracture because surgery may be necessary in some cases with a diastatic skull fracture [4].

(d) *Spontaneous intrauterine skull fracture:* During the intrauterine period, the skull of the baby is very soft and malleable compared to the adult skull, but fracture of the baby skull, frequently a linear or depressed fracture, may occasionally occur during a normal intrauterine gestation and/or uncomplicated delivery in which the use of instruments (application of forceps or vacuum extractors) is not required and it is impossible to determine the exact cause of such a spontaneous intrauterine fracture that will often require neurosurgical evaluation and treatment [17, 19]. In contrast to infantile skull fractures caused by the use of instruments, during the delivery and when such use was considered negligent or malpractice, the skull can fracture naturally, with or without the use of instruments [1, 16, 17, 19, 20]. Even today, delivery and birth are fraught with risks despite modern advances in obstetrics because the physical pressure that an infant is under during labor and delivery can be intense [1]. It should be kept in mind that natural external compression in utero may rarely cause a skull fracture, if the head of the baby is caught on the mother's pelvis or gets stuck in the birth canal, resulting in chronic remodeling of the skull [1, 16–21]. Merhar et al. suggested that the vast majority of these fractures, including ping-pong skull fractures, will remodel over time without any kind of intervention in the presence of intact skin [4].

Nowadays, it is well-known that spontaneous depressed skull fractures may be encountered in cases with an uneventful normal spontaneous vaginal delivery or CS delivery, without any significant predisposing factor [1, 19]. Even today, both etiology and appropriate management of spontaneous intrauterine depressed skull fractures still remain controversial [19, 21]. However, a consultation by a neurosurgeon is vital for the initial evaluation of these non-iatrogenic fractures, and surgical treatment is indicated for large defects and/or traumatic intracranial lesions [19].

It has been reported that fetal skull fracture is associated with existence of difficult delivery or extrinsic trauma [20]. Unlike local molding depressions of the calvarium related to long and complicated labor or delivery, linear intrauterine skull fracture associated with uncomplicated, spontaneous vaginal delivery is extremely rare [20]. In 1996, Heise et al. reported a case of spontaneous intrauterine linear skull fracture in which the fracture occurred in spite of a normal spontaneous vaginal delivery without any extrinsic cephalopelvic disproportion or traumatic event [20]. In their case, follow-up disclosed normal development without any focal neurologic deficit or epileptiform activity [20]. Based on their experience, they concluded that normal spontaneous vaginal delivery without any complication or history of instrumentation may cause a traumatic injury resulting in a linear fracture of the skull, despite the absence of any definitive etiology for such a fracture [20].

(e) *Basilar skull fracture:* A break of a bone of the base of the skull, called a basilar skull fracture, can occur because of trauma during labor or shortly after birth [2, 17]. Owing to the location of the break, they can be very serious, and they may require surgery and/or rehabilitation and leading to additional medical care [17]. However, such fractures are related to the skull base, and they will be excluded from the scope of this chapter since the scalp and calvarium are not primarily affected.

29.2.1.2.1.3 Symptoms

Clinically, depending upon the localization, type of a skull fracture (as noted above in detail), and the severity of any resulting brain damage, mild symptoms (bruises, cuts, bumps or dents, lethargy, vomiting, a lump on the skull, unnaturally pale skin, etc.) or alarming symptoms associated with brain injury (deformation of the skull, bleeding inside the skull, loss of consciousness, paralysis of a portion of the body, bruising behind the ear or around the eyes, bleeding or clear fluid draining from the ear or the nose, seizure, motor dysfunction, inability to speak, and loss of vision, hearing, taste, intellectual capabilities, etc.) may develop in newborns [2, 15, 17].

As a rule, children should be carefully monitored because severe complications may develop quickly, and consequences may be severe or even fatal. Therefore, a careful neurological examination and radiological studies such as X-ray, US, CT scan, or MRI scan will provide an accurate diagnosis [15]. From a surgical point of view, a small skull fracture will resolve on its own without major intervention, but a child may need surgical intervention if a fracture is more extensive. Fortunately, a skull fracture during childbirth usually does not cause serious harm to the health of the infant. As a simple rule, a medical error must have occurred during labor and delivery, if there is a fracture requiring surgical treatment. Unfortunately, however, even a successful surgical intervention may not completely resolve the negative effects of a skull fracture related to applying excessive force when using surgical equipment such as forceps or vacuum extractors during delivery [2, 15, 17]. In such malpractice cases, parents can seek compensation for the surgery and medication costs incurred in treating permanent disabilities of their child through the lawsuit.

29.2.1.2.1.4 Diagnosis and Treatment

Today, various imaging studies like X-ray and CT scan are the most common tests used to diagnose head injuries, but they can be deleterious for newborns because of the radiation exposure required, whereas an MRI scan or an US may be the safest option for diagnosis of infant head injuries. Although there is not a consensus regarding the best imaging choice for diagnosis of the skull fracture of the newborn, X-ray, CT scan, or MRI scan is indicated to determine the location and type of the fracture and/or the severity of the cerebral damage, when any infant skull fracture is suspected [1, 2]. If the brain is not involved, observation and close monitoring are sufficient in infants with skull fractures, even in those with depressed fractures [2]. Severe injuries might require surgery, breathing assistance, sedation, and monitoring for IICP caused by brain swelling. Even today, there is not a consensus about the length of the observation period for infants with skull fractures [2, 4].

29.2.1.2.2 Extra-axial Hemorrhage

Various kinds of extra-axial hemorrhage and epidural or subdural hematoma may develop from rupture of meningeal arteries or bridging veins or from the edges of the fractured skull. Fortunately, the vast majority of these hematomas related with skull fractures are ≤2 mm. As a rule, however, repeat CT of the brain for monitoring of the hemorrhage is indicated within 12 h if the thickness of the hematoma is >2 mm on the initial CT scan [4]. Clinically, new neurological symptoms and signs requiring surgical evacuation of the hematoma can develop; therefore, close monitoring is vital in such cases [4]. There is no doubt that repeat imaging studies and laboratory tests will be also useful to confirm the need for a surgical indication.

29.2.1.3 Birth Injury Involving the Brain

Intracranial injury during delivery, an uncommon occurrence, ranges from the mildest cases to very severe ones, with an incidence of about 3 per 100000 live births. Unfortunately, early diagnosis of intracranial hemorrhage in newborns is difficult because of the unfused sutures and open fontanelles in addition to an unstable clinical condition [2]. It has been reported that there are several risk factors for intracranial injury during delivery: Fetal macrosomia, precipitous (rapid) labor, and assisted delivery with forceps or vacuum extractors [2]. Theoretically, intracranial vessels (meningeal arteries, bridging veins or leptomeningeal collaterals) can rupture when the applied external forces are greater than the degree that can be compensated for by shaping the baby's head [2]. Clinically, various symptoms and signs including those of IICP and seizures may develop in cases of intracranial injury. Imaging of intracranial hemorrhage in newborns with US, CT or MRI provides an accurate diagnosis. As a treatment method, surgical intervention such as craniotomy or shunting may be necessary for cases with significant mass effect or hydrocephalus, respectively.

29.2.2 Craniosynostosis and Positional Plagiocephaly

Craniosynostosis, early fusion of one or multiple sutures of the skull with restriction of its growth perpendicular to the involved suture, is seen with a frequency of 1/2000–2500 births worldwide, resulting in growth of the skull parallel to the affected suture [3]. The visible skull deformity usually represents a ridge along the affected suture of the cranium, abnormal head shape, and slow head growth over time as the newborn grows, irrespective of the type of craniosynostosis [3, 22]. In almost all cases, definitive diagnosis of craniosynostosis is based on findings on both the physical examination and imaging studies such as X-ray and CT [3, 22]. Complications of craniosynostosis include signs of symptoms of IICP (headache, vomiting, papilledema, and altered mental status that varies from drowsiness to coma, etc.), delayed cerebral development, cognitive dysfunction, and feeding difficulty [3]. Management of craniosynostosis begins with a primary healthcare provider recognizing the skull deformity and referring the child to neurosurgeon or plastic surgeon for further radiological evaluation and treatment of craniosynostosis to prevent IICP [3]. The timing of surgery depends upon the severity of the skull deformity where surgical intervention for craniosynostosis is generally performed at 8–12 months of age in most centers in the world when the total volume of the intracranial cavity is sufficiently large and the child can tolerate having the surgery [3]. Outcome of the children with craniosynostosis depends on number of cranial sutures affected and the general health condition of the child, where patients with craniosynostosis who underwent surgical intervention frequently improve without any sequela [3].

Positional plagiocephaly, called deformational plagiocephaly, is the formation of a flat area of one side of the head of a child or on the back of the head. The deformation occurs when the child sleeps in the same position most of the time or due to problems in the neck muscles that result in a preference for turning the head [22]. This pathology is a condition that should be kept in mind in the differential diagnosis of cases with craniosynostosis, and a 3D CT examination should be performed as part of the differential diagnosis [22]. There is no doubt that a malpractice situation will occur if a case of positional plagiocephaly is misdiagnosed as craniosynostosis and operated on unnecessarily, or if a delay or mistake is made in the appropriate treatment of cases with skull abnormalities such as craniosynostosis and positional plagiocephaly.

29.2.3 Hair Transplantation

From a medical perspective, hair restoration surgery is an elective and nonessential aesthetic procedure involving the scalp, and an estimation of the risk-benefit ratio is important in this procedure [23, 24]. Complications related to the hair transplantation procedure generally originate from scar tissue development in the surgical site, low hair density in the donor area, defective graft implantation, etc. [23, 24]. Unfortunately, tolerance of the patients is low for any possible complication caused by a hair transplantation procedure, because the surgery performed by plastic surgeons is not a life-threatening procedure [24].

29.3 Medicolegal Aspects of Medical Conditions Involving the Scalp and Calvarium

"Instrumental" Birth Injuries

Medicolegally, it is important to know that there is a potential for permanent impairment as a result of a birth injury. Birth injuries may arise from errors or negligences by healthcare personnel, including midwifes and physicians, who use certain medical instruments such as forceps or vacuum extractors to assist the baby to come out of the birth canal, whereby, you might have grounds to file a medical malpractice claim. For example, improperly using the labor-assistive devices described above can cause an infant to suffer skull fractures. Despite modern advances in obstetrical practice, these medical tools are the most common cause of skull fractures in infants and such cases are often considered negligent or represent malpractice.

Currently, most obstetricians are realizing that instrumental vaginal births carry more risks than benefits, as given above in detail, and CS delivery seems to be safer than an instrumental birth for mother and baby. There is no doubt that the reason for an infantile skull fracture is usually the wrong application of surgical instruments (forceps or vacuum extractors) during childbirth, resulting a permanent cerebral damage and other medical complications. Primarily, infants who suffer skull fractures and severe neurological injuries might require extensive medical care, therapy, and rehabilitation. In clinical practice, injuries to the brain from a severe skull fracture can result in difficulty speaking, hearing loss, vision loss, inability to taste, intellectual impairments, behavioral problems, learning disabilities, and motor dysfunction. Unfortunately, there might be valid grounds to file a medical malpractice claim to recover compensation of the losses that the injured baby and his/her parents have incurred and might continue to incur in the future, if an infant suffered a skull fracture caused by the negligence of a physician, nurse, midwife, or other healthcare personnel. From a medicolegal point of view, a medical malpractice case involving an infant skull fracture is definitely possible, if there is concrete evidence confirming that the management of the healthcare personnel fell below the accepted standard of care and that the deviation from the standard of care caused an injury to the infant.

Legally, infants who suffer various forms of head injury during birth, in particular those involving the brain, might suffer permanent disabilities, and some children will require ongoing lengthy rehabilitation, medical or surgical therapy, and other interventions. In cases of an infant head injury during delivery, financial compensation will be required for the following types of damages: past and future all medical expenses, therapy expenses associated with necessary medical equipment (wheelchairs, braces, etc.), rehabilitation costs, lost wages, loss of earning capacity as a permanent disability, emotional distress, physical pain and suffering, mental health counseling costs, loss of enjoyment of life, and permanent scarring or disfigurement.

Differential Diagnosis of Natural Versus Iatrogenic Causes for Infant Skull Fractures

Before falsely claiming malpractice against healthcare personnel including midwives, obstetricians, neurosurgeons, plastic surgeons, radiologists, or pediatricians, some natural causes for infant skull fractures and/or scalp defects should also be considered. As given above in detail, it is well-known that the skull of the infants can fracture naturally without the use of surgical tools, called "spontaneous skull fracture," due to intense natural physical pressure upon the head of the fetus in the birth canal during a "long and complicated labor and delivery" [1, 16, 17, 19–21]. In such circumstances, there is no doubt that such a labor or delivery is an important risk factor for skull fracture of the baby. From a medical point of view, use of such instruments by the midwife or physician is indicated in the presence of a difficult birth, resulting in an inevitable high risk of skull fracture. Furthermore, the presence of asphyxiation of the baby, high birth weight (macrosomia), large head, and unusual presentation of the baby within the birth canal such as the breech position are additional natural risk factors for a long and complicated labor and delivery [1, 16, 17, 19, 20]. It is well-known that all of these risk factors can put more pressure on the skull of the child and increase the risk of a fracture during labor or delivery. There is no doubt that the healthcare personnel should act quickly when they suspect the presence of asphyxiation in the child; thus such a forced delivery may unavoidably cause a skull fracture in the newborn [16].

Differential Diagnosis of Accidental Fetal Scalp Lacerations from Congenital Skin Defects

Another issue that is very important from a medicolegal perspective is that, as previously reported in the literature, the entity "congenital skin defects" such as aplasia cutis congenita, which is accidentally reported as forceps or vacuum extractor-related trauma, called "instrumental fetal laceration" involving the scalp, should not be forgotten [25–27]. Medicolegally, therefore, it is suggested that such a possibility should be considered in such cases before a definitive decision regarding the source of the fetal scalp defects.

Differential Diagnosis of Craniosynostosis from Positional Plagiocephaly

Today, various medical entities such as craniosynostosis and positional plagiocephaly, sometimes referred to as deformational plagiocephaly, are among the medicolegal issues associated with the calvarium [22]. Recently, Gong et al. (2023) reported a total of nine cases of malpractice litigation regarding infantile skull deformity (craniosynostosis and positional plagiocephaly) in the US over three decades and importantly all cases involving jury verdicts or settlements resulted in compensation being awarded to the plaintiffs where the vast majority of causes for litigation regarding infantile skull deformity were related to the difficulty in diagnosis or misdiagnosis ($n = 4$) and medical negligence ($n = 3$) [28]. Thus, as found in their series, it is apparent that malpractice lawsuits involving infant skull deformity are very few, but almost all of them were ruled against the medical staff or hospital administration, and a very significant amount of compensation was awarded by the court.

Importance of Informed Consent for Hair Transplantation

In hair transplantation procedures, informed consent consisting of a detailed explanation of the etiology, all treatment options, and the outcome of the hair loss treatment is very important for satisfying the patient and is a method to reduce the potential for any unfair accusations against the healthcare personnel [24]. In today's medical environment where malpractice cases are increasing in number, it has been reported that providing better information to patients and having a better understanding of legal principles by healthcare personnel are very critical issues [29–31]. It is therefore imperative for physicians such as plastic surgeons or other healthcare personnel that perform hair transplantation to be knowledgeable in forensic legal issues regarding hair restoration techniques [24]. Legally, there is no doubt that ignorance of these conditions is not an acceptable defense in court [24]. At present, the overwhelming majority of malpractice claims in the field of plastic surgery originates from inadequate or nonexistent communication between the plastic surgeon and patient as well as wrong patient selection and are not related with any surgical error [24, 29, 32].

29.4 Basic Legal Concepts Regarding Lesions Involving the Scalp and Calvarium

As described in detail above, most of the lesions affecting the scalp and calvarium and their related medicolegal problems concern the fields of neurosurgery, obstetrics, and plastic surgery. These surgical disciplines represent the top three subspecialties listed with the highest numbers of malpractice cases in all around the world [33, 34]. Therefore, it is not possible for the vast majority of neurosurgeons, obstetricians, and plastic surgeons to avoid a malpractice claim at some point during their careers [33]. Unfortunately, it has been reported that the average time until a claim is resolved is at least 2 years and that the average annual possibility of a malpractice suit is about 20% [35]. In fact, physicians are not insured against the indirect expenses of litigation related with the loads such as time, intense stress, additional work, and loss of reputation, although they may be partially protected against potential compensation payments by malpractice insurance [34, 36]. Undoubtfully, there are concerns that have also been expressed about the impact of increased liability on tax practices such as "defensive medicine," resulting in high hospitalization charges [37].

Legally, there is no doubt that physicians and other healthcare personnel are responsible for the development of such damages caused by a lack of care in their efforts to achieve an anticipated result [38–41]. It is well-known that physicians and or other healthcare personnel are responsible for their smallest errors [40]. As a legitimate request, patients and their relatives have the right to expect that their physicians and other healthcare personnel will be meticulous and conscientious at every stage of the management of patients with lesions involving the scalp and calvarium. In particular, it is critical that patients and their relatives be informed by physicians or other healthcare personnel regarding the possible risks and benefits of surgical procedure. As a fundamental principle, the two main questions must be considered in resolving any medical malpractice case involving negligence claim: (1) did the conduct of the physician or other medical personnel violate the standard of medical care? and if the answer is believed to be positive, (2) did the negligence of the physician or other healthcare personnel cause harm to the plaintiff patient? [42]. In most medical malpractice cases, the main debate centers on whether the physician or other healthcare personnel were negligent, and the issue of patient injury has generally been accepted. However, the type of harm claimed by the plaintiff requires additional attention because it is uncommon to put it simply.

Medical Negligence

In accordance with the principles of "tort law," "medical negligence" defines a condition in which the accused healthcare personnel such as the doctor should or should not do in certain circumstances [43, 44]. To show that a case of "negligence prima facie" has occurred, a patient has to provide the four components ("four Ds") of medical malpractice-"d"uty, "d"ereliction (deviation from the standard of care, negligence), "d"amages, and "d"irect cause [43]. The physician has a trusting relationship with his/her patient as a requirement of his/her duties toward the patient [29]. In clinical practice, a dereliction (breach) of duty results if the physician provides services below the accepted standard of care, such as when the patient is given insufficient informed consent. It is accepted that in the case of an inadequate informed consent, a breach of the patient rights regarding his/her health and self-determination is in question because of a dereliction of duty where a patient suffers postoperative complications or damages [23]. Finally, the damages related to the complications should have a "direct causal link" with the dereliction of duty [23, 29]. It is important to remember that there is no intention in medical negligence, and it results when a healthcare provider mistakenly causes harm to a patient, either from not realizing something (ignorance) or from the inability to take action when and where it is needed [23, 44]. Although the act or omission is certainly medical negligence, it is not considered as a medical malpractice because the medical supplier did not perform the action with the intent to harm or with the ability to predict that the patient may be harmed [38, 44].

Medical Malpractice

Unlike medical negligence, in the case of "medical malpractice," the healthcare personnel are aware of the possible consequences of their actions or inaction. Malpractice is considered intentional not because the patient wants to be harmed but because the individual performs such an action or action knowing that there is a risk of harm [23, 38, 39]. The patient files a lawsuit alleging malpractice in the presence of low standard of medical practice as in violation of the acceptable medical standard(s) [23, 39]. In a previous study, Studdert et al. found that about 40% of claims were not related to any medical error [45]. At present, some authors maintain that the valid legal regulations have a significant role to increase the quality of care, while others strongly believe that it fails to compensate many patients who have medical injuries that can be prevented and harms some healthcare personnel such as physicians for unwanted conditions that are not caused by their medical negligence [36, 38, 39, 46]. No matter which is true, prominent increases in malpractice premiums observed in recent years and the significant increases in the number and multitude of claims awarded to plaintiffs have caused an increased interest in the malpractice liability organization, resulting in an imbalance between the cost of malpractice liability and the quality of care [33, 36, 47].

Patient Interview

The "patient interview or consultation" is an adequate communication with the patient that is necessary for understanding the patient's distress and for obtaining patient satisfaction, because the expectations of the patient may be different and apparently greater than anticipated [23]. After a careful examination of the patient, also known as part of the patient interview, a physician can communicate his or her assessment to the patient and outline any applicable treatments, keeping the patient's concerns and expectations in mind [23]. During the consultation, the physician may become aware of the patient's comorbid medical diseases such as diabetes mellitus, hypertension, and cardiac diseases, whereby the patient should be referred to the relevant specialist(s) for further treatment without delay, even though it can be extremely difficult in some patient cases [48].

Informed Consent and the Parents' Right to Information

"Informed consent" is legally a prerequisite for all medical procedures including surgical procedures for lesions involving the scalp and calvarium. Indeed, failure to obtain informed consent constitutes medical negligence in and of itself [49]. Informed consent involves ensuring that patients fully understand their condition and the possible solutions for these conditions, the scenic course and outcome of the condition, the nature of the proposed options for proper treatment, and any necessary additional treatment options required, alternative methods of management available, the approximate expense of the treatment procedure, possible risks of other alternative treatment methods or procedures recommended to the patient by the physician, likely outcome of the treatment and chances of success or failure, timeline of events, and pre- and postoperative services [49]. Essentially, obtaining consent from the patient carries the meaning of entering into a contractual obligation that covers a duty of care to the patient, but the fact that the patient has given consent for the procedure(s) to be performed and signed such a comprehensive consent form does not mean that the patient and his/her relatives will be protected against malpractice claims against the physician in case things go bad and a medicolegal problem develops in the future [49]. Even if a complication develops, the neurosurgeon or plastic surgeon must prove that it occurred despite strict adherence to medical standards and that there was no deviation from the work and procedures that an average physician should do [49].

29.5 Conclusion

Today, a lesion involving the scalp and calvarium may be treated erroneously due to the high frequency of misdiagnoses, leading to delayed or inappropriate management. Clinically, therefore, malpractice regarding the management of lesions involving the scalp and calvarium is a common occurrence. In terms of forensic medicine, physicians and other healthcare personnel frequently recognize that any medical negligence and carelessness at any stage of treatment will result in different forms of medical malpractice in the management of cases of various lesions involving the scalp and calvarium. In the future, large multicenter prospective randomized controlled trials and evidence-based medicine will be required to provide strong conclusions regarding this topic.

Acknowledgments The author would like to thank Atty. Hüsamettin İşcan for his guidance and support in legal interpretation of the potential problems regarding various lesions involving scalp and calvarium.

References

1. Abbassioun K, Amirjamshidi A, Rahimizadeh A. Spontaneous intrauterine depressed skull fractures. Childs Nerv Syst. 1986;2(3):153–6.
2. Chong S. Head injury during childbirth. J Korean Neurosurg Soc. 2022;65(3):342–7.
3. Mathijssen IMJ. Guideline for care of patients with the diagnoses of craniosynostosis: working group on craniosynostosis. J Craniofac Surg. 2015;26(6):1735–807.
4. Merhar SL, Kline-Fath BM, Nathan AT, Melton KR, Bierbrauer KS. Identification and management of neonatal skull fractures. J Perinatol. 2016;36(8):640–2.
5. Nakahara K, Shimizu S, Kitahara T, Oka H, Utsuki S, Soma K, Kan S, Fujii K. Linear fractures invisible on routine axial computed tomography: a pitfall at radiological screening for minor head injury. Neurol Med Chir (Tokyo). 2011;51(4):272–4.
6. Orman G, Wagner MW, Seeburg D, Zamora CA, Oshmyansky A, Tekes A, Poretti A, Jallo GI, Huisman TA, Bosemani T. Pediatric skull fracture diagnosis: should 3D CT reconstructions be added as routine imaging? J Neurosurg Pediatr. 2015;16(4):426–31.
7. Schifrin BS, Cohen WR. The effect of malpractice claims on the use of caesarean section. Best Pract Res Clin Obstet Gynaecol. 2013;27(2):269–83.
8. Dessole S, Cosmi E, Balata A, Uras L, Caserta D, Capobianco G, Ambrosini G. Accidental fetal lacerations during cesarean delivery: experience in an Italian level III university hospital. Am J Obstet Gynecol. 2004;191(5):1673–7.
9. Esposito C, Escolino M, Paternoster M, Buccelli C, Graziano V, Falco M, Alicchio F, Cerulo M, Settimi A, Savanelli A. Fetal laceration during caesarean section and its medico-legal sequelae. Med Sci Law. 2015;55(2):97–101.
10. Gajjar K, Spencer C. Fetal laceration injury during cesarean section and its long-term sequelae: a case report. Am J Obstet Gynecol. 2009;201(4):e5–7.
11. Wiener JJ, Westwood J. Fetal lacerations at caesarean section. J Obstet Gynaecol. 2002;22(1):23–4.
12. Lee SJ, Kim JK, Kim SJ. The clinical characteristics and prognosis of subgaleal hemorrhage in newborn. Korean J Pediatr. 2018;61(12):387–91.
13. Firlik KS, Adelson PD. Large chronic cephalohematoma without calcification. Pediatr Neurosurg. 1999;30(1):39–42.
14. Högberg U, Fellman V, Thiblin I, Karlsson R, Wester K. Difficult birth is the main contributor to birth-related fracture and accidents to other neonatal fractures. Acta Paediatr. 2020;109(10):2040–8.

15. Ciurea AV, Gorgan MR, Tascu A, Sandu AM, Rizea RE. Traumatic brain injury in infants and toddlers, 0-3 years old. J Med Life. 2011;4(3):234–43.
16. Dupuis O, Silveira R, Dupont C, Mottolese C, Kahn P, Dittmar A, Rudigoz R-C. Comparison of "instrument-associated" and "spontaneous" obstetric depressed skull fractures in a cohort of 68 neonates. Am J Obstet Gynecol. 2005;192(1):165–70.
17. Bonfield CM, Naran S, Adetayo OA, Pollack IF, Losee JE. Pediatric skull fractures: the need for surgical intervention, characteristics, complications, and outcomes. J Neurosurg Pediatr. 2014;14(2):205–11.
18. Brittain C, Muthukumar P, Job S, Sanka S. 'Ping pong' fracture in a term infant. BMJ Case Rep. 2012;2012:bcr0120125631.
19. Veeravagu A, Azad TD, Jiang B, Edwards MSB. Spontaneous intrauterine depressed skull fractures: report of 2 cases requiring neurosurgical intervention and literature review. World Neurosurg. 2018;110:256–62.
20. Heise RH, Srivatsa PJ, Karsell PR. Spontaneous intrauterine linear skull fracture: a rare complication of spontaneous vaginal delivery. Obstet Gynecol. 1996;87(5 Pt 2):851–4.
21. Acevedo M, Ojeda V, Kim Y, Meislin R, Bautista J, Tsai MC. Spontaneous fetal skull fracture in an apparently uncomplicated vaginal delivery. Austin J Obstet Gynecol. 2014;1(4):2. ISSN: 2378-1386
22. Flannery AM, Tamber MS, Mazzola C, Klimo P Jr, Baird LC, Tyagi R, Bauer DF, Beier A, Durham S Lin AY, McClung-Smith C, Mitchell L, Nikas D. Congress of neurological surgeons systematic review and evidence-based guidelines for the management of patients with positional plagiocephaly: executive summary. Neurosurgery. 2016;79(5):623–4.
23. Paras M, Delbon P, Conti A. Cosmetic surgery: medicolegal considerations. Open Med (Wars). 2016;11(01):327–9.
24. Sattur SS, Sattur IS. Patient counselling and medico-legal aspects of hair transplant surgery. Indian J Plast Surg. 2021;54(4):441–5.
25. Dunn PM. Litigation over congenital scalp defects. Lancet. 1992;339(8790):440.
26. Kjaer M. Congenital skin defects. Acta Derm Venereol. 1968;48(6):608–11.
27. Marcovici I. Aplasia cutis congenita presenting as vacuum-extractor-related trauma. Int J Gynaecol Obstet. 2015;129(3):267–8.
28. Cong JH, Soliman L, Sobti N, Mehrzad R, Woo AS. Medical malpractice litigations involving infant craniosynostosis and deformational plagiocephaly in the United States. Cleft Palate Craniofac J. 2023 Mar 2:10556656231165591.
29. Michaels BD, Del Rosso JQ, Momin SB. Avoiding the legal "blemish": medicolegal pitfalls in dermatology. J Clin Aesthet Dermatol. 2009;2(12):35–43.
30. Park BY, Kim MJ, Kang SR, Hong SE. A legal analysis of the precedents of medical disputes in the cosmetic surgery field. Arch Plast Surg. 2016;43(03):278–83.
31. Shah AK. Newer implications of medico-legal and consent issues in plastic surgery. Indian J Plast Surg. 2014;47(02):199–202.
32. Yalcin Balcik P, Cakmak C. The evaluation of malpractice cases arising from aesthetic intervention in Turkey based on Supreme Court case law. Int J Health Plann Manag. 2019;34(01):e885–95.
33. Bekelis K, Missios S, Wong K, MacKenzie TA. The practice of cranial neurosurgery and the malpractice liability environment in the United States. PLoS One. 2015;10(3):e0121191.
34. Jena AB, Seabury S, Lakdawalla D, Chandra A. Malpractice risk according to physician specialty. N Engl J Med. 2011;365(7):629–36.
35. Seabury SA, Chandra A, Lakdawalla DN, Jena AB. On average, physicians spend nearly 11 percent of their 40-year careers with an open, unresolved malpractice claim. Health Aff (Millwood). 2013;32(11):111–9.
36. Baicker K, Fisher ES, Chandra A. Malpractice liability costs and the practice of medicine in the Medicare program. Health Aff (Millwood). 2007;26(3):841–52.
37. Studdert DM, Mello MM, Sage WM, DesRoches CM, Peugh J, Zapert K, Brennan TA. Defensive medicine among high-risk specialist physicians in a volatile malpractice environment. JAMA. 2005;293(21):2609–17.
38. Bal BS. An introduction to medical malpractice in the United States. Clin Orthop Relat Res. 2009;467(02):339–47.
39. Hakeri H. Distinction between malpractice and complication in medical law (in Turkish). Toraks Cerrahisi Bülteni. 2014;1:23–8.
40. Kök N. Malpractice and complication distinction. In: Kalkan E, Serel TA, Yilmaz EN, editors. Legal guide for physicians (in Turkish). Turkish Neurosurgery Academy Publications No: 1. Ankara: Sage Publishing; 2018. p. 109–39.
41. Marcus P. Book review of medical malpractice law: a comparative law study of civil responsibility arising from medical care. Hastings Int Compar Law Rev. 1981;5:235–43.
42. Berlin L. Proximate cause. AJR Am J Roentgenol. 2002;179:569–73.
43. Preskorn SH. Clinical psychopharmacology and medical malpractice: the four Ds. J Psychiatr Pract. 2014;20(05):363–8.
44. Sohn DH. Negligence, genuine error, and litigation. Int J Gen Med. 2013;6:49–56.
45. Studdert DM, Mello MM, Gawande AA, Gandhi TK, Kachalia A, Yoon C, Puopolo AL, Brennan TA. Claims, errors, and compensation payments in medical malpractice litigation. N Engl J Med. 2006;354(19):2024–33.
46. Brennan TA, Leape LL, Laird NM, Hebert L, Localio AR, Lawthers AG, Newhouse JP, Weiler PC, Hiatt HH. Incidence of adverse events and negligence in hospitalized patients. Results of the Harvard Medical Practice Study I. N Engl J Med. 1991;324(6):370–6.
47. Mello MM, Studdert DM, Brennan TA. The new medical malpractice crisis. N Engl J Med. 2003;348(23):2281–4.
48. Gilbert M. Agreements, coercion, and obligation. Ethics. 1993;103(04):679–706.
49. Kapoor L. Informed consent in aesthetic surgery. J Cutan Aesthet Surg. 2015;8(03):173–4.

Index

M. Turgut et al. (eds.), *Lesions of the Scalp and Cranial Vault*,
https://doi.org/10.1007/978-3-031-88244-9

MIX
Papier aus verantwortungsvollen Quellen
Paper from responsible sources
FSC® C105338

If you have any concerns about our products,
you can contact us on
ProductSafety@springernature.com

In case Publisher is established outside the EU,
the EU authorized representative is:
Springer Nature Customer Service Center GmbH
Europaplatz 3, 69115 Heidelberg, Germany

Printed by Libri Plureos GmbH
in Hamburg, Germany

MIX
Papier aus verantwortungsvollen Quellen
Paper from responsible sources
FSC® C105338

FSC
www.fsc.org

If you have any concerns about our products,
you can contact us on
ProductSafety@springernature.com

In case Publisher is established outside the EU,
the EU authorized representative is:
Springer Nature Customer Service Center GmbH
Europaplatz 3, 69115 Heidelberg, Germany

Printed by Libri Plureos GmbH
in Hamburg, Germany